handbook of PSYCHIATRY

2
Edition

handbook of
PSYCHIATRY

Edited by

PHILIP SOLOMON, MD
Clinical Professor of Psychiatry
University of California at San Diego
Medical School

VERNON D. PATCH, MD
Assistant Professor of Psychiatry
Harvard Medical School, and
Clinical Director, Psychiatry Service
Boston City Hospital

Lange Medical Publications
Los Altos, California

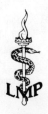

1971

A Concise Medical Library for Practitioner and Student

Current Diagnosis & Treatment 1971 M.A. Krupp, M.J. Chatton, S. Margen, Editors	$11.00
Current Pediatric Diagnosis & Treatment, 1970 C.H. Kempe, H.K. Silver, D. O'Brien, Editors	$11.00
Review of Physiological Chemistry, 13th Edition, 1971 H.A. Harper	$8.00
Review of Medical Physiology, 5th Edition, 1971 W.F. Ganong	$8.50
Review of Medical Microbiology, 9th Edition, 1970 E. Jawetz, J.L. Melnick, E.A. Adelberg	$7.50
Review of Medical Pharmacology, 2nd Edition, 1970 F.H. Meyers, E. Jawetz, A. Goldfien	$8.50
General Urology, 6th Edition, 1969 D.R. Smith	$8.00
General Ophthalmology, 6th Edition, 1971 D. Vaughan, R. Cook, T. Asbury	$8.00
Correlative Neuroanatomy & Functional Neurology, 14th Edition, 1970 J.G. Chusid	$7.50
Principles of Clinical Electrocardiography, 7th Edition, 1970 M.J. Goldman	$7.00
Handbook of Psychiatry, 2nd Edition, 1971 P. Solomon, V.D. Patch, Editors	$7.50
Handbook of Surgery, 4th Edition, 1969 J.L. Wilson, Editor	$6.00
Handbook of Obstetrics & Gynecology, 4th Edition, 1971 R.C. Benson	$6.50
Physician's Handbook, 16th Edition, 1970 M.A. Krupp, N.J. Sweet, E. Jawetz, E.G. Biglieri	$6.00
Handbook of Medical Treatment, 12th Edition, 1970 M.J. Chatton, S. Margen, H. Brainerd, Editors	$6.50
Handbook of Pediatrics, 9th Edition, 1971 H.K. Silver, C.H. Kempe, H.B. Bruyn	$6.50
Handbook of Poisoning: Diagnosis & Treatment, 6th Edition, 1969 R.H. Dreisbach	$6.00

Preface

Handbook of Psychiatry is offered in the hope that it will serve as a practical and pertinent review and discussion of the problems of our specialty. It is aimed primarily at the medical practitioner and psychiatric resident, but it is hoped that medical students will use it as an authoritative source of psychiatric knowledge and that psychologists, clergymen, social workers, nurses, school administrators, teachers, and psychiatric aides will be able to find in this volume what is useful to them in the daily exercise of their skills.

This *Handbook* really started some years ago when I served as Chairman of the Committee on Psychiatry and Medical Practice of the American Psychiatric Association. One of our chief interests was (and is) sponsoring postgraduate courses in psychiatry for nonpsychiatrist physicians, and one of our chief problems was the unavailability of a readable, practical, and authoritative text.

Those of our readers who are familiar with the First Edition will note some striking changes. All of the chapters have been reordered, reorganized, or combined, and the factual data and references have been updated.

The capsules at the beginning of the chapters are not meant to be introductions, or summaries, or evaluations, although they contain some features of each of these. They are more like highlights, or a bird's-eye view for a traveler about to descend and explore the terrain. Uniformity in these capsules has not been sought from one chapter to another. Some have turned out more like an overall picture, some like a road-map, some like a miniature guidebook. One or two, I suspect, say things that are not even in the chapter. The intention is to give the reader a quick insight into the editor's perspective of the subject.

We are gratified by the response this book has received and are pleased to announce that Spanish and Italian translations are in preparation.

We should be glad to hear from our readers regarding their opinions, disagreements, areas of controversy, and worthwhile data that we have omitted. We hope to improve the book in each subsequent edition and make it more nearly the mature work that is needed in the field.

Philip Solomon, MD

La Jolla, California
June 1971

Contributors

Keith Akins, MD
Formerly Assistant Clinical Professor of Child Psychiatry, University of British Columbia

David Anderson, MD
Chief of Service, Q Division, St. Elizabeth's Hospital, Washington, DC

Colin F. Bolton, MD
Psychiatrist to London Education Authority; Private Practice, Tunbridge, Wells, Kent

Carl N. Brownsberger, MD
Assistant Professor of Psychiatry, Harvard Medical School; Associate Visiting Physician in Psychiatry, Boston City Hospital

Jacob Christ, MD
Clinical Director, Georgia Mental Health Institute; Clinical Associate Professor of Psychiatry, Emory University Medical School, Atlanta, Georgia

Hikmet N. Emmanuel, MD
Clinical Assistant in Psychiatry, Harvard Medical School; Assisting Visiting Physician in Psychiatry, Boston City Hospital

Henry Everett, MD
Clinical Instructor in Psychiatry, Harvard Medical School; Assisting Visiting Physician in Psychiatry, Boston City Hospital

Saul Glasner, MD
Graduate and Member of Affiliated Staff, New York Psychoanalytic Institute; Lecturer in Psychiatry, Faculty of Social Work, Columbia University, New York

Jack Green, MD
Clinical Assistant in Psychiatry, Harvard Medical School; Associate Visiting Physician in Psychiatry, Boston City Hospital

Marion Heath, RN, MS
Associate Professor of Nursing, Boston College School of Nursing; Nursing Consultant, Psychiatry Service, Boston City Hospital

Louisa P. Howe, PhD
Assistant Clinical Professor of Sociology in the Department of Psychiatry, Harvard Medical School

Robert L. Kelley, MD
Clinical Instructor in Psychiatry, Harvard Medical School; Associate Visiting Physician in Psychiatry, Boston City Hospital

Nasir A. Khan, MD
Director of Geriatric Service, Massachusett Department of Mental Health; Clinical Assistant in Psychiatry, Harvard Medical School; Assisting Visiting Physician in Psychiatry, Boston City Hospital

Susan Kleeman, MD
Assistant Clinical Professor of Psychiatry, University of California at San Diego Medical School

William F. McCourt, MD
Director, Alcohol Unit, Boston State Hospital; Senior Clinical Instructor, Tufts Medical School

Patrick H. McDonagh, MD
Attending Staff, Department of Psychiatry, St. Vincent's Hospital, Bridgeport, Connecticut; Fellow, Division of Community Psychiatry, College of Physicians and Surgeons, Columbia University, New York

Audrey Mealia, RN, MS
Nursing Supervisor, Psychiatry Service, Boston City Hospital

Frederick H. Meyers, MD
Professor of Pharmacology, University of California School of Medicine, San Francisco

Emanuel Mirel, MD
Clinical Assistant in Psychiatry, Harvard Medical School; Assisting Physician in Psychiatry, Boston City Hospital

Lawrence B. Mutty, MD
Executive Director, Warren-Washington County Mental Health Center, Glen Falls, New York; Clinical Assistant Professor in Psychiatry, Albany Medical College

Peter E. Nathan, PhD
Professor of Psychology and Director of Clinical Training in Psychology, The Graduate School; Adjunct Professor of Psychiatry, The Medical School, Rutgers, The State University of New Jersey

Albert S. Norris, MD
Professor of Psychiatry, University of Iowa; Chief, Outpatient Department, State Psychopathic Hospital

Vernon D. Patch, MD
Assistant Professor of Psychiatry, Harvard Medical School; Clinical Director, Psychiatry Service, Boston City Hospital

Donald Pugatch, MD
Clinical Assistant in Psychiatry, Harvard Medical School; Assisting Visiting Physician in Psychiatry, Boston City Hospital

Anthony E. Raynes, MD
Clinical Assistant in Psychiatry, Harvard Medical School; Clinic Director, Drug Detoxification Unit, Boston City Hospital

Michael Rossi, PhD
Assistant Professor of Psychology in the Department of Psychiatry, Harvard Medical School; Chief Psychologist in the Department of Psychiatry, Boston City Hospital

Lionel A. Schwartz, MD
Clinical Instructor in Psychiatry, Harvard Medical School; Visiting Physician in Psychiatry, Boston City Hospital; Associate Consulting Psychiatrist, Wellesley College, Wellesley, Massachusetts

David E. Seil, MD
Clinical Instructor in Psychiatry, Harvard Medical School; Assisting Visiting Physician in Psychiatry, Boston City Hospital

Juliana Sustento Seneriches, MD
Senior Psychiatrist, Medfield State Hospital, Medfield, Massachusetts

Nathan T. Sidley, MD
Clinical Assistant in Psychiatry, Harvard Medical School; Associate Visiting Physician in Psychiatry, Boston City Hospital

Philip Solomon, MD
Clinical Professor of Psychiatry, University of California at San Diego Medical School

John B. Sturrock, MD
Clinical Instructor in Psychiatry, Harvard Medical School; Research Fellow in Psychiatry, Boston City Hospital

Anthony P. Vettraino
Supervisor, Psychiatric Social Work, Boston City Hospital

Paul W. Yost, MD
Clinical Fellow in Psychiatry, Harvard Medical School; Chief Resident in Psychiatry, Boston City Hospital

Table of Contents

PART II. PSYCHIATRIC ILLNESS

PART III. PSYCHIATRIC TREATMENT

Notice

1...
Introduction

Introductions are for those who can take the time in a busy world to stop and chat with the author a bit before proceeding to the serious business of the book. Make it a 2-way chat if you care to—your views would be welcome.

Encyclopedia, Textbook, and Handbook

A handbook should be differentiated from an encyclopedia and a textbook. An **encyclopedia** of psychiatry, whether it is called that or not, serves as a storehouse of all important information in the field. It makes available in one large volume (or several smaller ones) complete and authoritative material on any aspect of psychiatry that a student, scholar, or practitioner is likely to be interested in. A lengthy history of psychiatry is usually included, and many developments (eg, insulin shock and lobotomy) are discussed which have little pertinence to modern practice. An encyclopedia is essentially a reference or source book to which one turns, when he has plenty of time, to get a broad picture of the particular phase of psychiatry in which he is interested.

A **textbook** of psychiatry is intended to serve as an aid in teaching the subject. The principles of psychiatry are presented in a systematic and lucid fashion, and enough theory and clinical data are given to enable the student to learn, understand, and develop a scientific and therapeutic attitude toward psychiatric problems. Numerous examples (case histories) are helpful—especially if clear-cut and dramatic. Rare, vague, obscure, and trivial matters are avoided. There is no attempt to be all-inclusive or to cater to the needs of the expert psychiatrist. Nevertheless, all practical aspects of the field must be covered. The textbook is a manual of instruction. A good one can act as a supplement to a series of lectures, or even replace lectures altogether.

A **handbook** of psychiatry is intended for ready consultation when psychiatric problems arise. It is a storehouse of information of current practical importance and serves the student as a source of carefully organized knowledge with emphasis on practice rather than theory. Its chief function is to aid the physician who faces a psychiatric problem and wishes to review relevant material in the field. It should be small, compact, factual, and reasonably devoid of speculative or controversial data.

Bearing all this in mind, it is easy to see why this *Handbook of Psychiatry* has been difficult to prepare. Psychiatry is the youngest of the major medical specialities. It deals with the mind, emotions, and behavior of man—scientifically, the least understood aspects of the human animal. Much that is known in the field is still descriptive, pragmatic, and empiric. The task of the authors is to winnow out the chaff of conjecture and dogma from the wheat of useful truth.

The Reader

The practicing physician must deal with his psychiatric patient on the basis of what he knows or can find out here and now. The medical student must prepare himself for examinations in psychiatry on the basis of what is known or thought to be known today. The psychiatrist-in-training must have at his fingertips the full extent of modern psychiatric information and accepted doctrine. A handbook of psychiatry, therefore, while small enough to fit the hand, should be large enough to serve the immediate professional needs of a physician, medical student, and psychiatrist-in-training.

Most nonpsychiatrist physicians practicing today received little or no training in psychiatry at medical school. Many entered general practice or their own specialty with a repugnance for psychiatry based on uneasiness about their inadequate knowledge, distrust or dislike of "insane" patients, vague misgivings about their own emotional status, or simply a disdain for the "unscientific" subject itself. These physicians may tend to overlook or minimize the importance of emotional factors in their patients' illnesses—much to the detriment of the patients. They may fail to appreciate the value of their own personalities as a therapeutic tool. They may resist recommending a psychiatric consultation until it is unavoidable and perhaps too late. All of this is bad medical practice and is unbecoming to the profession at large. Every physician should practice psychiatry to some extent—at least in his "bedside manner." This book attempts to talk to the nonpsychiatrist physician in clear language from which most of the jargon has been removed and to offer him the kind of information and advice that he can and should use in his practice.

Medical students—although each year the incoming class seems to be smarter than the one before—do not have time to be omnivorous readers. Particularly in psychiatry, where the literature is so voluminous, they must pick and choose carefully. The encyclopedic works can be used only rarely, for special purposes. The textbooks tend to be long on theory and often heavily weighted with the authors' favorite school of thought. It is not easy to find well organized and clearly presented information that has immediate practical application—either to a clinical case in question or to sectors of the general field that one is scanning in preparation for an examination. This *Handbook* attempts to satisfy the needs of the conscientious student.

The psychiatrist-in-training is an advanced student. Wide reading is expected to supplement his clinical experience and supervised therapy. He will read historically important books, classical articles, biographies of the psychiatric giants, excerpts from their collected works, and current articles in the psychiatric journals. When he is confronted with an unfamiliar clinical problem and does not have time to go to the library, and when he is preparing for board certification examinations, he needs readily assimilable information quickly. This *Handbook* contains the help he needs, and if he knows the material in it thoroughly and can apply his knowledge under stress he need have no fear of examinations at any level.

Psychiatry

In these days of marked differences among the many schools of psychiatric thought, the reader of a handbook of psychiatry deserves a statement regarding the particular orientation of the authors. The contributors to this book share a conviction that psychiatry is first of all a branch of medical science. Although it is true that the clinical practice of psychiatry is still more of an art than a science, a young and imperfect science is still a science. Psychiatry, like other branches of medicine, has benefited from many kinds of human activity—imagination, speculation, missionary zeal, evangelism— but by none so much as by scientific investigation.

The essence of science consists of the systematic observation of nature for the purpose of understanding its laws and principles. Experimentation, measurement, reproducibility, controlled variables, statistical evaluation—all of these are difficult to apply to human behavior, but imprecise measurement of shifting variables and $< 100\%$ reproducibility of "same" procedures in "same" patients are problems in physiology and surgery as well as psychiatry. Freud was a scientist, although he speculated much and measured little; he was an honest observer who carefully recorded and systematized his findings to broaden our understanding of human nature and the workings of the mind. "Encounter" and "sensitivity" group enthusiasts who scoff at screening participants and refuse to require training qualifications of group leaders or to keep records cannot be called scientists. Some may be noble innovators, altruistic healers, or well-meaning visionaries, and it is conceivable that their work may lead to important advances—but scientists they are not, and as medical scientists we prefer not to support or contribute to this kind of work.

This book is built around a core of accumulated knowledge about mental illness and its treatment (Sections II and III). Background data (Section I) are included from related areas, and special fields in psychiatry are described in Section IV.

In covering a growing field such as psychiatry, many decisions must be made about what to include and what to omit. We have included new material only when we are reasonably confident that it will survive (eg, lithium treatment for affective disorders is included, but many new phenothiazines are not). We favor the practical over the theoretical (although we try to provide enough theory for intellectual satisfaction and student needs). We document some of the material, but not all—usually by references at the end of each chapter. (References are chosen for historical or classical value as well as to guide the reader to interesting recent work.) We try to strike a balance between exhaustive and condensed presentations (all that is important for clinicians and students, yet brief enough to be practicable).

We recognize that psychiatry overlaps with many other specialities in medicine (to some extent with all of them) and with many other areas of learning. Where the overlap is sufficient to be of practical importance to the clinician or student, we have taken special expository note of it. Our conviction that psychiatry is firmly rooted in **neurology** is shown in Chapters 3 and 15, as well as by the emphasis on organic factors throughout the book. The overlap with **internal medicine** dominates Chapter 18 and is prominent in Chapter 2 and in all the chapters of Sections II and III. Concern with **surgery** occupies a sizeable portion of Chapter 18 and a part of Chapter 15; **pediatrics** is predominant in Chapter 32 and is also involved in Chapters 7, 8, 31, 33, and 34. **Geriatrics** occupies Chapter 36 and is involved in Chapters 15 and 18.

The overlap of psychiatry with **psychology** is great since, in the broadest sense, psychiatry can be considered a branch of psychology known as psychopathology. In this book, psychologists have written Chapters 6, 7, 11, 12, and 28 and have influenced our thinking in places too many to mention. **Sociology** is also a basic science of psychiatry. A sociologist wrote Chapter 39 and a social worker Chapter 29. Reference to contributions of social workers to the practice of psychiatry will be found throughout the book. The overlap with the **law** is unavoidable in any field of human behavior. Forensic psychiatry is presented in Chapter 37, and medicolegal matters are also mentioned in Chapter 4. The **genetics** of psychiatric disorders is discussed in Chapter 8, **nursing** in Chapter 30, **epidemiology** in Chapter 9, **pharmacology** in Chapter 24, **administration** in Chapters 9, 10, 22, and 23, and **history** in Chapter 12.

Miscellaneous Comments

The preparation of a book of this kind gives one a perspective on the field not easily achieved in any other way. One sees brilliant accomplishments, areas of hopeful prospects, and vast regions of woeful ignorance. The most grievous unknowns surely lie in the field of etiology. Heredity, infection, endocrine pathology, dynamic psychopathology, and others have had their ups and downs. Each has claimed too much and proved too little, though there is probably some truth in each. Time and scientific investigation will be necessary before a more complete picture can be drawn.

We have tried to present plausible etiologic data from all useful sources. If it seems that too much space has been devoted to psychodynamic considerations, this is not because we believe that psychodynamics ranks preeminently high in the etiology of psychiatric disorders but because, if the subject is to be presented at all, it should be presented thoroughly enough to be intelligible. We believe that psychodynamic theory is of considerable value in the understanding and treatment of the neuroses, personality problems, and behavioral disorders; of some value in the management of psychosomatic conditions; and of little value for the psychoses or for predictive validity anywhere.

Authors and editors who pride themselves on the brevity and compactness of their book usually take great pains to avoid overlap and repetition.

We do not. In many places brevity has been deliberately sacrificed in the interests of usability and continuity of presentation. Certain practical aspects in the management of the suicidal patient, for example, will be found in several places in the book. Repetition is also prominent in the evaluation of depression and anxiety and the explication of psychodynamic principles. A measured amount of redundancy, as in spacecraft circuitry, has its safety value.

Certain topics have been barely mentioned or omitted altogether. There are fashions, short-lived enthusiasms, and oddities in psychiatry as there are in other branches of medicine. One need not take cognizance of all of them even though some may eventually turn out to be important. Psychodrama, poetry therapy, general systems theory, and existentialism have adherents among psychiatrists of stature but have not attained sufficient general acceptance to warrant extensive comment here.

Certain contemporary problems that have psychiatric implications have been touched upon at several places in the book. Among these are the current wars on the international scene; national problems such as pollution, the draft, racial unrest, riots, crime in the streets, and decay in the cities; and violence on the campus, youth protests, and incipient unrest and rebellion everywhere. It is hoped that most of these, though highly relevant today, will be of only fleeting interest.

A few comments on individual chapters are in order. Chapter 6, on differential diagnostic symptoms and signs, presents a unique approach to the diagnostic process in psychiatry. Students in psychiatry are usually taught how to elicit data from patients via the history and examination and then the chief characteristics of the most important clinical entities. How to match up the one with the other in an individual patient, what weights to put where, what level of confidence to attach to which possible diagnoses—these are matters left essentially to that will-of-the-wisp called "clinical judgment." Clinical judgment is the result of experience, and experience presumably must be accumulated slowly at the expense of one's patients. Chapter 6 makes a first attempt to show how to proceed from symptoms and signs to a likely diagnosis without resorting to anything mystical. It is not yet a computerized system, but it may be a useful beginning which can be used while clinical judgment is maturing.

Chapter 11 (Statistics in Psychiatry) gives the reader what we believe is available nowhere else in the literature in such nontechnical and practical form—an understanding of what he should (and can) know about the value of the data in the articles he reads.

Chapter 20 offers a framework for the understanding and management of the chronic alcoholic patient (social, neurotic, or psychotic) which appears for the first time in a volume on general psychiatry.

The inclusion of material on psychoanalysis (Chapter 31) in a book designed for general practitioners and medical students as well as for advanced students of psychiatry may seem surprising. We feel that there is nothing esoteric or forbidding about this subject and that there is no good reason for reserving it for a specially chosen few. Here as elsewhere in medical science, when specialists find something that can be helpful to patients, they are obliged to present it to all medical practitioners to use as they choose.

The **Psychiatric Emergency Routine** presented at the end of this book is an attempt to make readily available the information that a physician needs when dealing with a patient in a psychiatric emergency. It is condensed and frankly oversimplified in the interests of quick and ready usability. Those who wish more knowledge and guidance about psychiatric emergencies may refer to Chapters 22 and 23.

PART I.
PSYCHIATRIC BACKGROUND

2 . . .

The Doctor-Patient Relationship

The good physician treats not only the disease but the person who has the disease. To do this he takes a history of feelings as well as events, examines for emotions as well as physical signs, and prescribes for peace of mind as well as body. His most important therapeutic tool is his own personality, and he uses this consciously, wisely, and benevolently, with full knowledge of his own weaknesses and fallibilities.

The physician who wishes to serve his patients to the fullest extent cannot limit his objectives to accurate diagnosis based on objective evaluation of signs and symptoms followed by implementation of some standard treatment plan. He must consciously address himself to the *person* in whom the disease process occurs. A completely impersonal approach is not possible in medicine since the doctor and the patient react to each other as persons whether they wish to do so or not. Thus, since subjective factors cannot be eliminated, they must be recognized and understood and their therapeutic potentialities used for the patient's benefit. This is another way of saying that the doctor-patient relationship plays a definite and at times crucial role in the outcome of the treatment program. The physician must understand and guide this relationship, not only because he wishes to be more effective and bring about a cure but also because, unless he is aware of the emotional interaction between him and his patient, he may precipitate an iatrogenic illness.

EMOTIONAL ATTITUDES IN THE PATIENT

The patient's personality is the totality of the characteristic ways in which he deals with internal and external stresses, ie, his methods of maintaining emotional equilibrium. His signs and symptoms are inextricably bound up with different facets of his personality, and true communication is impossible unless the physician is alert to all that this implies.

The patient's attitudes and emotional responses toward his illness, his doctor, the hospital staff, etc mirror his earlier interactions with his family, friends, teachers, other doctors, and other significant people in his life. His peculiarities and "unusual reactions" are easier to understand and to handle therapeutically if something about his past experiences is known and understood. *Empathic* understanding is usually more useful than intellectual awareness and is often therapeutic in itself.

The Patient's Family

Knowing the patient's family is especially important in understanding him. A person who has had a genuinely motherly mother usually has a basic feeling of trust in people (and in life generally) that helps him to cope with an unpredictable and at times unfriendly world. A woman who is inconsistent and emotionally incapable of mothering is apt to send her child out into the world with a wary and hostile attitude toward what he will find there. Such a person may misinterpret a friendly and helpful gesture (eg, on the part of the medical staff) as an attempt to hurt or maneuver him or to "help" him only in ways that serve the helper's own convenience. Thus the doctor who tries to help may be perceived as doing so only because he wants to be rid of the patient or keep him solely for monetary gain.

The individual who was disliked by his mother will often grow up unconsciously disliking himself. This dislike is projected onto parental figures such as doctors and paramedical personnel, so that anything the doctor does is taken as "evidence" of his dislike. The physician who understands this mechanism of "self-hate" will be able to deal more adequately with the problems it causes.

A positive, loving, and adequate father, in addition to helping the mother (directly and indirectly) to fulfill her responsibilities to her children, provides goals, standards, and conditions that help the individual to orient himself realistically to life. Such an individual, when he ventures from home, is prepared to adjust emotionally and socially to his fellow man. The child who has had an immature or maladjusted father is often left with conflicting loyalties. To "honor" his father may involve living life according to the disordered pattern the father presented. The patient who somehow always seems to be at odds with his doctors and nurses may be trying to live up to his father's code of behavior, perhaps trying to convince himself that his father was right and the world wrong. The physician can avoid proving this false thesis by adopting an understanding attitude toward the patient's painful dilemma.

Siblings

Siblings usually play an important role in the development of personality. Feelings of jealousy toward other patients and the need to win status in the doctor's eyes may be related to childhood sibling rivalries. Valuable insights can be drawn from remarks like the following: "I came from a large family, doctor, and I was pretty much lost in the shuffle." "I was the oldest and had to take a lot of responsibility for things going right in the house." "I was the only girl in a family of six boys, and when mother died I became the family maid. Now that I am married, I am still the family maid. Honestly, doctor, if I could get rid of this pain in my back, I wouldn't complain so much." "When I was a baby I was the cutest thing and everyone's darling. Then when I was three, my brother was born. He was always sick and my mother spent all her time with him. My father was quite old and didn't like children. I felt alone and lost. The only time my mother paid any attention to me was when I got sick."

The "only child," and "youngest child," the "unexpected child" born to older parents whose other children are grown, and the child who felt like "nothing" because he wasn't the oldest or the youngest and wasn't the sex his parents wanted—all have special problems that play an important role in their behavior when they become ill. The patient who unconsciously feels guilty about sibling rivalries may report to his family doctor with cardiac symptoms several weeks after his brother dies of coronary heart disease. A patient who actually (or in fantasy) was partly responsible for a sibling's death (eg, in a boating accident) may feel a need to punish himself for the rest of his life with chronic symptoms.

Social and Other Factors

The patient's social, cultural, economic, geographic, racial, and religious background all play a role in his feelings toward his illness and his behavior toward the people whose help he seeks. A Chinese patient may feel more comfortable with a Chinese physician. A Jewish patient may be apprehensive about being in a Catholic hospital. A person who has not been exposed to physicians of foreign background may be convinced that only American physicians can give competent care. The elderly patient may be unable to develop confidence in a young doctor. Feelings of prejudice and superstition are often deeply ingrained and can only be overcome with great effort. When a person is ill, his apprehension makes him even more vulnerable to unreasonable emotions. At such times he may revert to beliefs which in less anxious times he knows to be false. The physician who understands all this will resist reacting with impatience and anger and will attempt to give the reassurance needed. Bringing the patient's fears into the open and discussing them with him in an accepting and empathic manner can go a long way toward minimizing their effect.

Troublesome Patients

Some patients seem to fall into categories which make them difficult or unappealing to deal with. Behind the unattractive facade, however, there is usually a troubled and emotionally confused person who is asking for help in the only "safe" way he knows. The "obnoxious patient" may be seeking attention in the only way he believes possible. He may be completely unable to receive affection from anyone without experiencing emotional discomfort and fear. He is so lonely that he decides unconsciously that negative attention is better than none. Some chronically guilt-ridden patients cannot tolerate a "pleasant" doctor or being made well. The "uncooperative patient" may prove to be an overly dependent individual who is expressing his resentment that he cannot have the doctor all to himself and completely under his control. The outwardly "angry patient" may be trying to ward off anxiety about his illness or his fear about becoming dependent on the doctor. The "overly affectionate patient" may be fighting his unconscious hostility, which is particularly dangerous when directed toward someone whose help is being sought.

Some patients seem to be always shopping around for new doctors. As soon as they establish a relationship with one physician, they feel compelled to seek out another. In many cases these are people who feel so unworthy that they are sure their doctors will come to dislike them sooner or later. Both for self-protection and for revenge, they abandon the doctor first.

EMOTIONAL ATTITUDES IN THE PHYSICIAN

Good medical practice dictates that treatment be based (whenever possible) on evaluation of symptoms and signs, formulation of a diagnosis, and understanding of etiologic factors. The physician must make his observations, conduct the necessary examinations, order diagnostic tests, evaluate and correlate the data, and finally come up with an interpretation of the patient's problem and what to do about it. The doctor's ability to do this competently is enhanced by an understanding of his own emotional reactions toward his patients.

Before He Sees the Patient

The doctor may begin to react toward the patient even before he sees him, and should make a habit of noting these reactions and their possible therapeutic implications. For example, his attitude may be different in anticipating an appointment with a patient referred by the dean of the medical school than in approaching an intoxicated vagrant brought in by the police or in responding to an "emergency call" in the middle of the night.

The First Meeting

When the patient and physician meet, the doctor automatically gains a series of impressions. What type of person does the patient appear to be? Is he in physical distress? Is he relaxed, calm, or apprehensive? Does he seem depressed, apathetic, or elated? What of his dress and posture, tone of voice, and manner of relating to the doctor?

Now comes a most crucial observation: *How is the doctor relating to the patient?* Why does he relate in this way? By asking himself these questions repeatedly, the physician obtains information about the patient that is not available from any other source. At the same time, he gradually becomes aware of the characteristic ways that he (the doctor) uses in dealing with his own internal and external stresses. By gaining insight into his own personality patterns, the physician can learn to rely on what his *feelings* tell him about his patients and to know when his seemingly objective observations are being colored by his own emotional bias.

The Physician's Motivations

It will help the physician to know as much as possible about the conscious and unconscious motives that influenced him to choose medicine as a career. These motives are often related to emotional factors during childhood development. The developmental history of every individual, from infancy onward, is a constant struggle between negative (destructive) and positive (constructive) drives. Some people greatly fear that their primitive aggressive impulses may overwhelm the other parts of their personalities. To cope with this anxiety, the individual may undertake a "healing" and "reparative" career to assure himself that he can mend and put together that which is broken or "sick." The emotional need to fight disease may be either a help or a hindrance to the well-balanced, effective, and mature practice of medicine or surgery.

Other unconscious ambitions of all sorts may play a role in the choice of medicine as a career. The choice of specialty may be related to repressed desires that can have great influence on the doctor's life without his being aware of them. The "motherly" physician may be replacing his own lost or emotionally defective mother. The "fatherly" or authoritarian doctor often has an emotional need to create this type of figure in his own life and in the lives of his patients.

The physician should recognize that his direct or indirect choice of patients might be related to emotional needs within himself. Why does he seem to get along well with certain types of patients and not with others? The doctor may subtly encourage his patients to act in ways that serve his emotional needs. Some physicians seem to be always fighting with their patients; others have only "obedient," extremely cooperative, or even submissive patients. An awareness of how he contributes to these situations will help prevent inappropriate emotional responses and keep him from using his patients as scapegoats and eventually alienating them. Such situations are bound to lead to low self-esteem and feelings of failure in the physician.

The doctor who unconsciously harbors strong feelings of inadequacy and boosts his self-confidence by looking down on patients because they are sick and in his mind "inferior" to him should not be surprised to find that these patients do not like him and tend not to regain their health fully while under his care. He is likely to attract precisely the type of patient who will unconsciously cater to his needs and will remain ill so that he will always have something to complain about.

Influence of Past Experience and Environment

The doctor's work with his patients is bound to be influenced by events in his personal life and his relationships with his fellow workers and supervisors, the hospital staff, and the community as a whole. The overambitious physician whose personal life is unsatisfactory may be tempted to make "fantastically brilliant" diagnoses and institute dramatic treatment procedures which do more for his own morale than for his patients' welfare. The young physician in financial distress may unconsciously project his problems onto his patients and avoid ordering valid diagnostic tests or prescribing necessary medication for fear that the patient could not tolerate the expense as well as he is presumably tolerating his illness. Unfortunately, it occasionally happens that a physician will charge high fees and order tests that profit him more than the patient, either because he feels he has to keep up with the medical Joneses or because he needs to bolster his feelings of insecurity by becoming a "financial success." The doctor who is afraid of his longings to depend on others may present himself as a "rebel" in the hospital or community and may fail to seek the help of consultants as often as he should. In these and similar circumstances, the physician should repeatedly ask himself whether his handling of the patient is in keeping with the patient's needs or his own.

In spite of extensive training, the physician may unconsciously harbor unrealistic attitudes toward illness. The emotionally immature physician often clings to a secret myth that all misfortune in life can be neutralized or prevented if people only try hard enough. He cannot tolerate the idea that there are things over which we have no control. When he sees an individual who is ill, he consciously or unconsciously holds someone responsible. This might be the patient himself, his family, or the "incompetent doctor" who saw him last. These emotions can usually be traced back to angry feelings toward parents who somehow failed to make him all-powerful and superhuman. Thus the innocent patient, his family, or his previous doctor may become the objects of hostile feelings the physician unconsciously harbors toward his parents.

A doctor may have inappropriate attitudes, again originating in his childhood, toward patients who don't seem to respond to treatment. He may feel that such patients don't "love" him—if they did, they would get well. In dealing with a patient with a chronic illness, he may tell himself, "Why tie myself down to a losing battle? I'll only make a token effort so that the outcome won't be so disappointing." With a patient who is dying, he might feel, "He's abandoning me; I may as well abandon him first." It takes years of emotional struggle and maturation to come to terms with life and death as they are and to reject unrealistic rationalizations whose only function is to make oneself feel more comfortable.

Self-Appraisal

The doctor should evaluate his ability to deal adequately with the patient who is hostile or pleasant, suspicious or submissive, evasive or cooperative, depressed or overactive, ungrateful or overly grateful, seductive or cold, etc. The awareness that he has difficulties with certain types of people will lead him to approach them with greater thoughtfulness and will help prevent conflicts which drive the patient away or make him uncooperative. Some physicians, for example, cannot tolerate a pleasant, cooperative patient. Their own life experiences have convinced them that when someone is friendly—or for that matter, whenever anything good comes along—the invariable outcome is disillusionment, hurt feelings, and disappointment. Thus they regard the patient's smile with suspicion, thinking, "What is he after?" The more the physician understands his own emotional attitudes and comes to accept *himself*, the less likely will he be to project his problems onto his patients and to treat them incompetently.

A special situation to be considered is the possibility of illness, physical or emotional, in the physician himself. It is very difficult to see oneself objectively. Psychologic *denial* to avoid unpleasant truths—especially about oneself—is a common phenomenon. The most difficult problem the physician may have is to admit to himself that he has a problem. Whether this problem is some physical infirmity, an emotional disorder, chronic alcoholism, or progressive incapacitation due to advancing age, the prudent practice of medicine demands that the physician courageously seek help for his problem and arrange his work in such a way as not to betray his patients' trust in him.

PSYCHOLOGIC ASPECTS OF
THE DOCTOR-PATIENT RELATIONSHIP

When the patient presents himself to the physician, he automatically gives up some of his independence and to some extent surrenders many of his obligations and responsibilities.

He submits himself to the authority of the doctor in somewhat the same way that a child submits to the authority of his parents and for the same reason—so that he may be properly cared for. This situation usually reactivates many of the emotional struggles that existed in the child-parent relationships. Dormant dependency feelings are reawakened.

The cardiac patient who has been a "lionheart" in the courtroom or on Wall Street may become a meek, bleating lamb who attempts to prolong every visit from his doctor or nurse. His feelings are easily hurt; he cannot tolerate even minimal frustrations; and everything frightens him. He expects those who attend him to shield him from every stress, no matter how slight, and when they fail to do so he reacts with the rage of the helpless child.

Many patients believe that it is the *right* of a sick person to throw temper tantrums.

The Patient's Reactions to the Doctor

The patient may try to control his doctor by being either a "good boy" or by subtly refusing to cooperate until his wishes are granted. A symbiotic emotional relationship may develop between the physician and the patient which would mirror the situation that existed in the patient's childhood. Unless the physician is aware of the existence of such a relationship and its implications for both himself and the patient, obstacles to good treatment may arise. Such a situation may leave both patient and doctor completely frustrated and even incapacitated, for they end up reacting only to the negative aspects of each other's personalities and become blind to the positive features. The excessive demands and expectations of the patient may so threaten the physician as to awaken similar desires (mostly unconscious) within himself. He may be tempted to punish the patient for feelings he unwittingly harbors within his own mind. These secret feelings may at times be condoned and enjoyed and at other times violently disapproved of. Good results cannot be expected if the physician alternately spoils and punishes his patients in order to satisfy his own emotional needs.

An undesirable situation is created when the doctor unconsciously disapproves of himself but perceives this disapproval as coming from the patient. He will then fight with the patient instead of with himself. When a practitioner is too zealous in seeking approval from his patients, he may be trying to neutralize his own self-disapproval.

A patient's hold on reality may at times be quite tenuous, and if his situation becomes intolerable he may retreat into fantasy. The physician who is sensitive to this possibility will try to make the "reality world" as palatable as possible to the patient. Small acts of kindness, adequate attention to relieving pain, and meeting the patient's needs for reassurance, acceptance, and understanding will effectively prevent the easy retreat into the world of unreality. Unfortunately, the patient is often unable to communicate his fears and despairs verbally. The physician should be alert to the patient's attempts to communicate with him on a symbolic level by way of his symptoms or behavior. The patient who is cranky, uncomfortable, and seemingly refractory to treatment may be saying, "Doctor, could you please put your hand on my brow and show me somehow that you like me, even just a little?" The desperately sick man who insists on signing out of the hospital may be saying, "I feel I'm just a number here. Nobody cares and nobody needs me. I'll have my revenge. I'll show you that I don't need you either. It's so unbearably lonely to be so unimportant to you busy doctors that perhaps if I provoke and annoy you I will get to matter more to you, even if it is in a negative way." The worst possible response the physician can make is, "We don't care if you stay or leave. You're only hurting yourself." The patient who refuses to give permission for an important test may be saying, "Don't take me for granted. Coax me a little. You have so much power over me, let me enjoy a moment of power over you." Patients who are always silent, those who appear to be unrealistically carefree, or those who chatter on compulsively about nothing are usually trying to "say" something to the physician, who will get the message only if he listens for it. "Sure 'tis easy to see when you look with the heart" is as scientific as it is sentimental.

The First Interview

The circumstances that bring the patient and the doctor together and the situation and setting of their contacts with each other play an important role in their relationship. The physician who is unaware of the importance of these factors will run into misunderstandings and blocks in communication. As has been suggested earlier, the physician is bound to feel differently toward the patient he sees in a noisy, crowded clinic plagued by administrative difficulties than toward the socially prominent patient who consults him in his private office. All patients are emotionally gratified by their physician's concern for their immediate comfort even in "small" matters. Has the doctor offered him a comfortable chair as he listens to his history? Are there frequent telephone interruptions and other distractions? Does the doctor seem to be in a hurry, or overburdened by too heavy an office or clinic schedule? Is the waiting room crowded, small, and dirty, with last year's half-torn magazines strewn about in disorder, or has some thought been given to the patient's comfort as he anxiously awaits his turn in the consultation room? There are also waiting rooms that are too grand and too lavishly decorated, with luxurious chairs that are more uncomfortable than plain ones because they remind the patient of the size of his coming bill.

The patient learns much about the doctor by evaluating his office, his receptionist, the response to his call for an appointment, the doctor's reputation, his hospital affiliations, and the diplomas and pictures on his walls. When they finally meet, the doctor's greeting, his handshake, whether he smiles or not, and his bearing in general make a great impression on the patient. The doctor's manner during the history taking and the physical examination is carefully and anxiously watched. The doctor who says to the patient, "I can tell you nothing until these tests are completed and the results come back," may in fact have already told his patient a great deal. The physician's treatment has already begun whether he planned it or not.

The doctor's evaluation of the patient may begin long before he actually examines him. Is the patient himself calling for the appointment, or has someone else done it for him? Is the patient's voice over the telephone timid, whimpering, apologetic, or aggressive and demanding? Does he arrive too early for his appointment (probably because of anxiety) or too late (because he is angry, depressed, or disorganized)? What is his appearance and manner as he greets the doctor? Each word, expression, and gesture conveys important information. How is the patient "put together"? Are different parts of him and his clothing "fighting" with one another, or is there a sense of harmony about him? What seems to be out of place? Or is everything perhaps too much in place—too perfect? What is he hiding? The answers to many of these questions can be very important for correct diagnosis and treatment. To obtain these answers, the physician must ask the right questions not only of the patient but of himself as well. Many of the answers can be learned only by recognizing and understanding his own emotional responses to the patient.

Specialty Roles

Although the doctor-patient relationship is at work for good or ill between all doctors and their patients, different specialties have become associated with special facets of their relationship. Next to the psychiatrist, the *general practitioner* probably makes greatest therapeutic use of the doctor-patient relationship whether he knows it or not. More so than other physicians, he knows his patients and their families and can see how many of their medical problems may be related to the emotional, social, economic, and other stresses in their lives. He observes directly how different patients perceive him in different ways, and learns that the approach he uses in evaluating one patient's gastrointestinal symptoms is not adequate for another patient's needs even if the symptoms are similar. His decisions to order certain tests, to refer to a specialist, to institute certain medical regimens, or to ask the patient to return next week, next month, or next year are often based as much on his knowledge of the patient as a person as on the medical data gathered from the examination. He also knows his "bedside manner" or 15 minutes spent simply talking with the patient may prove to be more effective in diagnosis and treatment than the tests he orders or the prescription he writes.

The *psychiatrist* is usually in the fortunate position of being able to offer himself as a person for the patient to relate to for substantial lengths of time and at relatively frequent intervals. Most psychiatrists agree that all forms of psychiatric treatment (including the somatic therapies) depend a great deal on the doctor-patient relationship. In some forms of psychotherapy, it is used primarily for emotionally supportive purposes. In others, it is permitted to develop along particular lines so that it can itself become the subject of study by the patient and the doctor. The intricacies of such a relationship can reveal unique evidence of the vital connection between the patient's disordered psychophysiologic or psychosocial functioning and his interactions (past and present) with significant figures in his life.

The *surgeon* often plays a special role in the life of his patient. The patient may be intellectually convinced, when he submits to being operated upon, that his doctor's reputation, integrity, skill, and desire to help will all be working on his behalf and that many of his fears are illogical. However, the patient's emotional sense of helplessness, his fears of what could be done to him while under anesthesia, the awareness of the great power the surgeon has over him before, during, and after the operation, and the knowledge that operations usually have painful and dangerous aspects serve to arouse a great deal of anxiety even though he may not express it or may try to hide it from himself. There are few people who are not tempted to put off a visit to the doctor if they are convinced that surgery will be recommended. Many patients unconsciously view a surgical procedure as a kind of punishment for real or fancied transgressions, and some actively seek surgery for mitigation of emotional conflicts or atonement for conscious or unconscious guilt. The surgeon may be seen as a godlike figure who prescribes and administers the necessary corporal punishment or penalty. After the offensive "bad" part has been removed and penitential pain endured, the patient may feel that he is "wholesome" once again and that he can now become a fit recipient of the authoritative and powerful surgeon's love.

The *obstetrician and gynecologist* should be particularly aware of how a woman may emotionally perceive a hysterectomy as the removal of something that made her a "good" or "bad" person or a "complete" or "incomplete" woman. The *urologist* too, should not underestimate the emotional trauma that is usually associated with surgery related to the genital and reproductive organs. Patients often have a self-image that they feel must remain intact if they are to be able to deal with life's problems. They fear that surgery might destroy something that is vital to this self-image. Consequently, the apprehension about becoming emotionally incapacitated may be just as great as the fear of physical crippling.

The *fear of death* is universal. Whether it is realistic in a particular instance or not, the physician should not respond with impatience or ridicule when such a fear is expressed. If he does, he will make his patient feel ashamed, unworthy, and frightened of revealing other important things about himself. Unconsciously the patient will sense that in the future he should protect the doctor from painful truths that might prove upsetting.

The *pediatrician* who forgets that he cannot treat children as if they were adults creates unnecessary problems in his dealings with his patients.

Getting along well with children is an art that some doctors have great difficulty mastering. The following basic points should prove helpful: The infant and young child is frightened of anything unfamiliar. Introducing anything or anyone new should always be done gradually. For years after children learn to talk, they attach literal meanings to words. The child may misinterpret the doctor's fanciful joke in a concrete way and misunderstand his meaning. It is best to speak to children simply and clearly and, whenever possible (in medical matters at any rate), not to leave things to the imagination. The child's knowledge of the world is still limited, and when the doctor says, "Oh, you have such a nice big tongue," the child may be quite impressed with this information and attach an importance to the statement that was not intended. Children are especially sensitive to losses of any kind. Loss of a parent, loss of the tonsils or appendix, or any injury to his "perfect body" is tolerated poorly during emotional development. The doctor who is aware of this will be better prepared to accept and deal with the child's anxiety (and the child's attempts to deal with it). The adolescent patient takes a great deal of understanding since he is still a child in some ways and an adult in others. He is unsure of how he will deal with the challenge of adult life but believes that accepting advice from adults is a sign of weakness or dependence. He is struggling with powerful sexual drives and maturational processes. He seems exhausted one day and full of boundless energy the next. In a sense, he tries on different identities "for size," as it were, to help him deal with particular crises. As a result, his attitude toward the doctor may change from day to day. The wise physician will think back to his own adolescence and avoid treating the patient of this age group as if he were completely either a child or an adult.

Relationship Therapy

The relationship between the doctor and patient can be a powerful therapeutic tool. The same medication or operative procedure in the hands of a physician who inspires trust and positive feelings in his patients will have better results than those achieved by a doctor who is mistrusted and feared. No physician can practice good medicine who is unaware of the "placebo effect" and its implications. There is still much to be understood about this phenomenon, but what we already know may be used to good effect.

There are some situations in which the outcome of the patient's illness will be crucially affected by the physician's being able to practice some "relationship therapy." This involves the following:

(1) The physician must make a deliberate effort to *accept* the patient and his need for individuality and status.

(2) The physician must express *emotionally supportive attitudes,* such as giving the patient some praise and some recognition of the pain, sorrow, and fear that are often associated with illness. Understanding the patient's resentments and feelings of guilt can often bring dramatic relief.

(3) The physician must give the patient an opportunity to *identify* with his doctor. This will enable the patient to borrow some strength from the person whom he usually regards as powerful, all-knowing, and confident.

The patient feels more comfortable when he is able to think, "My doctor and I are fighting this disease in me. As I get to know how my doctor thinks and feels, I can fight this in myself with a measure of his wisdom and strength."

(4) The physician must use the doctor-patient relationship to provide *emotionally corrective experiences.* The chronically fearful patient can, by observing his doctor's attitude and manner toward him, learn that his mind and body are not quite so delicate as, for example, his mother (probably because of her own anxieties) led him to believe. If the patient breaks down and cries in the presence of the doctor and is obviously embarrassed about his longing for emotional support, it is helpful for the physician to indicate directly or indirectly that this is normal under the circumstances. The doctor should make it clear that he understands such behavior and that, if the roles were reversed, he would not be ashamed of having to receive such help.

Secondary Gain

The problem of "secondary gain" is frequently encountered in sick people, and the physician should be prepared to deal with it firmly and effectively but with understanding and sympathy. It is natural that sick people should treasure the attention and kindness they get when they need these supportive responses so desperately; however, if they cling to the role of the sick one after the physical sickness is gone, then they have entered the realm of emotional invalidism and need help of a different sort. Attention must now be gradually diverted into giving them insight (gently) into their emotional needs and exploring the possibilities of satisfying these needs by healthy means.

The Doctor as Instrument of Therapy

The physician can and should use his own self as an instrument with which to understand and evaluate the patient. By asking himself how each patient makes him feel, he may gain a better insight into the patient's problems and behavior than can be obtained solely from the usual methods of observation and deduction. Human beings are not always trusting and candid. They may carry grudges, particularly against doctors. They may have trusted doctors once but were so hurt emotionally or physically that they resolved never to trust them again. The physician cannot do his best work unless he knows everything about the patient that should be known, and the patient who keeps secrets from his doctor is impairing his chances of getting well. The doctor should note his own feelings and give as much credence to what he senses about the patient as to what he can measure and photograph. This must be done with discretion, balance, and reason, and not with the fear that one is not being scientific or "objective."

REFERENCES

Books and Monographs

Becker, A.: *The General Practitioner's Role in the Treatment of Emotional Illness.* Thomas, 1968.

Fink, P.J., & W.W. Oaks: *Psychiatry and the Internist.* Grune & Stratton, 1970.

Usdin, G.L. (editor): *Practical Lectures in Psychiatry for the Medical Practitioner.* Thomas, 1966.

Zabarenko, L., Pittenger, R.A., & R.N. Zabarenko: *Primary Medical Practice: A Psychiatric Evaluation.* Warren H. Green, Inc, 1968.

Journal Articles

Bogdonoff, M.D., & others: The doctor-patient relationship. JAMA 192:45–48, 1965.

Bonime, W.: Some principles of brief psychotherapy. Psychiat Quart 27:1–18, 1953.

Davis, M.S., & R.L. Eichhorn: Compliance with medical regimens: Panel study. J Health Hum Behav 4:240–249, 1963.

Francis, V., Korsch, B.M., & M.J. Morris: Gaps in doctor-patient communication: Patients' response to medical advice. New England J Med 280:535–540, 1969.

Frank, J.D.: The dynamics of the psychotherapeutic relationship: Determinants and effects of the therapist's influence. Psychiatry 22:17–39, 1959.

Hofling, C.K.: The place of placebos in medical practice. GP 11:103–107, June 1955.

Kaufman, R.M.: Psychiatry for the nonpsychiatrist. M Clin North America 51(6), 1967.

Korsch, B.M., Gozzi, E.K., & V. Francis: Gaps in doctor-patient communication: Doctor-patient interaction and patient satisfaction. Pediatrics 42:855–871, 1968.

Lowinger, P., & S. Dobie: What makes the placebo work? Arch Gen Psychiat 20:84–88, 1969.

Preuss, H., & P. Solomon: The patient's reaction to bedside teaching. New England J Med 259:520–525, 1958.

Riffenburgh, R.S.: Doctor-patient relationship in glaucoma therapy. Arch Ophth 75:204–206, 1966.

Szasz, T.S., & M.H. Hollender: Contribution to the philosophy of medicine: Basic models of the doctor-patient relationship. Arch Int Med 97:585, 1959.

Veith, I.: The physician-priest: Craftsman or philosopher? California Med 113:20–26, Sept 1970.

3...

The Mind & the Brain

Sigmund Freud once said he was convinced there would one day be an organic explanation for all psychic processes. That day has not yet arrived, but considerable progress has been made toward the goal. This chapter does not attempt to present the work that has been done or the results achieved. It offers a point of view, admittedly oversimplified and partly hypothetical, but one that ties together a welter of information into a usable framework for thinking about the mind in terms of the brain.

The brain contains billions of cells arranged in over 100 histologically distinct areas and 12 different lobes. How it functions remains a mystery in spite of years of intensive and ingenious work by scientists in many fields. Some communications engineers, computer experts, and imaginative workers with scanning and programming devices think that with a roomful of the most advanced and miniaturized equipment they could reproduce a small portion of what the ordinary human brain can do. Only the barest beginnings have been made in understanding the mechanisms of memory storage and retrieval, of thought, reasoning, creativity, and emotion—let alone judgment, insight, or consciousness. Yet almost everything that occurs in human behavior, normal and abnormal, can be attributed to brain and CNS function and thus to the activity of brain cells and related groups of cells.

Clinically, the brain may be considered to operate roughly on 2 levels which may be called the lower and higher levels. *The lower level* (primitive and sensorial) encompasses conscious awareness and reactivity to both the body and its instincts and the outside world and its stimuli. Thus, feelings and emotions reside here alongside the sensorium (sensation and perception). This primitive "creature" portion of the mind is better developed in some other animals than in man. Psychologically, the id (instincts) and parts of the ego (awareness) are included in this lower level.

The anatomic parts of the nervous system that subserve the lower level of the brain are the brain stem and the autonomic nervous system; the limbic system; the sensory, auditory, visual, and motor cortices; and connecting pathways, spinal cord, and peripheral nerves.

Normal functioning of the brain at this level permits enormous adaptability to changing internal or external conditions of the environment from moment to moment. Consciousness, for example, is not an all-or-none phenomenon. Under circumstances of great excitement or intense outer interest (dramatic events, great danger), consciousness can become extremely acute, as though focused down to a searing small point. Awareness of non-relevant stimuli at such times may virtually cease. If the stimulation arises from within (thirst, hunger, erotic desire, fear), consciousness can be strong but broadened to sweep the surroundings in an eager, searching manner.

At the other end of the spectrum, consciousness can dim until most of it goes into abeyance in sleep. In deepest sleep, only forceful sensory stimuli may register and produce waking. In light sleep, a change in illumination (observed through the closed eyelids) or the slightest noise or touch may awaken the sleeper. Drowsiness, with reduced consciousness, may precede or follow sleep. Conditions that normally favor it are reduction of stimuli from within (satiety) or from without (sensory deprivation, isolation, monotony), or fatigue.

In the waking state, consciousness usually fluctuates well within the extremes discussed above but can switch rapidly to adapt to changing conditions. A drowsy or lightly sleeping mother will respond immediately with sharpened faculties at the sound of her baby's cry. A bored student in the lecture room will come alert abruptly if his name is called.

Emotions and mood are equally variable and responsive to internal and external situations. A single word (such as "no") can dash one's spirits from eager expectation to deep disappointment. In a marital quarrel, an intelligent, civilized man can talk and act like a brute and then, in sudden realization of what he is doing, react with shock and consternation to his own behavior. Normal feelings and mood can run the gamut from the extremes of misery to joy, but they remain appropriate to the existing situation. There are allowable individual differences within normal limits (temperament, disposition) from excitable and sensitive to phlegmatic and stolid, but lack of reaction when events call for it is abnormal and so is prolonged, inappropriate mood—usually depression, elation, excitement, anger, or suspicion.

The higher level (intelligent and judgmental) of the brain is the intellect. This is the level at which we think, remember, compare, consult our experience, understand, reason, solve problems, symbolize, put things into words, and make decisions. Included here also are integration and classification of perceptual impressions, factual information, memory storage and retrieval mechanisms, the cognitive processes (including learning), and psychologic "mechanisms of defense" such as repression, displacement, and projection—thus, much of the conscious ego or personality. Man's superiority to other animals depends largely on the integrity of this level. Intelligence probably operates as a function of many parts of the brain, but predominantly the temporal, parietal, and frontal lobes. The *quantity* of normal brain available (eg, after injury) is perhaps as important as its particular anatomic location in determining the amount and degree of intelligence remaining.

Intelligence is an operational term, signifying the ability to "use one's head." Although it encompasses a wide array of mental skills and there is no uniform agreement on priority among them, psychologists do agree about ways of measuring it. This is done by comparing performance on various tests with the results obtained in large standardized populations. (See Chapter 7.) For example, a mental age (MA) of 9 means that the individual's performance (intelligence level) is equal to the performance average of 9-year-olds in the population. A mental age of 9 in a 6-year-old child therefore implies an intelligence quotient (IQ) of $9 \div 6 = 1.50 = 150$ ("genius"); a mental age of 9 in a 12-year-old implies an IQ of $9 \div 12 = 0.75 = 75$ ("borderline"). Little attention is paid in these tests to the quality of intelligence; but, in industry, the arts, social life, and the world at large, people recognize the difference between "horse sense" or "common sense" and "book learning" or "school learning."

People also distinguish between having intelligence and using it, which brings up the interrelatedness of the levels of the mind. An old adage states that, "You cannot teach a hungry child." Educators also say you cannot teach a sick or frightened one, or any child whose intelligence and learning ability are not available to him for whatever reason. The functional capacity of both levels of the mind depends on such factors as oxygenation, hydration, temperature, electrolyte balance, pH of body fluids, blood supply, CSF pressure and drainage, and other physicochemical conditions. In addition, the higher level depends on the functional integrity of the lower level and the emotional status of the individual. It is no surprise that a delirious patient thinks poorly even though there is nothing irreversibly wrong with his intellect. The same is true of a deeply depressed patient, whose thinking may be characterized by "psychomotor retardation."

At the top of the higher level is man's ability to think in terms of abstract as well as concrete things and thus to be able to think about thinking, think about himself, judge his own behavior, and plan consciously for the future. These functions, unavailable to other animals,* are the roots of sagacity and wisdom, of programmed behavior, of the ability to pace activity, maintain goals, and adhere to principles and to ethical, philosophic, and religious ideals. This is the source of man's highest achievements: philanthropy, altruism, spiritual aspirations, imagination, and artistic and scientific creativity. Psychologically, judging oneself (conscience) in terms of the past and present and setting ego-ideals for the future constitute that aspect of the mind called the superego.

The frontal lobes, whose functions have become known only in recent years, are the anatomic loci for much of man's higher level mental activity. Ordinary intelligence is not damaged by their loss. But here each individual man is unique, much as in his fingerprints and electroencephalograms. If the lower mental level determines much of his personality (the sum total of his familiar patterns of behavior as seen by others), then the higher level may be said to determine his character (the sum total of his familiar attitudes, principles, and ideals as seen by himself). Shame (mental discomfort at being ill thought of by others) is a function of the lower mental level; but guilt (mental discomfort at being ill thought of by himself) probably began when man developed frontal lobes.

*Rudimentary forms of these functions may operate in primates and dolphins and perhaps other animals.

The activity of the higher mental level depends on the functional integrity of the lower level. A delirious person (disturbed at the lower mental level) could hardly do well at evaluative or judgmental tasks. Conversely, however, illness or disorganization at the higher level may leave the lower level quite unaffected—eg, a severely paranoid person may be alert, well oriented, well behaved, and even quite bright and logical within the framework of his paranoid system.

Normal persons differ as widely in their mental attributes as they do in their physical ones. The potential difference at the lower mental level ranges from lethargic to excitable or from callous to sensitive; at the higher level the difference is perhaps a magnitude greater—mentally subnormal to genius; and at the top of the higher level perhaps a second magnitude greater—foolish to wise, egoistic to altruistic, amoral to saintly. Much depends on the anatomic endowment, how it is used physiologically, how its use is understood psychologically, how the understanding can be fed back for cybernetic modification, how the resulting behavior can be controlled and modulated to adapt to the environmental situation, and how the resulting social adjustment can be made meaningful and directed toward spiritual values, future goals, and ideals.

REFERENCES

Books and Monographs

Adrian, E.D.: What happens when we think. In: *The Physical Basis of Mind.* P. Laslet (editor). Blackwell, 1952.

Association for Research in Nervous and Mental Disease: *The Brain and Human Behavior.* Proceedings, vol 36. Williams & Wilkins, 1958.

Cobb, S.: *Foundations of Neuropsychiatry.* Williams & Wilkins, 1952.

Eccles, J.C.: *Brain and Conscious Experience.* Springer-Verlag (New York), 1966.

Eccles, J.C.: *The Neurophysiological Basis of Mind: The Principles of Neurophysiology.* Clarendon Press, 1953.

Hamburg, D.A., Pribram, K.H., & A.J. Stunkard (editors): *Perception and Its Disorders.* Williams & Wilkins, 1970.

Hebb, D.O.: *The Organization of Behaviour: A Neuropsychological Theory.* Wiley, 1949.

Hess, W.: *The Biology of the Mind.* Univ of Chicago Press, 1964.

Himwich, W.A. (editor): *Developmental Neurobiology.* Thomas, 1970.

Magoun, H.W.: *The Waking Brain,* 2nd ed. Thomas, 1969.

Penfield, W.: *The Excitable Cortex in Conscious Man.* Liverpool Univ Press, 1958.

Penfield, W., & T. Rasmussen: *The Cerebral Cortex of Man: A Clinical Study of Localization of Function.* Macmillan, 1950.

Sherrington, C.S.: *The Integrative Action of the Nervous System.* Cambridge Univ Press, 1947.

Sherrington, C.S.: *Man on His Nature.* Cambridge Univ Press, 1940.

Solomon, P., & others (editors): *Sensory Deprivation: An Investigation of Phenomena Suggesting a Revised Concept of the Individual's Response to His Environment.* Harvard Univ Press, 1961.

Journal Articles

Cobb, S.: On the nature and locus of mind. Arch Neurol Psychiat 67:172–177, 1952.

Elithorn A.: Intelligence, perceptual integration and the minor hemisphere syndrome. Neuropsychologia 2:327–332, 1964.

Gerard, R.W.: The biological roots of psychiatry. Am J Psychiat 112:81–90, 1955.

Gerard, R.W.: Physiology and psychiatry. Am J Psychiat 106:161–173, 1949.

Geschwind, N.A.: Human deconnection syndrome. Neurology 12:675–685, 1962.

Jasper, H.H.: Evolution of conceptions of cerebral localization since Hughlings Jackson. World Neurol 1:97–112, 1960.

Penfield, W.: Memory mechanisms. Arch Neurol Psychiat 67:178, 1952.

Pirenne, M.H.: Descartes and the body-mind problem in physiology. Brit J Philosoph Sc 1:43–59, 1950.

Sperry, R.W.: Cerebral organization and behavior. Science 133:1749–1757, 1961.

Szilard, L.: On memory and recall. Proc Nat Acad Sc 51:1092–1099, 1949.

4 . . .

The Psychiatric Examination

The psychiatric examination searches for abnormalities in thinking, feeling, and behavior. These register on the examining instrument, the mind of the physician, which must be kept alert and sensitive. Just as the various elements of the neurologic examination can be interdigitated with the routine physical examination, a good deal of the psychiatric examination may be routinely incorporated into ordinary history-taking.

There is no standard psychiatric examination, just as there is no standard physical examination. A thorough and comprehensive psychiatric (or medical) examination can be performed when needed, but it is not necessary or efficient to gather all available data in every case. In practice, there is seldom enough time to do everything for every patient; the busy practitioner soon finds that there is often no need to do everything. With experience and clinical judgment, the physician learns when it is safe to confine his examination to essentials, being careful to err only on the side of caution. In general, it is sensible to *match the field of investigation to the presumed extent of the problem*, bearing in mind that the investigation can be expanded later if it seems justified to do so.

For purposes of exposition, psychiatric examinations may be divided into (1) comprehensive, (2) circumscribed, (3) in depth, and (4) special purpose examinations. In practice, there are frequent overlaps and modifications.

THE COMPREHENSIVE PSYCHIATRIC EXAMINATION

Patients should receive a full-scale psychiatric examination if they are referred for psychiatric consultation or if there is any reason to believe that psychiatric illness may be present. Wherever possible, the regular mental status examination should be made. A few suggestions on one's approach to the patient may be helpful.

(1) Talk person-to-person, not interrogator-to-person or scientist-to-person. If you are informal, with a minimum of pomposity and austerity, the patient may open up to you.

(2) Be good-humored. Avoid looking grim and determined even if you feel that way. A pleasantry or two may help you both to relax.

(3) Suit your manner to your patient. You can be direct and straightforward with the rough and ready type, but must be gentle and delicate with the sensitive. Don't be high-brow to the low-brow or vice versa.

(4) Trust yourself. Develop whatever technic comes natural to you. There is no right or wrong way; no 2 interviewers act the same. In general, it is well to take it easy, not focus too sharply, but sort of see out of the corners of your eyes. Be aware of the patient's behavior, speech nuances, and hesitations. If you feel like asking a question or making a remark even if you are not sure why, go ahead. Exclaim if you like; if you show some human feelings, the patient is more likely to follow suit.

With rational and cooperative patients, it is often best to begin with routine questions that carry little emotional charge, such as identifying data (name, address, telephone number, etc). As the patient settles down, one can say, "Now tell me your problem." The problem, or "present illness," may occupy the remainder of the session and may even call for one or more additional sessions.

During the discussion of the presenting problem, mention is usually made of a parent, sibling, or other family member. This is a good opportunity to interrupt and inquire about the "family background." Similarly, when an incident in the past is mentioned, the examiner may interrupt to inquire about the "past history" and "medical history."

Many items of the mental status examination will now have been covered. The remaining ones may be checked individually, preferably by tactful introduction.

For example, to check orientation: "Is your memory pretty good?" "Oh, yes." "Well, do you remember what day it is today?" "Wednesday." "I mean, what day of the month and year?" Etc.

To check delusions: "Do you ever get nervous? All of us do, I suppose." "Sure." "Do you ever get so nervous that you almost imagine things? That people have a grudge against you? That they talk about you? That you have a special role to play in life?" Etc.

Also: "Do you believe that supernatural things can sometimes happen? Have you ever experienced something supernatural, or something that was hard to understand?"

About hallucinations: "You think deeply, don't you?" "Yes." "Do you sometimes think so deeply you can almost hear your thoughts out loud? Or do you ever hear a voice when there is nobody there?" Etc.

About suicide: "Have you ever felt so low you almost wished you were dead?—And did you think that you might do something about it?—What?—How?—Did you take any steps to prepare for it?—What? Tell me about it."

Other useful questions are the following: "Do you sometimes feel that you know things nobody else knows?" "Do you ever have thoughts that bother you?" "Do you think that your emotions are normal?" "Are you ever afraid of things more than you ought to be—or depressed or empty inside?" "Do you cry a lot?"

When the interview is about to deal with potentially emotionally charged material, keep these points in mind:

(1) Your best attitude is to be keenly interested but nonjudgmental. You can laugh with the patient, but never cry with him. A moderate degree of sympathetic concern is all right, and also something like: "Let's look into this a little and see why it upsets you so much."

(2) As long as new material continues to appear, be nondirective. Let the patient keep the lead.

(3) When progress stalls and you begin to see why, wait until you are sure and then point out the block. If that doesn't eliminate it right away, keep after it. Try to study its origins, its possible causes, its different modes of expression. Show little interest in anything else until you have worried it into extinction. When it returns, attend to it again promptly. Then turn your attention to the next block; there will always be another.

(4) Don't let silences disturb you. It is a good idea to let a silence develop at least once in every interview. Let the patient break it, since what he then says spontaneously may be of special interest. If silences seem to embarrass the patient, you can say something like, "You don't have to talk every second. This isn't like ordinary conversation. If you want to stop and think for a while, it's all right." If you think the patient could use a little help, you can say, "What are you thinking of?" or "Just say whatever comes to your mind." If the silences become troublesome, you can investigate their possible meaning. "Is there something that you find difficult to say?" Or you may wish to be more specific: "Are you silent because of some feeling toward me that you don't want to express?" Or even, "Are you angry with (or disappointed in, or upset about) me?"

(5) Don't avoid your patient's feelings toward yourself, but don't let them disturb you either. If they get so intense as to constitute a block, treat them like any other block.

The major components of the **mental status examination** are the following:

(1) General appearance and behavior.

(2) Characteristics of speech.

(3) Mood or affect.

(4) Content of thought (hallucinations, faulty perceptions, delusions and misinterpretations, obsessive and phobic ideas).

(5) Sensorium functions (orientation, memory, learning, attention and concentration, fund of information and intelligence).

(6) Insight and judgment.

1. GENERAL APPEARANCE AND BEHAVIOR

Appearance

Much may be gleaned from the patient's physical appearance: his dress, state of body hygiene, and grooming. Are they appropriate to his position? The banker who comes from his office unshaven and dirty and who does not seem to recognize the inappropriateness of his appearance must be evaluated differently from the construction worker with similar appearance.

Observe facial expressions, body and limb movements, and mannerisms—and note particularly how they change with the topic of conversation. Staring into space or through the examiner, as if preoccupied, with sudden head or body movements, may be the first hint of hallucinations and may give the examiner the opportunity to inquire if the patient is listening to something. Strange postures, stereotyped movements such as grimacing, tics, and athetoid movements, apparently spontaneous emotional outbursts, rigidity of expression, and physical withdrawal should be noted.

When a patient is mute, all inferences of mental status may depend on these observations alone.

Behavior

Observe the general manner in which the patient approaches and reacts to the interview. Is he cooperative, frank, open, fearful, hostile, reticent? Does his general attitude change during the interview? A certain initial anxiety is to be expected. Is it unusual in intensity or duration? Observe the congruence of the patient's general manner with the demands of the situation. Does he "take over" the interview in an inappropriate way?

2. CHARACTERISTICS OF SPEECH

Of concern here is the form of talk rather than its content, which is discussed separately below.

Abnormalities of speech may be quantitative or qualitative or both. Quantitative abnormalities range from incessant speech, as if there is a pressure of ideas to be expressed—the so-called "flight of ideas" in manic illnesses—to scant, almost monosyllabic talk, as found in some forms of depression, and mutism. Qualitative abnormalities include circumstantiality (needless peripheral detail), talking past and around the point, perseveration (repetition of and constant return to some particular idea), irrelevance (a statement rational in itself but not germane), incoherence (a statement without sense in any context), word salading (a meaningless jumble of words), jargon talk, neologisms, slang associations, senseless punning, and mere animal-like sounds. More general abnormalities of form such as affectations, talk that is incongruent with the patient's level of education, and strange inflections and impediments such as stammers, stutters, and lisps should be noted. Whenever possible, record adequate samples of abnormal talk verbatim. Change in form of speech is often a valuable guide to progress in certain illnesses such as the manic phase of manic-depressive psychosis.

3. MOOD OR AFFECT

The level of and changes in feeling are a sensitive index of emotional illness. There are many possible moods: depression, elation, euphoria, anger, suspicion, fear, anxiety, panic, hostility, calm, happiness, sadness, grief, and combinations of these. The aim is to be able to describe in a precise way how the patient is feeling and not be content with conventional one-word labels such as "depressed" or "anxious."

Two factors must be evaluated to determine the patient's feeling state: (1) Is the mood appropriate to the thought content? (2) Is it at the expected level of intensity?

Bizarrely inappropriate moods may be observed in some patients suffering from schizophrenia. Depressed patients may show a mood appropriate in direction but excessive in degree. Patients with organic brain damage may show wide fluctuations in mood in response to seemingly trivial stimuli—so-called "mood lability." "Blunted" or "flattened" affect may be seen in a wide range of conditions, including simple schizophrenia, some types of brain damage (especially to the frontal lobes), and, in a particular form called *la belle indifférence,* in hysteria.

While the mood of some patients may be quite obvious, careful technic is required to elicit the true state of affect in others. "Smiling depression," for example, will be missed unless the examiner specifically inquires about feelings of sadness, depression, and ideas of suicide, as the patient may wear a "euphoric facade." Anger, rage, and hostility are often well concealed by patients for fear of rejection by the examiner.

4. CONTENT OF THOUGHT

In recording abnormalities of thought, it is necessary to distinguish between what is directly presented and what is inferred, noting in the latter the bases for the inference. Delusions or hallucinations should be described, eg, "The patient believes the Chinese communists have planted a bomb in his cellar and intend to destroy him"—rather than, "Patient has paranoid delusions."

While thought content abnormalities may be bizarre and obvious, they may also be quite subtle and not readily revealed by the patient, particularly if he has encountered a hostile or incredulous response upon previous attempts to say what is in his mind. The patient's general attitude and behavior may offer clues. A patient who appears to be listening to something or who speaks as if in reply to a voice may be asked, "Could you tell me what the voice just said to you?"—ie, a deliberately leading question should be asked, rather than, "Are you hearing voices?" which often prompts a false negative reply.

Hallucinations and Faulty Perceptions

These may affect any of the senses. Describe their vividness and degree of reality, and note the circumstances when they are most and least prominent. Does the patient develop delusional explanations to account for them? Can he start them or stop them voluntarily? Do they have "out-there-ness," or does the patient recognize their inner origin? Illusions or faulty perceptions are often recognized as such by the patient; but insight is rare in true hallucinations, which are almost always pathologic.

If auditory hallucinations are prominent, schizophrenia should be suspected; visual and tactile hallucinations are most often encountered in toxic states such as delirium tremens, drug intoxications, and deliria. Hallucinations of the other senses are relatively rare and suggest the possibility of organic brain disease such as temporal lobe epilepsy or tumor.

Delusions and Misinterpretations

The distinction between frank delusions and the attribution of false, specialized, or exaggerated meanings to events is often a matter of degree. The latter are often due to personality characteristics rather than mental illness. Delusions are described as paranoid (ideas of persecution or suspiciousness), megalomanic or grandiose, depressive (ideas of guilt and unworthiness), or somatic (ideas of bodily changes, eg, internal organs turned to stone, bowels dissolved away, insects eating up brain). Ideas of reference or of influence may fit into any of the above categories according to their content. An encapsulated delusion may be very difficult to elicit unless the topic it relates to (eg, religion, politics) is explored. Some care should be taken in interpreting the delusional nature of logically possible ideas (eg, unfaithfulness of the spouse).

Obsessive and Phobic Ideas

These terms are defined and discussed elsewhere in this book. Note whether the patient feels the idea arises within his own mind or from outside (a delusion). How distressed is he? Is their inappropriateness recognized? Distinguish between compulsiveness and punctiliousness; in the former, the patient makes no differentiation between trivial and important matters and feels excessive anxiety in either.

5. SENSORIUM FUNCTIONS

Disorders of the sensorium are most often a sign of organic brain disease. They may be transient, as in toxic states, or more or less permanent, as in dementia. However, it may be impossible to assess the status of the sensorium in an extremely excited, hostile, depressed, or psychotic patient because of the functional disorganization of other mental processes mentioned above. An acutely paranoid patient may be quite well oriented but will refuse to answer questions; a manic patient may have an excellent memory but be unable to concentrate long enough to achieve recall.

Orientation

Three areas of orientation are classically tested: person, time, and place. The sense of personal identity is usually the last to be lost in organic brain damage, but its loss is the presenting complaint in hysterical amnesia. The quality of orientation should be noted and the mode of inquiry varied if it is suspected that the patient—as often happens in a hospital setting after repeated examinations—is merely reciting by rote something he has just been told. (To avoid this difficulty in future examinations, do not correct the patient's mistakes.) Distinguish between practical orientation—eg, the ability to find one's way in familiar surroundings, awareness of the passage of time sufficient to eat and sleep appropriately—and what, for a retired person leading a simple life, may have no "survival value"—eg, the name of the city or state. Many old people appear much more disoriented in unfamiliar surroundings (eg, when first admitted to the hospital) than they would in their usual situations.

A fourth area of orientation that may indicate some mental disturbance is often called *situational orientation*. Does the patient sense his circumstances and surroundings? Is he able not merely to say where he is, who he is, and when it is but also to behave congruently with his replies?

Memory and Learning

Memory may be by rote or by a process of logic. Rote memory of heavily overlearned material (multiplication tables, nursery rhymes, familiar prayers, etc) may persist long after the ability to grasp the point of a story or to abstract the meaning of proverbs is lost. Some patients, aware of defects in memory, will attempt to mislead the examiner by recitations of such material. The patient's account of his life, especially when it can be compared with that given by others, will be a general guide to past memory. In general, events that had no personal consequence for the patient will be forgotten before those that did, and recent events will be forgotten before remote ones. If the examiner uses a name and address or other items of personal information to test grasp, retention, and recall, he should do so consistently and thus develop his own norms. Note gaps in memory and how the patient deals with them, eg, by falsely filling them in (confabulation).

A simple memory test consists of asking the patient to repeat after you numbers of 3 digits, 4 digits, etc. Say the digits slowly, about one second apart. Then ask the patient to repeat numbers backwards, and illustrate what you mean. Most people can repeat numbers of 5 or 6 digits forwards and 3 or 4 backwards.

Attention and Concentration

Can attention be aroused and sustained? Note what seems to distract the patient. Making change mentally and serially subtracting 7 from 100 (or the simpler 4 from 25) are useful tests of concentration, but the examiner must make certain that inability to do mental arithmetic is not the cause of failure or slowness. Telling the months of the year or the days of the week in reverse order are better tests of concentration for poorly educated patients.

Fund of Information and Intelligence

Tests of general information should be geared to the patient's experiences, interests, and level of education. As with memory tests, the examiner ought to develop standard questions, eg, "Can you name the President?" "Who was President before him?" "And before him?" "Who is the

Governor?" "What are the capitals of France, Germany, Italy, Spain, England?" "Name 5 large cities in the USA." "Five large rivers?" "What can you tell me about . . . [any item of current interest in the news]?" A gross measure of the patient's intelligence can be derived from his account of his history, general knowledge, and reasoning powers. For greater precision, a standardized test must be used (see Chapter 7) when indicated, eg, if a question of mental retardation arises or if there is disparity between educational performance and apparent ability. Patients with borderline intelligence when under great strain may manifest anxiety, frustration, and fear, with behavior that resembles psychosis.

6. INSIGHT AND JUDGMENT

Insight as used here does not necessarily mean deep understanding of the unconscious processes that cause symptoms. In the context of the mental status examination, a patient has insight if he sees himself as "sick"; as having "mental," "nervous," or "emotional" problems; as needing some sort of help or treatment; or if he understands that his symptoms or difficulties may be based, at least in part, on concerns and disturbing emotions within himself. Note the degree of awareness of test mistakes, gaps in the personal history, and inconsistencies of thought and behavior.

As tests for judgment you may ask, "What would you do if you were lost in the woods?" ". . . if you were in a movie theater and you were the first to see a fire break out?" ". . . if you found a letter on the street, and it was addressed, sealed, and stamped?" Lack of sound judgment does not necessarily indicate mental illness. However, deterioration in judgment is an important diagnostic clue, and the level of judgment may influence treatment programs and the prognosis.

THE CIRCUMSCRIBED PSYCHIATRIC EXAMINATION

With the increased public awareness that psychologic causes are often as important as somatic causes in bringing about various kinds of miseries, more and more problems of relatively minor severity are brought to the attention of psychiatrists. Many of these problems do not require a full-scale investigation. They do require that attention be directed toward the presenting problem, which in these instances often concerns matters less in the patient than in his environment.

With respect to the patient himself, the examiner, whether he be a psychiatrist, other physician, clinical psychologist, psychiatric social worker, or other ancillary professional worker, will look for abnormalities largely of 2 sorts: disorders of mood and disorders of thought.

Special note should be taken of whether or not the patient's mood is appropriate to his circumstances. For example, a patient who seems to overreact to a recent bereavement may be dangerously depressed and may be a suicidal risk; yet in some Mediterranean cultures, extremely demonstrative behavior (eg, at funerals) may be within the range of normal. Marked withdrawal or apathy may be suggestive of psychotic dissociation; yet in some northern cultures, remarkably stoic behavior would not be regarded as schizoid. Similarly, the examiner will note elevation of mood, overoptimism, and extravagant actions, bearing in mind the possible implications for hypomania.

Observation of disorders of thought does not require a formalized testing procedure. In discussing the patient's problem with him it will usually be obvious if there is something wrong with his thinking. It does not take a complete mental status examination to see that a patient is flagrantly irrational, deluded, hallucinating, paranoid, or demented.

Although most information is obtained through conversation, a great deal may also be learned by observing the patient's behavior. Hyperactivity, lethargy, vivacity, lugubriousness, purposeless or repetitive movements, suspiciousness, theatricality, impulsiveness, violence, or bizarre and inappropriate actions may be indicative of serious mental illness.

If abnormalities are detected, a comprehensive psychiatric examination is indicated.

Common presenting problems that can be investigated in a circumscribed way are discussed in the following paragraphs.

Crisis Situations

Crises occur in every life, and some may be considered as essentially normal happenings which test the ability to rebound: health problems, environmental changes, developmental staging, minor failures at school, at work, or in interpersonal relations, marriage, sex experiences, etc. Any of these may be so emotionally disturbing to some people as to threaten the stability and integrity of the personality and paralyze the capacity to react in a useful way.

More serious crises regularly act in this disturbing way—eg, bereavement, divorce, abortion, serious illness, natural catastrophes, personal disgrace, rape, and financial ruin. The normal reactions of shock, grief, fear, etc may threaten to progress to emotional collapse, despair, profound depression, mental dissociation, and schizoid and paranoid states. Assistance is often sought from psychiatrists, other physicians, social workers, ministers, and other professionals.

The psychiatric examination in crisis situations usually consists of a quick, informal evaluation of the mood and thinking. Individual modes of reaction to crises are highly variable; it often takes great experience and mature judgment to differentiate normal and pathologic responses. A woman whose husband has just died in a car accident may throw herself about, screaming that she is going to kill herself, and a few hours later, after a mild sedative and with her relatives around her, may quietly inquire about realistic concerns such as insurance and other family matters. On the other hand, a man who has just lost his fortune may seem silently grim but resigned and the next morning may be found dead by suicide.

The examiner who is in doubt about the immediate outcome will play safe in his management of the patient, making sure that he is not left alone and arranging to see him again that day or the next. If a crisis reaction persists beyond what are considered normal cultural limits, a more extensive psychiatric and mental status examination is indicated.

Children's Problems

Common childhood problems such as thumbsucking, nailbiting, nightmares, poor appetite, and other behavior disorders often come to the attention of physicians with a request for psychiatric evaluation (see Chapter 32). The examination may begin with a talk with the mother in which identifying data are recorded and the presenting difficulty discussed (perhaps 15—20 minutes). The child should then be seen briefly also. If he is young (under age 6), he is given some toys to play with. His intelligence and temperament can be estimated roughly by his behavior, attitude, and responses to simple remarks or questions about the toys, his clothes, or about himself.

A bright boy of 4 might say, "My cousin Johnny has a yellow dump truck just like that." An unhappy or frightened 2-year-old might cry, suck his thumb, and refuse to leave his mother's side. A dull 8-year-old might be pleasant and cooperative but say, "I don't like school. I don't know how to read."

The mother is then seen again. The impressions gained thus far may permit the examiner to inquire specifically about the emotional climate of the home, parental attitudes toward the children, the siblings' roles in the patient's problems, matters pertaining to physical health (illness, diet, sleep disturbances), development, and schooling. The mother's ideas about the problem should be heard. Any one of these areas can be explored more fully if suggestive leads are uncovered. Further visits probably will be necessary for more complete examination and treatment. For example, a 7-year-old nailbiter is much more tense and nervous after he has spent a weekend with his father. The father is brought in and interviewed and his attitudes toward the child are discussed. The child is seen again and chatted with as he plays with a mommy doll, daddy doll, and baby doll.

Children with serious psychiatric problems (bizarre or autistic behavior, school phobia, extreme cruelty toward animals, repeated running away, etc) should be observed and examined thoroughly in repeated interviews. The history may be taken by a social worker (who often makes a home visit), and a battery of psychologic tests should be administered by a clinical psychologist. In some instances, EEG, x-ray, or other laboratory procedures should be requested.

College Problems

The common problems of this group and of adolescents generally are often situational, and the psychiatric examination (and treatment) can then be confined largely to the current difficulties and handled in one or 2 visits. Common problems have to do with studies, examinations, roommates, sex, religion, morals, politics, emotional reactions to physical illness, and money. More severe problems are discussed in this chapter in the sections on Comprehensive and In Depth Psychiatric Examination and in Chapter 35.

In the psychiatric examination, the student is encouraged to describe his problem in detail. Specific inquiry should be made regarding his emotional reactions to elements of the problem and the people involved. A formal mental status examination is usually not necessary, and inquiries about family background may often be brief. Similar problems in the past should be inquired about, and the student should be allowed to discuss any matters he feels are relevant. If there are no indications of psychotic, neurotic, or other psychopathologic traits—or if there are but the student has them under control—treatment may proceed without further psychiatric examination.

For example, a bright freshman in a college for women was having trouble preparing for final examinations. She could not concentrate and was not sleeping well. She realized that the trouble was related to her boy friend, a senior at a nearby college, who was insisting that she sleep with him. She thought she might be in love with him, and certainly didn't want to lose him; but she was a virgin and wanted to stay that way for the present. She was a tense, high-strung girl and had a number of phobias. The therapist confined himself to the presenting complaints and offered simple reassurance and reinforcement of her attitudes.

Marital Conflict

Psychiatrists and family physicians are frequently asked to offer help in marital conflicts. One or both partners may accuse the other of mental illness, or the couple may agree to an impartial arbitrator as a last resort.

Physicians differ about what they consider their proper role in instances of marital discord. Some state flatly that they are physicians for people and not for institutions and will not try to doctor a marriage. They will examine either or both parties and render an opinion regarding mental health and the need for therapy.

Other physicians, including more and more psychiatrists, consider that marital conflict is a reflection of personality problems and that a sick marriage is a legitimate object of their concern. They will see husband and wife individually and together, and will focus their attention on the history of the marriage and the personalities involved. Such psychiatric examination as they do will be incidental to their probing into the marital relationship, but it will necessarily disclose any abnormalities in mood or intellectual functioning. If anything suggestive of mental illness is uncovered, the physician will go further in the psychiatric examination.

THE IN DEPTH PSYCHIATRIC EXAMINATION

In the phrases "depth psychology" and "psychotherapy in depth," the word "depth" means that the investigation aims to uncover factors operating below the surface of consciousness or in dim awareness. Conscious material can be obtained from patients directly, through their statements and through their answers to questions. Unconscious material must be obtained indirectly. Patients differ in the ease with which they divulge unconscious material, and an individual patient may himself vary greatly in this matter from one time to another as "resistance" to releasing unconscious material fluctuates. The examination in depth usually continues over the entire period of treatment in depth.

Information from the patient's unconscious is obtained by the process of free association and by examining the patient's dreams, daydreams and fantasies, parapraxias ("slips"), and peculiarities of behavior, posture, diction, etc.

Free Association

Free association has been called the "basic rule" of psychoanalysis. The patient is instructed to say anything that comes to his mind as uncritically and unselectively as possible. He may speak of thoughts, feelings, and fantasies and of the past, present, or future. There is no need for him to be logical, systematic, or even coherent. Utterances may involve memories, fragments of dreams, bodily sensations, feelings concerning the therapist, fears, plans, temptations, anything at all. The patient may be told that he should especially watch for fugitive thoughts and things that are hard to say, embarrassing, or disturbing. Although this sounds easy, in practice it is often difficult.

A few examples will demonstrate how free association helps to uncover unconscious material.

(1) **Recovery of a repressed memory**: A man in his 40's was in the second year of analysis. One of his symptoms was a persistent fear that he might develop epilepsy. One day he was speaking of his young son, who was ill. Suddenly he said, "Did I ever tell you I once had a younger sister?" No, he had always referred to himself as an only child. "Well, I did, but she died in infancy when I was about 5 years old." After a long pause, he said, "What I have just realized appalls me. She died of convulsions."

(2) **Realization of repressed feelings**: A mother was speaking of a recent scene with her young daughter, who had screamed at her, "You hate me! You hate me!" The mother said, "She's such a hateful child, maybe I do hate her. But that's ridiculous—a mother can't hate her own child." After a long pause, she went on: "I suppose I wouldn't have said that unless there was some truth in it. Maybe part of me really does hate her, at least sometimes. She reminds me of my little sister when she was a brat."

(3) **Uncovering unrecognized plans**: A young rabbi, about to leave the rabbinate, was in his final session of psychotherapy. He talked eagerly about his new career in social work and said, "It occurs to me just now that in all the 3 years with you I took it for granted that you would never let me conclude therapy until I got out of the rabbinate. Now I realize this was my own goal for the future right along, and I imputed it to you."

Dreams

Freud said the dream is "the royal road to the unconscious." The study and interpretation of dreams can throw great light on buried conflicts and hidden motivations.

After narrating a dream, the patient is asked to associate freely to the elements mentioned in the dream. Usually he can remember material from the preceding day that entered into the fashioning of the dream (the "manifest content"). The free associations and the knowledge of the patient's background, life experiences, and mental makeup help the therapist understand the "latent content" of the dream. A few examples (greatly condensed) follow.

(1) "We were being attacked. Bullets flew everywhere. One of the enemy chased me with a huge sharp ramrod. I could hear him getting closer and closer behind me. I woke up in panic."

Associations (manifest content). "I was watching TV before I went to sleep—an old movie in which they were storming the castle. Arrows and spears filled the air. They finally rolled up an enormous battering ram and smashed the gates in. . . . I had a letter from my older brother yesterday. It made me mad. He wants to borrow money from me."

Interpretation. "In the dream you were being attacked, especially from behind. In the letter, your brother attacked you in a way. What about you and your brother?"

Latent content. "I remember once when we were little he tried to put his penis in my rear end. I was too scared to let him."

(2) "I was shopping in a department store. I couldn't find what I wanted. I looked and looked. The saleslady was rude to me."

Associations (manifest content). "I did go shopping yesterday with the children, and we bought a lot of things for the summer camp. We had lunch in the store, but it wasn't good."

Interpretation. "A department store is a place where you expect to be able to buy anything you want. All you did yesterday was buy things for others. Even the lunch you got wasn't good. Do you think you may have felt a little deprived?"

Latent content. "You know how aimless and unrewarding I think my life is. I suppose the saleslady is my mother who never gave me the love I wanted and always scolded me."

Daydreams and Fantasies

Daydreams are imaginary events in the past or future, more or less consciously and voluntarily indulged in. *Fantasies* or reveries are similar but involve activities imagined as happening in the present, with insight that they are not actually happening. Daydreams and fantasies can usually be started and stopped at will. Though they are largely conscious, they often contain unconscious material, and they can provide valuable insights in much the same way that sleep dreams do.

(1) **Daydream:** "I often relive things that happened at Boy Scout camp, especially the ball games and swimming and track meets, where I did great things and won prizes."

Interpretation. "Is this reliving the time of your life of greatest triumph? Maybe just before a letdown?"

Insight. "Letdown indeed. Right after that was when I began to feel like such a social failure, such a flop with girls. I was scared to go near them and I couldn't dance."

(2) Daydream: "Ever since I became a big girl I have had secret daydreams that I never told anyone. In them I am a slave girl being sold at an auction. A handsome rajah buys me and I have to do anything he wants. But he falls in love with me and I become his favorite."

Interpretation. "Making yourself a slave girl relieves you of any responsibility for the interesting things you then do. Is having sex fun such a sinful thing to you?" (The oedipal implications are left for another time.)

Insight. "Yes. Ever since my mother caught me touching myself and shamed me horribly."

(3) Fantasy: "I enjoy pretending that I can fly. I see myself soaring over the crowds, and the people must prostrate themselves before me because they consider me a god."

Interpretation. "Could this sense of power be a special need of yours because you've had so little of it?"

Insight. "I guess you don't get much sense of power when you have a mother and father like mine and ten brothers and sisters!"

Parapraxias

Parapraxias are often called "Freudian slips." They include slips of the tongue, certain inadvertent oversights, errors, and significant blunders. They have in common the unexpected appearance of a bit of action that is not voluntarily wished for by the individual but that somehow finds its way into being when the guards are down. Something hitherto repressed gets by the "censor"* and finds outlet for expression.

Conditions in the therapist's office are especially conducive to the patient letting down his guards. The room is soundproofed, and privacy and confidentiality are assured. The therapist is sympathetic, objective, nonjudgmental, and keenly interested in the patient's welfare. Sometimes the truth pops out. Some examples will show how it may happen:

(1) "So I decided to take my mother and children to the circus—I mean my wife and the children. I often refer to her and the children as 'mother and the children.' "

(2) "I registered for the 5-week live-in summer seminar at the university, without my wife." "Five weeks?" "Did I say 5 weeks? It's 5 days—I suppose I would like to get away from her for 5 weeks. I'm surprised I didn't say 5 months."

(3) The patient is a research physician who has been irritated by an article written by a colleague: "I misplaced the reprint he sent me and searched all over for it. Finally I sat down, defeated and exasperated, and there it was on the desk right in front of me!"

---

*The censor in psychoanalytic theory is a hypothetical part of the mental apparatus that determines what psychic material must be repressed and to what degree.

(4) The patient has arrived for her appointment on the wrong day: "I was sure it was today, though now that I look at the card I see it is tomorrow. I guess I couldn't wait. I've got a lot on my mind."

Peculiarities of Behavior, Etc

Peculiarities of behavior, diction, posture, and the like may be signs of deepseated unconscious reaction patterns. The therapist may permit weeks or months to go by before he feels sure enough of the meaning to make a timely and useful interpretation.

(1) A young physician in analysis always picked up one of the small pillows on the couch and held it clasped to his chest during his sessions. After many months, he came in one day in great jubilation at a singularly gratifying triumph in his professional life. That day he did not touch the pillow. Therapist: "You didn't hug the pillow today. You must be feeling stronger." (Thus to discussion of infantile longings and frustrations.)

(2) A college girl, small and dainty, was very bright and popular but secretly unhappy. She had an unusually high-pitched, girlish, often querulous voice. After working through some of her severe emotional conflicts with her mother and her older brother's idolatrous attitude toward her, she began being less an "ideal daughter and little sister" and more a source of disturbance at home. In this phase of her treatment her voice began to sound in a lower register. Therapist (who had not mentioned her voice before): "Have you noticed that even your voice is growing up?"

(3) A businessman with a stooped posture spoke a great deal about his overpowering mother. One day the therapist remarked that his attitude toward her sounded remarkably submissive and ingratiating. The patient thought about this, agreed, and then asked if he had ever mentioned the story of his mother's harassment of him because of his posture. She had scolded, nagged, and mocked, often saying, "Well, did you find any nickels on the sidewalk today?" Repeated visits to orthopedists were of no avail. Therapist: "And you're not standing up to her even today, are you?"*

(4) A patient constantly came late to his appointment, giving all sorts of excuses. One day the therapist said, "I think you want to come when you want to, rather than when you are supposed to." The patient first objected vehemently, then admitted he hated rules and regulations and often subverted authority secretly.

---

*The use of "organ language" by the therapist may not have scientific validity but it sometimes is remarkably effective in its lasting therapeutic impression on the patient. If the interpretation is appropriate and is carefully preserved until a timely moment, the dramatic impact can produce "gut feelings" that deepen the therapy and open up new areas of unconscious material for study. The following are examples: "Is it your husband who is the chronic headache to you?" "Perhaps it is your boss who gives you the pain in the neck." To a vomiter: "You can't stomach your mother-in-law?"

SPECIAL PURPOSE
PSYCHIATRIC EXAMINATIONS

There are many situations in which a psychiatrist is called upon to examine a patient primarily for the benefit of someone other than the patient himself. In these situations, an answer is wanted to some specific question. For example, with respect to a man's mental condition: Is he able to stand trial, prepare a will, sell his property, serve in the armed forces, have custody of his children, or even live in the ordinary community (rather than a mental institution)? The psychiatrist must usually perform a comprehensive psychiatric examination, often in more than one visit, and, in addition, direct special attention to the specific question at hand. He must not only elicit sufficient information to make up his own mind; he must also gather evidence sufficient to convince a nonmedical authority. He must keep in mind that in court he may be asked questions about the conduct of the examination, including how often and for how long he examined the patient.

In the usual doctor-patient relationship, the patient engages the doctor in his interests, expects to pay for his services, and assumes that the doctor will do the best he can for him. In examinations that are arranged and paid for by someone else, the patient will not be so sanguine about the doctor's attitudes and intentions. Therefore, the patient's cooperation cannot be taken for granted but must be actively sought. The patient should be told at once why he is being examined and why a full understanding of his mental condition will be helpful to others in making a just and proper decision in his case. The correct decision will usually be of benefit to the patient also, though indirectly. If he does not cooperate, his refusal will surely be taken into account in judging his case. Finally, the doctor should stress that he is serving only as a professional consultant and that he will simply report his findings as he sees them.

MEDICOLEGAL PSYCHIATRIC EXAMINATIONS

A psychiatrist's opinion may be requested by the court, attorney general, prosecutor, defendant's counsel, plaintiff's counsel, or other interested persons. In such cases, the patient is usually aware of the reason for the psychiatrist's visit. Nevertheless, the psychiatrist should begin by explaining the situation and his role in it. He may then proceed with the complete psychiatric examination, beginning either with the current problem or with background material, whichever seems more suitable. At some time he will focus on the particular area for which the psychiatric examination was requested. The various ways in which he will do this depend on the kind of legal problem that is under investigation. The major legal problems for which psychiatric help is sought are discussed below.

Criminal Responsibility

To be legally responsible for one's acts, one must be able to be aware of his environment, to reason and judge what is morally right, and to control his own behavior. The psychiatrist in his comprehensive psychiatric examination should focus on consciousness, judgment (especially sense of right and wrong), rationality, and impulsiveness. If any of these is impaired by virtue of mental illness or defect, criminal responsibility may be seriously questioned.

Consciousness, in the clinical psychiatric sense of the word, is a state of wakefulness and awareness of the outside world and of one's own position in it. It may be impaired as a result of epilepsy, fever, head injuries, anemia, vascular, neoplastic, or metabolic brain disease, toxic states, trance states, fugues, stupor, and in certain forms of intoxication with alcohol, barbiturates, marihuana, LSD, heroin, and other drugs, especially when hallucinations or comatose states are involved. The possibility that any of these conditions are present must be investigated in detail, since crimes committed under their influence may be mitigated by lack of full criminal responsibility.

Simple questioning may help identify these conditions or cause them to be suspected. "Have you ever lost consciousness? Do things get hazy sometimes for a few moments so that you might miss a few words if someone is talking? Do you ever have blackouts or blank periods when you suddenly don't know how you got where you are? Dream-like states when you are awake? Strange feelings in which things seem to happen automatically? How do you act when you drink too much, or take drugs?" An EEG should be done in suspected cases.

Rationality is an extension of consciousness and overlaps it. Consciousness implies perception of the real world; rationality, the ability to think and reason about the world in a normal manner. It is impaired in mental retardation, the organic conditions listed above, and in functional mental illnesses, especially when delusions are involved—schizophrenia, paranoia, and manic-depressive states. Impaired rationality should be recognized in the comprehensive psychiatric examination, but in legal cases it is often wise to have a clinical psychologist examine the patient as well and administer appropriate psychologic tests. (See Chapter 37.)

Judgment is an extension of rationality and overlaps it. It is the ability to understand and appreciate the values of things one thinks and reasons about. It is one of the higher functions of the brain and includes the power to discriminate and compare and to see an event or situation of the here and now in the light of the elsewhere and past. It utilizes memory, knowledge, education, training, and experience. In questions of criminal responsibility, it concerns matters of morality, law and order, good and bad, and right and wrong as currently prevalent and accepted in the patient's community. It may be impaired in any of the conditions mentioned above under consciousness and rationality. Because of its more complex and more vulnerable nature, it may be the first and perhaps, for a time, the only mental function to be affected; and in recovery it may be the last to return to normal or the only one that never returns. It is tested routinely in the comprehensive mental status examination, but in legal cases, as with rationality, it is well to have an additional opinion from a clinical psychologist.

Impulsiveness occurs in pathologic degree (the "irresistible impulse") in some cases of mental retardation, in certain forms of organic brain disease (especially those involving the temporal lobes), character disorders (anti-social, passive-aggressive, paranoid), manic and hypomanic disorders, and some schizophrenic reactions. A history of impulsive behavior (violence in any form) is important: unusually frequent fights in childhood, cruelty to animals, battered children, physical attacks, excessive aggressiveness in driving a car (with frequent acidents), and antisocial behavior (including inciting to riot, rioting, rape, arson, or—if a policeman—brutality and viciousness in the exercise of official duties). In addition to the impulse to attack, there may be an abnormal degree of (or lack of control of) the impulse to take and enjoy things, as shown in sexual assaults, rape, larceny, looting, and burglary. Isolated instances of the foregoing can occur in essentially normal persons, especially if still immature; under great emotional stress; under the influence of alcohol; or if the CNS is otherwise organically impaired. Repeated instances suggest a basic lack of responsibility. In obscure or puzzling cases, neurologic studies (for example, EEG with temporal lobe leads) may be illuminating. Slow or dysrhythmic brain waves may be diagnostically important and very convincing to a nonmedical authority.

Ability to Stand Trial

In order to stand trial, a defendant must be in sufficiently good physical and mental health to be able to withstand the rigors of the experience and to cooperate properly in his defense. He may be excused (temporarily) if the public exposure or the interrogation produces such a severe emotional reaction that he becomes incapacitated for further participation. The psychiatrist may judge that a patient would react in such a way on the basis of the patient's previous performances in similar situations.

The ability to cooperate properly in the trial requires that the defendant understand what he is charged with and the methods, procedures, and significance of the trial; also that he be able to answer questions rationally and coherently in his defense. Delusions and impairment of intellectual processes usually are disqualifying. The psychiatric examination should cover these points specifically in the general mental status.

Commitability

A patient may be judged to be legally commitable to a mental hospital if he is, by virtue of mental illness or defect, a danger to himself, to others, or to property. To be psychotic is not enough. To be psychotic and to have made threats are also not enough. The psychiatrist must be reasonably sure that the patient is dangerous, and this usually requires that the patient shall have already made some actually dangerous move or gesture.

Sometimes a relative—usually a wife—begs for protection from a menacing man and a psychiatrist is called in for an opinion. He may recognize paranoid trends, but if the man has a negative history, if the threats cannot be corroborated, and if the man adamantly denies his threats or passes them off as joking or as simple attempts to intimidate, nothing much can be done. One must wait for him to act, and then it may be too late. However, most threateners do not carry out their threats, and civil liberties must be preserved.

The psychiatric examination may be brief and the opinion positive for commitment if it is obvious that the patient is suicidal, homicidal, unmanageable, or otherwise unable to take care of himself in the community. The psychiatrist may judge not only by his first-hand impressions of the patient (whom he must see on the very day of the commitment in most states), but also by information furnished to him by others. In cases where the situation is not obvious, a comprehensive psychiatric examination must be done, preferably in several repeated visits. A second psychiatric opinion may be necessary.

Testamentary Capacity

In order to be legally able to make a will, a person must know in a general way the nature and extent of his property, who his relatives are and what the relationships mean, and what it is to make a bequest. He may be quite psychotic in other areas and still be able to make a valid, lawful will. The psychiatrist, in examining a patient for testamentary capacity, should check the points mentioned above but should also do a comprehensive psychiatric examination. He thus protects his patient properly and may spare himself the embarrassment of being asked by a cross-examining attorney such questions as, "Yes, but doctor, didn't you know that Mr. Doe considered himself a saint?"—or owned 20 cats, or always wore 4 suits of underwear and 3 overcoats at a time, etc.

It is always well to inquire carefully why a psychiatric examination is wanted in the particular case.

Contractual Capacity

In order to buy or sell property, get married or divorced, or engage in any valid contract, a person must be able to understand the circumstances involved in the contract and the natural consequences of the transaction. Similar considerations are involved in matters of business competency and in the appointment of conservators or guardians. As in the case of wills, the psychiatric examination should cover the special points in detail but should also be comprehensive. As with wills, inquire in detail why someone thought it desirable to have a psychiatric examination in the case.

Therapeutic Abortion

A psychiatric examination is frequently requested in connection with the indications for a therapeutic abortion. In spite of greatly liberalized statutes in some states of the USA, in many states and in many foreign countries abortion may be performed only if the continuation of the pregnancy threatens the life or "physical or mental health" of the woman. The psychiatrist must add to his complete psychiatric examination special emphasis on the patient's attitudes toward her pregnancy, and, in the case of the unwed woman, the putative father, the unborn baby, and the possibilities of marriage or of having the child out of wedlock and keeping it or placing it for adoption. In evaluating the depth and danger of depression or schizoid symptoms, the psychiatrist must keep in mind the possibility that the patient may be exaggerating her symptoms or frankly malingering in the interests of obtaining a recommendation for abortion. In formulating his opinion, the psychiatrist must weigh the psychiatric dangers to the patient of the abortion as opposed to the dangers of the alternatives.

Custody

The legal custody of children in a divorce case may hinge on the psychiatric status of one or both parents. In making the examinations for the court, the psychiatrist will do comprehensive psychiatric examinations, usually of both parents, and will show special interest in the parents' attitudes toward their children, their own parents, siblings, and children generally. The psychiatrist may wish to supplement his own examination material with additional data obtained by a psychiatric social worker after a home visit and discussions with relatives.

Civil Suits

In tort cases, where the plaintiff alleges damage to his mental health, a psychiatrist may be called in by the plaintiff's lawyer to attest to the seriousness of the damage and another may be called upon by the defendant's lawyer to testify that the plaintiff has minimal or no damage. The deplorable differences of opinion that may result are often ascribed by the public to monetary considerations. All too often, they are the consequence of incomplete psychiatric examinations.

The psychiatrist must be scrupulous in conducting a comprehensive psychiatric examination with special attention to the possibilities of malingering or exaggeration of symptoms on the part of the patient. In order to arrive at an accurate, unbiased opinion, he should insist on seeing all relevant medical records, including the laboratory data. In doubtful cases he should see the patient repeatedly, interview relatives or other individuals with special knowledge of the case (perhaps with the help of a psychiatric social worker), and get additional supportive information by referring the patient to a clinical psychologist.

PSYCHIATRIC SCREENING EXAMINATIONS

Psychiatric screening is being done increasingly in a variety of situations. In most cases a group of some kind is screened to exclude those who are psychiatrically unfit for the particular task or goal, or a group may be screened to identify those who should have psychiatric treatment. Occasionally, a group of psychiatric patients are screened to determine which are well enough for some special decision in their behalf.

Exclusion

A. **Military Service**: Probably the largest-scale psychiatric screening of any type is done in induction examinations for military service. These examinations vary considerably depending on the urgency and the numbers of recruits that must be screened. For example, at the onset of World War II, the US Navy required an individual psychiatric interview with all recruits for the purpose of identifying those whose emotional makeup was sufficiently suspect to warrant a period of observation on a psychiatric ward. As the number of recruits increased, the duration of the screening interview decreased until it averaged about 30 seconds. Six or 8 questions were fired at the recruit as he stood naked on his way from one type of medical specialist to another. The questions varied among the different examiners, and, depending on the answers, not all were asked of every recruit, but they were approximately as follows: Where are you from? How far did you go in school? What work have you done? What do you do for fun? What is your favorite sport? Do you go out with girls? Have you ever had any nervous trouble? Have you ever seen a psychiatrist? If the recruit's behavior or answers were aberrant, he was questioned a bit more and then either passed or tagged for admission to the psychiatric ward. About 8% were tagged, and half of these were subsequently discharged from the service as unsuited for military duty.

When the recruiting urgency is not so great, psychiatric screening interviews are longer and more thorough. Sometimes they are supplemented (or replaced) by a written psychiatric questionnaire.

B. **Other Government Organizations**: Psychiatric screening has been done on applicants to other government organizations (eg, Peace Corps, Diplomatic Service, astronauts, police). It is desired especially to exclude those who are likely to become incapacitated with a psychiatric illness and those who have a character problem that could interfere with the applicant's proper discharge of his duties or cause danger or embarrassment to the government. Where successful candidates are to be given secrecy clearance or positions of unusual trust, particular emphasis must be placed on homosexuality and other sexual abnormalities, illnesses that may have paranoid features, alcoholism, drug dependency, and impaired judgment and reliability. Screening in these instances must include a comprehensive psychiatric examination with special attention to these areas. Psychologic testing may be added.

C. **Special Organizations**: A number of public and private organizations are finding it worthwhile to screen applicants psychiatrically. Some use written psychologic tests; others prefer individual clinical examinations. The psychiatrists or psychologists who do the examinations must keep in mind the selection inherent in the positions that the candidates are applying for as well as the special hazards of the work the successful candidates will be called upon to do. For example, candidates for the ministry, priesthood, or rabbinate may have been attracted to the life of the clergy because of inner psychologic problems involving schizoid traits, asocial tendencies, or pathologic sexual development; yet the life of the clergyman demands unusual social ability, personal integrity, and maturity. Similar considerations apply to screening for teaching positions, nurse training, executive positions in business, etc.

D. Medical and Surgical Procedures: Psychiatrists are frequently called upon to advise on the performance of such procedures as cosmetic surgery, transplants, use of artificial kidneys, operations on the sexual organs, surgery in hysterical patients, and various investigative or emergency procedures in unwilling patients. In most of these the psychiatrist must evaluate the patient's emotional stability and the likelihood of serious mental breakdown. In the unwilling patient, the psychiatrist may recommend (to the relatives, or to the court if necessary) that the patient, by virtue of his mental condition, is unable to make vital decisions regarding his own welfare. The psychiatrist should do as complete an examination as the circumstances warrant and should focus on the realistic or deluded attitude of the patient toward his immediate situation.

Identification

It is sometimes desirable to know which members of a group have psychiatric conditions that should be treated. An important example is the demographic survey conducted for epidemiologic and public health purposes (eg, Manhattan Mental Health Survey, Wellesley Mental Health Survey). In this case the huge numbers of people who must be screened make it necessary to use relatively unskilled workers who go from door to door and interview whomever they can. Interview questions and questionnaires are prepared in advance and made suitable for machine scoring and computer analysis.

Examples of smaller groups are hospitalized tuberculosis patients (psychiatric disorders, especially chronic alcoholism, are present in more than half) and unwed mothers awaiting delivery in special institutions. The psychiatric examinations in these groups are usually brief interviews that attempt to explore the major areas of possible disorder. They naturally focus on the patient's emotional reaction to the current situation.

Discharge

Screening may be done to exclude the mentally healthy. In large mental hospitals, periodic checks are made to determine which patients are well enough to be transferred to a ward with greater freedom, given weekend passes, allowed trial visits at home, or fully discharged. Since one psychiatrist may be responsible for dozens (or even hundreds) of patients in his screening decisions, he must rely heavily on behavioral data obtained from nurses, social workers, and ancillary personnel.

Patients who are obtaining disability assistance from a welfare agency on the basis of chronic psychiatric illness must be examined periodically to determine whether they are still too sick to do gainful work. Although these patients are all incapacitated and often live a wretched and miserable existence, they rarely receive treatment for their condition since they are considered incurable. Unfortunately, the "disability assistance" psychiatric examinations are usually done by an overworked psychiatrist or psychiatric resident and are fast and perfunctory, involving little more than checking on the patient's continuing symptoms and inability to work.

FOLLOW-UP PSYCHIATRIC EXAMINATIONS

Patients who have been discharged from a mental hospital usually require continued psychiatric supervision for weeks, months, or years afterward. Some remain in ambulatory psychotherapy with the psychiatrist who treated them when they were inpatients, although few public mental hospitals have sufficient professional staff to permit extensive outpatient care. A few discharged patients seek care by private psychiatrists or mental hygiene clinics in their home community, but most have to turn to their family doctor.

General practitioners should be competent to do follow-up psychiatric examinations on discharged mental hospital patients. They should have a copy of the patient's hospital discharge note and should take pains to have a telephone conversation (if not a personal visit) with the patient's psychiatrist at the hospital. They will then know what behavior and which factors in the mental status examination to look for when they see the patient. They will also have advice on medication, indications for repeated hospitalization, and general recommendations for follow-up management.

REFERENCES

Books and Monographs

Appel, K.E., & E.A. Strecker: *Practical Examination of Personality and Behavior Disorders.* Macmillan, 1936.

Bird, B.: *Talking With Patients.* Lippincott, 1955.

Deutsch, F., & W.F. Murphy: *The Clinical Interview.* Internat Univ Press, 1955.

Garrett, A.: *Interviewing: The Principles and Methods.* Family Welfare Association of America, 1942.

Gill, M., Newman, R., & F.C. Redlich: *The Initial Interview in Psychiatric Practice.* Internat Univ Press, 1954.

Kahn, R.L., & C.F. Cannell: *Dynamics of Interviewing.* Basic Books, 1963.

Preu, P.W.: *Outline of Psychiatric Case Study,* 2nd ed. Hoeber, 1943.

Reik, T.: *Listening With the Third Ear.* Farrar, Straus & Giroux, 1948.

Reports in Psychotherapy: Initial Interviews. GAP Report No. 49. Group for the Advancement of Psychiatry, 1961.

Ruesch, J., & G. Bateson: *Communication: The Social Matrix of Psychiatry.* Norton, 1951.

Stevenson, I.: *Medical History Taking.* Hoeber, 1961.

Sullivan, H.S.: *The Psychiatric Interview.* Norton, 1954.

Journal Articles

Aring, C.D.: Sympathy and empathy. JAMA 167:448, 1958.

Bartemeier, L.H.: The attitude of the physician. JAMA 145:1122–1125, 1951.

Burstein, A.G., & R.J. Leider: Teaching and evaluation of diagnostic skills. Arch Gen Psychiat 24:255–259, 1971.

Carter, G.H.: History-taking and interviewing technique. J M Educ 30:315–326, 1955.

Diethelm, O.: The evaluation of a psychiatric examination. Am J Psychiat 105:606–611, 1949.

Finesinger, J.E.: Psychiatric interviewing. 1. Some principles and procedures in insight therapy. Am J Psychiat 105:187, 1948.

Hall, B.H., & W. Wheeler: The patient and his relatives: Initial joint interview. Social Work 2:75–80, 1957.

Hendrickson, W.J., Coffer, R.H., & T.N. Cross: The initial interview. Arch Neurol Psychiat 71:24, 1954.

Meyer, A.: The aims and meaning of psychiatric diagnosis. Am J Insan 74:163–168, 1917.

Reider, N.: The reaction of psychiatric patients to physical and neurological examinations. Bull Menninger Clin 3:73–81, 1939.

Reisman, D.: Some observations on interviewing in a state mental hospital. Bull Menninger Clin 23:7, 1959.

Saul, L.J.: The psychoanalytic diagnostic interview. Psychoanal Quart 26:76–90, 1957.

Solomon, P.: The medical psychiatric examination. New Physician: 27–29, June 1958.

Stevenson, I., & R.A. Matthews: The art of interviewing. GP 2:59–69, 1950.

Sullivan, H.S.: The psychiatric interview. Psychiatry 14:361–373, 1951; 15:127–141, 1952.

Whitehorn, J.C.: Guide to interviewing and clinical personality study. Arch Neurol Psychiat 52:197–216, 1944.

5...

Common Psychiatric Symptoms

The most frequent and troublesome psychiatric symptoms are anxiety, depression, grief, paranoid ideation, delusions, hallucinations, and thought disorders. Normal people have the first 4 at times (mildly); neurotics have them severely; psychotics have the remainder.

ANXIETY

Everyone is anxious at one time or another. Anxiety is a normal response to threats directed towards one's body, possessions, way of life, loved ones, or cherished values. It is normal during extreme effort or in a life situation that changes rapidly and demands continuous adaptation. Parents and teachers as well as psychiatrists agree that "normal" anxiety spurs the individual to useful action and plays an important role in beneficial change and personality growth. In contrast, excessive anxiety not only makes a person unhappy but has a deleterious effect on his performance.

Anxiety is primarily a conscious subjective state, variously described as an emotion, affect, or feeling. It is expressed by certain kinds of behavior and is accompanied by characteristic physiologic changes. In psychoanalytic theory, the term "anxiety" has an additional, more abstract meaning. In this sense it can also be said to be unconscious as well as conscious. The concept of anxiety in psychoanalytic theory will be discussed below.

Whether anxiety is normal or abnormal depends upon its intensity and duration and the circumstances that cause it. In current usage, fear and anxiety are often differentiated by regarding fear as the response to a realistic danger and anxiety as the result of obscure or irrational causes. This distinction is hard to maintain consistently and has only limited practical value.

Severe, disorganizing anxiety is commonly called "panic."

THE SUBJECTIVE EXPERIENCE OF ANXIETY

The experience of anxiety is described differently by different individuals, but its essential feature is the unpleasant anticipation of some kind of

51

misfortune, danger, or doom. This apprehension is accompanied by tenseness, restlessness, and the feeling that something must be done. When what.is feared is perceived dimly or not at all, the anxiety is called "free-floating." If anxiety continues, it leads to a feeling of helplessness and the fear of collapse.

Anxious people usually have disagreeable sensations in their bodies. Most of these can be ascribed to psychophysiologic mechanisms (see below); others are more difficult to explain, eg, precordial pain and bizarre feelings in the head such as swelling, cracking, or a trickling sensation. The anxious person may or may not recognize that his physical symptoms are due to emotional causes. If he does not, he characteristically decides that he is physically ill and makes the symptoms the basis of his fear and worry.

BEHAVIORAL AND PHYSIOLOGIC MANIFESTATIONS

Anxiety often makes a person hyperalert, irritable, and uncertain. He may fidget or hold himself tensely immobile. He may be overdependent, hanging on the doctor's every word, or so preoccupied with his worries that he can scarcely pay attention. He is likely to talk too much. He sleeps poorly. Sexual interest and function are usually impaired.

Severe anxiety constricts the scope of the individual's daily activities and lessens his productivity at work. It can impair concentration, memory, abstract reasoning, calculating ability, and psychomotor efficiency. The nonverbal subtests of the Wechsler Adult Intelligence Scale (WAIS) are sensitive to anxiety, and an anxious subject will score lower on these than on the verbal subtests. Anxious people given tranquilizers may perform better on simple arithmetic tests, whereas less anxious controls become sedated and do less well than before.

Anxiety is associated with a wide variety of physiologic alterations. When these cause physical symptoms, they are usually called psychophysiologic disorders. Why different organ systems are involved in different patients remains poorly understood.

Common somatic manifestations of anxiety are the following:

(1) **Excessive perspiration.**

(2) **Skeletal muscle tension:** Tension headache, constriction in the back of the neck or chest, quavering voice, backache.

(3) **Sighing respirations.**

(4) **Hyperventilation syndrome:** Dyspnea, dizziness, paresthesias.

(5) **Functional gastrointestinal disorders:** Abdominal pain, anorexia, nausea, foul taste in the mouth, distention, diarrhea, constipation, "butterflies" in the stomach.

(6) **Cardiovascular irritability:** Transient systolic hypertension, premature contraction, tachycardia, fainting.

(7) **Genitourinary dysfunction:** Urinary frequency, dysuria, impotence, pelvic pain in women, frigidity.

PATHOLOGIC ANXIETY

Anxiety is regarded as pathologic (1) when it seems to be triggered by some minor event or occurs without known cause or (2) when it is unusually severe and persistent. Persistence (chronicity) of anxiety is evidence that the anxiety is no longer serving as a signal of danger but has become a danger and a burden in itself.

There are constitutional differences in the tendency to become anxious; the wide differences in observed autonomic reactivity and other measures of temperament among newborn infants must have a genetic or, at least, a congenital basis. Furthermore, every adult has his own history of different experiences. To one man, the sight of a clerical collar may provoke the anxious anticipation of hell and damnation; to another, the same cue elicits a gratifying fantasy of kindliness and comfort.

Dynamic psychiatric theory holds that a man can be made anxious by all sorts of stimuli without his being aware of it. For example, a woman's perfume may trigger forbidden sexual impulses which cause conscious anxiety even though the subject may not be aware of either the perfume or the sexual impulses. Both the sexual impulse and the contravening conscience are mental processes, and they are in conflict with each other. If either the desire or the proscriptions of conscience are absent, anxiety does not occur. According to psychoanalytic theory, continuing conflict between inner temptation and inner prohibitions is the fundamental explanation of chronic pathologic anxiety. Psychoanalytic theory further states that if the anxious patient were made aware of this conflict and were able to resolve it by conscious decision, the anxiety would be diminished even though he might remain unhappy. Anxiety is caused not so much by lack of gratification of sexual or aggressive drives as by continuing conflict about them. Deprivation causes unhappiness, but it is conflict that causes anxiety.

A Pavlovian theorist would offer a different explanation for the anxiety aroused by the perfume, ie, that the perfume had become a conditioned stimulus for anxiety by prior conditioning. Perhaps the perfume is associated in the subject's mind with a woman who in the past has repeatedly served as an unconditioned stimulus for anxiety. The conditioning history is regarded as crucial, and conflicting motives, even if present, are regarded as irrelevant.

Psychologists studying experimental neuroses can generate anxiety-like behavior in animals. In an experimental situation where the animal has learned that specific behavior will prevent painful stimuli, the psychologist can create anxiety by presenting problems in discrimination that are too difficult to solve or simply by changing the rules too often.

None of these theories about how chronic anxiety is generated are altogether satisfactory because they all fail to account for the chronicity, ie, they do not explain why some people stay anxious for so long. There must be self-perpetuating mechanisms or vicious circles that keep things going.

One such mechanism of clinical importance is as follows: The patient becomes anxious for unknown reasons; the anxiety produces frightening physical symptoms; the fright produces continuing physical symptoms; and the circle is complete. The clinical importance of understanding this process is obvious, since in mild anxiety reactions the cycle can be interrupted if the patient can be convinced that his physical symptoms are benign.

Anxiety has a central place in the psychoanalytic theory of neurosis. It is said that when the demands of the id conflict with those of the environment or superego, the resultant anxiety triggers the defensive operations of the ego. Some defenses, such as sublimation and repression, control the demands of the id in a relatively healthy way. Less adaptive defenses such as denial and displacement lead to neurotic symptom formation. When defense mechanisms are put into action without any conscious appreciation of anxiety, the anxiety is said to serve as a preconscious or unconscious signal of danger (unconscious anxiety).

Cultural factors are important in the causation of anxiety. Received values, educational and religious institutions, the legal framework, and the individual's own degree of sociocultural integration all help to determine the incidence of guilt and mutually exclusive goal-seeking behavior (conflict) that cause anxiety. Whether ours is truly the Age of Anxiety, as has been said, is not an easy question to answer. Certainly the rules of living seem to be changing rapidly, and man's realistic capacity for self-destruction is increasing.

The question for the clinician will always be somewhat apart from these larger problems about the health of our culture. For him the question must always be, Why is my patient more anxious than most people? What in particular has got him so upset?

DIAGNOSIS

It is useful to differentiate acute anxiety from the less dramatic but persistent chronic forms.

Acute anxiety (anxiety attack). The patient begins to feel very sick and frightened during the course of a few minutes or hours. He may recognize that he is having an emotional experience, but more commonly he does not know what is wrong or assumes that his body has suffered some catastrophe such as a heart attack. Physical symptoms are usually the presenting complaint—especially dyspnea, palpitations, chest or abdominal pain, faintness, trembling, or paresthesias.

Upon physical examination, restlessness, sighing or rapid respiration, tachycardia, excessive perspiration, hyperactive deep tendon reflexes, and systolic hypertension are usually present. The patient may have to interrupt the examination to urinate. The hypertension is usually transient, and the patient should not be told he has high blood pressure.

Relatives or friends often know what the precipitating event was although the patient may not. It is therefore useful to talk to someone besides the patient, assuming that he gives permission. If he does not give permission, it often means he has an idea about what is wrong, and the discussion about consulting other informants gives the therapist good opportunity to draw him out.

Chronic anxiety. The chronically anxious patient usually establishes the diagnosis himself by complaining that he is nervous, worried all the time, jumpy, tired, and unable to relax or sleep properly. He may recognize that he is irritable, but the most dramatic impact of his irritability is likely to be on those around him. His account of himself is usually confirmed by his uneasy, tense behavior, his difficulty in keeping to the point, and his complaints about physical ailments with no physical disease present to explain them. The most common physical complaints are tension headaches, gastrointestinal disorders, and fatigue.

The physical examination may reveal the same signs as in acute anxiety, but usually it is unremarkable. When signs of anxiety are present, it may be that the physical examination has caused superimposed acute anxiety.

The diagnosis of chronic anxiety is more difficult when the patient is unaware that he is emotionally upset and complains of physical symptoms alone. In such a case the diagnosis can be established only after a medical work-up that is complete enough to rule out primary physical disorders that cause similar symptoms. It is a venerable clinical dictum that a psychiatric disorder must be "ruled in"; it is not sufficient that physical disease be "ruled out." The reasoning is that all physical disease can never be ruled out, so that diagnosis by exclusion may lead to error. By the same token, however, the presence of an abnormal personality or distressing life events is only circumstantial evidence for a psychiatric explanation of physical symptoms. Psychiatric illness is no easier to "rule in" than physical disease is to "rule out." Both possibilities have to be thoughtfully considered, and there are no general rules of inference on which to base a diagnostic decision.

The differentiation will be easy in a healthy looking young person who arrives at the emergency service highly agitated and obviously hyperventilating after an upsetting life experience. It will be much more difficult in a middle-aged man in an apparently normal life situation who has suffered a gradual and progressive loss of well-being with headaches, dizziness, and fatigue.

As with all psychogenic physical complaints, there may be coexisting or interacting physical disease.

DIFFERENTIAL DIAGNOSIS

In the differential diagnosis of anxiety, one should consider both the variety of physical disorders that cause the same physical symptoms as anxiety and the several psychiatric disorders in which anxiety may be a principal symptom.

Anxiety Neurosis
One makes the diagnosis of anxiety neurosis in the presence of anxiety and the absence of other findings that would indicate some other medical or psychiatric disease. It is largely a diagnosis of exclusion.

Anxiety and Organic Disease

Patients with senility, general paresis, or other organic brain disease may suffer from anxiety before clinical signs of dementia become apparent. Hyperthyroidism is a well recognized mimic of anxiety reaction; until reliable laboratory tests of thyroid function became available, the 2 were frequently confused. Most physical disorders which cause marked anxiety in normal people, such as pulmonary or cardiac insufficiency, are severe and not difficult to recognize.

Anxiety and Drugs

Impending delirium tremens and many drug intoxications or withdrawal syndromes may begin with anxiety. Ingestion of hallucinogens and withdrawal from narcotics, barbiturates, meprobamate, or chlordiazepoxide are common examples.

Anxiety Symptomatic of Other Psychiatric Disorders.

Among the functional psychiatric disorders, the most important disorder to be differentiated from anxiety is agitated depression. This should be considered especially when severe anxiety develops in middle or late life. Feelings of hopelessness (as contrasted to helplessness), low self-esteem, and irrational protestations of guilt indicate depression. Nihilistic, hypochondriacal, or guilty delusions signify depression of psychotic degree and are often an indication for immediate hospitalization. In assessing the danger of suicide in the patient with severe anxiety, the degree of anxiety is probably more critical than the degree of depression. The patient who says, "I feel so nervous I will climb out of my skin!" or, "I just can't stand it!" is more worrisome to the physician than the one who says, "I am just no good. I have wasted all my opportunities."

Patients with schizophrenic illnesses often have severe anxiety early in their disease. Many of them have a discouraging history of repeated medical consultations in search of relief from the physical symptoms of anxiety before the appearance of overt schizophrenic symptoms makes the diagnosis obvious. A good rule for all physicians is that any patient with progressive unexplained anxiety symptoms over a period of weeks or months should receive a careful psychiatric examination to rule out early schizophrenia.

Homosexual panic is a commonly used diagnostic term with an ambiguous meaning. It is applied to young men in panic following homosexual experience or temptation or fear of these. It is also applied (improperly) to young men with acute schizophrenic reactions—whether or not homosexuality is a factor in their premorbid personality—simply because they mention homosexuality along with other confused or delusional concerns. The most misleading use of all is to assume that latent (unconscious) homosexual impulses are the primary cause of anxiety in any young man who presents with severe acute anxiety. This concept of latent homosexuality is of questionable validity and even less utility. Furthermore, there is no valid evidence that homosexuality regularly plays a role in the etiology of any kind of schizophrenia. Therefore, only the first, purely descriptive use of the term "homosexual panic" is defensible. It too should probably be abandoned to avoid confusion.

TREATMENT

The treatment of anxiety principally involves giving appropriate attention to the disorder of which it is a symptom—eg, psychoneurosis, intolerable life situation, agitated depression, hyperthyroidism, delirium tremens. Some degree of symptomatic relief is often obtainable with the use of tranquilizers regardless of the basic cause. If anxiety has caused an uncomfortable physiologic disorder, this can also be treated directly, eg, treat hypocapnia in hyperventilation by rebreathing; control diarrhea with diphenoxylate (Lomotil). Symptomatic relief in psychogenic anxiety is often sufficient to cause lasting remission because it breaks the vicious circle of staying anxious because of being frightened by the symptoms of being anxious.

In the symptomatic treatment of anxiety it is useful to help the patient discover that he is not continually anxious but rather has periods or "attacks" of more severe anxiety. Tranquilizers, supportive phone calls, and special office visits should be focused upon these bad times, with the strong suggestion that they are temporary and can be overcome by a variety of means within the patient's power. Gradually, the patient discovers that these attacks are benign and safe although uncomfortable. At about this time they disappear, because safety and anxiety are incompatible.

For the symptomatic treatment of neurotic or situational anxiety it is usually best to use a sedative (including the so-called minor tranquilizers), eg, chlordiazepoxide (Librium), diazepam (Valium), and meprobamate (Miltown, Equanil). When the anxiety is associated with psychosis or organic brain disease it is usually more effective to use a major tranquilizer—a phenothiazine or butyrophenone.

With any tranquilizer, the dose varies widely according to how anxious the patient is. Mild anxiety does not require sedatives. Moderate anxiety is benefited by small to moderate doses of sedatives, and the placebo effect is important. Panic requires major tranquilizers, often in massive doses for effective control, and massive doses at these times will not oversedate the patient. The most common errors are to use doses too small to relieve anxiety when the patient is upset and to continue to administer the drug during remissions.

A final consideration in the treatment of anxiety is a reminder that anxiety is not always pathologic. One should permit a person to worry enough to help himself but not so much as to become disorganized and ineffective.

PROGNOSIS

When anxiety presents acutely as a dramatic attack, one can expect that the attack will pass within a few minutes or hours or 1—2 days, depending largely on the aptness of treatment. The frequency of anxiety attacks can generally be gratifyingly reduced even with less than optimal treatment.

Chronic anxiety is a more difficult matter. Here the prognosis depends on several interrelated factors: the duration of symptoms, the personal strengths of the patient, the difficulties of his life situation, the possibility of support from others, secondary gain considerations, and the availability of psychiatric care. In general, the shorter the duration of symptoms, the better the prognosis regardless of severity. Among other factors, perhaps the most important is the patient's capacity to change his behavior even before his feelings have greatly changed. The patient who can do this alters the feedback he receives from his environment. His new behavior, if well conceived, may help him avoid meeting the originally pathogenic stimuli and lead to improvement without basic personality change.

DEPRESSION

Depression rivals anxiety as the most important and inclusive category in psychopathology. It is a neurotic symptom and is the salient feature of 3 psychoses: manic-depressive psychosis, involutional melancholia, and psychotic depressive reaction. Even in other psychiatric conditions, depression is commonly a significant part of the symptomatology and a principal focus of therapeutic effort.

Depression regularly accompanies serious physical illness and can be considered a normal response to the misfortunes of life. Nevertheless, much as pathologic anxiety can be contrasted with realistic fear, it is useful to contrast pathologic depression with normal disappointment, sadness, and grief.

SYMPTOMS OF DEPRESSION

Mild depression manifests itself largely by a loss of pleasurable interest in the usual affairs of life. Spontaneity is gone. Everything requires extra effort and provides less gratification than before. One does not feel physically ill but neither does one feel comfortable and well. Fatigue is excessive. Realistic worries and ordinary bodily discomforts are prominent in awareness, while encouraging memories, hopes, and plans are hard to keep in mind. A person with a mild depression such as this does his work, meets his obligations, and appears normal to acquaintances. To himself and his intimates, however, something has changed.

In more severe depression the patient is frankly despondent or feels physically ill (or both). He is usually gloomy, hopeless, helpless, and bereft of self-esteem. His thinking, speech, and movements may be slowed (psychomotor retardation), or he may be tense, hypervigilant, and restless (agitation, anxiety). The agitated depressed patient is likely to complain endlessly about aches and pains, fatigue, feelings of unworthiness, or guilty fears. If the depression is of psychotic severity, the patient may actually believe things are as bad as he feels they are and he may have elaborate delusions, often hypochondriacal in nature.

Of the numerous physical symptoms, insomnia is the most prominent. EEG studies of depressed patients confirm that they tend to have a higher proportion of light or restless sleep and a shorter period of total sleep. In severe depressions, patients commonly awaken early after only enough sleep to take the edge off their exhaustion. These lonely vigils in the early morning hours are often the times of deepest despair.

There are neurotic syndromes involving depression in which hypersomnia is a problem. In severe depression, however, the opposite is the rule.

Anorexia and weight loss are also characteristic. Involuntary weight loss of 7 lb or more in a month has been suggested by some writers as a diagnostic criterion for severe depression. Many other somatic complaints commonly occur in depression, particularly obscure pain, gastrointestinal symptoms, menstrual irregularities, and the whole range of psychophysiologic disorders. Sexual disinterest or incapacity ("loss of libido") is described as a classical symptom. To put it briefly, the 4 major appetites are impaired: food, sleep, sex, and activity.

CLASSIFICATION OF DEPRESSION

Although depression has been recognized as a clinical syndrome since ancient times, debate continues about whether it is a single well defined entity of varying severity or a mixed category of qualitatively different disorders.

The difference between neurotic and psychotic depression is quantitative in the sense that both lie on a continuum with no precise distinction in the middle. From the viewpoint of planning therapy, however, a mild depressive neurosis differs so greatly from a severe depressive psychosis that it is practical to think of the 2 as qualitatively different. The differentiations made in the current nomenclature among the affective psychoses still rest upon shifting sands of unproved theoretical tradition; they have no implications for therapy.

PSYCHOANALYTIC AND PSYCHODYNAMIC VIEWS OF DEPRESSION

The concept of a resemblance between grieving and pathologic depression has been important as a starting point for contemporary psychodynamic explanations of depression and also as a landmark in the development of psychoanalytic theory. Freud's essay on *Mourning and Melancholia* (1917) presaged the "structural" postulate about the psyche with its tripartite conception of id, ego, and superego.

In normal grieving (eg, after the death of a spouse, parent, or child), there is dejection, diminished interest in the outside world, loss of capacity to love, inhibition of activity, a feeling of hopelessness, and a tendency to ruminate about different aspects of the lost person.* Freud noted that the same picture characterizes pathologic depression except that the patient seems to be grieving over an inner loss (or absence) rather than the loss of an external love object. The patient ruminates not about a lost person but about himself—specifically, about those real or imagined aspects of himself that destroy his security or self-esteem. He may be very hostile toward himself, ie, belittling, accusatory, and even reviling.

Freud believed the depressed patient's anger against himself was originally directed toward another person who had been symbolically taken into himself (introjected) by a kind of identification process. The psychic mechanism of introjection contributed to the subsequent psychoanalytic formulation of the superego as part of the psyche that is acquired by internalizing the rival parent at the resolution of the oedipal conflict.

Modern psychodynamic formulations emphasize dependency as a primary issue in people prone to depression. Such people have exaggerated needs for nurturing, support, or approval. Some require special foods and bodily attentions from specific other people; others can get by if they have plentiful general conversation and companionship; for others, simple assurances that they are morally worthy or vocationally competent suffice, but they cannot get along without those assurances.

A very dependent person is always vulnerable to disappointment. Since he needs too much, he can never get enough. Because his needs are chronically unfulfilled, he has feelings of frustration and anger. Such a person is in a serious bind because expressing his anger will drive away or make hostile the very people he is dependent on. Therefore, he must hold in his anger, which seems to eat away at his insides, leading ultimately to feelings of helplessness and self-reproach. It is significant that the vicissitudes of anger and hostility remain part of every dynamic account of depression. It usually comes as a surprise to discover how angry the patient is, because superficially and consciously he blames no one but himself.

The anger becomes apparent when one attempts to reassure a depressed person by asking him to be realistic or even optimistic about himself. Secondary gain in depression may be considerable. By being so miserable, the patient not only gains reassurance and sympathy from his friends but also makes them feel sad and guilty, thus gratifying his anger.

Psychoanalytic literature offers competing dynamic explanations of depression, and one can only conclude that no single account is universally applicable. Different kinds of depression are to be understood in different ways. That there are indeed several kinds of depression is confirmed by descriptive psychiatry. Some depressions are characterized by guilt, others by grief; some by anxiety, others by apathy; some mainly by physical symptoms, others purely by mental ones. In general, one can summarize the

---

*This subject is discussed more fully in the following section.

psychodynamic understanding of depression in this way: All of the mental symptoms of depression are correlates of a loss of self-esteem, no matter how it came about. The patient experiences hopelessness, guilt, or bodily discomfort in varying proportions. At one time or another, he reveals considerable anger which he has directed largely toward himself. What made him angry is a loss, actual or symbolic. He is particularly vulnerable to loss because of excessive needs for nurturing or because his conscience is exceptionally vigilant, cruel, and unreasonable.

SOMATIC VIEWS OF DEPRESSION

Physiologic and biochemical investigations have disclosed a variety of physical alterations in depression. Among these are increased urinary 17-hydroxycorticosteroid excretion, sodium retention, and changes in sleep EEG patterns. These abnormalities are of uncertain significance, but some psychiatrists have inferred that the etiology of depression is primarily physical and that secondary psychologic factors, although they may determine the mental content of the symptoms, are not their cause. The major arguments cited in support of the somatogenic hypotheses of depression are (1) the hereditary pattern of manic-depressive psychosis; (2) the occurrence of depression antecedent to or coincident with physical illness; and (3) the frequent occurrence of severe depression without any clear psychologic precipitant.

Psychiatrists who tend to favor organic explanations of psychic events do not search diligently for psychologic precipitants but call the depression "endogenous." They postulate some subtle physicochemical misadventure in the archipallium and upper brain stem.

DIAGNOSIS

The diagnosis of depression is easy when the patient understands that he is despondent and talks freely. The difficulty occurs when the patient's symptoms are predominantly physical, or he is uncommunicative.

When a depression manifests itself principally as physical symptoms, pain, insomnia, anorexia, and easy fatigability are the most common. Although the patient's description of his symptoms may suggest a psychiatric illness, the most reliable clue is the apparent absence of organic disease. An antecedent depressing life event adds circumstantial evidence. Often such an event is obvious to the family but not to the patient himself. Clearly, a medical work-up is essential before the physical symptoms can be said to be due to depression. The identification of a precipitating event or the presence of mental symptoms of depression is not conclusive evidence that physical disease is absent.

When the patient is totally uncommunicative, the differential diagnosis is among (1) organic disease causing stupor, (2) functional psychosis, and

(3) a social situation (of which the examiner is unaware) that has made the patient acutely angry and uncooperative. Organic brain syndrome must be considered first, since immediate medical treatment may be indicated. The final diagnosis in the uncommunicative patient is most frequently functional psychosis. A sad face or a history of depressive ideation before the patient became mute suggests depressive psychosis rather than schizophrenia, but the 2 may occur together (schizo-affective disorder).

In the communicative patient whose depression is evident from what he says about himself, the diagnostic problem is to differentiate between neurosis and psychosis and between primary depression and depression as a secondary symptom of some other psychiatric disorder.

The recognition of depressive psychosis is important because hospitalization is usually necessary to effect prompt treatment and lessen the danger of suicide. In depressive psychosis, as contrasted with depressive neurosis, the mood disturbance is much more profound. It interferes with concentration and subjectively with memory. The patient often has guilty or hypochondriacal delusions. The insomnia is usually of the early morning type, and weight loss is often considerable. The patient is unable to function normally, and family or friends at work are almost always of the opinion that he is definitely sick, although they may not recognize the sickness as depression.

The kind of depressive psychosis that involves the greatest risk of suicide is that in which agitation is a major symptom. Physical restlessness, hand wringing, or the expressed feeling that "something must be done" or that "I will jump out of my skin" are urgent indications for supervision and sedation, and perhaps hospitalization.

An unresolved problem in the diagnosis of depression is that of "masked depression," "smiling depression," or "depressive equivalent." Disorders that can be successfully treated as depressions may appear in the guise of unusual somatic complaints or other psychiatric syndromes. In either case, the mood disturbance characteristic of depression is either absent or very hard to observe. The concept is valuable as a reminder that certain patients with pain or other obscure physical complaints have been dramatically relieved by ECT or other antidepressant therapy. It is also true that certain types of behavior, eg, unusual sexual activity or voluntary overwork, may be a substitute for or defense against depression. Nevertheless, the concept of "depression *sine* depression" will always be difficult to handle systematically. It tempts those who are overenthusiastic about some particular form of treatment for depression to regard almost any disorder as requiring their favorite treatment. The possibility of significant organic disease must always be considered.

TREATMENT

A plan of therapy should be based on the evident problems and assets of the patient. The doctor must decide where he can effectively intervene in a process of interaction among many factors. If an organic treatment such as a mood-elevating or sedative drug can ease the pain of bereavement, then it should be used. However, even if an organic constitutional factor makes a patient vulnerable to depression, a psychologic approach still may be most helpful. It is generally agreed that the therapist must be relatively active, since severe depressive symptoms make it impossible for the patient to take the responsibility for initial steps toward getting well. He is inclined to be discouraged and helpless. If psychotic, he may believe he deserves to be sick or dead.

If the patient can accept reassurance and kind attention, these can be very helpful. In some types of depression, however, every gesture of affection or kind regard can "twist the knife" in the wound of the patient's guilty self-contempt. In such cases it may help to confront the patient sternly with his cruelty toward himself. The disapproving sternness gratifies his self-hate and at the same time helps him realize cognitively that he is not so bad as part of him claims he is.

The traditional goal of psychotherapy in depression is to help the patient achieve insight into the nature of the precipitating loss, usually symbolic, which has activated a cruel, arbitrary conscience. But whether or not much insight can be achieved, supportive psychotherapy can often shorten the course of a depression and lessen its pain and danger.

In recent decades most of the innovations in the treatment of depression have been in the development of somatic therapies. The use of ECT, antidepressant drugs, and lithium carbonate is discussed elsewhere in this book.

Suicide risk (see Chapter 22) must be evaluated in all cases of depression and in all illnesses associated with depression. Errors in the direction of underestimating the danger of suicide usually occur when the doctor has been hesitant to question the patient directly about his inclinations and intentions. In the course of treating a patient with a suicidal depression, special periods of danger occur after a setback—especially rejection by or loss of another person (including the doctor); when agitation develops; when a patient with motor retardation becomes more active; and soon after going home after a period of hospitalization.

PROGNOSIS

One of the characteristics that has traditionally defined depression as a discrete clinical entity is its well defined onset and tendency toward eventual remission. Most patients recover completely from acute episodes. The duration of an attack depends, of course, on the treatment available, but most often is 3−8 months. Acute onset, younger age, and milder symptoms favor a shorter duration. Little is known about the incidence of recurrence in depressive neurosis, but recurrence is fairly common in the affective psychoses. A small minority of patients with an affective psychosis demonstrate frank schizophrenia upon subsequent attacks.

ACUTE GRIEF REACTION

Acute grief reaction ("mourning," "normal depression," "simple depression") is the grief that occurs in response to the loss of a loved one by death. It is different from the pathologic depressive reactions described elsewhere in this book in which the loss may be real or fancied, may be precipitated by various causes, and where self-esteem is drastically lowered and regressed behavior occurs. Just as family and community celebrations and festivals may be regarded as within normal limits in the direction of mania, grief may be considered the normal counterpart of pathologic depressive states.

MANIFESTATIONS OF GRIEF

The loss of a loved one leads to a behavioral syndrome with the following well defined manifestations.

(1) A sensation of somatic distress, occurring immediately and recurring in waves lasting for 20 minutes to an hour at a time. There is tightness in the throat, choking and shortness of breath, sighing, an empty feeling in the abdomen with lack of muscular strength, and intense subjective distress, all precipitated by any mention or memory of the deceased. The intensity of the suffering fluctuates but diminishes with time, usually subsiding within a month. Mild "echoes" may occur indefinitely, especially at anniversaries ("anniversary syndrome").

(2) Intense preoccupation with the image of the deceased, accompanied by a sense of vagueness, a feeling of unreality, and an increased emotional distance from other people.

(3) Feelings of guilt. The patient searches the time before the death for instances of failure to behave properly toward the lost one.

(4) Disconcerting loss of warmth in relationships with other people, with either an aloof manner or irritability and anger.

(5) Loss of normal patterns of conduct, with restlessness, inattentiveness, absentmindedness, and a painful lack of capacity to initiate and maintain organized patterns of activity.

GRIEF REACTIONS IN CHILDREN AND IN THE ELDERLY

Grief reactions in childhood are a highly controversial topic. Melanie Klein states that there is no difference between mourning by an adult and by a child. Rochlin asserts that the child's ego is not sufficiently developed to feel grief and that children use narcissism, indifference, or anxiety instead. Furman feels that a child as young as 3½–4 years old can mourn as an adult and that this capacity can be assisted and sustained by adult support.

Elderly people respond to bereavement with a relative paucity of overt grief or of conscious guilt feelings; a readiness to channel material into somatic illness and identify with the dead person rather than feel guilty; and a tendency to deal with ambivalence by "splitting the image" in such a way that the hostile component is transferred to a living person while the deceased is idealized.

GRIEF WORK

Grief work is the term used to indicate the internal process of gradual emancipation from bondage to the lost person. It involves a painful review of the bereaved person's memories of the deceased and of his current relationships in such a way that the present situation can be comprehended and accepted in the light of the lost person's absence. At first, there is tearful denial and angry protest and an urge somehow to recover the lost person. The latter goal is also achieved in fantasy by an intense preoccupation with memories of the lost person, and identification with him manifested by a tendency to adopt his mannerisms and ideals or even (fleetingly) the symptoms of his last illness.

The bereaved person repeatedly tests reality and is repeatedly disappointed in the psychic wish for reunion. Despair may set in, and behavior may become temporarily disorganized.

In time, ties with the lost person are loosened and memories fade. The survivor becomes gradually free to seek new attachments.

COURSE

The intensity, duration, and course of grief reactions are determined by the following factors.

(1) The type and duration of the relationship with the lost person. An extremely ambivalent relationship can make grief reaction complicated or pathologic. (See Chapter 16.) It is as important to review and accept one's negative feelings toward the lost person as one's positive feelings.

(2) Earlier losses and reactions to them.

(3) The extent to which the sufferer has prepared himself for the loss.

(4) The sufferer's view of the world as a safe place to live without the lost person.

The habituation and extinction of grief are seldom complete, and there are great cultural and individual variations. In some parts of India, for example, the Hindu widow must remember her dead husband all her life by having her head shorn every month, by not wearing any ornaments, and by participating in no form of amusement; while the Dhimar, a caste of fishermen, customarily "mourn" only one day for children whose ears are not pierced.

PATHOLOGIC GRIEF REACTIONS

Although grief is normal and an essentially healthy restitutive process, some individuals are unable to experience it properly. The following pathologic reactions can occur:

(1) Persistent absence of emotion following the death of a loved one represents an effort to avoid the intense distress of grief. In such cases, grief will be expressed in clearly pathologic or disguised ways. It may be displaced, as in an obsession with the deceased's life work; transformed into a neurotic identification, as when the mourner, avoiding activity and the joys of living, lives as one dead; or delayed for many years, as in some patients who undergo acute bereavement on the anniversary of the death of a loved one.

(2) Unduly prolonged grief reactions tend to become ends in themselves in the survivor's effort to deny the loss. One form of this is idealization of the lost person so that unpleasant features of the relationship will remain repressed.

(3) Exaggerated grief reactions may be due to guilt, with a need for punishment. The survivor may respond with somatic symptoms (often those of the lost person's last illness) or hostility and irritability.

ILLNESSES PRECIPITATED BY BEREAVEMENT

The stress of grief has been said to precipitate a wide variety of disorders: (1) psychiatric illnesses, eg, anxiety states, hysteria, obsessional reactions, depressive reactions, manic-depressive states, or schizophrenia; or (2) somatic illnesses, eg, asthma, Raynaud's disease, hyperthyroidism, functional uterine bleeding, rheumatoid arthritis, ulcerative colitis, osteoarthritis, diabetes mellitus, pernicious anemia, leukemia, lymphoma, and tuberculosis. (See Chapter 18.)

MANAGEMENT

The physician should encourage grief work, with its full expression of feelings. In the process, he may have to absorb hostile reactions from the patient. Mourning rituals, as in eulogies and memorial services, are to be encouraged.

With a patient in whom grief is particularly intense or in whom grief seems to be playing a role in the precipitation or aggravation of illness, the physician can be helpful as follows: (1) At the crisis stage, he can administer a sedative or hypnotic (eg, a barbiturate or chloral hydrate) and make sure that relatives or friends will watch over the patient. The possibility of a suicidal attempt may have to be considered. (2) In the early stages following the crisis, the patient should be seen frequently, perhaps once a day for a week, for interviews of 15–60 minutes. Emotional ventilation is the chief goal, and the physician need say very little. Mild tranquilizers may be prescribed (eg, meprobamate or chlordiazepoxide). (3) In the late stages, if symptoms do not abate satisfactorily, more extensive efforts at psychotherapy should be attempted. Visits should be 2 or 3 times a week for a half hour or more each, and the patient's entire emotional past and present should be explored. Medication should be tapered off.

A number of community organizations have sprung up in recent years to help the bereaved. An example is the "Widow to Widow" program in Boston, sponsored by the YMCA, synagogues, churches, and the Harvard Laboratory of Community Psychiatry. Some hospitals have special teams that deal with the family of dying patients in an attempt to foster normal grief and prevent mental breakdown.

PARANOID IDEATION

Paranoid ideation occurs in a number of psychiatric states. It is characterized by persecutory thoughts and feelings which are not subject to modification by logic or experience. A basic feature is the individual's belief that some one person or group is intent, directly or deviously, on causing him harm. The actual content is strongly influenced by the individual's social and cultural history. (*Examples:* A Negro from a rural and fundamentalist southern community may be "persecuted by the devil" or pursued by a "flaming cross." An individual in a position of high political authority, perhaps a senator, sees Communists behind every bush and desk.)

Types of Paranoid Ideation

Mild forms of paranoid ideation occur in everyone at times. It is a normal inclination to blame others sometimes for one's own misfortunes and failures, eg, the wife who burns the dinner may blame the husband for coming home late; a husband who is arrested for drunken driving blames his wife for having nagged him to drink.

Psychiatrically significant paranoia may be classified as follows:

A. Paranoid Personalities: While remaining integrated and functioning, these people exhibit traits of excessive rigidity and suspiciousness in their dealings with others.

B. Classical Paranoia: This term, which once meant just "insanity," is now restricted to a fairly rare state in which an encapsulated delusional system exists though the patient remains otherwise well integrated. (*Example:* A student from an emerging African country found increasing difficulty in keeping up with his courses at an American university and was lonely and isolated. He attributed his difficulties with his studies to distractions caused by "political enemies" who interfered with the heating system in his room, producing "noises" and "overheating" which prevented him from working. He had no other symptoms, and functioned well at a part-time job.)

C. Paranoid Schizophrenia: Here the contact with reality is much more tenuous, the ideation more bizarre, and the personality more disintegrated. There may be accompanying hallucinations. Other characteristic features of schizophrenia are usually present, such as thinking disorders or impoverished affect.

D. Depressive States: Especially in psychotic depressions, paranoid delusions can be extremely troublesome.

E. Toxic and Organic Brain Syndromes: An example is alcoholic hallucinosis, in which paranoid ideas are accompanied by hallucinations and an appropriate degree of fear. (*Example:* A young Negro who had been drinking heavily for several weeks began to hear voices saying they were out to get him. He thought he heard shots. Three men in the street seemed to be waiting to kill him. He cowered behind the consulting room door as a motorcycle passed, thinking it was machine-gun fire.)

Organic brain syndromes also occur as a result of trauma, hormonal deficiency (myxedema), or senile degeneration. (*Example:* A 72-year-old woman developed itching of the skin on her face. She claimed this was due to the activities of her son-in-law, who slipped a rubber tube over her bedroom door every night and blew clouds of a poisonous powder into her room. She resorted to wearing a mask.)

In both toxic and organic brain syndromes, preexisting personality trends determine the presenting picture to a considerable degree.

Etiologic Factors

A. Sex, Marital Status, Age: Paranoid states are more common in women than in men, and the proportion of people in this group who are unmarried is higher than the population average. There is no typical age of onset, but paranoid schizophrenic reactions occur, on the average, years later than other types of schizophrenic reactions.

B. Social Factors: Social and cultural isolation predisposes to the onset of paranoid states, eg, it is more common among immigrants than among native-born members of a given population.

C. Premorbid Personality Traits: Prominent premorbid personality traits are mistrust, insecurity, high levels of anxiety, secretiveness and seclusiveness, inability to comprehend others, and continuous hostility.

D. Underlying Psychologic Mechanisms: The basic psychoanalytic explanation of paranoia was first elucidated by Freud in the famous Schreber case. Freud analyzed Schreber and noted that he had homosexual impulses that remained unconscious because they were unacceptable. The impulses were projected, reversed, and elaborated until Schreber became crazed with fear of being murdered by homosexuals. In projection, inner unconscious perceptions become more acceptable in their external and conscious form.

E. Precipitating Stress: In predisposed personalities, stressful situations may precipitate the paranoid picture—eg, cultural and social isolation, excessive demands at work or in personal relationships, physical illness or injury.

Treatment

Treatment depends on accurate diagnosis and, in general, consists of treating the underlying condition—eg, phenothiazine tranquilizers for paranoid schizophrenics, electroshock or antidepressants for psychotic depressives, milieu therapy in hospitalized cases, psychotherapy in ambulatory cases.

Since paranoid ideas are rarely responsive to direct challenge, it is better to avoid trying to argue against the patient's distorted image of reality in the early stage of the therapeutic relationship. Failure to observe this precaution may relegate the therapist to the ranks of the persecutors in the patient's mind, in which case his ability to help his patient will be severely impaired and he actually may become personally endangered. However, the therapist should not agree with the patient's paranoid interpretations but should take the neutral position of the interested observer who wishes to be helpful: "I think I understand how you feel. Tell me more about . . ."

Late in therapy, when a position of trust has been established between the patient and the therapist, attempts may be made to make the patient face up to reality. The therapist may frankly suggest that, even if the patient cannot relinquish his paranoid notions altogether, he can trust the therapist's version of things and act as though he believed him. "Sure, I know you keep suspecting every little thing your wife does, but I'm glad you've stopped haranguing her about it. You've got to take my word for it that she's being honest with you, and, as I've told you over and over, time will eventually prove to you that I'm right."

Time, assisted by medication and psychotherapy and perhaps a bit of luck on the outside, often does wear down paranoid ideas to extinction, or at least to the point where they can be tolerated with reasonable ease.

DELUSIONS

A delusion is a false belief, usually unique to the individual, which is not susceptible to modification or correction by logical persuasion or by compelling contrary evidence. At times, as in *folie à deux,* a delusion may be shared with another person who is dominated by the delusional patient, typically the spouse.

A delusional system is an elaborate complex based on the delusional premise, eg, a person who falsely believes he is being persecuted develops a delusional system which consists of the reasons for his being singled out, the identity of his persecutors, the means they use, and "evidence" to support his convictions.

The explanation of delusions in their purest form, as in the paranoid states, is not clearly established. Two main theoretical views are prevalent. One is that a specific biochemical or physiologic dysfunction underlies the disease process and that the delusion results from faulty perceptions or interpretation caused by this dysfunction. The alternative view is that delusion formation is a psychologic defense mechanism that enables the patient to cope with painful or threatening impulses, needs, or conflicts even at the cost of loosening his contact with reality. According to this view the patient is using the same mechanisms of denial and projection that everyone uses at times, but to an exaggerated and pathologic degree.

CLASSIFICATION

Some of the commonest forms of delusions are the following:

Paranoid Delusions
Ideas of persecution, of being followed, watched, slandered, having one's mind controlled or influenced, of being harmed physically, or of plots against one's life. The weapons of the persecutors are not readily amenable to confirmation or repudiation, eg, electronic devices or telepathy.

Depressive Delusions
Ideas of guilt, poverty, incurable disease, having no feeling, being dead, the world having ceased to exist.

Grandiose Delusions
Ideas of having great wealth, influence, or power or of being an outstanding, famous, or notorious person or a historic or religious figure.

Erotic Delusions
Ideas, most commonly paranoid, of infidelity, sexual molestation, or change of sex; but sometimes grandiose, such as being loved by someone, often a movie star who is constrained from making his or her feelings known.

Diffuse Delusions
Confused and poorly defined beliefs that oneself or one's surroundings are strange, unreal, or different. They may vary in content and in the earnestness with which they are held.

CONDITIONS IN WHICH DELUSIONAL IDEATION OCCURS

Psychoses
Delusions may occur in any psychotic state. The most common are the following:
A. Paranoid States and Paranoid Schizophrenia: Delusional ideation with persecutory content is typically found in these conditions. The delusional ideation may be circumscribed and interfere only slightly with the patient's adjustment, only becoming apparent when the subject it involves is touched on; or it may be expanded into an elaborate delusional system which affects every aspect of the patient's functioning.

B. Psychotic Depressive States: These conditions are commonly manifested by delusional ideas with depressive content which often lead to suicidal attempts (eg, having committed the "unpardonable sin," being totally worthless).

C. Manic-Depressive Psychosis: Delusional ideation is common in both phases of this condition. Grandiose delusions are particularly common in the manic phase.

D. Schizophrenia: In addition to delusions of persecution observed in paranoid schizophrenia, delusional ideation—often bizarre—is common in all types of schizophrenia. In acute schizophrenic states, delusions are often diffuse.

Toxic Conditions
A. Infections: Exhaustive illnesses, often with high fever.

B. Drug Intoxication: Delusional ideation may occur during the acute stage or for a variable period afterward. Intoxications frequently associated with delusional ideation include those due to amphetamines, LSD, alcohol, atropine, bromides, barbiturates, and corticosteroids.

C. Physiologically Altered States: Sleep deprivation, sensory deprivation, postoperative states, electrolyte imbalance.

D. Metabolic Disorders, Endocrinopathies, and Vitamin Deficiencies: Many types of psychiatric disturbances sometimes occur as a manifestation of these disorders. Delusional ideation may be included in the general psychotic picture. Examples are porphyria, myxedema, Cushing's syndrome, pellagra, and pernicious anemia.

Central Nervous System Disorders
A. Senile Dementia: Paranoid or depressive delusions may be the earliest symptoms of senile degeneration.

B. Cerebral Arteriosclerosis: Paranoid or depressive delusions may occur, particularly when the onset is insidious and the progress of the condition is slow.

C. General Paresis: Grandiose delusions are often said to be characteristic, but any type of delusions may occur.

D. Huntington's Chorea: Paranoid delusions may precede the neurologic manifestations.

E. Others: Brain tumor, Friedreich's ataxia, multiple sclerosis, and a wide variety of other neurologic conditions.

CLINICAL EVALUATION AND SIGNIFICANCE

Evaluation of the premorbid personality, a history of alcoholism or drug dependence, past syphilitic infection, and recent unusual stress such as sleep deprivation may help to establish the cause. Physical examination and routine laboratory tests may lead to a diagnosis of organic conditions which may account for the psychiatric symptoms.

Delusional ideation with a clear sensorium is usually associated with functional psychoses. Disorientation, confusion, and memory impairment suggest toxic or organic conditions. In the schizophrenias, delusions are usually associated with other indications of thought disorder. In depressive and manic states, the corresponding abnormal affect is present.

In paranoid conditions, if the patient's thought processes and social adaptation are well maintained, the delusion or delusional system may be the only manifestation of illness. Considerable skill and judgment may be required to elicit the delusional ideation if the patient has learned that his belief is not acceptable to others. Similarly, if the delusional belief is not obviously pathologic and the facts cannot be easily established—eg, in delusions of marital infidelity—the diagnosis may be difficult. The patient's affective responses to being interviewed—whether he talks freely or is reticent and evasive—are helpful clues.

The possibility that the patient might act on his delusional belief must be considered. Some patients dissociate their ideation and behavior, so that a patient who believes himself to be omnipotent may nevertheless submit meekly to direction. On the other hand, a patient who believes himself to be threatened may take violent action in self-defense. In assessing these possibilities, the past history of behavior and the intensity of the affect associated with his belief are helpful factors.

MANAGEMENT OF THE DELUSIONAL PATIENT

In interviewing a patient with delusions, an attitude of noncommittal respect and willingness to listen to the patient's ideas without prejudgment is desirable. Expressions of incredulity or amusement or a patronizing pretense of agreement must be avoided. An empathic recognition of the patient's affective response to his beliefs should be maintained. No attempt should be made to argue with the patient or persuade him of the falsity of his ideas, since any such attempt interferes with rapport and may cause the patient to incorporate the interviewer into his delusional system.

Specific treatment for underlying organic disorders should be given as indicated. No special treatment is required for the delusions; they usually disappear as the underlying mental illness abates. Rarely, they may continue in circumscribed form in an otherwise well-recovered patient; in these instances, the patient has at least partial insight and does not permit the delusions to affect his behavior.

HALLUCINATIONS

Hallucinations are spontaneous, unwilled sense perceptions, experienced as arising outside the self, for which there is no external basis. Awareness of the unreality of the perception (ie, insight) may or may not be present. Volition and consciousness are essential considerations in distinguishing hallucinations from certain other mental phenomena. Volition, as here used, refers to mental activity that is voluntary and willed as opposed to that which is involuntary, spontaneous, and uncontrolled. In the former, there is a sense of the mental experience occurring inwardly; in the latter, a sense of "out-thereness" about the experience. Dreams are sometimes cited as examples of hallucinations in normal experience, but they probably should not be so considered since they occur during sleep, when consciousness is largely absent. Daydreams are usually voluntary and controllable. However, since neither consciousness nor volition is absolute, a sharp distinction between hallucinations and these other mental phenomena is frequently impossible.

Any sensory modality may be involved in hallucinations, ie, hearing, vision, taste, smell, touch, and proprioception. These may occur singly or in combination. Hallucinations vary in clarity, vividness, intensity, and associated affect according to the varying circumstances in which they occur. The significance of hallucinations depends on many factors to be discussed below. They are not necessarily indicative of a mental disorder.

The mechanism for the production of hallucinations is unknown. Various theories stress psychologic or physiologic factors, peripheral or central factors, sensory or motor factors, and cortical or subcortical mechanisms.

In the normal waking state, the brain is bombarded by a constant stream of changing stimuli from within the body and from the outside world. This input of stimuli serves to inhibit earlier perceptions from emerging into consciousness. If the input is impaired or absent, as it is in some normal and pathologic states (eg, sensory deprivation, hallucinogenic drugs), preconscious or unconscious material may be released in the form of hallucinations.

The meaning and dynamics of hallucinations are usually suggested by their content, which may reflect wish fulfillment or psychologic needs, especially efforts to master anxiety.

Normal individuals may have *hypnagogic hallucinations* in the drowsy state before going to sleep and *hypnopompic hallucinations* while awakening. (These hallucinations are more common in hysterics.) They are usually visual but may include voice sounds (usually indistinct) or paresthesias, particularly of the mouth and hands. They are usually momentary experiences, and differ from dreams in that the individual is partially aware of his surroundings. In these states of partial sleep the individual is often terrified by his inability to move (*sleep paralysis*). After what seems like hours (actually it is only a few moments), the spell may be broken by return of the ability to make the slightest movement, even of a little finger.

Hallucinations are among the psychopathologic phenomena that occur during prolonged periods of *sleep deprivation*. These hallucinations are usually visual, but Berger and Oswald describe a subject who heard voices when a water tap was running and stopped hearing them when the tap was turned off. Luby and Gottlieb point out that visual hallucinations are usually preceded by burning, itching eyes and blurred or diplopic vision. These symptoms are followed by illusional misinterpretation of actual objects and, finally, by hallucinations. These authors describe one subject in a sleep deprivation study who saw complex geometric visual hallucinations; another who saw "smoke" seeping out from under a door, and a third who reported seeing flashes of light that appeared to shoot out of the walls.

Fleeting visual hallucinations may be part of the clinical picture associated with prolonged extreme *physical exertion* or *starvation*. Factors such as sleep deprivation and electrolyte imbalance probably play a role.

Hallucinatory experiences in persons subjected to *prolonged isolation,* such as shipwrecked sailors and polar explorers, have long been recognized. In recent years, many investigators have reported the occurrence of hallucinations in volunteers subjected to isolation and *sensory deprivation.* Visual, auditory, and somesthetic hallucinations have been described. In different studies, visual phenomena have ranged from flashes of light and geometric designs to complex scenes. Seven of 28 subjects in a study by Solomon and Mendelson had visual hallucinations; and 3 of the 7 had, in addition, somesthetic hallucinations. One of the 3 described the experience as follows: "I feel as though I were at the bottom of a big football pileup, crushed down by weight and unable to move."

Hallucinations may be part of a *delirious state after surgery* in persons who exhibited no sign of mental illness preoperatively. The cause of such delirious states is obscure; the anesthetic agent used, infection, and electrolyte imbalances are among the possibilities. The possibility of a functional reactive psychosis should also be kept in mind.

Hallucinatory states following cardiac surgery may be particularly complex both because of the intense emotional stresses involved and because various types of physiologic shocks are unavoidable.

Hallucinations, usually visual, are common among primitive peoples during *trance states.* They are benign in nature and disappear with the termination of the trance. Similar hallucinations occur in various delirious states, and as a symptom of drug-taking (LSD, mescaline, peyote, etc).

In some individuals during deep hypnosis, hallucinations may be produced by suggestion, depending in part on the expectations of the subject and the hypnotist and the rapport between them. A subject may see an object or hear a sound that is not actually present or have taste, smell, or touch hallucinations. "Negative hallucinations" may occur if the subject is asked not to see or hear an object or sound that is present.

HALLUCINATIONS IN THE FUNCTIONAL PSYCHOSES

Schizophrenia

Hallucinations are frequent symptoms of schizophrenia and may be vague or quite definite and realistic. Most common are auditory hallucinations, usually voices. It is not unusual for the patient to hear himself discussed. He often hears himself being threatened or called obscene names, and the voices may order him to perform specific acts. Many schizophrenics report hearing the voice of God or the devil, or hearing their own thoughts. The voices are occasionally pleasant, especially in patients with the hebephrenic type of schizophrenia.

Visual hallucinations, while not rare, are less common. When they do occur, they are often present throughout the waking hours. This is usually not so of the visual hallucinations of patients suffering from organic or affective psychoses.

Hallucinations of touch, smell, or taste sometimes occur, particularly if visual hallucinations are present. Cenesthetic hallucinations—peculiar visceral sensations—are often experienced by schizophrenics.

The following is an example of multiform hallucinations in a schizophrenic patient: A 53-year-old woman with paranoid schizophrenic reaction of 5 years' duration was admitted to a psychiatric ward shortly after her apartment had burned. In addition to hearing insulting voices, seeing obscene pictures on the walls of her bedroom, and experiencing the sensation of having her clitoris stimulated by a popular singer, this patient had an unusual and complex hallucination. She could feel a burning stick of wood in her back and could both see and smell the smoke.

Manic-Depressive Psychosis

Hallucinations are rare in the manic phase except in manic delirium, when auditory hallucinations are common. They occur rarely in the depressive phase and, when they do, tend to resemble illusions rather than clear-cut hallucinations. They generally relate to the depressed mood in that they are condemnatory and often call on the patient to harm or kill himself. They occur most often at night rather than throughout the day, as in schizophrenic patients.

Psychotic Depression

Hallucinations are rare and almost always auditory when they do occur. They have the same characteristics as those in the depressive phase of manic-depressive reactions.

Involutional Melancholia

In the depressive type, auditory hallucinations that support the nihilistic delusions may occur. The possibility of organic brain disease should be considered. Auditory hallucinations appropriate to the delusions occur in the paranoid type of involutional psychosis also.

HALLUCINATIONS IN HYSTERIA

Hallucinations (usually visual) may occur in conversion reactions, especially in trance states or fugues. They often involve complex scenes or fragments of action of a real past event of emotional significance to the patient.

HALLUCINATIONS IN CONVULSIVE DISORDERS

Simple hallucinations are frequently experienced during the auras that precede convulsive seizures. Discharges in the occipital lobe may be associated with sensations of light or color, eg, flashes, flames, prisms, or amorphous colors. Olfactory auras resulting from lesions of the temporal lobe have long been recognized. These so-called uncinate fits are associated with convulsive discharges in the uncal region and consist of odors described usually as unpleasant. Much less commonly, uncinate fits include or consist of hallucinations of taste. Lesions in the first temporal gyrus may cause auditory hallucinations such as ringing bells or buzzing sounds.

Complex hallucinatory experiences are rare manifestations of epileptic seizures; they consist of vivid auditory or visual hallucinations (or both). Even more rarely, they include olfactory, gustatory, or tactile sensations. The visual hallucinations are usually in color and 3 dimensions; and the scenes, sounds, and other sensations are completely realistic. They are described as a memory or reminiscence of a *déjà vu* or *déjà entendu* nature. At times, the patient experiences the hallucinations while fully aware of his actual environment, a condition Hughlings Jackson termed "mental diplopia."

Baldwin recounts the following repetitive hallucinatory experience of one epileptic patient: "I was walking up a gravel path toward a house and along a hedge. I had been there before. I could hear the gravel crunch under my feet and smell the cooking from the house. When I reached the porch, I blacked out."

HALLUCINATIONS IN ORGANIC BRAIN DISEASE

Hallucinations can occur in a wide variety of organic diseases of the brain. Among these are tumors, vascular disease, head trauma, senile dementia, febrile states, metabolic disease, electrolyte disturbances, deficiency states, toxic psychoses, pathologic alcoholic intoxication, delirium tremens, and acute alcoholic hallucinosis. In febrile, toxic, and delirious states, the hallucinations are characteristically visual; in alcoholic hallucinosis, auditory; in brain tumor, sometimes gustatory or olfactory.

ELICITING THE HISTORY OR PRESENCE
OF HALLUCINATIONS

In some cases it is quite apparent that patients are hallucinating. They appear to be listening to or seeing something not present, or they may voluntarily tell about their hallucinations. On the other hand, many patients will deny or withhold their hallucinatory experiences. The examiner should note repetitive eye movements, movements of the lips, and any other behavior that suggests that the patient may be responding to hallucinations.

Patients whose contact with reality is obviously disturbed may be asked directly if they hear voices or see strange things. Less direct inquiry may be called for with other patients. Frequently, they will say something that, if pursued, will bring out the presence of hallucinations. Questions such as the following are useful: "Do you ever hear your own thoughts out loud?" "Have you ever heard your named called when no one was there?" "Have you ever had what seemed like a dream when you were awake?" "Do you ever imagine things?"

It is important also to ask patients if they smell unusual odors, have peculiar tastes in their mouth, or feel things on their skin that they can't see.

EVALUATION OF HALLUCINATIONS

If the presence of hallucinations is established or strongly suspected, the following factors should be considered:

(1) What sensory modalities are involved?

(2) What is the intensity, clarity, realistic quality, and apparent source of the hallucinations?

(3) Under what circumstances do they occur? At night? While wide awake or only while drowsy?

(4) Can they be started or stopped at will?

(5) What is the content and associated affect? Are the voices or visions single or multiple? Of persons known or unknown? Are they pleasant or disturbing? What is the patient's reaction to them?

(6) Does the patient accept the hallucinations as real, or does he have some understanding of their true nature?

DISORDERS OF THOUGHT

Most mental illness is marked by some degree of disordered thought process, although schizophrenic thought is generally cited as the model (and most severe) example.

Thinking may become disordered from the standpoint of content, form, realism, progression, direction, quantity, and expression.

DISORDERS OF THOUGHT CONTENT

Disorders of thought content may consist of the presence of abnormal content or the absence of normal content.

Presence of Abnormal Thought Content*

(1) **Illusions:** Misinterpretation of actual sensory experience constitutes an illusion. Illusions are particularly apt to occur in response to ambiguous stimuli or under conditions of diminished discrimination, eg, at night. Mental states such as anxiety, fatigue, or intoxication predispose to illusions. Elderly people and the blind and the deaf are especially prone to illusions because of their diminished or absent sensory acuity. Unlike hallucinations, illusions can be corrected by providing collateral information. *Micropsia,* an illusion in which objects appear smaller than they are, may occur in hysterical neurosis or in temporal lobe epilepsy. *Macropsia,* in which objects appear larger than life, generally occurs only in hysterical neurosis. *Synesthesia* is a disorder in which visual stimuli are perceived as sounds or vice versa. It occurs in LSD intoxication, which may also be characterized by other illusions such as shimmering, multicolored halos around persons or objects.

(2) **Ideas of reference:** In conditions of egocentric preoccupation, particularly paranoid schizophrenia, the indifferent statements or gestures of others are interpreted as referring to the patient, most often disparagingly or threateningly.

(3) **Confabulations:** Patients with recent memory gaps unconsciously fill in these gaps with fictitious stories. They are not lies, since the patient does not realize the stories are not true. Korsakoff's psychosis is the classic example.

(4) **Phobias:** The recurrent experience of dread of a specific event or object (in the absence of objective danger) is called a phobia. The following prefixes (only a few are listed) are commonly used to specify the phobia: *acro-,* (fear of) heights; *agora-,* open spaces; *claustro-,* closed spaces; *xeno-,* strangers.

(5) **Neologisms:** Schizophrenic and manic patients (and others less often) tend to invent new words, frequently by combining other words of personal significance. Schizophrenic neologisms differ from new words invented by healthy people in that they have no general utility, ie, they convey only autistic meaning.

(6) **Circumstantiality:** This is the persistent and compulsive recitation of extraneous detail. It may be a feature of obsessive compulsive neurosis; but is more common in schizoid and schizophrenic individuals. Tangentiality, circumlocuity, and verbigeration are similar. All these must be distinguished from irrelevance and irrationality which imply greater breaks from reality.

(7) **Stereotypy:** Stereotypy is the compulsive and repetitive utterance of words or phrases, often meaningless ones, in a ritualistic way. The unvarying persistence and ritualistic quality distinguish stereotypy from perseveration (see below).

(8) **Other types of abnormal content:** It would not be useful to attempt to list and define all of the possible ways in which thinking can become disordered in association with psychiatric illnesses. A few more of the com-

*Delusions and hallucinations are discussed elsewhere in this chapter.

mon types of abnormal thought content are rhyming, punning, scolding, and declamation of a compulsive and persistent quality.

Absence of Normal Content

(1) **Disorientation**: In states of confusion or clouding of consciousness, as in organic brain syndrome due to drug intoxication, the patient may give the incorrect time, may not know where he is or who he is, and may not be able to recognize his own family and friends. Time, place, person, situation—any or all may be involved.

(2) **Amnesia**: Loss of memory can be categorized as follows: *Total* amnesia is usually due to organic causes, eg, trauma, epileptic fugue states, and intoxication. *Partial or selective* amnesia is often seen in functional disorders such as hysterical neurosis. Organic states that interfere with the initial registering of incoming stimuli produce *irreversible* amnesia. Functional amnesia may remit spontaneously, but intervention in such ways as amobarbital (Amytal) interviews or hypnosis is often helpful. Traumatic amnesia for events preceding injury is called *retrograde;* amnesia for events subsequent to injury is called *anterograde.* Amnesia of organic origin (eg, after ECT) is generally for *recent* events; functional amnesia may be either for recent or *remote* events.

Feigned amnesia may be detected by the internal inconsistencies of the patient's story or by external inconsistencies, eg, the patient may behave or speak in a manner that indicates accurate recollection of events that occurred during the interval he claims he can't remember.

DISORDERS OF THE FORM OF THINKING

Disordered forms of thought are logical errors or, more specifically, disruptions and distortions of the relationships between the symbols employed in thinking (syntactics). Schizophrenic thought has been most carefully examined in this regard, and *loosening of associations* was cited by Bleuler as its cardinal feature.

The observed similarities between the thinking of schizophrenic patients, persons living in primitive cultures, and children have led to the notion that schizophrenic thought represents a regression to earlier phases of intellectual development. Freud believed that the language of dreams was a manifestation of the persistence of such thought in normal individuals.

The following is a comparison of the terms used for primitive and advanced thought by Freud, Sullivan, Arieti, and Piaget.

	Primitive Thought	Advanced Thought
Freud	Primary process	Secondary process
Sullivan	Prototaxic, parataxic	Syntaxic
Arieti	Paleologic	Logical
Piaget	Syncretic, concrete	Abstract, categorical

At one time or another, every fallacy known to logicians has been detected in schizophrenic thought. Some have been cited as pathognomonic. However, the study of normal populations shows that—in part because of the vagaries of language itself—logical lapses and syntactic and semantic errors are universal. Moreover, factors such as anxiety and fatigue can temporarily disrupt thought processes. Pretentious erudition in the uneducated or unintelligent and, at times, even pronouncements of philosophers or mystics may yield a semblance of schizophrenic thought termed *benign paralogia.* What distinguishes schizophrenic thought is the quantity and persistence of disorders of form.

One must also distinguish the *aphasias* of organic etiology from functional disturbances.

Many terms have been used to denote the various aspects of disordered forms of thought. A few are still in use. Some are equivalent or overlap considerably: *Metaphoric thinking,* marked by the excessive use of metaphors or symbolic substitutes. *Concretism,* the inability to derive generalities or categories from specific instances. (May indicate organic or functional mental illness. The tendency to transform abstract ideas into visual images or plastic word representation is typical of schizophrenia.) *Condensation,* the compression or collapse of several different ideas into one phrase forming a collage of thought.

DISORDERS OF THE REALISM OF THINKING

In mental illness, especially schizophrenia, the semantic relationship of thought to reality is apt to be tenuous; or there may be no direct relationship, in which case the thinking is termed *dereistic* or *autistic.* Personal idiosyncratic symbols and logic underlie the disordered realism.

Ordinary logic demands that identity be based on likeness of subjects. The Von Domarus principle of schizophrenic thought cites the propensity for deciding identity on the basis of likeness of predicates. (*Example:* "General Taylor is a soldier. I am a soldier. Therefore, I am General Taylor.") Such mistaken identity may be based on like predicates of quality or of spatial or temporal contiguity.

DISORDERS OF THOUGHT PROGRESSION

The flow of thought may be too rapid or too slow, or may be interrupted. Too rapid thinking, termed *logorrhea,* may be called *pressured* or, if very severe, a *flight of ideas.* The latter occurs most typically in the manic phase of manic-depressive illness, in which ideas occur at such a great rate that they tend to impinge on one another and become cluttered.

Too slow (*retarded*) thinking in a person of normal intelligence is indicative of depression.

Thinking suddenly interrupted is said to be *blocked.* Bleuler believed that a high degree of blocking was pathognomonic of schizophrenia. This blocking is accounted for by the sudden intrusion of a highly charged theme or, frequently, by a hallucination.

DISORDER OF THE DIRECTION OF THINKING

The thinking of manic patients particularly tends to be *tangential* rather than *goal-directed.* Some normal or neurotic individuals think this way at times.

DISORDERS OF THE QUANTITY OF THINKING

Thinking becomes *impoverished* in chronic, deteriorated mental illness, most notably in patients institutionalized for many years. The quantity (and variety) of thinking may be markedly diminished in severe obsessive compulsive neurosis, schizophrenia, or senile dementia, in which one or a very few themes tend to dominate completely the content of consciousness. This phenomenon may be termed *fixed idea (idée fixe).*

DISORDERS OF THE EXPRESSION OF THOUGHT

The transformation of thoughts into speech may be disturbed in functional or organic mental illnesses. *Mutism,* the refusal to speak (speech negativism), must be distinguished from reduction (impoverishment) in thought content. Patients with catatonic schizophrenia, though frequently mute, may manifest a wealth of association when persuaded to communicate. *Perseveration* is either the repetition of a word or phrase several times or the *inability to switch themes.* Perseveration is not as persistent or ritualistic as stereotypy. *Echolalia* is a tendency to repeat verbatim what has just been said. It is typically a schizophrenic trait.

Central (syntactic) aphasia is easily mistaken for a functional thought disorder. Patients with lesions in the dominant temporoparietal region of the brain may manifest fluent speech marked by grammatical confusion and the utterance of nonexistent or incorrect words. Since the comprehension of speech is impaired, the patient does not recognize his own errors and may pour forth a stream of unintelligible nonsense. Reading and writing are usually less affected, though the patient may become confused if he reads aloud. The ability to comprehend written material and to communicate coherently in writing distinguishes this type of aphasia from functional thought disturbances. Furthermore, the systematic distortion in terms of a core of psychologic conflict that is present in schizophrenia is not present in the aphasic patient.

GLOSSARY OF TERMS DEFINED
IN THIS SECTION

Aphasias: A well educated patient is unable to read a page of newsprint, understand spoken language, or use language in the normal way. "May I have a glass of—" (unable to recall the word "water").

Autistic thinking: Absorbed in self-gratifying fantasies to the exclusion of reality. "There are little princes all around me and I am their queen."

Blocked thinking: "I must tell you, I—" (unable to continue even with great effort).

Circumstantiality: Patient describes every detail of his lunch; strains to recall exact dates when it doesn't matter; pauses at length to remember "who was there" at some event in his past life, correcting himself frequently and losing the thread of what he is trying to say.

Concretism: An old saying such as "A stitch in time saves nine" may be interpreted to mean *only* that repairing a tear in a garment before the tear becomes larger will save much more sewing later on.

Condensation: "I grew up—Fred love—now dead—no radio no TV"—summarizing a lifetime of deprived loneliness ending in a crowded home for old people where there is no private access to her favorite TV programs.

Confabulation: Patient relates an elaborate adventure with CIA agents in another city to account for the interval since hospitalization of which he has no memory.

Delusions: Patient believes the lining of his stomach is being dissolved by radio waves coming from TV, causing diarrhea and weakness.

Dereistic thinking: Lacking in logic or ties to reality. "I will be able to go to the moon tomorrow because I want to so much."

Disorientation: Asked his name and address, the patient may pause and say, "Philadelphia?" Asked if he knows where he is: "Some kind of building? Is this Fred's house?"

Echolalia: "What is your name, sir?" "What's your name, sir, name, sir?" "How do you feel?" "How do you feel?"

Fixed idea: Patient thinks of nothing but the threat of Communist takeover in South America, the decline of respect for older people, etc.

Flight of ideas: "Told her many times too much can't last getting tired getting old slow down no must keep going more more no rest no comfort fighting like this all the time."

Hallucinations: Patient sees God's finger beckoning to his wife; hears muffled laughter and shouted obscenities; feels mice scampering up and down his legs.

Ideas of reference: An outburst of laughter as a story is being told across the room is interpreted as a mockery of the patient's clothing or social manner.

Illusions: Patient feels searing pain when a cool stethoscope is applied to his back; interprets an actual spot of light as the sparkle from a fairy's wand.

Impoverished thinking: In spite of attempts to stimulate communication, the patient may ruminate continuously about the texture and fit of his bathrobe or the smell of the powdered soap in the washroom.

Logorrhea: Endless trivial talk.

Loosening of associations: "We went to see my sister and her children. I get a pension from the Coast Guard, you know."

Macropsia: A pet cat seems to fill the doorway.

Metaphoric thinking: "She was a leaf in the wind—free, but directionless; I, a reed broken by the same wind."

Micropsia: An apple lying on the table looks like a marble.

Mutism: The patient remains silent, staring at the interviewer, and may continue silent for
years.

Neologisms: Patient refers to his boss as "Twinkle-dee," his wife as "Loomaloony"; asks
for a "flim-flam jam-jam" when he wants a cigarette.

Perseveration: "I don't like doctors. I keep telling you I don't like doctors. Well, I don't. I
don't like doctors."

Retarded thinking: "I . . . know . . . I . . . feel . . . wrong. All wrong. It's no . . . use explain—"

Stereotypy: "I went to work I went to work I went to work work work."

Tangential thinking: In attempting to explain an argument with his wife, the patient
digresses frequently to describe and praise a pet dog who was whining by the door
to get out.

REFERENCES

Anxiety

Cameron, D.E.: Observations on the patterns of anxiety. Am J Psychiat
101:36–41, 1944.

Gellhorn, E.: Central nervous system tuning and its implications for neuropsychiatry. J Nerv Ment Dis 147:148–162, 1968.

Hulbeck, C.R.: The irrational and the nature of basic anxiety. Am J Psychoanal
30:3–12, 1970.

Janis, I.L.: *Psychological Stress: Psychoanalytic and Behavioral Studies of Surgical
Patients.* Wiley, 1958.

Leighton, D., & others: *The Character of Danger.* Basic Books, 1963.

Lesse, S.: *Anxiety: Its Components, Development and Treatment.* Grune & Stratton, 1970.

May, R.: *The Meaning of Anxiety.* Ronald Press, 1950.

Pitts, F.N., & J.N. McClure: Lactate metabolism in anxiety neurosis. New England J
Med 277:1329–1336, 1967.

Sarason, S.B., & others: *Anxiety in Elementary School Children.* Wiley, 1967.

Shipman, E.G., Oken, D., & H.A. Heath: Muscle tension and effort at self-control
during anxiety. Arch Gen Psychiat 23:359–368, 1970.

Tavel, M.E.: Hyperventilation syndrome with unilateral somatic symptoms. JAMA
187:301–303, 1964.

Wheeler, E.D., & others: Neurocirculatory asthenia. JAMA 142:878–889, 1950.

Whittenborn, J.R.: *The Clinical Pharmacology of Anxiety.* Thomas, 1966.

Depression

Anthony, E.J.: Two contrasting types of adolescent depression and their treatment.
J Am Psychoanal A 18:841–859, 1970.

Beck, A.T.: *Depression.* Hoeber, 1967.

Bibring, E.: The mechanism of depression. Pages 13–48 in: *Affective Disorders.*
Greenacre, P. (editor). Internat Univ Press, 1953.

Blinder, M.G.: Differential diagnosis and treatment of depressive disorders. JAMA
195:8–12, 1966.

Bradley, J.J.: Severe localized pain associated with depressive syndrome. Brit J
Psychiat 109:741–745, 1963.

Bunney, W.E., Jr., Hartmann, E.L., & J.W. Mason: Study of a patient with 48-hour manic-depressive cycles. 2. Strong positive correlations between endocrine factors and manic defense patterns. Arch Gen Psychiat 12:619, 1965.

Grinker, R., & others: *The Phenomena of Depressions.* Hoeber, 1961.

Kiloh, L.G., & R.F. Garside: The independence of neurotic depression and endogenous depression. Brit J Psychiat 109:451–463, 1963.

Lesse, S.: Masked depression: A diagnostic and therapeutic problem. Dis Nerv System 29:169–173, 1968.

McLaughlin, B., & others: Meprobamate-benactyzine (Deprol) and placebo in 2 depressed outpatient populations. Psychosomatics 10:73–81, 1969.

Mendelson, M.: *Psychoanalytic Concepts of Depression.* Thomas, 1960.

Thomas, F.B., & others: Apathetic thyrotoxicosis: A distinctive clinical and laboratory entity. Ann Int Med 72:679–685, 1970.

Tonks, C.M., Paykel, E.S., & G.L. Klerman: Clinical depression among negroes. Am J Psychiat 127:329–335, 1970.

Acute Grief Reaction

Averell, J.: Grief: Its nature and significance. Psychol Bull 70:721–748, 1968.

Bibring, G.L.: The death of an infant: A psychiatric study. New England J Med 283:370–371, 1970.

Bowlby, J.: Process of mourning. Internat J Psychoanal 42:317–340, 1961.

Hill, O.: Some psychiatric nonsequelae of childhood bereavement. Brit J Psychiat 116:679–680, 1970.

Kennell, J.H., & others: The mourning response of parents to the death of a newborn infant. New England J Med 283:344–349, 1970.

Lindemann, E.: Symptomatology and management of acute grief. Am J Psychiat 101:141–148, 1944.

Marshall, J.: Helping the grief-stricken. Postgrad Med 45:138-143, 1969.

McConville, B.J., & others: Mourning processes in children of varying ages. Canad Psychiat AJ 15:253–255, 1970.

Pollock, G.H.: Anniversary reactions, trauma and mourning. Psychoanal Quart 39:347–371, 1970.

Siggins, L.: Mourning: A critique of the literature. Internat J Psychiat 3:418–432, 1967.

Silverman, P.R.: The widow-to-widow program: An experiment in preventive intervention. Ment Hygiene 53:333–337, 1969.

Volkan, V.: Typical findings in pathological grief. Psychiat Quart 44:231–250, 1970.

Wolff, J.R., & others: The emotional reaction to a stillbirth. Am J Obst Gynec 108:73–77, 1970.

Yamamoto, J.: Cultural factors in loneliness, death and separation. Med Times 98:177–183, 1970.

Yamamoto, J., & others: Mourning in Japan. Am J Psychiat 125:1660–1665, 1969.

Paranoid Ideation

Cameron, N.: The development of paranoiac thinking. Psychoanal Rev 50:219–233, 1943.

Novey, S.: The outpatient treatment of borderline paranoid states. Psychiatry 23:357–364, 1960.

Salzman, L.: Paranoid state: Theory and therapy. Arch Gen Psychiat 2:679–693, 1960.

Waelder, R.: The structure of paranoid ideas: A critical survey of various theories. Internat J Psychoanal 32:167–177, 1951.

Delusions

Arthur, A.Z.: Theories and explanations of delusions. Am J Psychiat 121:105–115, 1964.

Retterstol, N.: Paranoid psychosis with hypochondriac delusions as the main delusion. Acta psychiat scandinav 44:334–353, 1968.

Hallucinations

Frieske, D.A., & others: Formal qualities of hallucinations: A comparative study of the visual hallucinations in patients with schizophrenic, organic, and affective psychoses. Proc Am Psychopath A 54:49–62, 1966.

Jansson, B.: The prognostic significance of various types of hallucinations in young people. Acta psychiat scandinav 44:401–409, 1968.

Kass, W.: The experience of spontaneous hallucination. Bull Menninger Clin 32:67–85, 1968.

Klüver, H.: *Mescal and Mechanisms of Hallucinations.* Univ of Chicago Press, 1966.

Rabkin, R.: Ego functions and hallucinations. Am J Psychiat 123:481–484, 1966.

Sedman, G.: A comparative study of pseudohallucinations, imagery, and true hallucinations. Brit J Psychiat 112:9–17, 1966.

Sedman, G.: Experimental and phenomenological approaches to the problem of hallucinations in organic psychosyndromes. Brit J Psychiat 113:1115–1121, 1967.

Solomon, P., & J. Mendelson: Hallucinations in sensory deprivation. Page 137 in: *Hallucinations.* West, L.J. (editor). Grune & Stratton, 1962.

West, L.J. (editor): *Hallucinations.* Grune & Stratton, 1962.

Disorders of Thought

Arieti, S.: *Interpretation of Schizophrenia.* Robert Brunner, 1955.

Atkin, S.: Psychoanalytic considerations of language and thought: A comparative study. Psychoanal Quart 38:549–582, 1969.

Freeman, T., & C.E. Gathercole: Perseveration—the clinical symptoms—in chronic schizophrenia and organic dementia. Brit J Psychiat 112:27–32, 1966.

Rapaport, D. (editor): *Organization and Pathology of Thought.* Columbia Univ Press, 1951.

Rimoldi, N.J.: Thinking and language. Arch Gen Psychiat 17:568–576, 1967.

Siomopoulos, V.: On form and similarity in mental functioning. Psychoanal Rev 56:415–424, 1969.

6...

Differential Diagnostic
Symptoms & Signs

Instead of going from disease to symptoms, this chapter does the reverse. It helps in suggesting diagnostic possibilities, but even computers cannot replace clinical judgment.

Most textbook discussions of psychiatric disorders, like the medical literature generally, are "disease oriented" in that they begin with an agreed diagnosis and proceed in an organized way to describe its etiology, symptoms and signs, treatment, course, and prognosis. However, the patient who comes to a general hospital emergency room or the admitting floor of a psychiatric hospital usually demonstrates a complex of symptoms that have not yet been given a formal diagnostic label but which require one. This "symptom oriented" chapter consists essentially of a glossary of psychiatric manifestations together with the diagnostic conclusions they suggest. First, we will summarize some of the special problems of psychiatric diagnosis to show the ways in which it differs from diagnosis in the other medical specialties.

Critics of the current status of psychiatric diagnosis usually justify their pleas for the abolition or radical alteration of current diagnostic practices by pointing to the low *reliability* (lack of consistency and reproducibility) of the procedures now in use. Among the major sources of low diagnostic reliability are the following typical events in psychiatric diagnosis.

Experienced psychiatrists frequently differ among themselves on which diagnostic labels should be affixed to the same set of symptoms, most often because they assign different weights to one or more of the symptoms than their colleagues do. Conversely, the same clinician may diagnose the same disease entity differently on different occasions because he himself does not necessarily weigh symptoms the same every time he sees them.

Objective diagnostic criteria are difficult to establish in psychiatry primarily because of unpredictable changes in a patient's symptomatic behavior during the natural course of his illness. These inevitable changes in symptoms, in turn, contribute to low diagnostic reliability by causing a diagnosis given a patient at one point in time to be inadequate or erroneous at another.

Moreover, patients who are ultimately given the same diagnosis often show such great differences initially in the frequency and intensity of symptoms that their common diagnoses may easily be missed.

Many of these problems of diagnostic reliability are serious enough to call into question the value of psychiatric diagnosis as it is presently accomplished. Even greater doubts are raised when one considers the unproved *validity* of psychiatric diagnosis (the fact that diagnostic statements often prove to be of limited value even when they are rigorously attained).

Thus critics of psychiatric diagnosis point out that, especially for treatment purposes, diagnostic labels are often less important than understanding the patient in more general, "dynamic" terms. Consequently, many clinicians in private practice make no attempt to assign diagnostic labels but attempt only to understand the presenting symptoms in terms of their relationship to the patient's total psychodynamic make-up. Accordingly, because psychiatric diagnoses, unlike medical diagnoses, are of such severely limited utility for determining etiology, planning treatment, predicting disease course, and estimating prognosis, many investigators consider the traditional "medical model" conception of diagnosis inappropriate for understanding emotional disability.

Traditionally, the medical clinician has assumed that a diagnostic formulation based on knowledge of the origin, signs, and symptoms of an illness ultimately permits its successful treatment. Since the origin and course of most functional psychiatric illnesses are not known, and diagnosis of these illnesses from signs and symptoms is both largely unreliable and of unproved validity, many investigators now propose radical changes in the manner of approaching diagnosis. Many of them emphasize the need for a broader conception of psychopathologic diagnosis than presently exists, one that emphasizes the pathology not only of the individual but also of the society and of the individual's unique relationship to that society. A number of these investigators base their efforts on hopes that effective diagnostic procedures can be evolved which will directly relate eventual therapeutic methods to assessment of the patient's current inappropriate behaviors and their controlling stimuli in the environment.

In spite of these criticisms and the attractiveness of potentially useful new diagnostic technics, not enough is known today to justify acceptance of any one of them in place of traditional "medical model" views. For one thing, continuing efforts are being made to maximize the reliability of diagnosis from signs and symptoms, based upon alterations of current procedures, to permit final definitive assessment of the validity of diagnosis. The bulk of this chapter, taken from a systems analysis of current diagnostic procedures in psychiatry, represents such an effort to increase the reliability of diagnosis.

THE PRINCIPAL DIAGNOSTICALLY USEFUL PSYCHIATRIC SYMPTOMS

For the purposes of professional communication and research, an agreed system of diagnostic terminology is both desirable and necessary. The American Psychiatric Association (APA) classification of psychiatric disorders is the most widely used today. An abridged version of the Standard

Classification of Psychiatric Disorders, taken from the *Diagnostic and Statistical Manual of Mental Disorders,* 2nd ed (DSM-II), is presented in the Appendix.

In the following alphabetical listing 40 diagnostically useful psychiatric symptoms and signs are described. Their significance for the assignment of specific diagnostic labels is indicated by identifying them as definitive, major, or minor cues to these specific labels. Thus, *definitive* cues are signs or symptoms which are always or almost always present in a particular psychiatric illness and are never or almost never present in any other. Observation of these symptoms is therefore tantamount to making a definitive diagnosis; they are equally useful in ruling out whole groups of other psychiatric conditions. In practice, the principal value of these cues is either in differentiating psychotic illnesses from other psychiatric conditions or in separating schizophrenic patients from other psychotic patients; with few exceptions definitive cues are cues to psychosis, often schizophrenic psychosis.

Since some definitive cues are difficult to observe reliably, the safest procedure is to base a firm diagnostic decision on more than one definitive cue (eg, as with inadequate mood and inappropriate mood in schizophrenic reactions).

Major diagnostic cues are symptoms which are often observed in particular psychiatric illnesses but are also occasionally observed in other illnesses. They strongly suggest the diagnosis, especially when they are observed in association with other symptoms having the same diagnostic significance. At least 2 major cues to a specific diagnosis, in the absence of other cues to different diagnoses, are usually required for a definitive diagnostic decision.

Minor diagnostic cues are symptoms which occur irregularly or infrequently in certain psychiatric illnesses and commonly in others, so that they do not strongly support a specific diagnosis. It may rarely happen that a sufficient number of minor cues justifies a specific diagnosis.

Ambivalence

Simultaneous, concurrent contradictory feelings toward the same object. (*Example:* A schizophrenic patient, in referring to her lover, states repetitiously, "You devil, you angel, you devil, you angel.")

A *minor* diagnostic cue to:

(1) Schizophrenia.

(2) The neuroses.

Amnesia

Loss of memory, especially for recent or remote events that one would be expected to remember. (*Example:* A patient who is recovering from an auto accident in which she suffered a concussion is unable to remember the events leading up to the accident.)

A *major* diagnostic cue to:

(1) The organic brain syndromes (often with disturbed consciousness and intellect).

(2) Hysterical personality.

Anxiety

A marked and continuous feeling of threat, especially of a frightening nature. (*Example:* A young man of 26, who shows an anxiety reaction, is overcome one day by attacks of anxiety, panic, and apprehension, accompanied by a "terrible sinking feeling inside," palpitations, sweating, and weakness.)

When present, although environmental or personal circumstances do not justify it, a *major* diagnostic cue to:

(1) The neuroses (when psychosis can be ruled out), especially anxiety neurosis (when anxiety is the principal symptom).

(2) The schizophrenias, involutional melancholia, and the major affective disorders (when psychosis is present).

When absent, although environmental or personal circumstances seem to justify it, a *major* diagnostic cue to hysterical neurosis, conversion type, and the personality disorders (when psychosis can be ruled out), especially antisocial personality.

Antisocial Behavior

A tendency to disregard usual social codes and often to come in conflict with them. (*Example:* A young man is arrested, convicted, and sent to jail for stealing from his employer. This is his 14th arrest for theft; he is only 19 years old.)

A *major* diagnostic cue to antisocial personality (when psychosis can be ruled out and anxiety is minimal or absent).

Aphasia

A primary disturbance of the reception (sensory aphasia), manipulation, or expression of language (motor aphasia). (*Example:* A young man who recently suffered brain damage in an auto accident shows expressive aphasia. He cannot find names for common objects in his spontaneous speech and cannot give names for familiar objects presented to him. Thus he calls a pen "what you write with," although he can link the object and the name when shown them together.)

A *definitive* cue to organic brain syndromes.

Autism

A strong and omnipresent tendency for thoughts and perceptions to be regulated by affective needs or desires rather than by objective reality. Autism represents a serious divorce from reality. (*Example:* A well-educated young woman whose schizophrenic illness is at first hardly noticeable suddenly moves her bowels before a whole social gathering and cannot comprehend the shock and embarrassment which she causes among her friends.)

A *definitive* diagnostic cue to schizophrenia.

Blocking

The associative activity of thinking seems to come to an abrupt and complete standstill. When it is resumed, ideas emerge which have very little (if any) connection with what went before. (*Example:* A hysterical woman complains of "losing" time and noticing gaps in her train of conscious thought. She often stops speaking in the middle of sentences, only to repeat her last words and continue talking.)

A *major* diagnostic cue to:

(1) Schizophrenia and psychotic depressive reaction.

(2) Hysterical neurosis, dissociative type, and anxiety neurosis (when psychosis and petit mal can be ruled out).

Catatonia

A condition characterized by marked motor anomalies—either generalized inhibition or excessive psychomotor excitement and activity. Patients may show catalepsy—waxy flexibility—during which limbs maintain whatever position another person imparts to them. (*Example:* One morning shortly after a catatonic schizophrenic patient is readmitted to a state hospital, he is found in a statuesque position with his limbs contorted. He appears to be unable to see or hear.)

A *major* diagnostic cue to:

(1) Catatonic schizophrenia (when stupor from organic causes can be ruled out).

(2) Severe anxiety neurosis (when psychosis can be ruled out).

Circumstantiality

Speaking and thinking which characteristically proceed indirectly to their target ideas, with many tedious details and parenthetical and irrelevant interpretations. (*Example:* A mentally retarded boy is asked his age. He replies that he was born Sunday, that today is Sunday, that it was just as warm then as now, and that he is probably 12, although he can't be certain.)

A *major* diagnostic cue to chronic undifferentiated schizophrenia (when psychosis is present, the organic disorders can be ruled out, and the patient's IQ is 70 or above).

A *minor* diagnostic cue to:

(1) The organic brain syndromes, especially the chronic brain disorders (when the patient's IQ is 70 or above).

(2) The mental deficiencies (when the patient's IQ is below 70).

Clouding of Consciousness

In clouding of consciousness, perceptions are not produced by sensory stimuli that ordinarily result in clear perceptions. (*Example:* Admitted to a hospital shortly after an auto accident, a young woman stares at persons she knows without recognizing them and clearly does not feel pain when her lacerations are sutured.)

A *definitive* diagnostic cue to the organic brain syndromes, especially acute brain disorders.

Compulsions

An insistent repetitive urge to perform an act contrary to ordinary conscious wishes. (*Example:* A patient feels the need to repeat over and over a certain kind of behavior such as handwashing for fear of impending, ill-defined disaster.)

A *definitive* diagnostic cue to obsessive compulsive neurosis (when psychosis can be ruled out).

A *minor* diagnostic cue to schizophrenia and the major affective disorders (when psychosis is present).

Confabulation

Inability to recall recent experiences, combined with a tendency to disguise the memory gaps with any material that comes to mind.

A *major* diagnostic cue to the chronic organic brain syndromes, especially Korsakoff's psychosis.

Confusion

A state characterized by bewilderment, perplexity, and environmental disorientation. (*Example:* A patient with toxic psychosis is brought to the hospital emergency floor. He does not know who he is or where he is, who the persons are who are ministering to him, or how he came to be where he is).

A *major* diagnostic cue to:

(1) The acute organic brain syndromes.

(2) Schizophrenia, especially acute schizophrenic episode (when organic determinants can be ruled out).

Conversional Behavior

A bodily symptom, often bizarre (eg, partial paralysis or paresthesia), which occurs as a result of psychic conflict. (*Example:* A hysterical young woman who suffers temporary loss of sensation in her left hand later remembers that she once struck her mother with this hand).

A *major* diagnostic cue to hysterical neurosis, conversion type (when psychosis can be ruled out and the symbolic meaning of the behavior can be determined).

A *minor* diagnostic cue to schizophrenia (when psychosis is present).

Cyclothymia

Alternating periods of elation and depression, increased and decreased psychomotor activity, excitement and apathy. (*Example:* A 22-year-old college student is considered very "moody" by her friends. No one can predict her moods, for she may be joyous and effervescent one day and in the depths of depression the next.)

A *major* diagnostic cue to:

(1) Manic-depressive psychosis, circular type (when the moods alternate infrequently).

(2) Cyclothymic personality (when psychosis can be ruled out).

A *minor* diagnostic cue to schizophrenia (when psychosis is present and the moods fluctuate frequently, eg, every day).

Decreased Psychomotor Activity

Retardation of the prevailing level of motor behavior; a general slowing down of the patient's usual activity level. (*Example:* A psychotically depressed young man lies motionless in bed, covering his head with the bedclothes; he confesses later that he does this to shut out the sights and sounds of the ward in order to reduce the intensity of his overwhelming fright.)

A *major* diagnostic cue to:

(1) Catatonic schizophrenia (when psychosis and catatonia are present).

(2) Manic-depressive illness, depressed type, and psychotic depressive reaction (when psychosis is present and catatonia is not).

(3) Depressive neurosis (when psychosis can be ruled out).

Delusions

A delusion is a belief held in the face of evidence normally considered sufficient to destroy it. (*Examples:* An illiterate, manic patient plans to run for President of the United States, falsely stating that he has received encouragement for his candidacy from many members of Congress. A paranoid schizophrenic patient comes angrily to his doctor's office, protesting the doctor's attempt to harm him by planning to publish details of his sexual history in the daily newspaper. A psychotically depressed patient plans suicide by self-immolation, considering herself the worst sinner in the world because she had not attended church the previous Sunday.)

In general delusions are *definitive* diagnostic cues to psychosis. There are several specific types of delusions.

A. Delusions of Grandeur: A *major* diagnostic cue to:

(1) The organic brain syndromes, especially general paresis (chronic brain syndrome associated with central nervous system syphilis).

(2) Manic-depressive illness, manic type (when organic disorders can be ruled out).

A *minor* diagnostic cue to schizophrenia.

B. Delusions of Persecution: A *major* diagnostic cue to schizophrenia, especially paranoid type. A *minor* diagnostic cue to:

(1) Manic-depressive illness, depressed type, involutional melancholia, and psychotic depressive reaction.

(2) The chronic organic brain syndromes, especially among elderly patients.

C. Delusions of Self-Accusation: (Sin, guilt, impoverishment, and illness.) A *major* diagnostic cue to involutional melancholia, manic-depressive illness, depressed type, and psychotic depressive reaction. A *minor* diagnostic cue to schizophrenia.

Depersonalization

Loss of conviction of one's own identity and loss of a sense of identification with and control over his own body. (*Example:* A patient in the early stages of schizophrenia compares his feelings to the way a counterfeit bill might feel on being examined by a banker who knows the difference between good and bad currency.)

Depersonalization may be present mildly at times in normal individuals, especially when they are greatly fatigued.

A *minor* diagnostic cue to:

(1) The acute brain syndromes.

(2) The psychoses.

(3) Neuroses (when psychosis can be ruled out).

Depressed Affect

A prevailing mood of sadness, despondency, or despair. Depressed mood has diagnostic significance only when it can be differentiated from normal grief and mourning.

A *major* diagnostic cue to:

(1) Depressive neurosis (when psychosis can be ruled out and depressed mood is the patient's chief complaint; or when depressed mood is accompanied by a variety of somatic complaints, such as insomnia, lack of appetite, constipation, fatigue, or weight loss).

(2) Involutional melancholia (when psychosis is present and the patient is elderly and has had no prior psychiatric history).

(3) Manic-depressive illness, depressed type, or psychotic depressive reaction (when psychosis is present and involutional psychotic reaction can be ruled out).

A *minor* diagnostic cue to schizophrenia.

Echolalia and Echopraxia

Echolalia is the involuntary and senseless repetition of a word or sentence just spoken by another person. Echopraxia is the automatic imitation of another's movements. The two often appear together. (*Example:* A severely disturbed schizophrenic patient, whenever he hears the ward nurse announce a meal, repeats over and over, "Lunch is ready, ready, ready, ready . . .," at the same time mimicking the nurse's posture and facial expression.)

A *definitive* cue to the psychoses.

Elevated Affect

A prevailing mood of euphoria, including an optimistic mental "set" and a feeling of well being and confidence when not justified by circumstances or experience.

A *major* diagnostic cue to:

(1) Manic-depressive illness, manic type (when organic disorders can be ruled out, psychosis is present, and no symptoms demonstrative of schizophrenia are seen).

A *minor* diagnostic cue to schizophrenia, especially hebephrenic type.

Flight of Ideas

Extremely rapid idea production without regard for logical processes. The patient rapidly expresses a thought and follows it quickly with another that is tangentially connected to it at some minor point or apparently not connected at all. (*Example:* A manic young man writes letters to friends and relatives in such volume that he uses more than 100 feet of paper a day in his efforts. He spends 18 hours a day writing. On reading from the letters, one can barely discern logical connections between sentences, although individual sentences more or less make sense.)

A *major* diagnostic cue to manic-depressive illness, manic type (when grossly illogical connections between thoughts are observed).

A *minor* diagnostic cue to schizophrenia (when no connections between thoughts are observed).

Hallucinations

False sensory stimuli in the absence of an actual external stimulus. (*Examples:* A schizophrenic patient reports that he hears voices which tell him to assault his wife and children. A patient in delirium tremens sees and feels insects crawling over his skin. An epileptic patient experiences rotten and burned smells and tastes whether he is eating or not.)

Hallucinations are *definitive* cues to the psychoses. There are several specific types of hallucinations.

A. Auditory Hallucinations: A *major* diagnostic cue to schizophrenia. A *minor* diagnostic cue to:

(1) Involutional melancholia, manic-depressive illness, depressed type, and psychotic depressive reaction (when no symptoms demonstrative of schizophrenia are seen).

(2) The organic brain syndromes.

B. Visual Hallucinations: A *major* diagnostic cue to the acute brain syndromes, especially delirium tremens and toxic psychoses. A *minor* diagnostic cue to schizophrenia (when the acute brain syndromes can be ruled out).

C. Olfactory Hallucinations: A *major* diagnostic cue to the organic brain syndromes, especially temporal and frontal lobe lesions and epilepsy. A *minor* diagnostic cue to schizophrenia (when the organic disorders can be ruled out).

D. Gustatory Hallucinations: A *major* diagnostic cue to the organic brain syndromes, especially temporal lobe lesions and epilepsy. A *minor* diagnostic cue to schizophrenia (when the organic brain syndromes can be ruled out).

E. Tactile Hallucinations: A *definitive* diagnostic cue to schizophrenia (when the tactile hallucination is of the sexual organs). A *major* diagnostic cue to the organic brain syndromes, especially delirium tremens (when the tactile hallucination is not of the sexual organs).

F. Kinesthetic Hallucinations: A *major* diagnostic cue to:

(1) The acute brain syndromes.

(2) Schizophrenia (when the sexual organs are involved).

A *minor* diagnostic cue to the schizophrenic reactions (when the sexual organs are not involved).

Hypochondriasis

Morbid and continual concern over the state of one's health, with exaggeration of trifling bodily signs and symptoms. (*Example:* A 68-year-old woman is constantly worried about her health, even though all her physical examinations have been negative. She thinks that pains in her arms mean arthritis, that rumblings in her stomach mean she is developing ulcers, and that the spots she occasionally sees before her eyes indicate beginning glaucoma. She takes 7 kinds of pills a day, including 3 different vitamin capsules.)

A *major* diagnostic cue to involutional melancholia (when psychosis is present and the patient is elderly, with no history of psychiatric illness).

A *minor* diagnostic cue to:

(1) Depressive neurosis (when psychosis can be ruled out).

(2) The major affective disorders and schizophrenia (when psychosis is present and involutional melancholia can be ruled out).

Ideas of Reference

The continual impression that the conversation, smiles, and behavior of other persons have reference to oneself. (*Example:* A patient later diagnosed as having paranoid schizophrenia reports that everyone on the subway is talking about him. When they smile in conversation with their friends, he thinks they are laughing at him.)

A *major* diagnostic cue to:

(1) Paranoid schizophrenia.

(2) Involutional melancholia, manic-depressive illness, depressed type, and psychotic depressive reaction (when no symptoms of schizophrenia are seen).

(3) The acute brain syndromes, especially incipient delirium tremens (when no symptoms of schizophrenia are seen and organic disease can be identified).

Illusions

A false perception misinterpreting an actual sense impression. (*Example:* A paranoid schizophrenic patient, on hearing a tree rubbing against the side of his house during a windstorm, believes that God is sending a sign to him that he will be crucified in the morning.)

A *major* diagnostic cue to:

(1) The acute brain syndromes.

(2) The psychoses.

Inadequate Affect

Emotional dullness, detachment, and insensitivity to stimuli in an environment that normally causes pleasure or pain. (*Example:* A schizophrenic boy shows continued "flat affect"; he neither smiles or frowns nor does he show any other facial expression of emotion no matter what happens around him. He speaks in a monotonous way, not accenting any words.)

A *definitive* diagnostic cue to schizophrenia.

A *major* diagnostic cue to involutional melancholia, manic-depressive illness, depressed type, and psychotic depressive reaction (when no other definitive cues to schizophrenia are seen).

Inappropriate Affect

Inappropriate emotional reactions, eg, the patient may act happy when he should be sad, and sad when he should be happy. (*Example:* A schizophrenic woman tells her therapist that she thinks her husband plans to kill her children, and she giggles with glee.)

A *definitive* diagnostic cue to schizophrenia.

A *major* diagnostic cue to involutional melancholia, manic-depressive illness, depressed type, and psychotic depressive reaction (when no other definitive cues to schizophrenia are seen).

Increased Psychomotor Activity

Acceleration of prevailing levels of motor behavior; a general dramatic increase in the patient's usual activity level. (*Example:* A manic patient is busy from early morning to late evening organizing his campaign for greater church attendance. He sleeps but 3 hours a night, spending the remainder of his time in constant motion, on the telephone, behind the wheel of his car, walking the downtown streets in search of friends, etc. He is a study in perpetual motion.)

A *major* diagnostic cue to:

(1) Manic-depressive illness, manic type (when psychosis is present and the increased activity has purpose, even if difficult to ascertain).

(2) Catatonic schizophrenia (when psychosis is present and the increased activity does not have clear purpose).

A *minor* diagnostic cue to the acute brain syndromes, especially delirium tremens.

Isolation

The state of excessively being or remaining alone by choice. (*Example:* A young woman reports that she much prefers being by herself to being with other people. She has no close friends, has refused offers of friendship from co-workers, and spends most of her waking non-work hours watching television alone in her apartment.)

A *major* diagnostic cue to:

(1) Schizophrenia (when psychosis is present).

(2) Involutional melancholia, manic-depressive illness, depressed type, and psychotic depressive reaction (when psychosis is present and no definitive cues to schizophrenia are seen).

(3) Schizoid personality (when psychosis can be ruled out).

Loose Associations

Lack of continuity in thinking; thoughts and speech proceed at random; no logical connection exists between contiguous elements of speech and thinking; "word salad." (*Example:* A chronic schizophrenic man writes: "I am here because he wants me there. Because I am helping God. And today

is the fifth which means that the Cardinals will lose and I will go swimming. She said she would see me again. I wonder when I can die and go free.")
A *definitive* diagnostic cue to the psychoses.
A *major* diagnostic cue to schizophrenia.

Mannerisms
Stereotyped body movements, often repeated over and over in a ritualized manner. These movements are often of the face and include grimaces, stereotyped frowns or smiles, and peculiar postures of the head and neck. Stuttering and stammering are not generally included within this category. (*Example:* A seriously disturbed schizophrenic man rocks back and forth in his seat all day, holding his left hand directly in front of his body as though to ward off a blow while his right hand firmly grasps his right ear. He continues his manneristic behavior through most of every day, although he does stop briefly to eat and use the bathroom.)
A *major* diagnostic cue to:
(1) Extrapyramidal reactions following phenothiazine medication; also other forms of parkinsonism.
(2) Schizophrenia, especially hebephrenic or catatonic type (when the symptom is not organic).
A *minor* diagnostic cue to obsessive compulsive neurosis and hysterical neurosis, conversion type (when psychosis and organic causes can be ruled out).

Mutism
Unwillingness to talk.
A *major* diagnostic cue to catatonic schizophrenia (when organic causes can be ruled out).
A *minor* diagnostic cue to:
(1) The chronic organic brain syndromes.
(2) Psychotic depressive reaction and manic-depressive illness, depressed type (when catatonia is not present and organic causes can be ruled out).

Neologism
A newly coined word, or an old word used in a novel, idiosyncratic way. (*Example:* A schizophrenic man refers to his wife as "Swordwar" because he thinks she is a "battleaxe.")
A *major* diagnostic cue to schizophrenia.

Obsessional Thinking
Persistent conscious preoccupation with a circumscribed set of unwanted words or ideas that cannot be shaken off. (*Example:* A young obsessive compulsive college student admits that he has frequent recurring thoughts of harming his father and mother, despite continuous conscious efforts to banish the thoughts. They keep him awake several hours each night and burden him daily when he is not otherwise occupied.)
A *definitive* diagnostic cue to obsessive compulsive neurosis (when psychosis can be ruled out).

A *major* diagnostic cue to neuroses, especially obsessive compulsive neurosis (when psychosis can be ruled out and when not accompanied by compulsions).

A *minor* diagnostic cue to the psychoses.

Perseveration

The tendency for activity (usually verbal) to recur without apparent external stimulus; often the repetition of one answer to several different questions. (*Example:* An elderly patient with arteriosclerosis replies to every question asked of him, "Well, I'll be damned!")

A *major* diagnostic cue to the chronic organic brain syndromes.

A *minor* diagnostic cue to schizophrenia, especially catatonic type (when chronic organic brain syndromes can be ruled out).

Phobia

Excessive fear of some particular object or situation; fear that is persistent and unfounded or without sufficient grounds. (*Example:* A young boy suddenly develops such an intense fear of horses that he will not leave his house to walk in the park across the street. He has never been harmed by a horse, nor has he ever seen a horse harm anyone.)

A *major* diagnostic cue to the neuroses (when psychosis can be ruled out), especially phobic neurosis (when phobias are the principal symptom).

A *minor* diagnostic cue to:

(1) The chronic organic brain syndromes.

(2) The psychoses (when the chronic organic brain syndromes can be ruled out).

Reality Testing, Loss Of

Impaired ability to perceive and evaluate events and situations. (*Example:* A psychotic man hallucinates and shows prominent and bizarre delusions. He is unwilling or unable to test the reality of his false perceptions and unrealistic thinking. He believes in his hallucinated voices and complex delusions implicitly.)

A *definitive* diagnostic cue to the psychoses.

Retardation of Thinking

Slow initiation and progress of thought. Often the patient will state that his thoughts come slowly or that he has difficulty in thinking.

A *major* diagnostic cue to:

(1) The chronic organic brain syndromes.

(2) Involutional melancholia, manic-depressive illness, depressed type, and psychotic depressive reaction (when psychosis is present and no symptoms demonstrative of schizophrenia or the chronic organic brain disorders are observed).

A *minor* diagnostic cue to:

(1) Schizophrenia.

(2) Depressive neurosis (when psychosis can be ruled out).

Stupor

Deadened or dazed sensibilities with little or no appreciation of surroundings. In profound stupor, the patient is unconscious. (*Example:* An elderly woman considered to be psychotically depressed is brought into the hospital after attempting to burn herself to death in her own furnace. She sits mute, does not eat, takes no interest in her surroundings and has to be bathed, dressed, undressed, and fed a liquid diet through a nasal tube.)

A *major* diagnostic cue to:

(1) The acute organic brain syndromes (when no symptoms demonstrative of schizophrenia are observed).

(2) Catatonic schizophrenia (when psychosis and catatonia are present).

(3) Psychotic depressive reaction.

REFERENCES

Books and Monographs

Ban, T.A., & H. Lehmann: *Experimental Approaches to Psychiatric Diagnosis: Psychometric, Conditioning, & Psychopharmacological Studies.* Thomas, 1970.

Nathan, P.E.: *Cues, Decisions and Diagnoses: A Systems Analytic Approach to the Diagnosis of Psychopathology.* Academic Press, 1967.

Journal Articles

Ash, P.: The reliability of psychiatric diagnosis. J Abnorm Social Psychol 44:272–277, 1949.

Beck, A.T.: Reliability of psychiatric diagnosis. 1. A critique of systematic studies. Am J Psychiat 119:210–216, 1962.

Beck, A.T., & others: Reliability of psychiatric diagnosis. 2. A study of consistency of clinical judgments and ratings. Am J Psychiat 119:351–357, 1962.

Chance, E.: Implications of interdisciplinary differences in case description. Am J Orthopsychiat 33:672–677, 1963.

Foulds, G.: The reliability of psychiatric, and the validity of psychological diagnosis. J Ment Sc 101:851–862, 1955.

Fowler, R.D., & M.L. Miller: Computer interpretation of the MMPI: Its use in clinical practice. Arch Gen Psychiat 21:502–508, 1969.

Gauron, E., & J.K. Dickinson: Diagnostic decision making in psychiatry. Arch Gen Psychiat 14:233–237, 1966.

Jones, N.F., Kahn, N.W., & D.G. Langsley: Prediction of admission to a psychiatric hospital. Arch Gen Psychiat 12:607–610, 1965.

Kanfer, F.H., & G. Saslow: Behavioral analysis. Arch Gen Psychiat 12:529–538, 1965.

Kety, S.S.: The heuristic aspect of psychiatry. Am J Psychiat 118:385–397, 1963.

Langfeldt, G.: The significance of a dichotomy in clinical psychiatric classification. Am J Psychiat 119:537–539, 1962.

Nathan, P.E., & others: Thirty-two observers and one patient: A study of diagnostic reliability. J Clin Psychol 25:9–15, 1969.

Nathan, P.E., & others: Syndromes of psychosis and psychoneurosis: A clinical validation study. Arch Gen Psychiat 19:704–716, 1968.

Nathan, P.E., & others: A systems analytic model of diagnosis. 1. The diagnostic validity of abnormal psychomotor behavior. J Clin Psychol 25:3–9, 1969.

Pasamanick, B.: On the neglect of diagnosis. Am J Orthopsychiat 33:387–388, 1963.

Rappaport, J., & J.M. Chinsky: Behavior ratings of chronic hospitalized patients: Cross-situational and cross-rater agreement. J Consulting Psychol 34:394–397, 1970.

Scheff, T.J.: Decision rules, types of error, and their consequences in medical diagnoses. Behav Sc 8:97–107, 1963.

Sletten, I.W., Altman, H., & G.A. Ulett: Routine diagnosis by computer. Am J Psychiat 127:1147–1152, 1971.

Ward, C.H., & others: The psychiatric nomenclature: Reasons for diagnostic disagreement. Arch Gen Psychiat 7:198–205, 1962.

Wilson, M.S., & E. Meyer: Diagnostic consistency in a psychiatric liaison service. Am J Psychiat 119:207–209, 1962.

7 . . .

Psychologic Testing *

This compares to important laboratory data in a medical work-up. The psychometrist can furnish accurate information on intelligence level and school achievement and sometimes helpful leads on personality, vocational aptitude, and psychopathology.

Psychologic testing as an aid to psychiatric diagnosis and the planning of treatment undertakes to measure the individual's capacity to interact intellectually and emotionally with his environment. In the hands of a skilled examiner, psychologic tests can often provide objective, meaningful data on psychopathology and intellectual functioning in a shorter time than can other means of individual assessment.

The main virtue of psychologic tests is that the nature and extent of a patient's deviation from established test norms permit the clinician to judge more accurately the components of his psychopathology. Norms for "standardized" personality tests are possible because it has been found that patients with comparable psychopathology often respond in similar ways to the same test stimuli.

The clinical usefulness of psychologic tests depends to a great extent on the skills of the examiner. The psychometrist is trained to administer, score, and evaluate measures of intelligence, personality, and psychopathology in terms of established norms; hence, he is less subject to the clinician's natural inclination to judge psychopathology solely against a background of his own accumulated clinical experience. Other mental health professionals can be trained to administer psychologic tests; but, since most of the training of the psychiatrist and social worker is clinical in nature, they may not consistently utilize the established norms of tests to best advantage.

CLASSIFICATION AND DESCRIPTION OF PSYCHOLOGIC TESTS

Psychologic tests may be either *group* or *individual* tests, and either *objective*, *subjective*, or *projective* tests (see Table 7–1). Technics of

*See also Table 33–4.

TABLE 7–1. Classification of psychologic tests.*

	Group	Individual
Objective tests	Otis Test of Mental Abilities Army Alpha and Beta Shipley-Hartford Abstractions Test Achievement tests Aptitude tests	Wechsler Adult Intelligence Scale Wechsler Intelligence Scale for Children Stanford-Binet Test Wechsler Memory Scale Graham-Kendall Test Bender Gestalt Test
Subjective tests	Minnesota Multiphasic Personality Inventory (group form) Rating scales Questionnaires Sentence Completion tests	Minnesota Multiphasic Personality Inventory (card form)
Projective tests	Figure-drawing tests	Rorschach and Holtzman Tests Thematic Apperception Test Figure-drawing tests Rosenzweig Picture-Frustration Study

*The tests listed are examples of a broad range of tests available in each category.

administration and evaluation commonly vary with the purpose for which a test is administered.

Group tests are "paper-and-pencil" tests that can be given to more than one person at a time. They are often designed to permit machine scoring. The value of *individual* tests depends largely upon the experience and skill of the administrator since they are given by one examiner to only one subject at a time. Most psychologists feel that individual tests of personality and intelligence are more reliable and valid than group tests; they are also much more costly of time and materials than group tests.

OBJECTIVE TESTS

Objective tests consist of questions of fact that cannot be interpreted differently by different subjects. Subjects' responses to objective test questions are usually in one of 2 directions (eg, true or false). These tests may measure intellectual capacity, extent of organic involvement in psychopathology, and scholastic aptitude and achievement.

TABLE 7−2. IQ distribution in USA standard sample population.

IQ	Description	Percentage of Population
130−above	Very superior	2.2%
120−129	Superior	6.7%
110−119	Bright normal	16.1%
90−109	Average	50.0%
80−89	Dull normal	16.1%
70−79	Borderline	6.7%
Below 70	Mental subnormality	2.2%

Intelligence Tests

There are both group and individual intelligence tests. Individual intelligence tests administered by experienced examiners are considered better measures of intellectual capacity than group tests, primarily because the administrator of an individual IQ test, unlike the group IQ administrator, can observe, record, and evaluate extra-test behavior.

An important disadvantage of these tests is that they are heavily influenced by sociocultural factors such as level of education and social status. They are probably grossly invalid as measures of intelligence for members of minority groups whose backgrounds differ markedly from those of the standardization groups.

The uncertain reliability and predictive validity of IQ tests make it inadvisable to inform a subject (or his parents) of the exact numerical result of his test. Every clinician knows intellectually slow persons whose drive and ambition have enabled them to achieve great success in life and, conversely, very bright individuals whose personality difficulties have severely limited their achievements. No practical purpose is served by telling a subject specifically how he did on any test.

The *Wechsler Adult Intelligence Scale (WAIS)* and the *Wechsler Intelligence Scale for Children (WISC)*, both individual tests, are widely used to measure the intellectual level (ie, current capacity to deal with verbal and symbolic demands of the environment) of adults and older children. Each of these tests is comprised of 11 subtests which together measure a variety of verbal and nonverbal components of intelligence. The Wechsler subtests measure a subject's general level of information, vocabulary, short-term memory, abstract thinking ability, and capacity to perform various psychomotor and perceptual tasks. These tests provide an IQ score based upon an extensive national standardization and hence permit valid comparison of one individual's intellectual functioning with another's provided they come from comparable backgrounds.

Tests of Organic Involvement

The *Graham-Kendall Test, Bender Gestalt Test,* and *Wechsler Memory Scale (WMS)* measure an individual's ability to remember and reproduce complex geometric designs. Consistent distortion of test patterns suggests malfunction due to neural injury or organic brain damage. The WMS also calls on the subjects to learn and recall a variety of verbal symbols (words and numbers), since these abilities are often impaired by organic brain damage. These tests also have psychopathologic diagnostic value.

These tests must be administered and evaluated by a trained examiner, who looks not only for specific performance deficits but also for the individual's characteristic approach to the problems and his methods of adjusting to psychomotor impairment.

Achievement Tests

Achievement tests (eg, some components of the *College Board Entrance Examination Tests*) are group tests that measure the individual's level of achievement in various subject areas for comparison with the performance of others of similar age and education. They are often used to measure the results of systematic education and training and to predict the chances for success in future education. They are given routinely on entry into the armed forces.

Aptitude Tests

Aptitude tests such as the *Differential Aptitude Tests* and the *Scholastic Aptitude Tests* of the College Boards measure potential abilities in specific fields such as law, medicine, stenography, or machine shop operation. Like achievement tests, aptitude tests are often administered to large groups, as at army induction centers. They do not have to be administered or scored by highly skilled examiners, although their value does increase with the experience and skill of the person who evaluates them. Because it is difficult to establish appropriate criteria for judging future success in a complex field, they are most useful in judging the ability to acquire skill in narrow fields (eg, typing rather than law).

SUBJECTIVE TESTS

The test stimuli (questions) of subjective tests, like those of objective tests, permit little differential interpretation by different subjects. Subjective tests differ from objective tests in that the answers to the questions may be subject to divergent interpretations by different examiners because the behavior they measure (ie, the personality components they undertake to describe) is so complex and ill-categorized. The questions generally tap "conscious" determinants of behavior ("I don't like girls because my mother betrayed me") and subjectively perceived mood states ("I am often depressed").

Questionnaires and Rating Scales

The *Minnesota Multiphasic Personality Inventory (MMPI)* and the *Vernon-Allport-Lindzey Scale of Values* undertake to measure a variety of personality traits and psychopathologic behavior in order to permit comparison with statistically established norms. These norms may be based upon traditional psychiatric classification (as in the MMPI) or on some other classification system (such as the Scale of Values norms, based upon Jungian classification).

The MMPI, one of the most widely used psychologic tests of personality, consists of 550 statements (eg, "I work under a great deal of tension," "I believe in a life hereafter") requiring a "true or false" answer. It measures an extremely broad range of potential psychopathology. Its 9 "clinical" scales of measurement (hypochondriasis, depression, hysteria, schizophrenia, psychopathic deviance, masculinity-femininity, paranoia, psychasthenia, and mania) were carefully standardized by comparing the test responses of a large number of psychiatric patients whose diagnoses were unquestioned with those of normal groups, and then selecting test items which consistently differentiated between the 2 groups on each of these scales. Therefore, the MMPI is felt by many to be more securely based on statistically appropriate norms than any other psychologic test.

Sentence Completion Tests

Sentence completion tests (eg, *Rotter Incomplete Sentences Test*) require the subject to complete a series of sentences whose first words are supplied (eg, "My mother was . . . "; "My favorite . . . "). They are designed to permit the subject to express in a systematic way some of his feelings about relevant features of his environment, particularly his interpersonal relationships with parents, siblings, and spouse. Because these are not well standardized, they must be interpreted quantitatively (ie, "More than . . . ") rather than simply qualitatively ("Yes, No").

PROJECTIVE TESTS

The test stimuli of projective tests are intentionally ambiguous and elicit divergent responses from different subjects; therefore, their evaluation depends on entirely different procedures from those used with other psychologic tests. Projective tests are thought to tap "unconscious" determinants of behavior and fantasy of which the subject himself is usually unaware.

Deliberately ambiguous test stimuli force the subject to bring his own order and meaning to seemingly unstructured and meaningless stimuli. In so doing, he is thought to reveal significant aspects of his personality—the characteristic manner in which he approaches the world, the means by which he orders it, and those elements of his environment which he chooses to deal with and those which he must avoid—things of which he himself may be unaware.

Unstructured Projective Tests

Projective tests such as the various figure-drawing tests require the subject to supply his own test stimuli and to apply all the order and form he perceives in the environment to the task. While such tests yield useful diagnostic data in the hands of the experienced examiner (eg, sexual identity, level of psychosocial adjustment), the absence of large-scale validation data on these tests renders them of unproved utility.

(1) Rorschach Test: The most widely used projective test is the Rorschach. Unstructured projective tests such as the Rorschach are useful because they are relatively less "leading" and thus less threatening to a disturbed patient than more structured tests of personality. They are utilized widely because they seem to tap areas of personality that are remote and otherwise inaccessible to all but intensive psychotherapy and psychoanalysis. The Rorschach test consists of a series of 10 cards on each of which is a design made from an inkblot. Five of the blots are black and white and 5 contain color. The subject views one card at a time in numerical sequence and tells the examiner what he sees in the card and where on the card he sees it. On completing all 10 cards, he is required to explain what it was that determined each "percept," ie, the respective influence of color, form, shading, etc on the organization of his responses. The interpretation of the subject's test behavior is based on an analysis of his responses to each card, the total number of replies, and their interrelationships in terms of accepted norms.

(2) Holtzman Inkblot Test: This test consists of 45 inkblots to each of which the subject gives but one response. Its proponents claim that it is more reliable and valid than the Rorschach.

Semistructured Projective Tests

Semistructured projective tests allow the subject to impose his own meaning and organization upon stimuli that already possess some of their own. Examples are the *Thematic Apperception Test (TAT)* and the *Rosenzweig Picture-Frustration Study (PF)*. The TAT consists of a series of 20 drawings of persons engaged in various activities. The subject is required to explain the activities portrayed by the people on the cards, and thus identifies himself partially with the characters in the stories as he imparts his own wishes, fears, and conflicts to the thematic material. The PF test consists of a series of 16 cartoons, each of which depicts a frustrating situation (eg, knocking over a valuable vase at a relative's house; being involved in a minor automobile accident). In supplying dialogue for the cartoons, the subject inadvertently throws light on the direction (intropunitive, impunitive, extrapunitive) and appropriateness of his characteristic reaction to similar real-life frustrations.

RELIABILITY AND VALIDITY
OF PSYCHOLOGIC TESTS

A test is *reliable* when it gives similar results on repeated administration to the same person or to persons with similar capacities or attributes. A test is *valid* when it measures what it sets out to measure (concurrent validity) or predicts correctly those aspects of future performance it presumes to predict (predictive validity). Clearly, a psychologic test can be reliable but not valid, but it can never be valid if it is not reliable.

In general, objective psychologic tests are more reliable and valid than projective tests.

RELIABILITY

The reliability of most psychologic tests has not been firmly established, although extensive test-retest studies have examined the intra-subject reliability of certain objective tests, most notably the WAIS. Thus, repeated administration of most psychologic tests to the same individual does not always provide the same diagnostic picture. Because the reliability and validity of these tests have not been established, batteries of psychologic tests rather than single tests are given routinely to psychiatric patients.

Some of the factors that determine the reliability of psychologic tests are described in the following paragraphs.

Subject Variables

In many psychiatric illnesses the patient may manifest different patterns of symptoms at different times. When the same psychologic test is given at different times to a patient with a changing pattern of symptoms, the test results should reflect this fact. Subjects may also respond differently at different times to the same test items even though their fundamental symptomatology remains the same.

Examiner Variables

When several examiners administer the same test to the same subject and elicit different results, the discrepancy may be a function of differences in their technics of administering, scoring, or interpreting the test. Hence, low test reliability may be due to examiner differences. Similarly, if the same examiner does not administer a test the same way at all times, he may himself be responsible for low reliability scores.

VALIDITY

Concurrent Validity

If the user of psychologic test information accepts as true the old maxim that, "Intelligence is what the intelligence test measures," he can be confident that the validity of psychologic tests of intelligence is high. However, most clinicians also use psychologic test results to give them a summary of a patient's current level of functioning, the amount of his present psychopathology, and the degree to which he utilizes specific psychologic defense mechanisms. In these cases, it cannot be proved that psychologic tests measure what they set out to measure, since it is not always clear how to define objectively or specify exactly the variety of personality and intellectual components of a person's behavior.

These criticisms, of course, apply also to the traditional psychiatric "mental status" examination (Chapter 4), which lacks normative sample data and is not reproducible by different examiners.

Predictive Validity

Numerous studies suggest that psychologic tests by themselves cannot consistently predict future behavior, response to treatment, or subsequent levels of psychologic functioning. In attempting to predict the future course of a patient's illness, it is important also to take into account his current and past behavior in society. In many cases, the past predicts the future at least as well as anything else does.

HOW TO ASK FOR PSYCHOLOGIC TESTS AND WHAT TO ASK OF THEM

Typically, the psychologist gives a psychiatric patient a battery of psychologic tests, usually consisting of an individual intelligence test, one or 2 projective tests, a subjective test of personality (usually the MMPI), and perhaps an objective test which measures organic involvement. A battery of tests is employed because each test measures well only a relatively restricted behavior element. However, although the WAIS is an intelligence test, it also frequently provides insight into psychopathology (eg, extent of cognitive disorder or difficulty in concentration); and, although the Rorschach is a test of personality, it also often gives valuable information on intellectual functioning (ie, the characteristic manner in which a person organizes his approach to the world). Similar comments may be made about most other psychologic tests.

Requests for testing should include more than just a patient's name, age, sex, and tentative diagnosis. They should also include information on his presenting symptoms; personal, medical, and psychiatric history; and relevant laboratory tests. Just as with other requests for consultation, the clinician requesting psychologic tests should assume that the consultant would like to have as much pertinent information about the patient as possible.

Psychologic tests are appropriately used in the following ways.

Measurement of Intellectual Level

(1) Comparison of present intellectual functioning with premorbid levels of functioning; realistic assessment of future educational goals as judged from present and premorbid levels.

(2) Judgment of the degree to which existing psychopathology interferes with intellectual functioning, and potential for improvement in intellectual functioning if the disease process abates.

(3) Prediction of chances for success in psychotherapy as a function of IQ level.

Differential Diagnosis of Psychopathology

(1) Differentiation among the psychoneuroses, psychoses, and organic pathology.

(2) In particular, differentiation of early or "ambulatory" schizophrenia, from mental retardation; of organic impairment (of an acute nature) from one of the psychoneuroses or psychoses; of manic-depressive psychosis from schizophrenia; of character disorder from schizophrenia, etc.

Although these differentiations are by no means always provided by psychologic tests, it is sometimes possible to base differential diagnostic statements on test results.

Evaluation of Separate Functional and Organic Components
of Psychopathology

Although few psychologists feel that psychologic tests consistently reflect the separate influence of organic and functional components of psychopathology, most psychologists agree that such distinctions can be drawn at times by using both objective tests of intelligence and specific tests for organic involvement. In particular, they think that these tests often provide information on the degree to which an individual's "verbal" and "psychomotor" capacities deviate from established norms in directions consonant with CNS disease, and that psychologic tests may reveal an organic component of psychopathology that may have eluded neurologic or laboratory examination.

Evaluation of Potential Response to Treatment

Certain intellectual and personality characteristics are considered essential for a successful psychotherapeutic relationship. Among these characteristics are adequate intellectual level, motivation to change inappropriate modes of behavior, and adequate capacity to feel and utilize emotions that may develop during close interpersonal relationships. To varying degrees, psychologic tests give the therapist some idea of the chances of success before a doctor-patient relationship is established. They may also enable him to shorten therapy by providing information he might otherwise have to elicit laboriously from the patient, eg, information on the patient's use of defense mechanisms to guard against frightening aspects of his own psyche; knowledge of these mechanisms may allow the therapist to anticipate sources of therapeutic difficulty.

Vocational Guidance and Rehabilitation

The therapist may use psychologic tests measuring intelligence, vocational aptitude and achievement, and personality integrity in attempts to determine future vocational objectives.

WHAT NOT TO ASK OF PSYCHOLOGIC TESTS

As with requests for consultation in other fields of medicine that require diverse competencies, requests for psychologic tests may be either appropriate or inappropriate. Appropriate requests for psychologic tests are those which ask for data that the tests can provide. Requests of this kind are detailed above. Inappropriate requests for psychologic tests include those that ask for the following:

"Psychologicals"

These nonspecific requests, usually made by persons inexperienced in the specific details of psychologic testing methods, do not tell the psychologist what kind of data are wanted. Consequently, the examiner is forced to provide a nonspecific report of test results which may not contain the information really needed.

Localization of Organic Lesions

Despite claims by some psychologists to the contrary, it has not been established that psychologic tests can localize brain lesions or other organic disease except in a very gross way. Although these tests often can determine whether an organic lesion is present or absent, they cannot localize the specific lesion.

Differential Diagnosis

Although some kinds of differential diagnosis are possible on the basis of psychologic testing, it is wrong to assume that these tests consistently make possible differential diagnosis of all forms of psychopathology, particularly the more exotic organic disorders, character disorders, and personality trait disturbances.

Prediction of Course of Illness, Outcome of Psychotherapy, or Response to Psychopharmacologic Drugs

Although tests can provide some information on variables thought to influence these events, many other variables that the tests do not touch are unique to each patient and interfere with the use of these tests for these purposes.

REFERENCES

Books and Monographs

Bennett, G.K., Seashore, H.G., & A.G. Wesman: *Differential Aptitude Tests.* Psychological Corporation, 1959.

DuBois, P.: *The History of Psychological Testing.* Allyn & Bacon, 1970.

Gough, H.G.: *California Psychological Inventory.* Consulting Psychologists Press, 1957.

Harris, D.B.: *Measuring the Psychological Maturity of Children: A Revision and Extension of the Goodenough Draw-A-Man Test.* World Book, 1961.

Hathaway, S.R., & J.C. McKinley: *Minnesota Multiphasic Personality Inventory,* rev ed. Psychological Corporation, 1951.

McReynolds, P. (editor): *Advances in Psychological Assessment.* Science and Behavior Books, 1968.

Murray, H.A.: *Thematic Apperception Test.* Harvard Univ Press, 1943.

Otis, A.S.: *Otis Self-Administering Tests of Mental Ability.* World Book, 1929.

Palmer, J.O.: *The Psychological Assessment of Children.* Wiley, 1970.

Rorschach, H.: *Psychodiagnostics: A Test Based on Perception.* Huber, 1942.

Rosenzweig, S.: *Rosenzweig Picture-Frustration Study.* Author, 1949.

Terman, L.M., & M.A. Merrill: *Stanford-Binet Intelligence Scale: Manual for the Third Revision, Form L-M.* Houghton-Mifflin, 1960.

Thorne, F.C.: *Principles of Psychological Examining.* Journal of Clinical Psychology Press, 1955.

Thorne, F.C.: *Clinical Judgement.* Journal of Clinical Psychology Press, 1961.

Tiegs, E.W., & W.W. Clark: *California Achievement Tests.* California Testing Bureau, 1957.

Wechsler, D.: *The Measurement of Adult Intelligence.* Williams & Wilkins, 1939.

Wechsler, D.: *Wechsler Intelligence Scale for Children.* Psychological Corporation, 1949.

Wechsler, D.: *Wechsler Adult Intelligence Scale.* Psychological Corporation, 1955.

Journal Articles

Goldberg, L.R.: Diagnosticians versus diagnostic signs: The diagnosis of psychosis versus neurosis from the MMPI. Psychol Monogr 79:1–28, 1965.

Kleinmuntz, B.: Profile analysis revisited: A heuristic approach. J Consult Psychol 10:315–324, 1963.

Luszki, M.B., & others: Long search for a short WAIS: Stop looking. J Consult Clin Psychol 34:425–431, 1970.

Rice, D.G., & R.J. Thurell: Teaching psychological evaluation to psychiatric residents. Arch Gen Psychiat 19:737–742, 1968.

Staudt, V., & J. Zubin: A biometric evaluation of the somatotherapies in schizophrenia. Psychol Bull 54:171–196, 1957.

Thorne, F.C.: Diagnostic classification and nomenclature for existential state reactions. J Clin Psychol 26:403–420, 1970.

8...
Genetics & Psychiatry

Farmers and breeders understand good seed better than psychiatrists do. Heredity operates importantly in intelligence (and mental subnormality), schizophrenia, manic-depressive psychosis, and various dementias; less so in personality, homosexuality, and criminality; probably not at all in neurosis.

The relation of genetics to psychiatry may be considered at a series of organizational levels: molecular, cellular, biochemical, neurophysiologic, psychopathologic, and demographic. In each of these there is continuous interaction between the organism and its environment. The study of genetics in psychiatry is concerned with the clarification of cause, effect, and interaction.

Each of these levels of interaction may be studied by means of laboratory studies (searching for chromosomal and biochemical abnormalities in individuals and in populations) and by statistical methods such as the following:

(1) **Pedigree method:** Involves single human family pedigrees. Pedigrees are of limited value and are not statistically representative of the population.

(2) **Census method:** Involves total population surveys and depends for its usefulness on the cooperation of the population.

(3) **Family risk studies:** Compare the expectancy of a condition developing among the relatives of an affected individual with its expectancy in the general population.

(4) **Twin-family method:** Compares monozygotic and dizygotic twins, siblings, and parents. This method provides an opportunity to examine intrafamilial variations with a minimum of uncontrolled variables.

Biochemical and chromosomal abnormalities are now known to cause some cases of mental retardation and a small but significant number of cases of criminality. No genetically determined biochemical abnormality or chromosomal aberration has been definitely identified as yet in other psychiatric disorders, but a number of possibilities are under intense study. Statistical studies suggest important genetic factors in the etiology of these diseases.

The gene carries the predisposition for development of a trait, and this trait materializes only in the appropriate environmental circumstances. The environment always plays an important role in the expression of any trait.

A gene is responsible for starting a long series of chemical reactions which may be modified at any point by environmental factors. Genetic effects vary in the degree of their expressivity and penetrance. A person with an abnormal gene that predisposes him to a psychiatric disease may appear clinically normal until he is subjected to unfavorable interpersonal or environmental circumstances, whereupon he may develop clinical manifestations of the disease, which is the degree of expressivity of the gene. This interaction is important when considering psychiatric illness in terms of genetic predisposition and environmental stress.

Mechanisms of Inheritance

There are 2 mechanisms of inheritance: single factor (single gene) and multifactorial (multiple gene) inheritance. Single gene inheritance is said to be *dominant* when the genetic effect (phenotypic expression) is produced in both the homozygous (ie, receiving the same gene from both parents) and heterozygous (ie, receiving different genes from the parents' corresponding chromosomal loci) forms and *recessive* when the genetic effect is produced only in the homozygous form. Huntington's chorea is an example of dominant single factor inheritance, and phenylketonuria of recessive single factor inheritance.

Multifactorial inheritance is produced by the interaction of multiple genes which individually have small or nonspecific effects but cumulatively act to product a continuous range of variation. This mechanism is probably responsible for whatever inheritance there is of such characteristics as intelligence, temperament, and personality.

Inheritance may also be *X-linked (sex-linked)* or *autosomal,* depending on whether the gene is situated on the sex chromosomes or on the others (autosomes). In X-linked inheritance, the distribution of a trait between the sexes is unequal; in autosomal inheritance, it is equal. Examples of X-linked inheritance are one form of Hurler's syndrome, Merzbacher-Pelizaeus disease, and Lesch-Nyhan syndrome (an X-linked recessive disease in which self-destructive behavior seems to be a prominent feature).

Chromosomal Abnormalities in Psychiatric Disorders

Each cell of the human body contains 23 pairs of chromosomes which carry the genetic material. There are one pair of sex chromosomes and 22 pairs of autosomes, which are further subdivided into 7 groups according to the size of the chromosome and the position of its centromere.

It has been found that among inmates of institutions for the criminally insane there is a higher incidence of XYY than in the general population or among mental defectives. This "YY" syndrome appears to represent an instance of specific mental disorder correlated, though weakly, with a highly specific genetic lesion.

Some types of mental deficiency and some organic sexual abnormalities are associated with chromosomal aberrations. Some patients with mental deficiency associated with abnormal karyotypes exhibit psychotic behavior, which suggests that genetic defects may contribute to the etiology of the psychosis.

Glossary of Genetic Terms
Used in This Chapter

Autosomes: The chromosomes (22 pairs of autosomes in man) other than the sex chromosomes (cp Sex chromosome).

Centromere (centrosome): The palely staining cross-over point or primary constriction that divides the chromosome into 2 arm lengths.

Chromosome: A small thread-like or rod-like structure into which the nuclear chromatin divides during mitosis. The number of chromosomes is constant for any given species (23 pairs in man: 22 pairs of autosomes and one pair of sex chromosomes). Each chromosome is composed of a linear arrangement of small bodies called genes, each of which occupies a specific locus on its chromosome.

Dominant: Designating a gene whose phenotypic effect largely or entirely obscures that of its allele (gene paired with it for an individual trait) (cp Recessive).

Gamete (germ cell): A cell that is capable of uniting with another cell in sexual reproduction (ie, ovum, spermatozoon).

Gene: A unit of heredity which occupies a specific locus in the chromosome and which, either alone or in combination, produces a single characteristic. It is usually a single molecule capable of self-duplication or mutation.

Genetics: The science concerned with the phenomena of inheritance and biologic variation.

Genotype: The hereditary constitution, or combination of genes, which characterizes a given individual or a group of genetically identical organisms (cp Phenotype).

Heterozygous: Having 2 members of a given hereditary factor pair which are dissimilar, ie, the 2 genes of an allelic pair are not the same (cp Homozygous).

Homozygous: Having 2 members of a given hereditary factor pair which are similar, ie, the 2 genes of an allelic pair are identical.

Karyotype: The chromosomal constitution of a cell, individual, or species.

Penetrance: The likelihood or probability that a gene will become morphologically (phenotypically) expressed. The degree of penetrance may depend upon acquired as well as genetic factors.

Phenotype: The visible characteristics of an individual or those that are common to a group of apparently identical individuals (cp Genotype).

Recessive: Designating a gene whose phenotypic effect is largely or entirely obscured by the effect of its allele (cp Dominant).

Sex chromosome: The chromosome or pair of chromosomes which determines the sex of the individual (cp Autosomes). (In the human female, the sex chromosome pair is homologous, XX; in the male, nonhomologous, XY. Unusual combinations of sex chromosomes that have been found are as follows: XO, XXX, XXY, XXXY, XXXX, and XXXXY. These variations may be associated with alterations of normal sex characteristics, physical abnormalities, and mental retardation.)

Sex (X) linkage: The influence of sex on transmission of hereditary traits. There are 2 main types of sex-linked inheritance depending upon whether the sex-linked inheritance genes are located in the X or the Y chromosome. Sex linkage may be absolute or incomplete.

Zygote: The cell formed by the union of 2 gametes in sexual reproduction.

Between Genes and Behavior

Between the genetic molecules and the behavior for which they are responsible lie a series of complex physical intermediaries. These may be enzymes, hormones, or neurons. The effects of genes on behavior must always begin with some enzymatically controlled metabolic effect of the genes within the cell, and the neuronal and hormonal intermediaries are the eventual result. For example, idiopathic spontaneous hypoglycemia, an autosomal recessive disease, produces irritability, negativism, behavioral changes, or even mental retardation through hypoglycemia, thought to be due to adrenal dysfunction.

A. Enzyme Pathways: Some kinds of mental retardation are now known to result from single enzymatic defects. Phenylketonuria is an autosomal recessive metabolic disorder that causes severe behavioral disorders. It is due to a missing enzyme that results in a block in the oxidative pathway of phenylalanine and leads to the accumulation of phenylketone and related substances in the blood. The intellectual deficit caused by the toxic action of the abnormal metabolites can be prevented or improved by the early and careful reduction of the amount of phenylalanine in the diet.

B. Hormone Pathways: Genetic effects on behavior can be mediated through hormones in 3 ways (the enzymes involved are as yet unknown):

1. Hormones are important in the normal development and maintenance of behavioral factors, and defective production of a hormone (deficiency or excess) may be responsible for serious behavioral abnormalities. For example, thyroid deficiency early in development causes the multiple psychologic defects found in cretinism.

2. Hormones may control behavior through stimulation of structures employed in specific response patterns. For example, the development of normal adult sexual behavior depends on the normal growth of the genital organs, which is under hormonal control.

3. Hormones may have some effect on the integrative functions of the CNS, and thereby play a part in behavioral mechanisms. An example is the pituitary-adrenal responsiveness to stress.

C. Neuron Pathways: The genetic determination of neuronal defects is little understood, and neither the enzyme nor hormone mediators are known. An example is neurofibromatosis, an autosomal dominant disease in which there may be behavioral changes and psychosis. Abnormal ectodermal and mesodermal elements are present in the CNS.

It would seem that the individual variation of the fine structure of the brain is as likely to be genetically determined as are the patterns of the dermal ridges of the fingers, which are known to have genetic origins. Monozygotic twins reared apart, for example, have a high concordance rate in their sleep EEG patterns.

GENETIC TRANSMISSION
OF BEHAVIORAL CHARACTERISTICS

Intelligence

The available data show that heredity is an important determinant of intellectual abilities. Twin studies have demonstrated the concordance rates (percentage similarity between pairs) for intelligence to be about 90% in monozygotic twins and about 52% in dizygotic twins. Moreover, monozygotic twins show greater qualitative similarities on most intelligence tests than do dizygotic twins; in fact, the monozygotic concordance rate is about equal to the test-retest reliability of a single individual.

Evidence from twins reared apart supports the role of a hereditary factor in the determination of intelligence. However, grossly unfavorable environmental influences on one twin can lower the high concordance rates of monozygotic twins.

Familial correlation studies have also shown that similarities in intellectual capacity between parents and children appear to depend more on hereditary than on environmental factors.

There are 2 main theories of the mechanism of genetic transmission of intelligence. Hurst postulated that a dominant gene is responsible for the transmission of average intelligence and recessive genes for low or high intelligence. Having the dominant gene in homozygous or heterozygous form would endow the individual with "normal" intelligence; lack of the dominant gene would produce either high or low intelligence. Pickford's theory involves the action of 10 equal and additive gene pairs in the determination of intelligence. Observations show that offspring regress below or climb above parental means toward the population mean. This implies recessivity of extremes and dominance of normality in a multifactorial mechanism.

Personality

Although some twin studies support the view that some testable dimensions of personality depend on inheritance, the weight of the evidence emphasizes the influence of environmental factors.

Very little is known about the mechanism of possible genetic transmission of personality traits, but multifactorial mechanisms are probably involved.

GENETIC TRANSMISSION OF
PSYCHIATRIC DISORDERS

MENTAL RETARDATION

The genetic basis of many types of mental retardation is becoming increasingly clear. Classical family patterns of inheritance, enzyme deficiencies, and chromosomal aberrations have all been found to be associated with subnormal mental development. The following are some of the known inherited causes of mental retardation:

Errors of Metabolism

A. Disorders of Amino Acid Metabolism: Among the autosomal recessive diseases are phenylketonuria, tyrosinosis, maple syrup urine disease, Hartnup's disease, histidinemia, homocystinuria, argininosuccinic aciduria, and hyperprolinemia. Lowe's oculocerebrorenal dystrophy is an X-linked dominant disease with incomplete penetrance which occurs only in males. There are many others, and new ones are being discovered all the time.

B. Disorders of Lipid Metabolism: This group of diseases causes mental retardation with deposition of abnormal lipids in the CNS. These include autosomal recessive disorders such as Tay-Sachs disease, Krabbe's disease, and metachromatic leukodystrophy.

C. Disorders of Carbohydrate Metabolism: Galactosemia, von Gierke's disease, McQuarrie's hypoglycemia, leucine sensitive hypoglycemia, and fructose intolerance are all autosomal recessive diseases.

D. Miscellaneous: Other autosomal recessive metabolic disorders which are known to produce mental deficiency are idiopathic hypercalcemia, pseudohypoparathyroidism, certain cases of goitrous cretinism, familial nonhemolytic jaundice, pyridoxine dependency, and most forms of Hurler's syndrome.

Chromosomal Anomalies

Many chromosomal anomalies are known to be associated with mental retardation. Down's syndrome (mongolism) may result from an extra chromosome 21 (trisomy 21), producing a karyotype with 47 chromosomes, or the extra chromosome may be attached to another chromosome producing a karyotype with 46 chromosomes. *Cri du chat* ("cat cry") syndrome is known to be caused by deletion of part of chromosome 5; Klinefelter's syndrome in the male has an additional X chromosome (XXY), whereas Turner's syndrome in the female has only a single X chromosome. However, mental retardation in both Klinefelter's and Turner's syndrome is relatively mild, and most people with these syndromes are usually able to function well outside institutions. In general, the autosomal anomalies and those involving 3X, 4X, and 5X chromosomes produce severe mental retardation.

About 1–2% of all cases of mental retardation are known to be due to the inheritance of a single abnormal gene, whereas in institutions for the mentally retarded only 5–8/1000 are due to chromosomal aberrations. Mental retardation due to abnormal polygenic inheritance accounts for 20–40% of cases in institutions for the subnormal.

Miscellaneous

There are many other forms of mental retardation in which no chromosomal aberration or biochemical abnormality has yet been found but for which a clear familial pattern of inheritance has been established.

Autosomal dominant diseases are dystrophia myotonica, epiloia, Recklinghausen's disease, Sturge-Weber disease, Lindau-von Hippel disease, Marfan's syndrome, Sjögren's disease, achondroplasia, and craniodysostosis. Autosomal recessive diseases or those whose mode of genetic transmission is unknown are anencephaly, hydranencephaly, porencephaly, microcephaly, macrocephaly, agenesis of the corpus callosum, and some cases of hydrocephaly.

SCHIZOPHRENIA

Incidence

The incidence of schizophrenia in the general population is 0.5–1%. Studies of the incidence of the disease in the families of schizophrenics have shown that it is 10 times more common in the siblings of schizophrenics and in children with one schizophrenic parent and 50 times more common in children with 2 schizophrenic parents. There is clearly a correlation between the magnitude of the risk and the closeness of the relationship to the schizophrenic. However, the husbands and wives or unrelated stepbrothers and stepsisters of schizophrenics have twice the risk of developing the illness as that of the general population. The evidence, therefore, is for a strong genetic predisposition and an additional (but lesser) role played by environment.

Twin studies have shown concordance rates as high as 76–86% for monozygotic twins and 6–12% for dizygotic twins (both lower in recent studies). Monozygotic twins reared apart have essentially the same incidence of becoming schizophrenic as when reared together. Higher concordance rates have been found in the more serious forms of schizophrenia than in the milder forms, and lower concordance rates are reported in paranoid illnesses than in catatonic or hebephrenic illnesses.

In carefully controlled studies investigating the children of schizophrenics (the experimental groups) reared away from their home environment, it was found that there was a significant increase in the incidence of schizophrenia in the experimental groups over that of the controls.

Kety has shown that patients who were nonbiologically adopted in the first few months of life and who later developed schizophrenia showed a significantly higher incidence of schizophrenia in their biologic families than a matched control series.

All this evidence indicates a significant genetic contribution to the etiology of this illness.

Theories of Genetic Transmission

There have been many attempts to demonstrate that schizophrenia is due to a defect in a single gene. The hypothesis of a single causative gene suggests the existence of an inborn error of metabolism, an enzymatic deficiency on which the disease is based. So far, the search for a possible abnormal biochemical mechanism has been suggestive but inconclusive.

Kallmann's original theory proposed that schizophrenia was due to a recessive gene which produced a schizoid personality in the heterozygote and schizophrenia in the homozygote. Other theories have proposed a more simple dominant mode of inheritance. Nevertheless, auxiliary hypotheses are needed to account for the data, and it is most probable that the genetic component in schizophrenia is multifactorial and recessive.

Schizophrenia and Reproduction

At the turn of the century the reproduction rate of schizophrenics was only half that of the general population. Over the last 60 years it has increased to almost 90% since, with modern treatment, schizophrenics are spending less time in hospitals. This tendency of the reproduction rate to approach that of the general population will eliminate any selective disadvantage schizophrenics may have had in terms of human evolution. There is a great need, then, for genetic counseling to prevent as many schizophrenics as possible from reproducing themselves. Children born into a home where one or both parents are schizophrenic not only have a much greater chance of becoming schizophrenic themselves but are also apt to have overwhelming developmental difficulties due to broken homes, separation from the parent during hospitalization, and the sometimes chaotic lives of their parents.

MANIC-DEPRESSIVE PSYCHOSIS

The incidence of manic-depressive psychosis in the general population is 0.4–0.5%. The incidence is at least 20 times as high among close relatives of manic-depressive patients. Family studies reported by Kallmann in 1950 showed that the expectancy rates for manic-depressive psychosis among half-siblings of manic-depressives was 17%; among full siblings, 23%; among dizygotic twins, 26%; and among monozygotic twins, 100%. This maximum concordance rate for monozygotic twins was considered to be artificial since only severe, hospitalized index cases were chosen for the study. Kallmann concluded that manic-depressive psychosis was due to an autosomal dominant gene with incomplete penetrance and variable expressivity. Stenstedt, investigating the morbidity risks in relatives of manic-depressives, postulated a similar genetic transmission.

Although in both studies there was a higher incidence of females in the index cases, the sex ratio among the siblings, parents, and children was no different from that of the general population. The unequal sex incidence in the index cases may be accounted for to some extent by the higher rate of successful suicide in males with manic-depressive illness. In more recent family studies, Reich has postulated a single or double X-linked dominant gene as responsible for the transmission of this illness.

INVOLUTIONAL PSYCHOSIS

The incidence of involutional psychosis among the parents and siblings of schizophrenics is increased 7%, whereas in manic-depressives there is no increase. Kallmann found that in the families of involutional twin index cases the risk of involutional psychosis was increased 6% for parents, 6% for siblings, 6% for dizygotic twins, and 61% for monozygotic twins. The risk of schizophrenia in the same sample was also elevated (6% in parents and 4% in siblings), but there was no increase in risk for manic-depressive psychosis. From these data, it appears that involutional psychosis is more closely associated (in genetic terms) with schizophrenia than with manic-depressive psychosis.

DEMENTIA

Several kinds of dementia are known to have familial or genetic backgrounds.

Senile Dementia

Metabolic, endocrine, and vascular factors are all involved in the etiology of this disease. Twin and family studies have shown that normal and pathologic phenomena of senescence have significant genetic components.

Pick's Disease

A significant number of families suffering from Pick's disease have been reported. In these families it is transmitted as an autosomal dominant. Sporadic cases also occur.

Alzheimer's Disease

This disease is not clearly a genetic disorder, but familial occurrence suggestive of hereditary predisposition has been reported.

Porphyria

This inborn error of metabolism occurs in 4 forms: (1) congenital erythropoietic porphyria (Ganther's disease), which is transmitted as an autosomal recessive; (2) acute intermittent or hepatic porphyria, characterized by a wide range of behavior disorders, which is transmitted as an autosomal dominant; (3) hepatocutaneous porphyria, which is autosomal dominant; and (4) porphyria variegata, also autososomal dominant.

Friedreich's Ataxia

This disease may be associated with paranoid delusions, confusion, depression, excitement, or dementia. It is transmitted as an autosomal recessive disease, but sporadic cases also occur.

Huntington's Chorea

Beginning in the 3rd–5th decades of life, this degenerative disease of the basal ganglia and cerebral cortex, presenting as chorea and dementia, is inherited as an autosomal dominant. Sporadic cases have also been reported.

Wilson's Disease

This is an autosomal recessive disease resulting from an abnormality of copper metabolism and a deficiency of ceruloplasmin and characterized by degeneration of the basal ganglia, cirrhosis of the liver, and a pigmented ring at the limbus of the cornea. Mild dementia is always present, and in adolescents a schizophrenia-like syndrome may develop.

EPILEPSY

Lennox divided epilepsy into "symptomatic" and "essential" forms, depending on whether or not a neuropathologic condition antedated the first seizure. He found concordance rates of 85% for monozygotic twins and 5% for dizygotic twins in the essential group and 14% for monozygotic twins and 0% for dizygotic twins in the symptomatic group. Although the manifestation of the disease is not inevitable even in identical twins, the predilection for it does seem to be inherited. On the basis of the EEG evidence, Lennox proposed that the cerebral dysrhythmia rather than the convulsions is genetically determined (autosomal dominance with incomplete penetrance). Investigations into centrencephalic epilepsy (ie, generalized rather than focal seizures) showed a higher incidence in the parents and siblings of those afflicted than in the general population. A significantly higher incidence of cerebral dysrhythmia was also found in the siblings of centrencephalic epileptics. It was concluded that this kind of EEG record is the expression of an autosomal dominant with highest penetration between ages 4 and 15. Other studies have found focal temporal EEG abnormalities which are inherited as an autosomal dominant.

The probability of children of one epileptic parent being epileptic is between 2.5% and 5% for each child as opposed to 0.5% in the general population. The probability is increased when both parents have the disease.

PSYCHONEUROSES

Slater found an increased incidence of similar neurosis and personality disorders among the relatives of obsessional neurotics, anxiety neurotics, and hysterics. He proposed a multifactorial mode of inheritance with continuous and probably multidimensional variations in traits. It appears possible that constitutional factors alone may be largely responsible for the obsessive-compulsive state, whereas hysteria and anxiety states depend more on environmental factors.

CRIMINALITY

Twin studies have shown concordance rates for criminal and delinquent behavior of 14% for opposite sex dizygotic twins, 54% for same sex dizygotic twins, and 65% for monozygotic twins. This suggests that unfavorable environmental conditions and basic personality structures are both involved in producing the criminal offender. It is possible that the genotype determines the particular physical and psychologic characteristics that predispose toward asocial behavior, eg, physical appearance and strength, aggressiveness, and intolerance for frustration.

The "YY" syndrome may also make a small but significant contribution to the delinquent population.

HOMOSEXUALITY

There was much early debate about whether male homosexuals were in fact genetic females. However, sex chromatin studies and karyotype analysis demonstrated that there are no abnormalities in sex chromatin or sex chromosomes in male homosexuals.

Slater found a high incidence of a later birth order and older maternal age in a group of 401 male homosexuals and suggested a chromosomal anomaly in some homosexuals. Kallmann found an almost 100% concordance rate for male homosexuality in monozygotic twins, whereas in dizygotic twins the concordance rate did not differ from the incidence of homosexuality in the general population.

Some monozygotic twins discordant for male homosexuality have been studied, but in these cases the nonhomosexual twins were found to have sexual confusion and body image distortion. It is possible, therefore, that in male homosexuality genes may play a part in the disarrangement of psychic sexual identification or personality structure. There is no evidence of any abnormality of the gonadal apparatus.

Genetic data on female homosexuality are not yet available.

REFERENCES

Books and Monographs

Beadle, G.W.: *Genetics and Modern Biology.* American Philosophical Society, 1963.

Clarke, C.A.: *Genetics for the Clinician,* 2nd ed. Blackwell, 1964.

Fuller, J.L., & W.R. Thompson: *Behavior Genetics.* Wiley, 1960.

Goodman, R.M. (editor): *Genetic Disorders of Man.* Little Brown, 1970.

Hamerton, J.L.: *Chromosomes in Medicine.* Little Club Clinics in Developmental Medicine No. 5. Medical Advisory Committee of the National Spastics Society, 1962.

Harvald, B., & M. Hauge: Hereditary factors elucidated by twin studies. Pages 61–76 in: *Genetics and the Epidemiology of Chronic Diseases.* Neel, J.V., Shaw, M.W., & W.J. Schull (editors). US Department of Health, Education, & Welfare, 1965.

Inouge, E.: Similarity and dissimilarity of schizophrenia in twins. In: *Proceedings of the 3rd World Congress of Psychiatry.* Vol 1. Univ of Toronto Press & McGill Univ Press, 1961.

Kallmann, F.J.: *Heredity in Health and Mental Disorder.* Norton, 1953.

Kallmann, F.J.: *Expanding Goals in Genetics in Psychiatry.* Grune & Stratton, 1962.

Kringlen, E.: *Heredity and Environment in the Functional Psychosis: An Epidemiological-Clinical Twin Study.* Universitsforlaget (Oslo), 1967.

McKusick, V.A.: *Medical Genetics: An Annotated Review, 1961–63.* Pergamon Press, 1966.

Rosenthal, D. (editor): *The Genain Quadruplets: A Case Study and Theoretical Analysis of Heredity and Environment in Schizophrenia.* Basic Books, 1963.

Slater, E.: *Psychotic and Neurotic Illnesses in Twins.* Her Majesty's Stationery Office (London), 1953.

Journal Articles

Alanen, Y., & others: Mental disorders in the siblings of schizophrenic patients. Acta psychiat scandinav (Suppl 169):168, 1963.

Baker, D., & others: Chromosome errors and antisocial behavior. JAMA 214:869–878, 1970.

Casey, M.D., & others: Sex chromosome abnormalities in two state hospitals for patients requiring special security. Nature 209:641–642, 1966.

Clark, G.R., & others: Sex chromosomes, crime, and psychosis. Am J Psychiat 126:1659–1663, 1970.

Dorzab, J., & others: Depressive disease: Familial psychiatric illness. Am J Psychiat 127:1128–1133, 1971.

Gregory, I. Genetic factors in schizophrenia. Am J Psychiat 116:961–972, 1960.

Kallmann, F.J.: The genetic theory of schizophrenia. Am J Psychiat 103:309–322, 1946.

Kallmann, F.J.: Comparative twin study on the genetic aspects of male homosexuality. J Nerv Ment Dis 115:283–298, 1952.

Kringlen, E.: Schizophrenia in male monozygotic twins. Acta psychiat scandinav, Suppl 178, 1964.

Kringlen, E.: Schizophrenia in twins: An epidemiological-clinical study. Psychiatry 29:172–184, 1966.

Lennox, W.G.: Sixty-six twin pairs affected by seizures. A Res Nerv Ment Dis Proc 26:15–19, 1947.

Lennox, W.G.: The heredity of epilepsy as told by relatives and twins. JAMA 146:529–536, 1951.

Pollin, W., & others: Psychopathology in 15,909 pairs of veteran twins: Evidence for a genetic factor in the pathogenesis of schizophrenia and its relative absence in psychoneurosis. Am J Psychiat 125:597–611, 1969.

Price, W.H., & others: Criminal patients with XYY sex chromosomes complement. Lancet 1:565–566, 1966.

Proceedings of the seminars of the Lesch-Nyhan syndrome. Vermont, October 1967: Fed Proc 27:1019–1112, 1968.

Raphael, T., & M.W. Shaw: Chromosome studies in schizophrenia. JAMA 183:1022–1028, 1963.

Reich, T., & others: Family history studies: The genetics of mania. Am J Psychiat 125:1358–1369, 1969.

Rasavi, L.: Time affects chromosome-crime link. Internal Medicine News & Diagnosis News 4:1, Jan 15, 1971.

Reich, T., & others: Family history studies: The genetics of mania. Am J Psychiat 125:1358–1369, 1969.

Rosenthal, D.: Sex distribution and the severity of illness among samples of schizophrenic twins. J Psychiat Res 1:26–36, 1961.

Rosenthal, D.: Some factors associated with concordance and discordance with respect to schizophrenia in monozygotic twins. J Nerv Ment Dis 129:1–10, 1959.

Rosenthal, D.: The offspring of schizophrenic couples. J Psychiat Res 4:169–188, 1967.

Slater, E.: Genetical factors in neurosis. Brit J Psychol 55:265–269, 1964.

Stabenau, J.R.: Heredity and environment in schizophrenia: The contribution of twin studies. Arch Gen Psychiat 18:458–463, 1968.

Tienari, P.: Psychiatric illnesses in identical twins. Acta psychiat scandinav, Suppl 171, 1963.

Winokur, G.: Genetic findings and methodological considerations in manic depressive disease. Brit J Psychiat 117:267–274, 1970.

XYY syndrome. Leading article. Lancet 1:583–584, 1966.

Zung, W., & others: Sleep and dream patterns in twins: Markov analysis of a genetic trait. Recent Advances Biol Psychiat 9:119–130, 1966.

9 . . .
Psychiatric Epidemiology

Epidemiologic data can contribute to the clinician's under-standing of his patients' diseases. The figures on mental illness have for years portrayed frustration and despair—only recently the beginnings of hope.

Epidemiology is the study of diseases or other health characteristics in populations. By studying the incidence of psychiatric phenomena in a population and other changes in psychiatric variables, information can be obtained which is of potential usefulness in several ways:

(1) Determining "causes" of illness.

(2) Identifying high and low risk groups.

(3) Ascertaining the effectiveness of treatment or prevention methods.

(4) Estimating the social cost of psychiatric disorders and arousing public interest in remedial measures.

Psychiatric epidemiologic research consists primarily of records surveys, along with a few field surveys, but almost no experiments. Reliable and valid data are hard to obtain, partly because of the ambiguity intrinsic in psychiatric nosology and—especially in records surveys—partly because epidemiologic records, as an incidental function of the record-keeping agency, are usually not kept carefully or in a standardized form. However, particularly with data in mental hospitals, the figures from year to year do not seem to fluctuate greatly, and some fruitful comparisons can be made. A step toward improving these statistics was taken in 1951 by the US Public Health Service in the formation of the *Model Reporting Area for Mental Hospital Statistics.* This imposed record-keeping standards and requirements on member states and encouraged uniformity of record-keeping.

The most basic epidemiologic data relate to 2 questions:

(1) How many people are index cases of the problem? (The "prevalence" of the problem, usually expressed as a rate per 100,000 members of the population of comparison.)

(2) How many people become index cases of the problem in a unit time? (The "incidence" of the problem, usually expressed as a rate per 100,000 per year.)

In addition, the following question is important:

(3) What are the characteristics that differentiate index cases of the problem from noncases? (A type of correlation question.)

Data from mental hospitals constitute a prime source of information. The chief rationale is that people who are inpatients in mental hospitals are mentally ill and that they are improved if and when they are discharged into the community. The data presented below pertain to the system of hospitals in the USA serving psychiatric patients. They are of 4 types: state and county mental hospitals, Veterans Administration hospitals, private mental hospitals, and psychiatric wards in general hospitals. From the standpoint of this system, the following questions are important:

(1) How many patients *are in the system* at the start of a unit period of time? What is the distribution of patients within the system according to age, sex, and diagnosis?

(2) How many patients *come into the system* during a unit period of time?

(a) A patient may be newly admitted to one facility within the system but not be newly entered into the system itself (eg, if he is transferred from a different facility within the system).

(b) Since figures for the system as a whole are obtained only from individual hospitals, each of which keeps its own records for each patient, there is some inaccuracy in obtaining system-wide figures. (An individual may be listed as a new admission by more than one hospital, eg, if he changes hospitals.)

(3) How many patients *leave the system* during a unit period of time?

(a) Discharge to another hospital outside the system (eg, a hospital outside the USA; this is a negligible consideration).

(b) Death.

(c) Discharge into the community. (This depends on the course of patients' illnesses, but it may also be influenced by administrative changes in discharge policies. When a hospital's discharge rates increase, it is not always a reflection of improved treatment.)

(4) What is the average duration of time an individual spends *within the system?* (Since it is impossible to know the average length of stay for any group of patients until they all leave the system, figures for patients in recent years can only be estimates.)

(5) What influences a patient's *readmission to the system* if he has been previously discharged?

(6) What are the *costs of hospitalization* per patient?

(7) What are the *changes in mental hospital figures* over a period of years?

General trends of the data will be discussed, and further information may be obtained in the tabular supplement at the end of this chapter.

BASIC EPIDEMIOLOGIC DATA: RECORDS SURVEYS

Examples of the kind of data obtainable from records surveys follow.

Mental Hospitals

In the USA* there are about 400,000 patients residing in mental hospitals on any given day—about 200 for every 100,000 Americans. (The rates vary considerably from one locality to another, sometimes by as much as an 8:1 ratio from highest to lowest.) Eighty percent of the patients are in state and county hospitals, 10% in Veterans Administration hospitals, and 10% in private or general hospitals.

In the period of a year, about 500,000 people enter the mental hospital system for the first time. Almost 60% enter for the first time through general hospitals, while only 14% enter through state and county hospitals and 10% through private hospitals. Another 250,000 enter a facility within the mental hospital system during a year as transfer patients from other facilities or as second (or higher) admissions to the system from the community. Most of these go to state and county hospitals.

Public and private hospitals tend to differ in their distribution of patients. Seventy percent of patients in private hospitals are psychotic or neurotic, while only 25% have personality or organic disorders. In contrast, less than 40% of patients in state and county hospitals are psychotic and neurotic, while 60% have personality or organic disorders.

Psychotics outnumber neurotics in both types of institutions. More psychotics and neurotics are women, while more patients with personality and organic disorders are men. In about 15% of first admissions, alcohol or—to a lesser extent—drugs are involved. Only rarely is first admission due to a suicide attempt. About half the patients admitted to hospitals because of personality disorders are addicted to drugs or alcohol.

For every 10 patients already in the *mental hospital system* (not those just admitted to the system), one dies each year. Approximately 90% of patients admitted to the system are released from it. The average length of stay per patient is about 1 year. Most releases occur within 6 months after admission to a mental hospital, but in 1967 over 20% of patients hospitalized in the Veterans Administration system had been there more than 10 years. Most of these were psychotic or had chronic brain syndrome. Fewer than 20% of neurotics or patients with personality disorders in the Veterans Administration system had been hospitalized longer than 1 year. Caucasians, married people, and females tend to be released earlier and more frequently than people of other races, people in other marital status groups, or males. Males who have committed at least one antisocial offense are released earlier from mental hospitals than other males, and, like females, have lower hospital death rates (as they improve mentally, many are quickly transferred to jails).

*Mental hospital data for London are in the same general ranges as in the USA.

As of 1952, only 20% of senile patients were discharged from hospitals, while almost 50% died within a year of admission. Not surprisingly, younger persons within the senile group did better than older ones.

About half the admissions to mental hospitals represent readmissions or intrasystem transfers. During a year, about 33% of cases treated within the system have been under the care of 2 or more inpatient or outpatient facilities. People discharged from mental hospitals are more likely to be readmitted shortly after their discharge than after a long period of time, ie, if they can manage the initial readjustment to the community, they are not likely to return to the hospital.

In the 10-year period ending in 1965, the number of patients admitted to state and county hospitals increased by almost 150,000 per year—an increase of 85%—while patients resident in them declined over 50,000 patients—a 10% decrease. (Prior to 1955, a psychiatric turning point, the resident population had been increasing.)

The average daily maintenance expenditure for state and county patients was less than $7.00 in 1965—a disgraceful figure. Veterans Administration hospitals spent $15.00 per patient per day, while private hospitals spent $22.00. General hospitals spent nearly $42.00 per day for their psychiatric inpatients (pro rata expenses for laboratories, x-ray departments, pathology resources, etc are included).

Hospitals for the Mentally Retarded

There are almost 200,000 patients in hospitals for the mentally retarded, and about 10% of that number enter each year. Half of those admitted are eventually released to the community and about one-fourth die. The population in such hospitals is still increasing.

Outpatient Clinics

Approximately 1.6 million psychiatric patients per year are seen in outpatient clinics in the USA.

Suicide and Homicide Data* (For basic information, see Table 9–1.)

A. Suicide:

1. Racial incidence—Nonwhite males exceed white males up to age 50.

2. Occupational considerations—The suicide rate for physicians is about 10% more than expected considering all occupations, while the suicide rate for psychiatrists is higher than for physicians as a group.

3. Geographical incidence—In the USA, metropolitan and nonmetropolitan counties tend to have similar suicide rates. Southern states (except Virginia and Florida) tend to have the lowest rates and western states the highest rates. In 1960, 5 of the 6 metropolitan areas with the highest rates

*Note that only a small fraction of suicides and homicides occur because of mental illness. Reported figures are underestimates because of reluctance to have deaths classified as suicide.

TABLE 9–1. Suicide and homicide: Basic information (USA).

	Suicide	Homicide*
Number in 1967	21,325	13,425
Rate per 100,000 in 1964	10.8	6.8
Highest rate since 1921	17.4 (1932)	9.8 (1933)
Lowest rate since 1921	9.8 (1957)	4.2 (1961)
Approximate ratio whites/nonwhites	11/5	1/9
Age-sex-race group: Highest rate per 100,000	White males over age 85: 56.3	Nonwhite males ages 20–39: 116.6
Sex-race group: Lowest rate	Nonwhite females	White females

*Note that in the last few years suicide rates have remained about the same, while homicide rates, especially among nonwhite males, have risen significantly.

(ie, more than 15 per 100,000 population) were in either California or Florida.

4. Method employed—Firearms are more frequently used than other means; next in frequency are hanging and strangulation. Drugs are used more by women than by men, and they constitute the least successful method of suicide.

5. Incidence of suicidal attempts—Attempts by men tend to be both more violent and more successful than those by women. Perhaps one-sixth of those who attempt suicide are successful, while one-seventh of those who succeed have made a previous attempt. (Different studies give somewhat different figures.)

6. Illness and alcoholism as factors in suicide—While probably not more than one-third of those who commit suicide have ever suffered from a major mental disorder, the suicide rates in mental hospitals are 3–5 times higher than in the general population. Most people who commit suicide after leaving a mental hospital do so within the first 90 days. Up to one-third of all who commit suicide suffer from serious physical illness. Alcohol is a contributing factor in less than one-fifth of suicides.

7. Climatic, demographic, and social factors—Suicides occur most frequently in spring, with the month of April tending to have the highest rate and December the lowest. Unlike crime and delinquency, suicide is not associated with poverty as such, and it tends to decrease in wartime periods and in concentration camp situations. About one-fifth of those who commit suicide were living alone at the time. Especially among middle- and upper-class groups, the incidence of suicide fluctuates with the business cycle, increasing during depression periods and decreasing during prosperity periods.

8. As with mental illness, suicide occurs less among married persons and more among those who are widowed, single, or divorced. The rate of suicide among married people decreases with the birth of each child until the sixth child is born, when it increases.

TABLE 9−2. Prevalence of mental disorder.
Review of 11 surveys (Plunkett & Gordon).

Survey	Total Mental Disorders Per 100,000 Population
Nassau County, 1916	3,640
Eastern Health District (Baltimore), 1933	4,450
Eastern Health District, 1936	6,050
Williamson County, Tennessee, 1935−1938	4,670
Hutterite Communities, Western USA, 1950	1,670
Hunterdon County, New Jersey, 1951−1955	13,800
Baltimore, 1953−1955	10,860
Salt Lake City (over age 16), 1955	33,300
Syracuse (age 65 and over), 1955	23,200
Syracuse (age 65 and over; serious incapacity), 1955	5,300
Midtown Manhattan (age 20−59; "psychiatric impairment"), 1952−1958	23,300

TABLE 9−3. Prevalence and incidence of mental disorder.
Review of 5 surveys (Lewis).

Survey	Prevalence
England and Wales (mental deficiency), 1929	860 per 100,000 population (total); 2560 per 100,000 population, ages 10−14
London suburb GPs' patients (nervous symptoms), 1940−1942	20−40% of all patient visits (depending on time of the year)
GPs' patients in England and Wales (400,000 patients, neurotic disorders), 1955−1956 (1 year)	457 per 100,000 population consulted their doctor for a neurotic complaint. (One of every 15 patients who consulted a GP during the year.)
Southeast London GPs' patients (psychiatric morbidity), 1956−1957 (1 year)	7% of all men and 11% of all women registered with the GPs consulted them for psychiatric problems. 5% more patients had nonconspicuously-disabling personality abnormalities. (Investigators stated that if they had included patients who had illness without physical cause and stress-induced "psychosomatic" disorders, the figure would have exceeded 50% of those consulting the GPs.)
Midlands (3000 engineering factory workers; neurotic illness and symptoms), 1947	10% had definite neurotic illness; 20% more had minor nondisabling neurotic symptoms.

9. Suicide rates in other countries—For men, the highest rate is in Hungary: 35.5 per 100,000 population. The rates in Austria, Sweden, West Germany, Japan, France, and Australia are all above 20 per 100,000, while in Italy the rate is only 7.1 per 100,000. For women, the highest rate is in Japan: 14.3 per 100,000 population. In Hungary, Austria, and West Germany the rates are above 10 per 100,000, while in Italy the rate is only 2.9 per 100,000.

B. Homicide: Among nonwhite men, the rate of homicide victims exceeds 100 per 100,000 in the age group 20—39 and is above 50 per 100,000 between ages 15—64. The highest rate of victims among white men is 7.2 per 100,000 between ages 25—29. The highest rate of victims among nonwhite women is 21.7 per 100,000 between ages 25—29.

Drug Production and Sales in the USA

In 1965, 779,000 pounds of barbiturates (an estimated 3.5 billion doses) and 1,573,000 pounds of tranquilizers (an estimated 7 billion doses) were produced in the USA. Sales were approximately 65% of production. (An unknown proportion of production was devoted to foreign markets.)

Costs of Mental Illness in the USA

The estimated annual cost of mental illness in the USA is $20 billion. The sources of this cost include expenses for hospitals and other treatment facilities, the loss of earnings of the ill, and expenses for assistance to the mentally ill and their dependents.

FIELD SURVEYS OF THE
INCIDENCE OF MENTAL ILLNESS

One way of estimating the magnitude of the overall mental health problem is the field survey, which usually consists of questionnaire interviews conducted by specially trained interviewers. In some of the studies reviewed below, physical examinations or psychologic tests were performed also. Final evaluation of the records (and the decision about whether or not mental illness was present) was done by a panel of experts including a psychiatrist.

It is recognized that populations and sampling procedures are highly variable features, but in the examples summarized below an attempt was made to obtain representative samples of the limited populations studied.

It is worth noting that different investigators working in different areas and with different age groups reported widely divergent estimates of the prevalence of mental illness (see Tables 9—2 and 9—3).

Note the extreme variation both among these rates and between these rates and those obtained from treatment records. Some variation probably results from difference in population, some from sampling error, some from method of investigation and evaluation. It is almost certain that the number of patients under treatment for diagnosed mental illness represents but a small fraction of the total number with symptoms and impairments attributable to mental illness.

CORRELATION STUDIES

The following are some of the generally agreed-upon findings.

Factors Positively Correlated With Mental Illness or Suicide

(1) Physical illness in childhood or adult life.

(2) Age and sex: See hospital tables, the trend of which is confirmed in other studies.

(3) Marital status: Single, divorced, and widowed persons have higher rates of disorder than married persons.

(4) Childhood broken homes (death of a parent or separation of parents; also parental quarreling).

(5) Perception of a parent's character as deficient.

(6) Geographical considerations.

(a) Urban dwellers have higher rates than rural.

(b) Area in the city: Mental disorder tends to decrease from the center of a large city to the periphery. Different disorders occur to a greater extent in different areas. For example, there is more paranoia in the rooming-house districts; more catatonia in districts with new immigrants (eg, from other countries or interstate, eg, Negroes moving north); and more arteriosclerosis and senile psychosis in districts with the lowest proportion of homeowners. The greatest rate of Boston's psychiatric rejections for the army in World War II came from poor neighborhoods.

Social isolation is regarded as an important correlation factor in mental illness rate differentials across districts.

(7) Economic factors: The lower classes tend to have relatively more mental illness, especially schizophrenia, general paresis, and alcoholic psychoses; the upper classes have relatively more affective disorders and neuroses.

(8) Ethnic factors: Different ethnic groups tend to have different patterns of mental illness incidences. However, after other factors such as age and marital status are partialed out, the differences are difficult to evaluate and the conclusions are unsatisfactory. In Texas, Anglo-Americans had the highest overall rates of psychosis, whereas Spanish-Americans had the highest rate of affective psychosis. Nonwhites had the highest rates of toxic and syphilitic psychoses. In Texas, the 3 ethnic groups had different relative rate distributions according to geographical area in the state.

(9) Major social changes: Non-Western people isolated from their place of birth and in contact with Western people (eg, tribal workmen imported for industrial work) tend to have higher rates of mental illness than the people who stay in the native locale (though the rates tend to be less than those of Westerners). Bomber crews (less so for pilots) became most upset from the 5th through the 12th dangerous bombing mission.

(10) People characterizable in terms of greater numbers of the above factors have proportionally higher mental illness rates than those characterizable by lesser numbers of them.

(11) The following factors have not been generally agreed on as important in relation to mental illness: occupation, immigration (but see ¶ [6b], above), major social events such as wars or depressions.

Factors Associated With Variation in Treatment

A. Age: Multiple psychiatric admissions to a hospital or clinic are more common among middle-aged adults than among the very old or the young. The use of psychiatric facilities is relatively high for nonwhite adult males but low for nonwhite children of either sex.

B. Ethnic Factors: In Texas, the only group using private facilities more than public facilities was Anglo-American females. (That datum is a few years old, and the situation may now be different.) In Texas, urban area nonwhites used public facilities 20 times as much as private facilities. The case was similar in rural areas. In Maryland, whites tend to use outpatient facilities more than nonwhites.

C. Social Class and Income Factors: Upper-class patients in a clinic are more likely to receive psychotherapy, especially by the more experienced therapists, and to stay longer in treatment than patients from other classes. Middle-class patients are more likely to have an emphasis on drugs. Lower-class patients tend to receive organic or drug treatment or no treatment (less commonly, group therapy).

1. Some probable reasons are that psychotherapy is more consonant with upper-class patients' expectations from psychiatry; they are verbally more adaptive to psychotherapy, find it easy to relate and be related to by conversation, and are more often self-referred. Lower-class patients are often referred at the instigation of others than the patient himself (eg, by a judicial officer, with some element of compulsion).

2. Not surprisingly, patients who make use of private psychiatric facilities tend to have higher incomes than those using public facilities.

Some Findings From a Major Interview Survey Regarding Adjustment and Mental Health (Gurin & others)

Happy people worry more than unhappy people (who have tended to give up hope for improvement). The major issues for most people regarding happiness and worry are economic security and family concerns.

More highly educated people tend to be more self-critical than those with lesser education. (Women are also more self-critical than men.)

Self-critical people are more likely to seek help than less self-critical persons. People who see a defect in themselves are more likely to see psychiatrists than those who see their problems as coming from others.

Older men are more satisfied with their jobs and report fewer work problems than younger men.

More highly educated people tend to react to stress with psychologic symptoms; less well educated people react with somatic symptoms.

One in 5 said "yes" to a question about present or previous concern over a nervous breakdown. (About half of those people saw a doctor at the time.) Most of these occurred at crisis times involving death or illness of a loved one, personal illness, or job and financial tension.

Sixty-five percent of people who consulted clergymen or nonpsychiatrist physicians said they were helped, while 46% of those who saw psychiatrists said they were helped. (One hopes it was the more serious cases that were seen by psychiatrists.) One person in 7 said he did not go for help because of the stigma of emotional problems. Only 28% of people who sought professional help mentioned that someone else referred them to the source of help.

Significance of the Foregoing

It must be acknowledged that unfortunately the data summarized above are of limited significance. Yet, despite this limitation, the findings are of considerable interest. For example, the case is made that treated patients comprise only a fraction of sick patients; however, in a given locality, the factors that influence the value of that fraction probably do not change greatly over a short time, and data concerning treated patients do bear some relation to "true incidence" and "true prevalence." These data thus probably represent not only the best estimate of incidence and prevalence available but also useful estimates of those parameters. Furthermore, correlation studies provide some basis for leverage for an attack upon various public aspects of mental illness control. Thus, suggestions about where to look for likely cases, where to concentrate educational programs, which agencies to focus on for collaboration in mental health efforts, etc can be found in available epidemiologic data despite their obvious limitations. Indeed, the nature of the field is such that no matter how much investigative effort is devoted to it, the conclusions arrived at will probably always have an irreducible amount of uncertainty. The wise approach would seem to be to refine technics as much as possible (as feasibly and as flexibly as can be done) and plan programs on the basis of the data, humbly realizing not only that the plans will be imperfect but that where the imperfections lie cannot always be known.

TABULAR SUPPLEMENT*†

USPHS MENTAL HOSPITAL DATA

Except as otherwise specified, the figures presented below are approximations based on extrapolations from data presented by the US Public Health Service for the years 1962 and 1964.

(1) Total patients resident in mental hospitals on a given day (1966):

	No.
State and county	386,190
VA	57,120
Private (estimated)	14,000
Total USA	457,310

(General hospital beds are not included, since psychiatric patients admitted to general hospitals stay a relatively short time. Later figures are not available, but totals for 1970 for the USA are estimated to be about 400,000 patients.)

(2) Average number of patients resident in state and county mental hospitals per 100,000 population:

	No.
USA	254.4
Highest state (New York)	489.3
Lowest state (Utah	60.8

(Comparison of highest and lowest states is inserted to indicate the range of variation from one locality to another.)

(3) New admissions to mental hospitals in a year:

	No.	%
USA	534,342	100
State and county (1965)	144,042	27
VA	17,600	3
Private	60,700	11
General (based on the assumption that 90% of psychiatric admissions are first admissions)	312,000	58

*Percentage figures have been rounded off and may not add precisely to 100.
†Figures for private and general hospitals are extrapolated from available data on the assumption that figures for nonreporting hospitals are not greatly different from those for reporting hospitals.

(4) First admissions by diagnosis, age, and sex:

(a) Grand total first admissions:

State and County Hospitals
Male   78,300
Female   60,000
                138,300*

Private Hospitals
Male   23,650
Female   38,500
                62,150

*Grand total first admission figures are not the same as those in previous tables because not all hospitals reporting first admissions also reported first admissions by diagnosis, age, and sex.

(b) Psychosis:

	Total: All ages		Under 24		25–54		55–74		Over 75	
	No.	%*	No.	%	No.	%	No.	%	No.	%
				State and County Hospitals						
Male	16,285	11.77	4430	3.22	9660	6.97	2110	1.52	85	.06
Female	20,120	14.57	3460	2.49	13,700	9.88	2865	2.07	95	.07
	36,405†	26.34	7890	5.71	23,360	16.85	4975	3.59	180	.13
				Private Hospitals						
Male	7799	12.55	1884	3.04	4500	7.25	1322	2.11	93	.01
Female	15,767	25.32	2320	3.73	10,540	16.95	2740	4.42	167	.03
	23,566	37.87	4204	6.77	15,040	24.20	4062	6.53	260	.04

*% refers to the fraction that category represents of *total first admissions* in either broad group—state and county or private mental hospitals.
†Marginal totals have been adjusted to be consistent with internal totals. There may be slight error because of decimal rounding off.

(c) Psychoneurosis:

	Total: All ages		Under 24		25–54		55–74		Over 75	
	No.	%	No.	%	No.	%	No.	%	No.	%
				State and County Hospitals						
Male	5563	4.08	1012	.73	3740	2.70	774	0.56	37	.03
Female	10,074	7.26	1970	1.42	6780	4.88	1256	0.91	68	.09
	15,637	11.34	2982	2.15	10,520	7.50	2030	1.47	105	.12
				Private Hospitals						
Male	6206	9.96	784	1.25	4220	6.77	1154	1.85	48	.08
Female	13,719	22.05	1940	3.12	9460	15.18	2197	3.53	122	.19
	19,925	32.01	2724	4.37	13,680	21.95	3351	5.38	170	.27

(d) Personality disorders:

	Total: All ages		Under 24		25–54		55–74		Over 75	
	No.	%	No.	%	No.	%	No.	%	No.	%
			State and County Hospitals							
Male	24,902	18.00	5660	4.09	16,560	11.97	2620	1.89	62	.04
Female	7110	5.14	2165	1.56	4470	3.23	459	.33	16	.01
	32,012	23.14	7825	5.65	21,030	15.20	3079	2.22	78	.05

(Of the total personality disorders first admitted to state and county hospitals, 55.77% involve alcohol and drug addiction.)

	Total: All ages		Under 24		25–54		55–74		Over 75	
			Private Hospitals							
Male	4934	7.92	918	1.48	3215	5.16	774	1.24	27	.04
Female	3650	5.86	868	1.39	2369	3.80	398	.64	15	.01
	8584	13.78	1786	2.87	5584	8.96	1172	1.88	42	.05

(Of the total personality disorders first admitted to private hospitals, 48.18% involve alcohol and drug addiction.)

(e) Acute and chronic organic mental disorders (except mental deficiency, birth trauma, and prenatal conditions):

	Total: All ages		Under 24		25–54		55–74		Over 75	
	No.	%	No.	%	No.	%	No.	%	No.	%
			State and County Hospitals							
Male	21,433	15.50	1118	.81	5540	4.00	7720	5.58	7055	5.10
Female	16,426	11.79	562	.46	2474	1.78	6005	4.38	7385	5.34
	37,859	27.29	1680	1.27	8014	5.78	13,725	9.96	14,440	10.44

(Of the total of organic mental disorders first admitted to state and county hospitals, 12.58% were acute, mostly under age 55. The rest were chronic brain syndromes.)

	Total: All ages		Under 24		25–54		55–74		Over 75	
			Private Hospitals							
Male	3630	5.82	186	.30	1188	1.90	1514	2.43	742	1.18
Female	4160	6.67	182	.29	1060	1.70	1387	2.22	1531	2.46
	7790	12.49	368	.59	2248	3.60	2901	4.65	2273	3.64

(Of the total of organic mental disorders first admitted to private hospitals, 18.4% were acute, mostly under age 55. The rest were chronic brain syndromes.)

(f) First admissions involving alcohol or drugs: (Not a separate category. All alcohol and drug admissions were listed under other categories. Over 80% involved alcohol. Most patients were under age 55. Only a very small fraction represents drug intoxication, as in suicide attempts.)

	No.	%
State and County Hospitals		
Male	20,560	15
Female	3890	3
	24,450	18
Private Hospitals		
Male	4145	7
Female	2294	4
	6439	11

(g) Comparison of state and county vs private mental hospital first admissions by proportions in broad diagnostic categories:

	State and County Hospitals	Private Hospitals
Psychosis	26%	38%
Psychoneurosis	11%	32%
Personality disorder	23%	14%
Organic disorder	27%	12%
	87%	96%

(5) Total admissions to mental hospitals in a year: (New admissions, readmissions, transfers, etc.)

	No.	%
USA	805,043	100
State and county hospitals	314,443	39
VA hospitals	38,300	5
Private hospitals	105,700	13
General hospitals	346,600	43

(6) Total mental hospital admissions per 100,000 population:

	No.
USA	416
State and county hospitals	164
Highest (Connecticut), 314	
Lowest (Hawaii), 72	
VA hospitals	20
Private hospitals	54
General hospitals	178

(7) Number of releases (alive) from mental hospitals in a year (and not entering other mental hospitals):

	No.	%
USA	699,039	100
State and county hospitals	286,989	41
VA hospitals	35,050	5
Private hospitals	99,100	14
General hospitals	277,900*	40

*Note that 71,300 releases from general hospitals (20% of psychiatric admissions to general hospitals) were released to other kinds of mental hospital facilities.

(8) Number of releases from mental hospitals (not entering other mental institutions) per 1000 total admissions to hospitals:

> State and county hospitals (USA): 913
> Highest (Hawaii), 1211*
> Lowest (New York), 754

> *The figure of 1211 releases per 1000 admissions implies that in that year more patients left the hospital system than entered it. The residual number of patients in the system at the year's end was less than at the beginning of the year.

(9) Total time on hospital rolls for different diagnostic groups: (US Veterans Administration, 1962; random sample from VA hospitals.)

Diagnosis	No. of patients	Under 3 months	3–5.9 months	6–11.9 months	1–1.9 years	2–9.9 years	10 years and over
Brain syndrome	12,455	2,470	1,130	1,245	2,020	3,900	1,690
Psychosis	31,680	5,125	2,375	2,540	3,030	8,425	10,185
Neurosis	4,405	2,705	620	380	400	280	20
Personality disorder	2,800	1,985	270	225	140	145	35
Total patients	51,820	12,455	4,420	4,425	5,615	12,855	12,050

(10) Daily maintenance expenditures per resident patient:

State and county hospitals (USA, 1969)	$12.59
Highest (Alaska) $38.93	
Lowest (Mississippi) $ 5.40	
VA hospitals	16.00 plus
Private hospitals	33.00 (approx.)
General hospitals	44.00 plus

(11) Changes in state and county hospital totals in 10 years:

	1955	1965
Total number of resident patients at one time	553,922	492,577*
Total admissions per year	178,003	314,443
Net releases per year	126,498	286,989
Deaths in hospital per year	44,384	44,270
Daily maintenance expenditures per resident patient	$3.06	$6.74

*The resident population has decreased in all age groups except under age 25, in which there has been an increase.

(12) Average stay in hospital: Because it is impossible to know the average length of stay of patients admitted in a given period of time until all those admitted during that time either die or are released, exact average stay figures cannot be determined for recent years. It can only be said that the average stay in the late 1950s and 1960s seems to be less than 1 year and that prior to that time it was greater than 1 year. (This conclusion is based on the simple observation that the number of resident patients increased until the 1950s and has been decreasing since then.) As of 1959 it appears that a person admitted to a mental hospital with a diagnosis of schizophrenia has a 4 in 5 chance of being discharged within a year. Note that the above figures list 805,043 admissions but only 699,989 discharges and 53,970 deaths (a total of 753,959 reductions of hospital rolls, while 51,084 were additions to hospital rolls), yet the total number of patients resident in mental hospitals is decreasing. (*Explanation:* Since the same individual may be the source of 2 admissions but only one discharge in a year if he is discharged from a mental hospital to which he was transferred from a general hospital, the total admissions figure is inflated relative to the discharges figure.)

(13) Outpatient psychiatric clinics (1967):

Cases terminated during year	703,000
Total patients treated (estimated)	1,600,000

(14) Public and private institutions for the mentally retarded (1966):

Resident patients at end of year	189,858
Admissions	14,998
First admissions	12,986
Live releases	9,202
Deaths in hospital	3,601

(The number of males generally exceeds that of females in hospitals for the retarded. In ages above 35, females exceed males.)

STATE OF TEXAS STUDY*

"Psychosis" included "functional," "organic," and "old-age" psychoses.

Annual incidence of psychosis (ie, occurrence of new cases): 73.3 per 100,000 population.

(1) By age:

Lowest rate:	Under 15 years
	1 per 100,000 population
Highest rate:	75 and older
	225 per 100,000 population

(Generally, rate increased with age increase.)

*Comprehensive record survey, including inpatient, outpatient, and private practice facilities, 1951 and 1952 (Jaco).

(2) By diagnosis:
Functional psychosis about 51 per 100,000 population.
Organic psychosis about 22 per 100,000 population.

STATE OF MARYLAND CASE REGISTER, 1962 (BAHN)

(1) Prevalence of treatment in psychiatric facility (1962): 1080 per 100,000 Maryland residents.

(2) Incidence of new cases entering treatment in psychiatric facilities in Maryland (1962): 440 per 100,000 residents.

(3) Of total cases both in treatment in July 1961, and entering treatment in 1962, 53% were treated in outpatient facilities and 47% in inpatient facilities.

(4) Approximately 30% of all patients (not on facility rolls in July 1961) receiving treatment during the following year either were admitted to 2 or more facilities or to the same facility 2 or more times; thus, the total number of admissions was multiplied by a correction factor of 0.7 to determine the number of persons receiving treatment.

(5) The figures above omit patients seen by privately practicing psychiatrists and are, therefore, underestimates.

REFERENCES

Books and Monographs

Causes of Mental Disorders: A Review of Epidemiological Knowledge, 1959. Milbank Memorial Fund, 1961.

Faris, R.E.L., & H.W. Durham: *Mental Disorders in Urban Areas: An Ecological Study of Schizophrenia and Other Psychoses.* Univ of Chicago Press, 1939.

Gurin, G., Veroff, J., & S. Feld: *Americans View Their Mental Health.* Basic Books, 1960.

Hoch, P.H., & J. Zubin (editors): *Comparative Epidemiology of the Mental Disorders.* Grune & Stratton, 1961.

Jaco, E.G.: *The Social Epidemiology of Mental Disorders.* Russell Sage Foundation, 1960.

Langner, T.S., & S.T. Michael: *Life Stress and Mental Health.* Macmillan, 1963.

Leighton, D.C., & others: *The Character of Danger: Psychiatric Symptoms in Selected Communities.* Basic Books, 1963.

Lewis, C.A.: Current field studies in mental disorders in Britain. Chap 11 in: *Comparative Epidemiology of the Mental Disorders.* Hoch, P.H., & J. Zubin (editors). Grune & Stratton, 1961.

Monroe, R.R., Klee, G.D., & E.B. Brody: *Psychiatric Epidemiology and Mental Health Planning.* Psychiatric Research Report No. 22. American Psychiatric Association, 1967.

National Committee Against Mental Illness: *What Are the Facts About Mental Illness in the United States?* Washington, 1966.

Norris, V.: *Mental Illness in London.* Chapman & Hall, 1959.

Outpatient Psychiatric Services, 1967. Public Health Service Publication No. 1982. National Institute of Mental Health, 1969.

Pasamanick, B. (editor): *Epidemiology of Mental Disorder.* American Association for the Advancement of Science, 1959.

Patients in Mental Institutions, 1964. Parts 2 & 3. US Public Health Service, 1964.

Person, P.H.: *The Relationship Between Selected Social and Demographic Characteristics of Hospitalized Mental Patients and the Outcome of Hospitalization.* American University (Washington, DC), 1964.

Plunkett, R.J., & J.E. Gordon: *Epidemiology and Mental Illness.* Basic Books, 1960.

Provisional Patient Movement and Administrative Data, State and County Mental Hospitals, United States, 1965. Mental Health Statistics Current Reports. US Public Health Service, 1966.

Pugh, T.F., & B. MacMahon: *Epidemiologic Findings in United States Mental Hospital Data.* Little, Brown, 1962.

Reissman, F., Cohen, J., & A. Pearl (editors): *Mental Health of the Poor.* Macmillan, 1964.

Rose, A. (editor): *Mental Health and Mental Disorder: A Sociological Approach.* Norton, 1955.

Sainsbury, P.: *Suicide in London: An Ecological Study.* Chapman & Hall, 1955.

Schneidman, E.S., & N.L. Farberow (editors): *Clues to Suicide.* McGraw-Hill, 1957.

Statistical Abstract of the United States, 1966. US Department of Commerce, 1966.

Stengel, E., & N. Cook: *Attempted Suicide: Its Social Significance and Effects.* Chapman & Hall, 1958.

Suicide in the United States, 1950–1964. Vital and Health Statistics, Series 20, No. 5. US Department of Health, Education, and Welfare, 1967.

US Monthly Vital Statistics Report: Annual Summary for 1961. Part 2, Vol 10, No. 10. July 31, 1962.

Veterans With Mental Disorders, 1963–1967. Public Health Service Publication No. 1934. National Institute of Mental Health, 1969.

Veterans With Mental Disorders Resident in Veterans Administration Hospitals, October 31, 1962. Publication No. 1223. US Public Health Service, 1962.

Vital Statistics of the United States, 1967. US Bureau of the Census, 1967.

Zubin, J., & others: Epidemiological aspects of prognosis in mental illness. Pages 119–142 in: *Epidemiology of Mental Disorder.* Pasamanick, B. (editor). American Association for the Advancement of Science, 1959.

Journal Articles

Bahn, A.K., & others: Services received by Maryland residents in facilities directed by a psychiatrist. Pub Health Reports 80:405–416, 1965.

Beiser, M.: A study of personality assets in a rural community. Arch Gen Psychiat 24:244–254, 1971.

Cerbus, G.: Seasonal variation in some mental health statistics: Suicides, psychiatric admissions and institutional placement of the retarded. J Clin Psychol 26:61–63, 1970.

Reifler, C.B., & M.B. Lipitzin: Epidemiological studies of college mental health. Arch Gen Psychiat 20:528–540, 1969.

10 . . .

Mental Hospitals

Modern practice trends strongly against hospitalizing the mentally ill. Nevertheless, certain exigencies (serious danger of suicide or other violence, unmanageability, catatonia) require hospitalization, and other classes of patients (some alcoholics, narcotic addicts, patients with extreme forms of obsessive compulsive, or phobic, or hysterical neuroses) do better if treatment begins with hospitalization. State mental hospitals, psychiatric wards in general hospitals, and private psychiatric hospitals each have their advantages and disadvantages.

THE STATE MENTAL HOSPITAL*

TRADITIONAL CONCEPT OF THE ROLE OF THE STATE MENTAL HOSPITAL

Until recent years, the major task of the state hospitals was the physical care and control of the inmates. Acute personnel shortages imposed a pyramidal system of authority in the interest of efficiency. The patients' direct contacts were principally with the aides, who reported to the nurses, who reported to the physicians, who reported to the superintendent. Orders involving all aspects of the patient's life came from the superintendent down through the various echelons and finally to the patient.

The new patient went to an admission ward where the best staff and the few available therapeutic facilities existed. This was his chance to get well. If substantial improvement did not occur within a few weeks or months, he began the descent through the ward system to ever more chronic and perhaps violent wards. With each step downward, there were fewer staff, less treatment, less privacy, more regimentation, and more hopelessness. The hospital usually had no outpatient services, and little assistance was available to the discharged patient.

Not all patients who remained in hospitals had such a bleak prospect. Many people who could not tolerate the stressful outside community were able to do well in the protected hospital environment. They obtained varying degrees of privilege and freedom. They usually ran the farm, maintained the

*Admission procedures are discussed in Chapter 37.

143

gardens, did the laundry, and cooked the food. For many patients, this environment represented their optimum social adjustment, and they were well served by a great many dedicated professionals working under difficult circumstances.

CURRENT TRENDS AND CONTEMPORARY STATUS OF STATE MENTAL HOSPITALS

The recent trend (in the last 10 years) has been toward decentralization of authority and toward the use of the hospital milieu as an integral part of the therapeutic experience. The most common method of decentralization has been the unit system. The hospital is divided into several autonomous sections, each responsible to a unit director. A 1200-bed hospital may thus function as four 300-bed units, each with its own treatment, eating, and sleeping facilities.

In some hospitals the patients in the units are divided into sections under a leader who may be a physician, social worker, registered nurse, or recreational therapist. Each section is subdivided into social units under the care of aides.

An essential feature of the milieu concept is that all personnel have therapeutic potential, ie, not only the usual professionals but also the aides and all others who have contact with the patient. Their therapeutic role is facilitated by team meetings where all can express their opinions, describe problems, and participate in their solution. Patient groups and patient government organizations give the patients themselves a voice in ward decisions.

The goal of milieu therapy is open and easy communication at all levels. The traditional hierarchical and authoritarian professional roles and relationships are minimized.

In addition to the change it implies in the hospital environment, the unit system encourages closer relations with the community. Each unit is usually responsive to a specific segment of the community. The particular unit becomes the mental hospital for this geographical area. Outpatient diagnostic and therapeutic services are provided for the same population by the same unit. Follow-up observation and care of discharged patients are carried out in the same manner.

Only a few state mental hospitals have fully implemented the changes in therapeutic approach mentioned in the foregoing paragraphs, but most have adopted at least some of the concepts of the therapeutic milieu.

Nationally, in spite of greatly increased numbers of admissions, the number of beds in use has declined. In the USA the overall decrease in the state mental hospital population has been over 12% from 1957 to 1970. A 50% decrease is common, and at least one state has reported an 80% decrease of patients in mental hospitals.

There has been a marked increase in public interest in and support for mental health programs, resulting in much more adequate staffing. Because of the lowered chronic population and improved staffing, the patient-staff ratio has moved in a much more favorable direction. This has permitted all personnel to exchange their custodial role for a therapeutic one.

Because better care is available in the hospital and because the public has learned to accept psychiatry as a method of solving problems, there has been a notable rise in the number of voluntary admissions. This has introduced an entirely new category of patients. Where at one time only "very sick" people entered mental hospitals—primarily psychotics and a few severe neurotics and alcoholics—the proportion of patients with neuroses and personality disorders has increased markedly in recent years. This has been a factor contributing to the improved milieu and increased optimism in state hospitals, since this new patient population demands a greater flexibility of treatment philosophy.

Organic therapies are still in use, but they no longer constitute the whole armamentarium. Tranquilizing and antidepressant drugs are the main therapeutic resource for the psychotic population.

Electroconvulsive therapy is employed less frequently than was at one time the case—usually only for severe suicidal depressions. It is now seldom used as a means of controlling behavior. Psychosurgery and insulin coma therapy have almost passed into history along with hydrotherapy, cold packs, and physical restraints. There is a trend toward transferring patients with chronic diseases such as schizophrenia and chronic brain syndrome to nursing and custodial homes, thus permitting the state hospital to focus therapeutically on more acutely ill patients.

Group therapy of the more formal, traditional type is still being used, although it appears that the therapeutic community is tending to replace group therapy. There is a greater emphasis also on recreational and occupational therapy, with particular attention to their role in fostering constructive social interaction.

Hospitalization now tends to be brief and flexible. The patient may receive treatment during the day and return home at night; a working man may maintain his job and receive treatment in the evening. The emphasis is on maintaining contact with the family and community and helping the patient to adapt to them more effectively. Social and other agencies in the community are being utilized as an extension of the treatment process. Some hospitals have utilized the space freed by the decreased patient population to provide onsite social agencies.

FUTURE THERAPEUTIC ALTERNATIVES TO THE STATE MENTAL HOSPITAL

The state hospitals have been severely criticized for the poor care they have traditionally offered the mentally ill, and have been blamed for the large numbers of chronic patients that exist. Many mental health professionals have urged the abolition of the state hospital.

A growing segment of the community psychiatry movement who espouse the social model state that the medical model, which defines mental disorders as illnesses, is outmoded and that it interferes with appropriate care. Advocates of this view believe that the sources of deviant behavior lie in the environment and in disturbed interactional processes. They go further and claim that the knowledge necessary to correct mental disturbances already exists and that we have only to learn how to deliver these insights to the community. In their opinion there is no further need for any mental hospitals.

The high discharge rate and decreased chronic population in some states does suggest that other states with less impressive records are not providing effective treatment. The difference between a 12% decrease in patient population in one part of the country and an 80% decrease rate in another certainly raises this question. However, in considering this accusation it must be remembered that discharge rates are not necessarily correlated with improvement. Follow-up studies on patients in the "progressive" states indicate that clinical improvement does not parallel statistical improvement and that the number of chronic patients remains about the same. Their behavior is less socially disruptive because they are receiving drugs, but it is questionable whether a withdrawn patient sitting at home watching television all day or rocking quietly in the corridors of a county home represents noteworthy improvement.

The methods of treatment that have proved most effective in mental illness are largely those of an organic nature derived from the medical model: penicillin to prevent general paresis, niacin for the dementia of pellagra, thyroid for myxedema madness, tranquilizers for a wide range of disturbed behavior, electrotherapy and antidepressants for depression, and lithium for mania.

Social engineering has not yet been demonstrated to be effective, although it may be in the future.

If all our attention turns to community mental health and if all our resources, financial and intellectual, are directed toward primary, secondary, and tertiary prevention of mental illness, the seriously ill and chronic patient will again be in danger of neglect. The major psychiatric problems are still with us and cannot be eliminated by new definitions of illness and administrative fiat. This means that the patients who are most in need of help are in danger of being left out of the mainstream of psychiatric effort and progress. It would be ironic indeed if the current "revolution" should again fill the "alms houses and county homes" with the mentally ill whom Dorothea Dix found in the 19th century and who stimulated her far-reaching reforms to obtain care for the neglected insane.

A progressive attack on the problems of the mentally ill will utilize *both* medical and social models. It will recognize that most psychiatric problems are still poorly understood but that their solutions are worth seeking. The state hospital and the chronic patient will not be rejected but will become a part of a comprehensive search for treatment based on a rational, scientific understanding of etiologic processes, whether they be organic, social, intrapsychic, or some combinations of these.

There are already examples of state hospitals having become integrated with the community mental health services. Mental health clinics and other social agencies can be located in the state hospital. Laboratories of many types can be based there, particularly those focused on the unresolved problems of chronic mental illness. This comprehensive facility can be the center of training in all aspects of mental illness—acute and chronic, organic and functional. Persons in a wide range of disciplines working together can recognize the contributions that each can make and can perceive the incredible complexity of the problems involved. Such a center for service, training, and research will attract the best personnel and have the best facilities available. All patients of whatever type will receive optimal care based on current knowledge and the latest research. In this way, the reality of mental illness, our progress, and our deficiencies will be constantly kept before us. Abolition of the state hospital can only have the unfortunate effect of denying our ignorance and encouraging yet another "cult of curability."

THE GENERAL HOSPITAL

PSYCHIATRY SERVICES IN GENERAL HOSPITALS

In the mind of the general public, there are many stigmas attached to being admitted to a mental hospital; and the usual rural and inconvenient location of mental hospitals, making visiting difficult and increasing the patient's sense of isolation, further deters the psychiatric patient from accepting admission. The psychiatry service of a general hospital is a much less frightening and more convenient place to receive short-term psychiatric hospitalization. The patient with early symptoms is more likely to seek or accept help sooner if general hospital admission is offered, and this has the effect of avoiding catastrophic emergencies, preventing deterioration, and facilitating early treatment and unembarrassed return to the community.

ROLES OF THE PSYCHIATRY SERVICE IN THE GENERAL HOSPITAL

The psychiatry unit of a general hospital should provide the following services: inpatient care, day care, outpatient care, emergency care, and consultation to the general wards.

The Inpatient Ward

The ward varies in size and complexity depending upon the size and needs of the hospital and the community. Although the idea of accepting "unmanageable" patients or those with severe mental illness in a general hospital is still resisted, the availability of psychotropic drugs now makes it possible to treat all types of patients in a general hospital. However, because the number of beds available is limited, the community cannot afford to allocate them for custodial care. The hospital must concentrate on the segment of the psychiatric patient population most amenable to short-term intensive care. Most of these patients are willing to enter hospital on a voluntary basis, and therefore the stigma of "commitment" is unnecessary. Similarly, locked doors and physical restraints are rarely needed.

The design of the ward should facilitate observation of the circulation areas by the nurses without sacrificing the patients' need for privacy. Single rooms tend to deprive patients of the stimulation necessary to maintain good contact with reality, and potentiate feelings of isolation and loneliness. Wards with too many patients may be very disturbing and interfere with privacy. Wards consisting of 4—6 screened beds seem to be ideal.

The circulation areas and dayroom should be bright and airy and comfortably furnished. A supply of newspapers and magazines encourages the patient to maintain interest in community and world affairs.

Visiting hours are usually the same as in the rest of the hospital. Telephone privileges and passes to leave the hospital for short periods may be granted depending upon the physician's view of the patient's needs.

Staffed by psychiatrists, nurses, psychiatric social workers, psychologists, and occupational therapists, the inpatient ward should provide a full range of therapeutic approaches, including ECT and milieu therapy. ECT can be given in the patient's own bed, or it may be more convenient to use a special room set aside for this purpose. Having diagnostic and laboratory facilities readily available promotes greater efficiency in treatment and shortens the period of hospitalization.

The cost of a psychiatric inpatient bed in a general hospital is the same as for other patients in the hospital. The cost is greater than in a large mental institution, but this may be balanced by the shorter period of hospitalization.

The Day Care Center

The creation of day care facilities in psychiatric units in general hospitals reflects the general trend away from custodial treatment of mental illness and toward the open ward with the objective of returning the patient to his community. The day care center provides treatment for patients who require only part-time hospitalization. It may serve as a primary treatment center for early therapeutic intervention, thus avoiding the necessity for inpatient care; or it may provide a transitional facility for patients being discharged from the inpatient service, facilitating earlier discharge. Full-time hospitalization isolates the patient from his family and community and encourages relatives and friends to abrogate their responsibilities to him. Day care minimizes dependency and regressive phenomena by maintaining contact between the patient and his family and community.

The day care center can offer most of the therapeutic facilities available on the inpatient service.

The Outpatient Department

Besides providing a follow-up facility for discharged inpatients and day care patients, the outpatient department receives patients referred from the other departments of the hospital, from the emergency service, and from agencies outside the hospital. Individual psychotherapy, family therapy, and group therapy are all managed in the outpatient department, as well as pharmacotherapy, social service casework, and evaluative services such as psychologic testing.

The Emergency Service

Many patients who come or are brought to the general hospital emergency service have psychiatric problems requiring emergency diagnosis and management. The immediate availability of psychiatric consultation on a 24-hour, walk-in basis facilitates care and referral. Early contact with the patient with emergency psychiatric problems makes possible early intervention and prevents deterioration and is an asset to a community mental health service.

The Consultation Service

An important function of the psychiatric service of the general hospital is to provide a consultation service to the rest of the hospital and to encourage a more comprehensive approach to patient care. The general management of disturbed, frightened, toxic, and confused patients and those with puerperal psychosis, anorexia nervosa, depressive illnesses accompanying physical disabilities, and psychosomatic disorders is greatly enhanced by interdepartmental cooperation in the general hospital. In particular, understanding of the toxic confusional state or delirium occurring in the course of medical or surgical illness has increased greatly with the advent of psychiatric units in general hospitals.

PRIVATE PSYCHIATRIC HOSPITALS

Private psychiatric hospitals occupy a very important and frequently unrecognized position in the treatment of psychiatric patients in the USA. Private psychiatric hospitals are active treatment institutions that admit patients with a wide range of psychiatric diagnoses, provide continuous 24-hour service, and have organized medical staffs. They are operated on a nonprofit or proprietary basis and, if associated in some way with a larger institutional complex, they have sufficient administrative or physical independence to be recognized as separate entities.

The National Association of Private Psychiatric Hospitals lists about 130 members, and there are 60 nonmember hospitals. The association encourages member hospitals to obtain accreditation from the Joint Commission on Accreditation of Hospitals of the AMA. Private psychiatric hospitals increased the percentage of accreditation from 57% in 1966 to 75% (101) in 1967, a much higher percentage of accreditation than among state hospitals.

Private psychiatric hospitals account for 15,000 beds (2% of the psychiatric beds of the nation) and average 40,000 first admissions and 30,000 readmissions per year. The average cost per day in a private psychiatric hospital is about half the cost of general hospital care. Third-party payments (such as commercial insurance, Blue Cross, and Medicare) pay for about 65–70% of the expense.

The length of stay varies with the therapeutic orientation of the hospital, but the acute patients' stay averages 3–5 weeks. The average stay for chronic patients is longer.

The types of psychiatric treatment available in private psychiatric hospitals are the same as in other psychiatric care facilities. Some private psychiatric hospitals still offer insulin treatment in selected cases, but in general the orientation is toward brief psychotherapy, drug therapy, electroconvulsive therapy, and activity therapy. Newer forms of therapy, such as lithium carbonate, unipolar ECT, day care only, night care only, family therapy, and conjoint marriage therapy, are being tried by some. A limited number of hospitals specialize in long-term, psychoanalytically oriented psychotherapy of patients with schizophrenic reactions and severe character disorders. The treatment of alcoholism is undertaken, particularly if there is an underlying emotional problem.

Most private psychiatric hospitals are reluctant to accept children or young adolescents.

Preferably, admissions to private mental hospitals are voluntary; however, all but a few will accept involuntary patients under the particular laws of the state. In some areas, private psychiatric hospitals serve as comprehensive community mental health centers, and others are participating actively in planning for future centers. Many offer beautiful and spacious grounds as well as elaborate rehabilitative, occupational, and recreational facilities.

The advantages of private psychiatric hospitals over public hospitals are as follows: (1) the greater acceptability to patients because of greater privacy and less stigma; (2) better patient-staff ratios; (3) the greater rapidity with which patients can be evaluated and treated; and (4) the fact that the referring physician may continue to care for his patient during hospitalization and following discharge, so that there will be no break in the patient-doctor relationship.

The advantage of private hospital care over treatment in a psychiatric ward in a general hospital is that the orientation of the entire hospital is toward the care of the mentally ill patient. More facilities can be offered than in most general hospitals, where psychiatry and psychiatric patients with their special needs are sometimes regarded as necessary evils.

REFERENCES

Books and Monographs

Brook, C.P.B., & D. Stafford-Clark: Chap 12, pp 111–118 in: *Trends in the Mental Health Services.* Freeman, H., & J. Ferndale. Pergamon Press, 1963.

Cummings, J., & E. Cummings: *Ego and Milieu Theory and Practices of Environmental Therapy.* Atherton, 1962.

Glasscote, R., & C. Kanno: *General Hospital Psychiatric Units.* Joint Information Service of the APA and NAMH, 1965.

Kaufman, M.R. (editor): *The Psychiatric Unit in a General Hospital.* Internat Univ Press, 1968.

Martin, M.: *The Mental Ward.* Thomas, 1962.

Journal Articles

Beahan, L.T.: Emergency mental health services in a general hospital. Hosp Community Psychiat 21:81–84, March 1970.

Caplan, M.A., & D. Blaine: Organizational obstacles to change in a large mental hospital. Am J Psychiat 126:1107–1114, 1970.

Detre, T., & D. Kessler: The role of the general hospital in modern community psychiatry. Am J Orthopsychiat 33:690–700, 1963.

Dunham, H.W.: Community psychiatry: The newest therapeutic bandwagon. Arch Gen Psychiat 12:303–313, 1965.

Fortin, J.N., & others: The evolution of psychiatry in the general hospital: Retrospective study and statistics. Un Med Canada 96:699–701, 1967.

Hammersley, D.W., & P. Vosburgh: Iowa's shrinking mental hospital population. Hosp Community Psychiat 106:166, 1967.

Herz, M.I., Wilensky, H., & A. Earle: Problems of role definition in the therapeutic community. Arch Gen Psychiat 14:270–276, 1968.

Kaplan, H.M., & D. Blaine: Organizational obstacles to change in a large mental hospital. Am J Psychiat 126:1107–1114, 1970.

Kraft, A.M., Binner, P.R., & B.A. Dickey: The community mental health program and the longer-stay patient. Arch Gen Psychiat 16:64–70, 1967.

Kubie, L.S.: Pitfalls of community psychiatry. Arch Gen Psychiat 18:257–266, 1968.

Linn, L.S.: State hospital environment and rates of patient discharge. Arch Gen Psychiat 23:346–351, 1970.

Mannuccii, M., & M.R. Kaufman: The psychiatric in-patient unit in a general hospital: A functional analysis. Am J Psychiat 122:1329–1343, 1966.

Mendel, W.M., & S. Rapport: Determinants of the decision for psychiatric hospitalization. Arch Gen Psychiat 20:321–328, 1969.

Messier, M., & others: A follow-up study of intensively treated chronic schizophrenic patients. Am J Psychiat 125:1123–1127, 1969.

Orwin, A.: The mental hospital: A pattern for the future. Brit J Psychiat 113:857–864, 1967.

Ozarin, L.D., & A.I. Levenson: The future of the public mental hospital. Am J Psychiat 125:1647–1652, 1969.

Persons, P., Harley, P., & R. Giesler: Psychiatric patients in general hospitals. Hospitals 40:64–68, 1966.

Pupostamon, P.A.: Psychiatric consultations in a general hospital. Psychosomatics 11:57–62, 1970.

Rond, P.C.: Psychiatry and the community general hospital. Ohio MJ 60:751–753, 1964.

Silverman, M.: Psychiatric units in general hospitals. Lancet 2:47–48, 1970.

Statistical Reports: Lunatic asylums in the United States. Am J Insan 2:46–68, 1845.

Tourney, G.: A history of therapeutic fashions in psychiatry, 1800–1966. Am J Psychiat 124:92–104, 1967.

Visher, J.S., & M. O'Sullivan: Nurse and patient responses to a study of milieu therapy. Am J Psychiat 127:451–456, 1970.

Wortis, J.: Physiological treatment. Am J Psychiat 117:595–600, 1961.

11...

Statistics in Psychiatry

Statistics are an essential part of scientific method. Psychiatrists (and all physicians) should understand the basic statistical concepts and be able to use them in evaluating data.

The subjective nature of many of the observations and interpretations in psychiatry makes it somewhat more difficult to apply statistical methods to psychiatry than to many other disciplines of clinical medicine. Perhaps for this reason, it is especially important to have a working familiarity with the statistical terms and reasoning that are most commonly used in psychiatry.

There are 5 major applications of the term statistics. The first is implied in such terms as actuarial, descriptive, vital, record-keeping, etc—the simple and straightforward counting and summarizing of data. It is applied to such questions as how many schizophrenics are hospitalized each year, what proportion of college students are under psychiatric care, etc.

Statistics are applied also to the problem of approximating an underlying constant of nature, eg, the speed of the nerve impulse. Because it is usually not possible to obtain a single direct, error-free measure of these constants, a number of measures must be gathered as a means of arriving at approximate values. Statistics are used to evaluate their accuracy so that the approximation of the constants can be continuously refined.

Statistical reasoning is used also in attempting to predict an event on the basis of knowledge about the potential influence of each factor involved. For example, a prediction about whether or not a college freshman will eventually graduate depends upon the relative importance of different factors for graduation (IQ, endurance, reading ability, etc) and the relative strengths of these factors within the student.

The fourth application of statistics is to explore for regularities in nature. This usage underlies the correlation coefficient (discussed below). The exploration for regularities or relationships is usually a prelude to further investigation to determine the nature of the relationships. For example, a study disclosing a relationship between emotional disturbance and criminal behavior would have to be extended to determine whether the emotional disturbance led to the criminal behavior, the criminal behavior (and its consequences) led to the emotional disturbance, or the criminal behavior and the emotional disturbance were both caused by a third factor such as social estrangement.

The fifth and most controversial application of statistics is to arrive at some judgment concerning data. Examples of such judgments are whether the results of a study confirm or reject a given hypothesis, or whether the results are accurate reflections of reality or not. This is the usage leading to statements of "statistical significance." The controversial nature of this usage arises from the fact that statistical significance is often erroneously equated with logical significance, so that it is often used as the judgment itself rather than as an aid to judgment.

The 5 uses of statistics briefly described above are not mutually exclusive, and any or all uses may be employed in a given data analysis.

BASIC STATISTICAL CONCEPTS

It will be of help in the discussion that follows to establish a set of measurements that can be used for reference purposes. Because measurements collected in an actual study are often too numerous and complex to be useful for brief illustrations, we will use a set of measurements that could have been collected in a hypothetical study of the effectiveness of a new drug, XX, in reducing the duration of alcoholic delirium tremens. Let us say that the study employed 2 groups of 7 perfectly matched alcoholics who were just beginning to show symptoms of delirium tremens: (1) an *experimental group* who received the new drug; and (2) a *control group* who did not receive the drug. The results show that symptoms of delirium tremens abated in the 7 alcoholics in the experimental group after 2, 3, 3, 4, 6, 8, and 9 hours; and in the 7 alcoholics in the control group after 12, 13, 13, 14, 16, 18, and 19 hours.

Central Tendency

When a number of different measurements has been collected, it is often useful to derive one value to represent them all. The value most commonly used for this purpose is the *central tendency,* or, as it is often called, the *average.* A common misconception is that there is only one average for a given set of data. In reality, there are 3 acceptable methods of arriving at an average, and each method may yield a somewhat different value.

(1) **Mode**: The mode is the most frequently appearing value in a series of values. In our hypothetical study, the modal average for the experimental group is 3 and for the control group 13.

(2) **Median**: The median is the midpoint in a series of measures, 50% of the measures falling above this midpoint and 50% falling below. In our hypothetical study, the median average for the experimental group is 4 and for the control group 14.

(3) **Mean**: The mean is obtained by a simple summation of all values divided by the number of values. In our hypothetical study, the mean average for the experimental group is 5 and for the control group 15.

These examples demonstrate how the average can fluctuate as a function of the measure of central tendency used. None of the 3 ways of measuring central tendency unfailingly yields the most representative value in a set of measures, yet all give "statistically accurate" values. Each has its advantages and disadvantages, and the choice of which is "best" for a given set of data is determined more by the purposes of the researcher than by statistical formulas.

Variation

One of the fundamental properties of measurements in psychiatry is that they often vary from one another even when they purport to measure the same phenomenon. This property is referred to as *variation,* and it arises from 2 major sources: *experimental influences,* associated with known and controlled variables; and *chance or error influences,* associated with unknown and uncontrolled variables. The experimental influences, of course, are usually the foci of interest in a study, and variations produced by their presence lead to greater stability, predictability, and understandability of the data; whereas variations produced by the presence of chance or error influences have the opposite effect. For this reason, statistical analyses are often concerned with determining the relative proportion of each source of variation in a given set of research results. In our hypothetical study, the variation of measures *within* each group would be considered due to chance or error influences (since all subjects were matched to control known sources of variation), and the goal of a statistical analysis would be to determine how much of the variation in scores *between* the groups was due to the experimental influence (ie, the new drug) and how much was due to chance or error.

(1) **Range**: The simplest statistic to use in describing the amount of variation is the range, which is given by the endpoint values. In our hypothetical study, the range for the experimental group is 2–9. The range is the least stable or informative description of variation and is of limited usefulness in statistical analyses.

(2) **Deviation**: The difference between an individual value and the mean value is termed a deviation.

(3) **Variance**: When all the deviations in a set of measures are squared, summed, and divided by the number of measures, the result is the variance. In other words, the variance is the mean of the squared deviations. The experimental group in our hypothetical study had a mean of 5; the variance, therefore, would be $(5-2)^2 + (5-3)^2 + (5-3)^2 + (5-4)^2 + (5-6)^2 + (5-8)^2 + (5-9)^2$ divided by 7, or 44 divided by 7, or 6.29. By a similar procedure, and by coincidence, the variance for the control group can be shown to be 6.29 also. Variance is a useful statistical concept because it has properties necessary for many different kinds of mathematical operations. For example, the mean of 2 or more variances will give the variance for all measures combined. In our hypothetical study, the variance for all 14 measures can be obtained by simply adding the variances for the 2 groups and dividing by 2 rather than by finding the mean of all 14 measures, computing the deviations, squaring them, and so on. This is being discussed not to provide a short-cut in statistical computations but to illustrate the important principle that variances are additive. This principle makes it mathematically possible to analyze the variation in a set of measurements into components attrib-

utable to *experimental influences* and *chance or error influences.* This is the goal involved in a frequently used statistical technic called *analysis of variance.*

Standard Deviation

The standard deviation is a measure of the constancy of data. It is the square root of *variance.* For our hypothetical experimental group, the standard deviation is the square root of 6.29 or 2.51. In this example, it would be the same for the control group and for both groups combined.

Standard Error

The standard error is a measure of the dependability of data. It is the standard deviation divided by the square root of the number of measures when the number of measures is 30 or above or by the number of measures *minus 1* when the number of measures is below 30. (The reason for different procedures associated with the number of measures need not concern us here.) Our experimental and control groups would each have a standard error of 2.51 divided by the square root of 6, or 1.02, The combined groups have a standard error of 2.51 divided by the square root of 13, or 0.69.

The standard error is assumed to approximate the standard deviation of the *mean* value in a set of measurements. The idea is that if a number of different sets of measurements were collected (eg, if an experiment were repeated many times), each set would probably yield a different mean because of chance or error influences on each set of scores. As these means were collected, they could be treated as a new set of scores which would yield a mean (the mean of the means), standard deviation, variance, and so on. The standard error is an approximation of the standard deviation of this hypothetical set of means, and, since it can be obtained from knowledge of only one mean and its standard deviation, it obviously is easier and quicker to use the standard error than to collect a whole set of means to determine its standard deviation. The importance of the standard error is that it represents the amount of *variation* in scores that can be expected from *chance and error influences.* It will be recalled that one of the goals of statistical analyses is to determine what proportion of the variation is due to *chance and error* and what proportion to *experimental influences.* The standard error gives an estimate of the proportion due to chance and error.

This discussion has limited itself to the standard error of the mean. The same conceptual basis underlies standard errors of other statistics.

Correlation

When 2 or more variables are related in such a way that a variation in one is accompanied by a lawful and consistent variation in another, the relationship can be expressed by a *correlation coefficient.* If the variations occur in the same direction (eg, if more education is always accompanied by more conventionality), the correlation coefficient is *positive;* if the variations occur in opposite directions (eg, if more education is always accompanied by less conventionality), the correlation coefficient is *negative.* If the variations occur in the same direction up to a point and in opposite directions thereafter (eg, if more education is accompanied by more conventionality up to the high school years and by less conventionality after that), the correlation coefficient is *curvilinear.*

The correlation coefficient is a measure of relationship and not cause and effect. In the above example, more education could be either the cause or the effect of conventionality, or both education and conventionality could be the effect of still another variable, such as dependency.

There are various correlation coefficients such as *rank-order, biserial, correlation ratio, multiple, partial* and others which differ mainly in method of computation (and underlying assumptions) and not in meaning.

Probability

The term probability refers simply to credibility. Mathematicians speak of establishing probabilities that an event will or will not occur, but what they are attempting to establish is the *credibility of the belief* that the event will or will not occur. There are no probabilities attached to events themselves: either they will occur or they will not. Weather bureau statisticians computing the probability of rain tomorrow are referring to the credibility of the belief that it will rain tomorrow and not to the actual occurrence of the rain, for either it will or will not rain.

Level of Significance

The object of a statistical test of significance is to arrive at a figure that will succinctly express the probability that obtained results are not artifacts due to chance or error but are really due to experimental influences. It is important to keep in mind that the statistical test of significance in these cases establishes only the *credibility of the belief* that the obtained results are due to experimental influences and not that they are in fact due to experimental influences.

Keeping in mind that a statistical test refers to the credibility of an interpretation of results makes it easier to avoid the confusion that arises from the extraordinary fact that *statistical tests invariably involve a double negative.* Tests of significance require that the belief to be tested be the one that states, "The results are not due to experimental influences." If the statistical test indicates that this statement has very low credibility, then the opposite of that statement, ie, "These results are due to experimental influence," is assumed to be credible. Furthermore, the credibility of the latter belief is assumed to be in inverse proportion to the lack of credibility of the former belief, ie, the less one can accept the former belief, *presumably* the more one can accept the latter belief.

Because this double negative aspect is so essential to understanding statistical tests of significance, it is worth restating: Generally speaking, *a statistical test does not lead to a confirmation of a positive statement about data but to a negation of a negative statement.*

"p," the probability figure usually used to indicate *level of significance,* refers to the credibility of the negative statement. Thus, a *p* value of 0.05

associated with a set of results indicates that chance or error influences alone would produce the obtained results 5 out of 100 times. In this case the statement, "The results are not due to experimental influences," would have low credibility (5 out of 100 chances of being true), whereas the opposite statement, "The results are due to experimental influences," would have high credibility (95 out of 100 chances of being true). The inverse relationship between the credibility of the 2 statements combined with the fact that p refers to the credibility of the negative statement explains why we say the smaller the probability figure, the more statistically significant the results. The point at which p indicates "significance" (eg, 0.01, 0.05, 0.1, etc) is determined by custom and not by mathematics. In psychiatric clinical studies, a p of less than 0.05 ($p < 0.05$) is generally regarded as impressive; in laboratory studies, $p < 0.01$ is more convincing and desirable. *F ratio* is the ratio of the variance of one set of scores with the variance of another set of scores. An F ratio significantly different from 1 indicates that different influences were present in the 2 sets of scores. One of the variances commonly used in the F ratio is an estimate of the variance that would be obtained by the sole influence of chance or error factors. A significantly greater amount of variance in a given set of scores over the estimated chance variance presumably is due to the influence of nonchance factors, ie, the experimentally manipulated factors.

Analysis of variance: Analysis of variance is one of the technics commonly used to analyze research data. The major advantage of the technic is that it makes possible multiple comparisons using the same basic data by regrouping the data in various ways and determining the *variance* of each different grouping. The *F ratio* is used in these comparisons. Another advantage of the analysis of variance technic is that it allows an evaluation of *interaction effects* between experimental variables. For example, in a study of the effect of sex and diagnoses on length of hospitalization, it may be found that males and females are hospitalized for equal lengths of time and that schizophrenics and manic-depressives are also hospitalized for equal lengths of time, but that males with diagnoses of schizophrenia are hospitalized significantly longer than other groups. Thus, the important determiner of length of hospitalization would be neither of the main variables alone, sex and diagnoses, but rather a particular combination (interaction) of the variables. The analysis of variance technic is one of the few methods of evaluating these interaction effects.

Critical ratio and *t* ratio: These ratios are used to determine whether obtained differences (eg, between 2 means) are larger than would be expected by the operation of chance or error influences alone. The ratios are of obtained differences to the *standard error* of the differences. The critical ratio is used when the number of subjects is 30 or more, and the *t* ratio is used when the number of subjects is less than 30.

Chi-square is used to determine whether an obtained distribution of scores differs significantly from the distribution expected by the operation of chance or error influences alone. The technic employs categorization of variables. For example, in a study of mental illness and intelligence, the former variable could be broken into the categories of normal, mild, moderate, and severe; and the latter variable could be broken into the categories of low, normal, high, etc.

REFERENCES

Books and Monographs

Armore, S.J.: *Introduction to Statistical Analysis and Inference for Psychology.* Wiley, 1966.

Blackwell, D.: *Basic Statistics.* McGraw-Hill, 1969.

Bross, I.D.J.: *Design for Decision.* Macmillan, 1953.

Downie, N.M., & R.W. Heath: *Basic Statistical Methods,* 3rd ed. Harper, 1970.

Freund, J.E., & F.J. Williams: *Dictionary Outline of Basic Statistics.* McGraw-Hill, 1966.

Games, P.A., & G.R. Klare: *Elementary Statistics: Data Analysis for the Behavioral Sciences.* McGraw-Hill, 1967.

Glass, G.E., & J.C. Stanley: *Statistical Methods in Education and Psychology.* Prentice-Hall, 1970.

Hammond, K.R., & J.E. Householder: *Introduction To the Statistical Method.* Knopf, 1963.

Herzog, E.: *Some Guidelines for Evaluative Research.* Children's Bureau, 1959.

Huff, D.: *How to Lie With Statistics.* Norton, 1954.

Klugh, H.E.: *Statistics: The Essentials for Research.* Wiley, 1970.

McCall, R.B.: *Fundamental Statistics for Psychology.* Harcourt, Brace & World, 1970.

McNemar, Q.: *Psychological Statistics,* rev ed. Wiley, 1955.

Psychiatric Research and the Assessment of Change. GAP Report No. 63. Group for the Advancement of Psychiatry, (Nov) 1966.

Some Observations on Controls in Psychiatric Research. GAP Report No. 42. Group for the Advancement of Psychiatry, (May) 1959.

Wallis, W.A., & H.V. Roberts: *Statistics: A New Approach.* Macmillan, 1956.

Journal Articles

Thorpe, J.G., & A.A. Baker: Statistics, science, and psychiatry. Arch Gen Psychiat 1:338–341, 1959.

12...

History of Psychiatry

Those who do not remember the past are condemned to relive it. —Santayana

I. GREEK, ROMAN, AND ARABIC INFLUENCES

(1) **Hippocrates** (460–377 BC) and the Hippocratic authors of *Corpus Hippocraticum* expounded the view that temperaments are based on a mixture of bodily humors. This doctrine was held by many physicians well into the 18th century, and treatment of abnormal temperaments was aimed at restoring the proper balance of humors. The *Corpus* includes descriptions of diseases recognizable as melancholia, postpartum psychosis, phobias, toxic delirium, senile dementia, and hysteria. This can be considered as the first attempt to classify mental diseases. The importance of the doctor-patient relationship was stressed.

(2) **Herophilus** (c 335–280 BC), considered to be the "father of anatomy," did not accept the doctrine of bodily humors and attributed mental abnormalities to defects within the brain.

(3) **Asclepiades** (c 150 BC) believed mental abnormalities to be the result of emotional disorders. He emphasized the distinction between acute and chronic diseases and differentiated illusions from delusions. He advocated psychologic methods in treatment.

(4) **Celsus** (25 BC–50 AD), in his medical textbook, *De Re Medicina,* advocated harsh treatment for mentally ill patients to shock them into health. This influential book was one of the first medical books to be printed (1478), and it provided a rationale for the brutal treatment of deranged persons for centuries.

(5) **Aretaeus** (50–130 AD), an insightful clinical observer, was one of the first to study premorbid personalities of the mentally ill and to conduct follow-up studies. He was the first to describe mania and depression as 2 phases of one illness. He advocated an eclectic approach in treatment.

(6) **Soranus** (93–138 AD) made many accurate, classical descriptions of mental illnesses. He also advocated an eclectic humane approach in treatment, emphasizing that harsh treatments are usually ineffective because of the defective reasoning of the mentally ill.

(7) **Galen** (c 130–200 AD) propagated the humoral theory of temperaments in a dogmatic fashion that hindered the development of knowledge concerning the roots of mental illness.

(8) **St. Augustine** (354–430 AD) wrote an influential self-analysis *(Confessions)* that illustrated the role of early memories, emotional conflicts, and irrational feelings in the mental life of man.

(9) **An asylum for the mentally ill** was built in Baghdad in 705 AD. One of the first recorded in history, it provided relatively humane treatment for the mentally ill.

(10) **Rhazes** (865–925 AD), called the Persian Galen, was physician-in-chief of the Baghdad Hospital, one of the first hospitals to have a ward for mentally ill patients. His views combined an organic cause of mental illness with psychologic methods of treatment.

(11) **Maimonides** (1135–1204 AD), in addition to describing depression in a detailed clinical manner, advocated a mental hygiene program for sound mental health.

II. THE DARK AGES (c 300–1500 AD)

Following the disintegration of the Roman Empire, there began a reversion to supernatural and demoniacal explanations for mental illness. Although the mentally ill were believed to be possessed by demons, their treatment was relatively humane for many centuries. In Europe, this treatment gradually became more brutal and punitive and reached its lowest point with the publication of the *Malleus Maleficarum* (c 1487), in which the prescribed treatment for mental illness was torture and death.

III. PRODROMES OF MODERN PSYCHIATRY

(1) **The first European hospital** devoted entirely to mentally ill patients was constructed in Valencia in 1409. The treatment of patients was relatively humane. The first separate unit for mentally ill children was added to this hospital in 1545.

(2) **Bethlehem Hospital** in London, founded as a priory in 1247, was given its charter as a "hospital for the cure of lunatics" in 1547 by Henry

VIII. Its name gave rise to the word bedlam as a synonym for madhouse and disorderly confusion. At times, the general public was allowed to visit the hospital for the entertainment of staring and poking fun at inmates.

(3) **J. Weyer** (1515–1588) was the first physician whose major interest was mental illnesses. He published *The Deception of Demons* (1563), which systematically refuted the view that demons were the cause of mental illness. He also provided accurate clinical observations on the verbalizations and behavior of mental patients.

(4) **F. Plater** (1536–1614) advocated reliance on observation rather than speculation in understanding mental illness. He attempted to classify mental illnesses on the basis of his own observations and believed that brain damage was the chief cause of mental aberrations.

(5) **R. Burton** (1577–1640) wrote *Anatomy of Melancholy* (1621), which remains a classic description of depressive states.

(6) **T. Sydenham** (1624–1689) provided a description of symptoms of hysteria that was so thorough and accurate that it would be difficult to improve on today. He was one of the first to note that males can be hysterics and that apparent organic impairments may be symptoms of hysteria.

(7) **G.E. Stahl** (1660–1734) is credited with being the first to make a distinction between organic and functional mental illness.

(8) **W. Cullen** (1710–1790) wrote a comprehensive text on nosology that was widely used. He believed that mental illnesses result from a breakdown in the nervous system. He was the first to use the term neuroses to denote diseases without fever or localized pathology.

(9) **R. Whytt** (1714–1766), Scotland's first neurologist, devised a nosology which divided the neuroses into hysteria, hypochondriasis, and nervous exhaustion (neurasthenia).

(10) **W. Battie** (1704–1776) wrote the first extensive treatise on mental diseases published in England, *Treatise on Madness*. He was one of the first to make a distinction between mental illnesses that arise from internal and external causes.

(11) **The Pennsylvania Hospital**, founded in Philadelphia in 1751, was the first hospital in the USA to accept mentally ill patients. The Eastern (sometimes called Williamsburg) Asylum, which opened at Williamsburg in 1773, was the first asylum in the USA to be established exclusively for the care of the mentally ill.

(12) **J.C. Reil** (1759–1813) cofounded *Magazin für psychische Heilkunde,* the first psychiatric periodical. He wrote *Rhapsodies About the Application of Psychic Therapy Methods to Mental Disorders,* which advocated a wide range of therapeutic programs including occupational therapy, music therapy, and drama therapy.

(13) **Franz Anton Mesmer** (1733–1815) developed "animal magnetism"– later called "hypnotism"–in Vienna about 1775.

(14) **J.G. Langermann** (1768–1832) wrote the first doctoral dissertation psychiatry, *On the Method of Diagnosing and Treating Chronic Mental Diseases.* His belief that organic malfunctioning can result from psychologic disturbances places him among the pioneers of psychosomatic medicine.

IV. EARLY MODERN PSYCHIATRY

(1) **Philippe Pinel** (1745–1826) ordered chains removed from mental patients at Bicêtre Asylum in 1793. His action is widely regarded as the symbolic beginning of modern psychiatry. Later, at La Salpêtrière, he instituted many other reforms in treatment, and the hospital remained as the psychiatric center of the world for a century.

(2) **Vincenzo Chiarugi** (1759–1820) instituted humane reforms at the Bonifacio Asylum in Italy (1788) 5 years before Pinel's historic order at Bicêtre Asylum, but he was less effective than Pinel in influencing others to humanize the treatment of the mentally ill.

(3) **William E. Tuke** (1732–1822), a merchant and member of the Society of Friends, founded the York Retreat (1792) in England in protest against the inhumane treatment of asylum inmates.

(4) **Joseph Guislain** (1797–1860) is considered the "Belgian Pinel" for his hospital reforms at Ghent.

(5) **Benjamin Rush** (1745–1813), considered to be the "father of American psychiatry," wrote *Medical Inquiries and Observations upon the Diseases of the Mind* (1812), the first systematic textbook on mental illness written by an American. His portrait is on the seal of the American Psychiatric Association.

(6) **Jean E.D. Esquirol** (1772–1840), outstanding clinician and hospital reformer, was a student of Pinel and a teacher of many influential psychiatrists of the 19th century. His book, *Medical, Hygienic, and Medical-Legal Aspects of Mental Illness* (1838), remained a standard text for half a century. He coined the term hallucination to differen-

tiate this phenomenon from illusions. He was one of the first to advocate treatment instead of punishment for the criminally insane.

(7) **Johann C. Heinroth** (1773–1843), a German psychiatrist, propounded many views that could be considered as forerunners of psychoanalytic theory. Among them was the belief that personality is the outcome of an inner struggle between instincts, the self, and the conscience. He was the first to use the term "psychosomatic."

(8) **Jean P. Falret** (1794–1870), a student of Esquirol and director of La Salpêtrière, developed psychiatric interviewing technics and carried out pioneer studies on suicide. He introduced the term *mental alienation* to rid patients of the social stigma attached to such terms as *dementia* and *insane*. The new term led to the appellation of *alienists* for physicians treating the mentally ill.

(9) **Jacques J. Moreau** (1804–1884), another student of Esquirol, developed conceptions of mental illness that were more dynamic than those of his predecessors, which were based on description and classification. He is credited with being the first to differentiate between primary and secondary thought processes and to recognize the importance of dreams in understanding mental illness.

(10) **Ernst von Feuchtersleben** (1806–1849), a Dean of the University of Vienna Medical School, is sometimes called the "father of psychosomatic medicine" for his writings stressing the indivisibility of the body-mind phenomenon, the role of the mind in producing physical illnesses, and the effectiveness of psychologic measures (psychotherapy) in treating some physical illnesses.

(11) **Benedict A. Morel** (1809–1873), a director of La Salpêtrière, focused on hereditary factors in mental illness, which he believed to be a degenerative process. He observed that a type of mental illness appeared to begin during adolescence and he named this illness *démence précoce*.

(12) **Wilhelm Griesinger** (1817–1868) held the post of Professor of Psychiatry and Neurology at the University of Berlin. He was influential in gaining recognition for psychiatry as a medical specialty, and is sometimes regarded as the "first genuine (full-time) psychiatrist." He promulgated an extreme materialistic, organic orientation toward mental illness in his teaching and in his widely read textbook, *Mental Pathology and Therapeutics* (1845).

(13) **Daniel H. Tuke** (1827–1895), a prolific English writer of dictionaries, manuals, histories, and treatises on psychiatry, did much to collect and synthesize available knowledge on mental diseases. He was a great-grandson of William E. Tuke, founder of the York Retreat.

(14) **Karl Kahlbaum** (1828–1899), a German nosologist, introduced the terms *symptom complex, cyclothymia* and *catatonia.*

(15) **Ewald Hecker** (1843–1909), a student of Kahlbaum, was the first to describe and name hebephrenia as a disease entity.

(16) **The M'Naghten Rule,** a legal criterion for insanity in English-American law, was established in 1843. The criterion is that the defendant "was labouring under such a defect of reason, from disease of the mind, as not to know the nature and quality of the act he was doing; or, if he did know it, that he did not know it was wrong." This rule was later supplemented by the "irresistible impulse" clause, ie, the concept that although he was aware that the act was wrong, the defendant was unable to control his behavior because of mental disorder.

(17) **The American Psychiatric Association** was organized October 16, 1844, as the Association of Medical Superintendents of American Institutions for the Insane. It was reorganized in 1892 as the American Medico-Psychological Association and obtained its present name in 1921.

(18) **Samuel Woodward** (1787–1850), the first president of the American Psychiatric Association, wrote *Essays on Asylums for Inebriates* (1838), which reflected his special interest in alcoholism.

(19) **Valentin Magnan** (1835–1916), a French psychiatrist, is considered to be the first to study alcoholism and narcotic addiction in a scientific manner. He was also one of the first to provide clinical demonstrations of mental illnesses in his courses.

(20) **Jean Martin Charcot** (1825–1893), physician-in-charge of La Salpêtrière, conducted pioneer studies on hysteria and the use of hypnosis in psychiatric treatment. Freud and Janet were his students.

(21) **St. Elizabeth's Hospital** in Washington DC was established in 1855 as the (first) United States Government Hospital for the Insane. It received its present name on July 1, 1916.

(22) **Hippolyte-Marie Bernheim** (1840–1919), a French physician, carried out extensive studies on posthypnotic suggestion which he believed demonstrated the power of unconscious motivation on behavior. Freud studied his technics and was strongly influenced by his views on hypnosis and hysteria.

(23) **Henry Maudsley** (1835–1918) published *The Physiology and Pathology of the Mind* (1867), which stressed his views that mental diseases were primarily of organic origin and that the classification of mental

diseases should be based on etiology. The publication of the book has been called the "turning point in English psychiatry" because of its influence in fostering scientific conceptual systems in place of romantic, philosophical systems.

(24) **Karl Wernicke** (1848–1905), a Viennese neurologist, published a classic work on aphasia (1874). His finding of specific memory losses with brain damage provided one basis of differentiating organic and functional psychosis.

(25) **Richard von Krafft-Ebing** (1840–1902), a German psychiatrist, published *Psychopathia Sexualis* (1886), a classical description of sexual aberrations. He also conducted original scientific research on syphilis.

(26) **Sergei Korsakoff** (1854–1900), a Russian neuropsychiatrist, described a common symptom of advanced alcoholism, Korsakoff's psychosis, which is characterized by marked disorientation and memory losses filled with confabulations.

(27) **Emil Kraepelin** (1856–1926) published *Psychiatrie: Ein Lehrbuch* (1883), a classic, comprehensive text that was the "psychiatrist's bible" for several decades. He developed a system of classifying mental illnesses on the basis of manifest behavior.

(28) **Eugen Bleuler** (1857–1939), director of a mental hospital and university psychiatric clinic in Zurich (Burgholzli), was the first influential academic leader to support the theory of psychoanalysis and its use for treatment purposes. C.G. Jung and A.A. Brill (the first American psychiatrist to practice psychoanalysis) were among his students and assistants. Bleuler withdrew his support of psychoanalysis in 1911 when he concluded that the theory was being transformed into dogma. He maintained a dynamic orientation toward psychiatry, believing it should concern itself with interpretation of abnormal behavior and not mere description. He coined the term schizophrenia to replace dementia praecox to reflect his belief that this illness is caused by splitting of the personality (ie, splitting of thought processes from emotional reactions).

(29) **Pierre Janet** (1859–1947), a French psychiatrist, started the movement to unite clinical and academic psychiatry. A systematic psychopathologist, he stressed the concept of personality integration and coined the term psychasthenia to indicate an illness in which there is a dissociation of ideas due to weak integration. He is perhaps best known for his description of the obsessive compulsive neuroses.

V. MODERN PSYCHIATRY

(1) **Sigmund Freud** (1856–1939) initiated a historic intellectual revolution in man's view of man with his development of psychoanalytic theory. He believed that unconscious forces were highly significant in the causes of mental and emotional illness. In developing psychoanalysis as a method of treatment and research, he placed great emphasis on infantile sexuality and amnesia; the pleasure and reality principles; psychodynamics; the Oedipus complex; penis envy; screen memories; sibling rivalry; the primal scene; the constructs of ego, superego, and id; libido theory; repression and the other mechanisms of defense; and the therapeutic use of the couch, free association, dream analysis, slips of the tongue, resistance, and transference.

(2) **Informal psychoanalytic societies** which met regularly were formed in Vienna and Zurich during the first decade of this century. In 1908, the Vienna Psychoanalytic Society became the first formally organized society. In 1910, the International Psychoanalytic Association was founded.

(3) **Carl G. Jung** (1875–1961), a Swiss disciple of Freud, developed a modified version of analytic theory which stressed inherited elements of the unconscious. He originated word-association tests and gave impetus to the use of such terms as *complex, introverts, extroverts,* and *archetypes.*

(4) **Alfred Adler** (1870–1937), a Viennese disciple of Freud, founded the Society of Individual Psychology in 1912. His view stressed the holistic, unique organization of psychic elements in each person; the central importance of inferiority feelings; of "the will to power"; and the emotional disturbances that arise from failure to adapt to organic inferiority.

(5) **Otto Rank** (1884–1939), another Viennese disciple of Freud, developed the concept that birth trauma was the prototype of all anxiety occurring later in life.

(6) **Karl Abraham** (1877–1925) was a German disciple of Freud whose main contributions were in the area of psychoanalytic understanding of character formation and early psychosexual development.

(7) **Ernest Jones** (1879–1958), an English disciple of Freud, is best known for his authoritative biography of Freud and his application of psychoanalytic concepts to art and literature.

(8) **Hermione von Hug-Hellmuth** (fl 1920), the first woman granted membership in the Vienna Psychoanalytic Society, stimulated the development of play therapy technics through her book, *A Study of the Mental Life of the Child* (1919).

(9) **Melanie Klein** (1882–1960), an English psychoanalyst who was the first to apply psychoanalytic methods extensively to the treatment of mentally ill children, stimulated work in this area with the publication of her book, *The Psychoanalysis of Children* (1932).

(10) **Adolph Meyer** (1866–1950) developed a theoretical system known as "common sense psychiatry" in which psychobiologic unity was stressed. He was considered the "dean of American psychiatry" for several decades.

(11) **Clifford W. Beers** (1876–1943) published *A Mind that Found Itself* (1908), an autobiographical account of treatment in "insane asylums." The book stimulated a wave of reform that swept throughout the world.

(12) **The (US) National Committee for Mental Hygiene** was founded in 1909 under the guiding hand of Clifford Beers. It was the first of many such associations established around the world.

(13) **Ernst Kretschmer** (1888–1964), a German psychiatrist, conducted studies on the relation between psychoses and body types (asthenic, athletic, and pyknic).

(14) **The American Orthopsychiatric Association**, dedicated to an interdisciplinary approach in the study, prevention, and treatment of mental illness, was founded in 1924.

(15) **The first psychoanalytic institute in the USA** was established in New York in 1931. There are at present 19 institutes and 3 training centers in this country.

(16) **Franz Alexander** (1891–1964) undertook the first systematic research on psychosomatic illness in the USA (1932).

(17) **Jacob Klaesi** (1883–) experimented with sedative-induced, prolonged sleep as a treatment for some types of mental illness (c 1922).

(18) **Julius Wagner von Jauregg** (1857–1940), an Austrian, received the Nobel Prize in Medicine (1927) for the development of malarial fever treatment in general paresis. He is the first psychiatrist to have received this honor.

(19) **Manfred Sakel** (1900–1957) developed the method of insulin shock in treating psychoses (c 1933, Austria).

(20) **Ladislas J. von Meduna** (1896–1964) experimented with the use of camphor and a synthetic camphor preparation, cardiazol (Metrazol),

to induce convulsions in the treatment of psychoses (c 1934, Hungary).

(21) **Ugo Cerletti** (1877–1963) developed the use of electroshock in the treatment of some types of mental illness (c 1938, Italy). The relative simplicity and safety of the method led to its general replacement of chemoshock therapies.

(22) **Antonio Caetano de Abrero Freire Egas Moniz** (1874–1955) pioneered in psychosurgery (lobotomy, lobectomy) in treating psychoses (c 1935, Spain), and was awarded the Nobel Prize (1955) for his work in this field.

(23) **S. and Rafat Siddiqui** isolated 5 alkaloids from the snakeroot plant (*Rauwolfia serpentina*), and Ganneth Sen and Katrick Bose experimented with the use of these alkaloids in the treatment of psychoses (c 1931, India). Derivatives of these tranquilizing agents were in widespread use within 2 decades.

(24) **Amphetamine derivatives,** first used clinically at the Boston City Hospital, began to be employed extensively in treating depressions during the late 1930s.

(25) **Albert Hoffman,** a chemist, discovered the hallucinogenic properties of lysergic acid diethylamide (LSD) by accident (1943, Switzerland).

(26) **Jean P.L. Delay** (1907–) pioneered with the use of a phenothiazine derivative (chlorpromazine) in treating psychoses (c 1952, France).

(27) **Frank M. Berger** (1913–) developed a synthetic compound (meprobamate) with mild tranquilizing properties (c 1952, USA).

(28) **The Durham decision,** by Judge David Bazelon–"An accused is not criminally responsible if his unlawful act was the product of mental disease or mental defect"–was handed down in 1954. Several states have adopted this criterion to replace the M'Naghten rule.

(29) **The English Homicide Act** (1957) incorporates the concept of gradations of criminal responsibility. This concept was rejected as unconstitutional by the United States Supreme Court.

(30) **J.F. Cade,** an Australian, introduced lithium as a successful treatment for manic excitement in 1949. Schou, in Denmark, subsequently demonstrated its effectiveness in preventing both manic and depressive attacks.

REFERENCES

Books and Monographs

Ackerknecht, E.H.: *Short History of Psychiatry*. Hafner, 1959.

Alexander, F.G., & S.T. Selesnick: *The History of Psychiatry*. Harper, 1966.

American Psychiatric Association: *One Hundred Years of American Psychiatry*. Columbia Univ Press, 1944.

Boring, E.G.: *History of Experimental Psychology*. Appleton-Century-Crofts, 1950.

Bromberg, W.: *The Mind of Man: The History of Psychotherapy and Psychoanalysis*. Harper, 1959.

Conolly, J.: *The Treatment of the Insane Without Mechanical Restraints*. Smith, Elder & Co., 1856.

Goshen, C.E.: *Documentary History of Psychiatry*. Philosophical Library, 1967.

Harms, E.: *Origins of Modern Psychiatry*. Thomas, 1967.

Hunter, R., & I. Macalpine: *Three Hundred Years of Psychiatry, 1535–1860*. Oxford Univ Press, 1963.

Lewis, N.D.C.: *A Short History of Psychiatric Achievement*. Norton, 1941.

Mora, G., & J.L. Brand (editors): *Psychiatry and Its History*. Thomas, 1970.

Roback, A.A.: *A History of Psychology and Psychiatry*. Philosophical Library, 1961.

Schneck, J.M.: *A History of Psychiatry*. Thomas, 1960.

Zilboorg, G., & G.W. Henry: *A History of Medical Psychology*. Norton, 1941.

PART II.
PSYCHIATRIC ILLNESS

13...

The Schizophrenias

The commonest of mental illnesses is characterized by faulty reality sense, disharmony and inappropriateness of thinking and feeling ("split"), and often hallucinations and delusions. The tendency is hereditary, perhaps via biochemical (enzyme) abnormalities, but psychosocial factors are contributory. Common types are paranoid ("persecuted," pathologic nonconformity), catatonic (mute, stuporous, waxy or bizarre, excited, frenzied), hebephrenic (shallow, silly, withdrawn), and simple (apathetic, regressed). Treatment is with antipsychotic drugs (phenothiazines in ample dosage) and psychotherapy, with minimal hospitalization.

The American Psychiatric Association defines schizophrenia as "a group of disorders manifested by characteristic disturbances of thinking, mood, and behavior. Disturbances in thinking are marked by alterations of concept formation which may lead to misinterpretation of reality and sometimes to delusions and hallucinations, which frequently appear psychologically self-protective. Corollary mood changes include ambivalent, constricted, and inappropriate emotional responsiveness and loss of empathy with others. Behavior may be withdrawn, regressive, and bizarre. The schizophrenias, in which the mental status is attributable primarily to a *thought* disorder, are to be distinguished from the *major affective illnesses*, which are dominated by a *mood* disorder. The *paranoid states* are distinguished from schizophrenia by the narrowness of their distortions of reality and by the absence of other psychotic symptoms."

Emil Kraepelin provided a detailed phenomenologic description of schizophrenic symptoms, but laid great stress on a prognostic criterion—tendency toward ultimate deterioration ending in a state of dementia—as a feature of the diagnosis. Although Kraepelin's term "dementia praecox" is used more or less synonymously with "schizophrenia," we no longer accept Kraepelin's gloomy prognosis as inevitable. In 1911, Eugen Bleuler named the syndrome "schizophrenia," emphasizing a splitting of the psychic functions rather than an inexorable downhill progression. He distinguished between fundamental and accessory symptoms, and considered the disorder of the associative processes the most important fundamental symptom. Adolph Meyer believed schizophrenia to result from an accumulation of faulty habits of reaction. He recommended study of the patient's entire life history, with attention to early environmental factors, and he attempted to correlate prepsychotic faulty habits with the full-blown schizophrenic symptoms. Sigmund Freud described how painful, unacceptable ideas can give rise to hallucinatory psychosis. The concept of regression to infantile or archaic levels of integration in schizophrenia replaced Kraepelin's concept of deterioration.

Authorities still disagree about whether schizophrenia is a disease in the classical medical sense, a group of syndromes, a maladjustment, or an aberrant style of life. At present, the term "schizophrenia" denotes a clinical constellation of signs and symptoms. It may be that continuing research will show that what we now call the schizophrenias are a group of specific conditions with diverse causes.

INCIDENCE OF SCHIZOPHRENIA

Worldwide Incidence

Schizophrenic reactions have been observed in all parts of the world and in all societies subjected to careful study. Estimates of the worldwide prevalence vary from an overall 0.3% to an estimate that as many as 1% of people experience a schizophrenic reaction at some time in their lives.

Prevalence of Schizophrenia in Mental Hospitals

Schizophrenics account for about 25% of first admissions to public mental hospitals in the USA. Because of the protracted length of hospitalization in the past, schizophrenic patients still make up more than half the population of most mental hospitals. Modern treatment, in avoiding "training for institutionalization," is producing more rapid discharge and a declining mental hospital population for the first time in history.

Latent Versus Overt Schizophrenia

Since Bleuler first called attention to the high incidence of latent schizophrenia, most authorities have agreed that the statistics for hospitalization of schizophrenics give a misleading (low) impression of the total. Vast numbers of schizophrenics manage to function in the community without ever being admitted to a psychiatric hospital. The incidence of latent schizophrenia probably exceeds that of overt schizophrenia.

Sex Ratio and Ordinal Position in the Family

In psychiatric hospitals, female schizophrenics slightly outnumber males. The importance of birth order appears to be different in different cultures. In small families in the upper social levels of American society, first-born men have a significantly higher incidence of schizophrenia than last-born. One reason may be the excessive parental expectations to which the first-born male is subjected at this social level. In large American families, schizophrenia is more common among later-born members, perhaps as a result of parental rejection and powerful competitive pressures.

In Japanese families, schizophrenia is most frequent in the oldest son.

Social Class and Schizophrenia
Hollingshead & Redlich report that in the lowest social class schizophrenia is 9 times as frequent as in the 2 upper classes. Perhaps the hardships to which lower class individuals are exposed make them more vulnerable; or perhaps defective genes result both in more "lower class-ness" and more schizophrenia.

CAUSES OF SCHIZOPHRENIA

There is no definite agreement concerning the fundamental causes of schizophrenia, and theories are most plentiful where the available data are least precise. Almost every conceivable physiologic or psychosocial variant has at some time been thought by someone to be an etiologic factor in schizophrenia. In general, the theories of etiology can be divided into those concerned with organic factors and those concerned with psychosocial factors.

Organic Factors
A. Genetic Predisposition: Franz Kallmann studied 500 pairs of fraternal twins in whom one twin had a diagnosis of schizophrenia. He found that 15% of the other twins were schizophrenic. In a similar study of 174 pairs of identical twins, one of whom was schizophrenic, he found a concordance rate of 86%. This suggested to Kallmann a genetic basis for schizophrenia. However, other investigators have reported a much lower concordance rate for identical twins with schizophrenia. The various twin studies have been subjected to conflicting interpretations. Some investigators consider the results of twin studies to be compatible with an environmental etiology.

Pollin & others reported a series of 15,900 pairs of male veteran twins, whose medical follow-up averaged 18 years, in which the concordance rate for schizophrenia in monozygotic twins was 3.3 times that in dizygotic twins. The comparable ratio for psychoneurosis was only 1.3—as low as the ratio for any of 8 other control nonpsychiatric diagnosis categories. Pollin felt that the findings suggest "the presence of a genetic factor in the pathogenesis of schizophrenia and its relative absence in psychoneurosis. However, the role of the suggested genetic factor appears to be a limited one."

Kety in recent years has directed a profound statistical study into the genetic aspects of schizophrenia. For his purposes he recognized only 3 types: chronic, acute, and borderline. Investigating the incidence of the "schizophrenia spectrum disorder" in the relatives of schizophrenics and of controls, and utilizing data obtained from the study of children placed for adoption shortly after birth from both schizophrenic and control families, he concluded that the genetic factors in schizophrenia are multiple and that what is transmitted is not schizophrenia as such but a vague personality characteristic that may move into the schizophrenia spectrum depending upon the particular constellation of affected genes and environmental factors. "If that is the case," he writes, "the transmission of intelligence with its genetic and environmental components, rather than the transmission of PKU, would seem to be the appropriate model for the transmission of schizophrenia, which lessens somewhat the likelihood that the schizophrenia is the result of a simple biochemical process. It may perhaps be just as difficult to find a biochemical test for schizophrenia as it might be to find one for high intelligence."

Ernst Kretschmer attempted to correlate body types with schizophrenia and claimed a preponderance of athletic, leptosomic, and dysplastic constitutions in schizophrenic patients. Kretschmer's conclusions have been challenged by others.

B. Biochemical Factors: The literature on schizophrenia is replete with reports of biochemical abnormalities. However, many such studies have not been confirmed by others; and even when a biochemical abnormality definitely appears in a group of schizophrenics, an intervening variable having nothing to do with schizophrenia may be responsible. One early study reported abnormal xanthine metabolism in a group of schizophrenics. Further study of the same group of patients showed that the schizophrenic patients were drinking much larger quantities of coffee than the control group, which meant that the abnormal urine levels of xanthine metabolites could be explained without reference to the mental illness.

1. Proteins—Heath and his associates reported extracting a psychotoxic factor called taraxein, which they believed resembled the copper-containing globulin, ceruloplasmin, though qualitatively different in some respects. Other investigators have reported elevation of serum ceruloplasmin in schizophrenics, but the specificity of this finding for schizophrenia and its etiologic significance await further investigation and confirmation.

Fessel reported elevation of S-19 macroglobulin levels in schizophrenic patients. Other investigators have been unable to confirm the specificity of this finding for schizophrenia.

2. Amino acid metabolism—Attempts have been made to relate schizophrenic symptoms to production of abnormal amines believed to be psychotogens, ie, a hypothecated conversion of tryptophan into a reported psychotogen, N,N-dimethyltryptamine (DMT). These findings have not been corroborated. Numerous variables (administration of drugs, gastrointestinal flora, diet, etc) must always be considered in interpreting the results of biochemical studies in schizophrenia.

There is some evidence that blood levels of serotonin are elevated during the first day of an acute schizophrenic episode and then fall below normal. These findings have been correlated with marked increases in urinary excretion of tryptamine and smaller increases in the excretion of other tryptophan metabolites.

It has been suggested that a disturbance in transmethylation results in the formation of psychotogenic substances. According to one theory, a small fraction of endogenous epinephrine or norepinephrine may be metabolized by an abnormal route in schizophrenic patients to form adrenochrome, adrenolutin, or some other possibly psychotogenic compound. However, doubts remain whether adrenochrome and adrenolutin are truly psychotogens and whether schizophrenic patients are indeed producing abnormal metabolites.

3. Carbohydrate metabolism—An anti-insulin factor has been reported in the blood and urine of schizophrenic patients. Reports of an increased ratio of lactate to pyruvate, an abnormal pathway of glucose metabolism, and a deficiency of hexokinase in schizophrenics all require confirmation.

C. Endocrine Factors: There is no convincing evidence that schizophrenia results primarily from an endocrine disorder, but the correlation of changes in adrenocortical steroids with changes in the clinical phase of schizophrenia is impressive. Sacher & others found marked elevations in urinary 17-hydroxycorticosteroid excretion—as much as 2–3 times normal—during periods of great anxiety or depression. Conversely, the output of corticosteroids dropped toward normal during "psychotic equilibrium" and "recovery" phases characterized by relative calm. Epinephrine excretion tended to follow a similar pattern, with elevations as high as 8 times normal during "turmoil" phases.

D. Toxic Factors: Observations of psychosis induced with mescaline and LSD suggested that schizophrenia might be the result of endogenous synthesis of a similar hallucinogenic substance. However, further research has tended to emphasize the differences (rather than the similarities) between schizophrenia and these drug-induced states. Most evidence fails to confirm the theory that LSD intoxication is really a model of schizophrenia.

Mandell & West critically review the significance of the claim that dimethyoxyphenylethylamine in the urine of schizophrenics is much higher than in normals. They find no evidence that dimethyoxyphenylethylamine even in large doses in man proves psychotogenic.

E. Neurologic Factors: Lauretta Bender developed a formulation for childhood schizophrenia emphasizing the schizophrenic child's developmental lag. Physiologic crisis, such as oxygen deprivation during childbirth, might be a precipitating factor in an infant with a constitutional predisposition toward schizophrenia. William Goldfarb & others were able to divide their schizophrenic child patients into 2 groups: one showing evidence of organicity or subtle neurologic abnormalities and one in which psychogenic factors appeared to be primarily responsible.

Heath and his associates reported specific septal spike patterns from deeply placed intracerebral electrodes. The significance of this finding has not yet been established.

Psychosocial Factors

A. Intrapsychic Conflict: The schizophrenic, like the nonschizophrenic, is driven by basic sexual and aggressive impulses and must contend with his ideals, ethical values, and social norms. Also like the nonschizophrenic, he must confront the external world and still try to satisfy his own needs. The schizophrenic differs from the nonschizophrenic in that his profound defects in mental functioning make it impossible for him to mediate successfully between the conflicting demands of instinctual impulses, conscience, and external reality.

1. Impaired ego function—The following ego functions have been noted as impaired in schizophrenia: relationship to reality and reality testing; regulation and control of drives; object relations (ability to form satisfactory relationships with other people and maintain object constancy); thought processes; defensive functions such as repression, sublimation, and reaction formation; cognitive functions such as perception, intention, thinking, and language; and synthesizing functions, which enable the individual to unite, organize, bind, and form meaningful configurations of his experiences.

Bellak & others have developed a profile for the study of ego functions in the schizophrenic syndrome in an attempt to delineate which were of prognostic value. Twelve ego functions were chosen as *necessary and sufficient* manifestations of overall ego functioning, especially in terms of ego strength and ego weakness. The ego functions are (1) reality testing, (2) judgment, (3) sense of reality, (4) regulation and control of drives, affects, and impulses, (5) object relations, (6) thought processes, (7) adaptive regression in the service of the ego; (8) defensive functioning, (9) stimulus barrier, (10) autonomous functioning, (11) synthetic-integrative functioning, and (12) mastery-competence.

They claim that a patient with fairly good scores in object relations and thought processes is apparently a good prospect for psychotherapy in conjunction with medication to control drives and mood and rehabilitation facilities for rebuilding self-esteem. Poor ratings on regulation and control of drives and poor defensive functioning are regarded by these authors as liabilities, and low autonomous and synthetic functions are a threat to the ultimate stability of improvement. Low scores for reality testing and judgment reflect acute disturbance, usually with hallucinations and delusions. An alternative way to evaluate the same results would be to note that the sicker patients do not do as well prognostically as those that are not so sick.

2. Withdrawal, regression, and restitution—The schizophrenic suffers so much disappointment, frustration, and loss of self-esteem in his attempts to deal with other people and the outside world that at some point he withdraws and becomes increasingly preoccupied with his own internal processes. Concomitant with this withdrawal is the tendency to regress to an earlier level of psychic functioning. Mechanisms appropriate to an earlier stage of life prove to be maladaptive in the present. In the earlier stages of psychosis, the world appears chaotic, fragmented, confusing, and terrifying. Some of the symptoms of schizophrenia may represent the patient's attempts to regain some sense of order—eg, a guilt-ridden paranoid schizophrenic may attribute his own omnipresent "voice of conscience" to an external voice making accusations against him. It is in this sense that hallucinations and delusions may be considered restitutive symptoms, as the patient tries to deal with his unbearable internal state by mentally constructing an unreal world.

3. Denial and projection of latent homosexual wishes—From his study of Schreber's *Memoirs,* Freud formulated an account of the development of paranoid ideation. It begins with a latent homosexual wish which is denied because it is too shocking. The initial thought, "I love men," is converted

into its emotional opposite, "I hate men," which is then projected as, "I don't hate men—it's they who hate me" (delusion of persecution).

B. Defects in the Mother-Infant Relationship: Anna Freud used the term "need-satisfying object" to describe the importance of the mother in providing the infant with his first predictably gratifying experience with an external object. In 1942 Kanner described a syndrome, "infantile autism," afflicting a group of infants who never seemed able to perceive the mother as a person.

Margaret Mahler described a second syndrome, "symbiotic infantile psychosis," in which the early mother-infant symbiotic relationship is marked but in which the infant encounters difficulty separating himself from the mother and achieving individuation. Children of the symbiotic group rarely show conspicuously disturbed behavior in the first year of life but manifest severe disturbances in the third or fourth year, when some measure of separation and independence from the mother normally occurs. The boundaries of self and nonself are blurred as the symbiotic infantile psychotic remains fixated at or regresses to the level of reality testing at which there was delusional omnipotence in the mother-infant relationship.

While the terms "schizophrenogenic mother" and "schizophrenogenic father" are frequently used, such concepts oversimplify to the point of falsification since they neglect the schizophrenic child's own contribution to the parent-child interaction. In any event, most parents of schizophrenics are already tormented by overwhelming guilt, and it is neither scientific nor kind to increase their guilt feelings by taking a judgmental attitude.

C. Pathologic Communication (the Double-Bind): Bateson, Jackson, and others described the breakdown in the individual's ability to discriminate properly in his logical thinking and hence to communicate or perceive reality effectively when exposed consistently over a long period of time to intense "double-bind" situations. A double-bind situation occurs when it is vitally important to discriminate accurately what sort of message is being communicated but the other person in the relationship expresses 2 contradictory messages. One message is often verbal and the other nonverbal. (See also p 410.)

(Example of double-bind situation: A mother says to her child, "Come here and give your mother a kiss." The child knows from past experience that if he does so his mother will simply push him away. If he disregards his mother's verbal command, he fears some punishment or loss of love. If he obeys the command and is rejected, he feels frustrated and worthless.)

It is theorized that frequent exposure to double-bind situations makes it impossible for the individual to trust any communication or to interpret reality accurately—hence the difficulty with reality relationships and thus psychosis. Granted the existence of double-binding in schizophrenic families, one problem with this theory is that double-bind relationships also occur frequently in the families of nonschizophrenics.

D. Pathologic Family Interactions: Lidz and Fleck & others described schismatic families in which the parents repeatedly threaten to separate or one spouse attempts to coerce the other to conform to rigid expectations. The relationship of the parents is characterized by recriminations rather than mutual support. In families where the parents derogate and undercut each other, the child cannot use one parent as a model for identification or as a love object without antagonizing the other parent.

Such families may show reasonable harmony on the surface, but in each marriage the serious psychopathology of the dominant parent is accepted or shared by the other. According to this theory, there is a transmission of irrationality from parents to children, causing the child great difficulty in establishing a satisfactory sense of his own identity. Lyman Wynne & others describe a constellation termed "pseudo-mutuality" in which the members are preoccupied with "fitting together" at the expense of individuation. Such a family is fearful that affirmation of the individual's personal identity will demolish the family relationship. The effort to maintain delusions of reciprocal fulfillment results in the persistence of inappropriate outgrown roles and stifles the mental development of the children.

SIGNS AND SYMPTOMS OF SCHIZOPHRENIA

Schizophrenic patients can present a veritable encyclopedia of symptoms, and psychiatrists often differ in the relative importance they assign to one symptom or another. Nevertheless, Bleuler's distinction between fundamental symptoms—those believed to be present to some extent in every case of schizophrenia—and accessory symptoms—those that may or may not be present—remains a useful point of departure.

Fundamental Symptoms (Bleuler's Four A's)

A. *A*ssociative Disturbance: The logical associations which normally lead from one thought to another appear loosened. The result is that thinking appears bizarre, illogical, and chaotic.

B. *A*utism: Autism is a form of thinking in which the major content is largely subjective or endogenous. The patient is preoccupied with ideas derived from daydreams and fantasies—even hallucinations and delusions. As autistic thinking increases there is a corresponding interference with reality relationships and reality testing.

C. *A*ffective Incongruity: Emotional responses may be inappropriate to the content of thought. Mood is often inconsistent or exaggerated. The affective disturbance may include indifference, shallowness, constriction, flatness, or blunted affect.

D. *A*mbivalence: The schizophrenic patient harbors contradictory feelings, attitudes, wishes, or ideas toward a given object, person, or situation, eg, he both loves and hates the same person at the same time. Ambivalence is a feature of other conditions also and may be present to some extent in normals, but in schizophrenia it is particularly intense.

Accessory Symptoms

A. Hallucinations: (Sensory perceptions which occur in response to no external stimulus.) Hallucinations may occur in any sensory modality—auditory (eg, God's voice), visual (eg, angels), tactile (eg, feeling crawling ants), gustatory (eg, bad taste), or olfactory (eg, bad smell); however, auditory hallucinations are the most common.

B. Delusions: A delusion is a false belief inappropriate to the patient's educational or social background and not influenced by logical contradictory evidence (eg, "The FBI is after me!").

C. Illusion: Misinterpretation of an actual sensory perception (eg, a spot on the ceiling is thought to be a spider descending upon the patient).

D. Ideas of Reference: A troubling impression that the conversation or gestures of other people have reference to oneself.

E. Depersonalization: The feeling of being alienated from one's own personality; the sense that one's identity or personality is being dissolved or lost.

F. Negativism: The patient does the opposite of what he is asked to do, eg, he closes his eyelids when he is asked to open his eyes.

G. Automatism: Actions are performed without the patient's conscious knowledge. The patient feels that it is not he that is performing his own actions.

H. Echolalia: Repetition of the speech of another.

I. Echopraxia: Repetition of the movements of another.

J. Mannerisms: Repetitive gestures or other forms of expression.

K. Stereotypies: Persistent senseless repetition of any action.

L. Impulsiveness: Actions that are performed unexpectedly without sufficient reflection and without consideration of the whole personality.

M. Benommenheit ("Benumbing"): Slowing of all psychic functions, with a resultant inability to deal with any relatively complicated or unusual situation.

CLINICAL TYPES OF SCHIZOPHRENIA

Simple Schizophrenia

Simple schizophrenia is characterized chiefly by reduction of interest in human relationships and the outside world, impoverishment of the personality, apathy, and indifference. Delusions do not often occur and hallucinations, if they occur, are rare and fleeting. Over a period of time the patient tends to regress to a lower level of functioning.

Hebephrenic Schizophrenia

In hebephrenic schizophrenia the emotional responses are shallow and inappropriate. Giggling and incongruous smiling and laughter are frequent. Fragmentary wish-fulfilling fantasies or delusions rather than elaborate, well organized systems are characteristic. Such patients are often markedly introverted and inaccessible to relationships with other people. The tendency to regress to a state of vegetation is probably greatest in this type of schizophrenia.

Catatonic Schizophrenia

In catatonic schizophrenia, motor abnormalities are the most conspicuous symptoms. They may take the form of generalized inhibition, thus presenting such symptoms as negativism, stupor, mutism, and waxy flexibility; or there may be excessive motor activity and excitement. In catatonic excitement behavior does not appear to be influenced by external stimuli but is stereotyped, apparently purposeless, impulsive, and unpredictable. The patient may run about aimlessly, go without sleep, refuse food, and become dehydrated and exhausted. Stereotypies, echolalia, echopraxia, mannerisms, grimacing, bizarre posturing, and catalepsy frequently occur.

Paranoid Schizophrenia

Paranoid schizophrenia, unlike other types, often begins in late life. It is characterized chiefly by delusions and often by hallucinations in addition to the usual schizophrenic disturbances of associations and affect, autism, and ambivalence. Persecutory themes often form the core of paranoid systems, and some element of grandiosity is frequently present. During the prepsychotic period the paranoid schizophrenic often reveals mistrust, excessive hostility, a "chip on the shoulder" attitude, emotional coldness, and a tendency to be resentful, litigious, and easily aggrieved. Ideas of reference and hypochondriasis frequently appear just prior to development of the full-blown delusional psychosis. The paranoid delusions may have a highly organized, pseudological quality or, with increasing personality disorganization, may appear fragmented.

Schizo-Affective Schizophrenia

This syndrome is characterized by marked mood disturbances, either elation or depression. Evaluation of the thinking processes shows that thinking is characteristic of a schizophrenic disturbance. The patient tends to disregard reality to a marked degree and to behave in a bizarre manner characteristic of schizophrenia.

Undifferentiated Schizophrenia

Patients often show profound disturbances of thinking, feeling, and behavior but insufficient specific symptoms to permit more precise classification. It often happens that the first (or early) schizophrenic attack will be undifferentiated and that as the reaction progresses it crystallizes into one of the definable types described above.

Less Malignant Conditions Related to Schizophrenia

A. Pseudoneurotic Schizophrenia: These patients present symptoms typical of the psychoneuroses—anxiety, conversion reactions, phobias, obsessive compulsive symptoms, depression—but there is excessive preoccupation with autistic thoughts and a tendency to withdraw from reality. Some patients may develop overt psychotic episodes of short duration, but many do not.

B. Ambulatory Schizophrenia: The ambulatory schizophrenic appears to be free of bizarre symptoms but, when exposed to stress, suddenly commits acts that reveal his underlying thought disorder. He may go through life without coming to psychiatric attention.

CLINICAL COURSE OF SCHIZOPHRENIA

Premorbid Schizophrenic Personality

It is rare for a schizophrenic illness to appear suddenly in a full-blown, fulminant form. Investigation usually reveals evidence of earlier symptoms or maladaptation. Most schizophrenic patients first appear ill enough to justify the diagnosis in adolescence or early adult life, but one can frequently find evidence of earlier emotional difficulties.

It is not known what relationship the schizophrenias of childhood bear to adult schizophrenia, or whether the childhood psychoses should truly be considered in the same nosologic category as schizophrenia. Schizophrenic symptoms in adult patients often seem to be correlated with childhood experiences of rejection, abandonment, loss of love, seductiveness on the part of parents, and other forms of psychic trauma. Although no one type of personality pattern is unique in people who later develop schizophrenia, the "schizoid personality" is frequent. Such individuals appear to have been emotionally cold, withdrawn, sensitive, and eccentric since childhood. They may do well academically, but their social adjustment is impoverished and they prefer solitary hobbies to the exclusion of interests which would require interaction with their fellows.

Another premorbid schizophrenic personality pattern is one Silvano Arieti terms the "stormy personality." Such people alternate between extreme aggressiveness and extreme submissiveness. Their lives are frequently a series of crises. Many stormy personalities have predominantly hostile and defiant traits which bring them into conflict with parents, teachers, and other authorities.

The paranoid personality frequently precedes paranoid schizophrenia. The paranoid is suspicious, mistrustful, and envious of others. While basically insecure and often troubled by feelings of inferiority, his outward manner may be overweening, condescending, and irascible. Paranoid personalities tend to collect grievances and are often litigious.

Prodromal Symptoms

During the prodromal phase a host of neurotic symptoms may appear. Although hypochondriacal or vaguely preoccupied with thoughts that something is not right with his own body, the patient has not yet reached the stage where he suffers overt somatic delusions (false and bizarre beliefs about the body). Depersonalization and derealization—the sensations that either his own body is not real or that the world around him is losing its real qualities— often herald the onset of overt psychosis. Common during this stage are feelings of strangeness, a vague sense of impending disaster, a searching for roots, and a preoccupation with abstract religious and philosophical ideas that formerly held little interest. During the prodromal phase, disturbances in sleep, appetite, and libido are common. The physician who sees a patient at this stage should be alert to the possibility of schizophrenia and should arrange for psychiatric consultation.

The onset of overt psychosis occasionally follows some precipitating event such as academic failure, death of a relative, loss of a job, or romantic disappointment, but often there seem to be no clearly precipitating circumstances and the onset is insidious.

Whether childhood schizophrenia is a prodrome of adult schizophrenia remains an unanswered research question. Goldfarb points out that the differential diagnosis of functional psychosis of childhood is a constant preoccupation in clinical practice and a frequent consideration in the literature, particularly because of the effort and skill required to differentiate childhood psychosis from mental deficiency, epilepsy, aphasia, brain damage, psychoneurosis, and responses to early psychologic deprivation and discontinuity.

Goldfarb & others make use of a 9-point diagnostic criterion developed by a British working group of 13 clinicians. No single symptom is diagnostic, but in practice the diagnosis is made after consideration of the total constellation of symptoms and behavioral characteristics.

The "9 points" for diagnosing the "schizophrenic" syndrome are as follows:

(1) Gross and sustained *impairment of emotional relationships* with people. This includes the more usual aloofness and the empty clinging (so-called symbiosis); also abnormal behavior towards other people as persons, eg, using them impersonally. Difficulty in mixing and playing with other children is often outstanding and long-lasting.

(2) *Apparent unawareness of his own personal identity* to a degree inappropriate to his age. This may be seen in abnormal behavior toward himself, such as posturing or exploration and scrutiny of parts of his body. Repeated self-directed aggression, sometimes resulting in actual damage, may be another aspect of his lack of integration, as is also the confusion of personal pronouns.

(3) *Pathologic preoccupation with particular objects* or certain characteristics of them, without regard to their accepted functions.

(4) *Sustained resistance to change in the environment* and a striving to maintain or restore sameness. In some instances, behavior appears to aim at producing a state of perceptual monotony.

(5) *Abnormal perceptual experience* (in the absence of discernible organic abnormality). This is implied by excessive, diminished, or unpredictable response to sensory stimuli—eg, visual and auditory avoidance, insensitivity to pain and temperature.

(6) Acute, excessive, and seemingly illogical *anxiety*. This tends to be precipitated by change, whether in the material environment or in routine, as well as by temporary interruption of a symbiotic attachment to persons or things. Apparently commonplace phenomena or objects seem to become invested with terrifying qualities. On the other hand, an appropriate sense of fear in the face of real danger may be lacking.

(7) *Abnormality of speech.* Speech may have been lost or never acquired, or may have failed to develop beyond a level appropriate to an earlier stage. There may be confusion of personal pronouns, echolalia, or other mannerisms of use and diction. Although words or phrases may be uttered, they may convey no sense of ordinary communication.

(8) *Distortion in motility patterns*—excess, as in hyperkinesis; immobility, as in catatonia; bizarre postures or ritualistic mannerisms, such as rocking and spinning (themselves or objects).

(9) *A background of serious retardation* in which islets of normal, near-normal, or exceptional intellectual function or skill may appear.

Overt Psychosis

To the outside observer, the patient demonstrates "deranged" thinking, feeling, and behavior. Not only are the form and content of thought likely to be disturbed, but the emotional response to thought content often becomes inappropriate. In the stage of fulminating psychosis there is a loosening or disorder in the process of associations. There may be blocking, irrelevance, tangentiality, circumstantiality, verbigeration, neologisms, and word salad. Response to questions may appear totally incoherent or bizarre. The patient's concept of his circumstances and the world may be fragmented. Any subject may be involved in delusion formation, but somatic delusions and persecutory delusions are particularly common—especially in paranoid schizophrenia. Hallucinations of any sensory modality may appear, but auditory hallucinations are especially common and often have an accusatory, persecutory content. A hallucinating schizophrenic may kill himself or others if he receives hallucinatory commands ordering him to do so. Fear, terror, and agitation are common early in the overt psychosis. Mood disturbances of almost any kind can occur. In this phase a schizophrenic patient may be depressed—perhaps suicidal. Communication and language may show idiosyncratic departures from the usual logical forms. Primary process thinking—disregard for time and space, condensation, displacement, identity of opposites, symbolization, part standing for the whole, etc—may be apparent. While the patient is preoccupied with his delusional material or autistic fantasies, he may not be able to pay attention to what is happening around him. Although intelligence, memory, and orientation may not be fundamentally disturbed, it may be difficult to enlist the patient's cooperation in testing for these functions.

Searles has described the impaired integration and differentiation of perception and thought in schizophrenia as an inability to distinguish fantasy and imagination from actual attributes of the real world. Similarly, the schizophrenic experiences memories of past events as literal reenactments of those events by the persons around him.

In *The Growth of Logical Thinking from Childhood to Adolescence,* Inhelder & Piaget present evidence that in the course of maturation the individual exists in a state of subjective nondifferentiation from the world about him in 3 successive phases leading to the development of adult thinking. These authors describe this "egocentrism" as occurring (1) in early childhood, at the "sensorimotor" level of thought development; (2) in later childhood, on the "representational" level; and (3) in adolescence, on the "experimental" level of formal thought or cognition.

Recovery and Remission

With proper treatment, symptoms may begin to subside almost from the very beginning. In other cases, several months may be required for significant remission of symptoms, and in a few cases, the patient may not respond to treatment at all. (See Prognosis of Schizophrenia, below.)

Apropos of the clinical course, Freeman emphasizes that the course of the illness cannot be considered apart from its treatment since the nature of the therapy radically influences the clinical expression of the disease. Unfortunately, treatment may have no effect and the symptoms will then remain unchanged in spite of the greatest efforts.

However, Freeman finds that the therapeutic community approach, group therapy, drug treatment, and encouragement and reinforcement of the nonpsychotic part of the patient's personality will prevent the development of the most dramatic and distressing manifestations of schizophrenia.

MANAGEMENT OF SCHIZOPHRENIA

The treatment of schizophrenia, as of any disease, attempts to be both specific and nonspecific. The former is handicapped by lack of knowledge of the etiology. The early views, established toward the end of the 19th century, involved a somatic model for the disease which failed to be borne out by extensive research in the neuropathology or neurochemistry that could be done at that time. As a result, perhaps, of this continued failure, and with the advent and popularity of psychoanalysis, a psychodynamic and sociopathic basis for schizophrenia began to predominate.

In the past few decades, treatment based on specific attempts to come to grips with the postulated underlying psychopathology in the schizophrenic has also failed. In spite of a voluminous literature and many claims of success, the data are unconvincing. Nonspecific help, yes. Kindness, good living conditions, and attention to the patient's personal problems will help anyone—just as rest in bed, a well chosen diet, etc may help many a patient with physical illness. But effect on any basic core of the schizophrenic illness has yet to be demonstrated.

Despite the lack of agreement about the causes of schizophrenia, effective nonspecific treatment methods are available. Most patients benefit from a combination of somatic therapy, psychologic intervention, and environmental manipulation. Hospitalization should be avoided unless the patient is so disturbed or dangerous he cannot be managed otherwise. The usual patient is started on medication and is seen frequently (2–4 times a week) in psychotherapy. Later, visits are reduced to once a week. The family is also seen by the psychiatrist or a psychiatric social worker.

Somatic Therapies

A. Phenothiazine Drugs: While the phenothiazine drugs are classified among the "major tranquilizers," there is much evidence that these drugs are not only tranquilizers but, more specifically, antipsychotic or antischizophrenic. Many drugs have been marketed, but it is usually sufficient to be familiar with one drug of each of the 3 chemical classes of phenothiazines: aliphatic, piperazine, and piperidine side chains. If large doses of any of the phenothiazines produce extrapyramidal dysfunction (eg, parkinson-like syndrome or torticollis), it is advisable to administer anti-parkinsonism drugs also. See Chapter 24 for a detailed discussion of the tranquilizers.

B. Shock Therapy: (See also Chapter 25.) The role of shock therapy in schizophrenia is controversial. Since the phenothiazines became available, drug therapy is generally considered the somatic treatment of choice. Nevertheless, certain indications for shock treatment for schizophrenia still exist. In certain catatonic states in which rapid intervention is required to prevent exhaustion, shock therapy may be lifesaving. Severe depression is also an indication for shock treatment.

C. Other: From time to time, various medicaments enjoy a brief vogue in the treatment of schizophrenia. Desperate parents and relatives of chronic patients will often grasp uncritically at any faint hope.

Recently, extravagant but unsupported claims have been made for "megavitamin" treatment, principally niacin in large doses. Greenbaum evaluated 57 schizophrenic children clinically and psychologically before and after a 6-month period of administration of niacinamide. They were separated into 3 groups: those given niacinamide, those given niacinamide plus a tranquilizer, and those given a placebo. There was no significant difference attributable to niacinamide.

Psychotherapy

Most schizophrenic patients will benefit from psychotherapy. In contrast to psychotherapy with neurotic patients, with whom a frequent therapeutic goal is to "make the unconscious conscious," psychotherapy with schizophrenics should generally have different goals. The schizophrenic patient is already overwhelmed by unconscious instinctual impulses that he cannot mediate, and psychotherapy must aim to strengthen his defenses. Psychotherapy of schizophrenia often does best to focus on the patient's difficulty with reality relationships. The aphorism that "the therapist must be the ambassador of reality" is particularly apt in this situation.

Frieda Fromm-Reichmann defined the essential skill of the psychotherapist in one terse sentence: "The psychotherapist must be able to listen." But psychotherapeutic listening demands an intense active effort.

At the beginning of psychotherapy the therapist may explain his purpose to the patient as follows: "I am here to try to help you understand yourself better." This may be the first time a fellow human being has treated him as someone whose thoughts deserve attention, as someone to be taken seriously, as someone who is capable of being understood.

The question, "How does the therapist promote an atmosphere of trust necessary for the psychotherapeutic enterprise with schizophrenic patients?" cannot be answered by mechanical precepts or rules of thumb, since so much depends on the therapist's sympathy, insight, and individual style of relating to the patient. Those few rules which are often helpful to beginning therapists are mainly negative injunctions:

(1) Do not exploit the patient for your own gratifications.

(2) Do not socialize with the patient, and avoid misleading or seductive behavior.

(3) Do not be a "district attorney." Therapeutic tact requires that the patient be allowed to tell his thoughts in his own way and in his own time. He should not leave therapeutic interviews feeling "psychologically raped."

(4) Do not derail the patient. Let him talk about what is important to him. In this sense, therapy is a matter of "follow the leader," and the leader here must be the patient. Do not run away from a topic because you are afraid of it.

(5) Do not use therapy as a forum to espouse your own private views.

(6) Do not make deep interpretations concerning instinctual impulses early in therapy. Such interpretations may increase the patient's guilt and anxiety levels to intolerable degrees. As in peeling the proverbial onion, one should proceed from the more superficial layers toward the deeper material, rather than the other way around. For example, the patient discusses a frightening dream in which someone kills his mother. The therapist might appropriately acknowledge how frightened the patient is of losing his mother and how dependent upon her he feels. It would probably be a mistake to offer the deeper speculation that the patient has a wish to murder his mother or to suggest still deeper oedipal feelings.

(7) Do not be too quick to give the patient what he consciously demands. Schizophrenic patients in particular require a therapist who is able to set firm, consistent limits.

Milieu Therapy

When hospitalization is necessary, the hospital chosen should be a therapeutic community. In such a setting, all aspects of the activities program (milieu)—recreation, vocational rehabilitation, patient government, patient-staff and intra-staff interactions—are planned to promote the patient's recovery. Since flexibility and individual consideration are the hallmarks of a therapeutic community, there can be few fixed rules. However, the following general guidelines are of value:

(1) Anything that tends to foster the patient's self-esteem can be considered desirable.

(2) An atmosphere where the staff members can reach agreement will be therapeutic for the patients. Stanton & Schwartz demonstrated that in a ward setting where the staff members can reach agreement the patients tend to do better; conversely, as the patients tend to do better, the staff members find it easier to reach agreement.

(3) It is important to provide a consistent structure that tends to facilitate reality testing rather than a confusing, unpredictable milieu for the patients.

(4) It is generally desirable to consider the patient in the context of his family and his community. Family therapy may be valuable, the type varying according to the particular situation.

(5) Early discharge to the home environment should be the acknowledged and generally sought goal of all. Transition to the home may be effectuated through the medium of day-night wards, half-way houses, and rehabilitation and after-care centers.

PROGNOSIS OF SCHIZOPHRENIA

With proper treatment, most schizophrenic patients will achieve some remission of symptoms after their first attack. However, one must distinguish between social recovery and complete disappearance of symptoms. Most patients hospitalized for the first time with the diagnosis of acute schizophrenic reaction can be .expected to make a social recovery in the sense that their chances are excellent for returning to their families and jobs. The ultimate prognosis depends to some extent on the quantity and quality of continued treatment, the stresses to which the patient continues to be exposed, and the severity of the disease. With the advent of phenothiazine drugs and other modern treatment methods, schizophrenia has become for many patients a disease of attacks and remissions. In clinical practice it is common to see patients decompensate to a psychotic level for 2—3 weeks and then recompensate well enough to function for 2 years before the next attack.

Many workers in this field distinguish between *process schizophrenia* and *reactive schizophrenia*. The process group are those who have an insidious onset of their disease, pursue a persistently chronic course, and seldom, if ever, make a social recovery that permits them to leave the hospital. The reactive group usually have a more sudden precipitating cause, and the course of their illness is usually briefer. The distinction is largely descriptive and post facto.

Clinical factors on the process (unfavorable) side: lowest socioeconomic group; unusually good deportment in school; widowed, divorced, or separated; gradual onset; long duration of illness prior to hospitalization; ectomorphic constitution; schizoid personality; apathy or flat, inappropriate affect; defiance; bizarre or referential delusions; prominent hallucinations; and paranoid or hebephrenic diagnosis.

Reactive (favorable) factors: upper socioeconomic group; good premorbid social, marital, or sexual adjustment; married; outgoing personality; sudden onset; short duration of illness prior to hospitalization; endomorphic constitution; psychogenic precipitating factors; marked affect component— manic, depressive, anxious, confused, or perplexed; self-reproachful or changing delusions; and catatonic diagnosis.

REFERENCES

Books and Monographs

Arieti, S.: *Interpretation of Schizophrenia.* Robert Brunner, 1955.

Artis, K.L. (editor): *The Symptom as Communication in Schizophrenia.* Grune & Stratton, 1959.

Auerback, A.: *Schizophrenia: An Integrated Approach.* Ronald Press, 1959.

Bellak, L. (editor): *Schizophrenia.* Logos Press, 1958.

Bellak, L.: *Schizophrenia: A Review of the Syndrome.* Logos Press, 1958.

Bellak, L., & L. Loeb: *The Schizophrenic Syndrome.* Grune & Stratton, 1969.

Bleuler, E.: *Dementia Praecox or the Group of Schizophrenias.* Internat Univ Press, 1950.

Burnham, D.L., Gladstone, A.I., & R.W. Gibson: *Schizophrenia and the Need-Fear Dilemma.* Internat Univ Press, 1969.

Cancro, R. (editor): *The Schizophrenic Reactions: A Critique of the Concept, Hospital Treatment, and Current Research.* Brunner/Mazel, 1970.

Cole, J.O., Goldberg, S.C., & J.M. Davis: Drugs in the treatment of psychosis: Controlled studies. In: *Psychiatric Drugs.* Solomon, P. (editor). Grune & Stratton, 1966.

Goldfarb, W.: *Childhood Schizophrenia.* Harvard Univ Press, 1961.

Hoskins, R.G.: *The Biology of Schizophrenia.* Norton, 1946.

Jackson, D.D. (editor): *The Etiology of Schizophrenia.* Basic Books, 1960.

Kallmann, F.J.: *Heredity in Health and Mental Disorder.* Norton, 1953.

Kasanin, J.: *Language and Thought in Schizophrenia.* Univ of California Press, 1944.

Scher, S.C., & H.R. Davis (editors): *The Out-Patient Treatment of Schizophrenia.* Grune & Stratton, 1960.

Searles, H.J.: The differentiation between concrete and metaphorical thinking in the recovering schizophrenic patient (1962). In: *Collected Papers on Schizophrenia and Related Subjects.* Internat Univ Press, 1965.

Solomon, P., & B.C. Glueck, Jr. (editors): *Recent Research on Schizophrenia.* American Psychiatric Association, 1965.

Journal Articles

Allen, M.G., & W. Pollin: Schizophrenia in twins and diffuse ego boundary hypothesis. Am J Psychiat 127:437–442, 1970.

Bellak, L., & others: Study of ego functions in the schizophrenic syndrome. Arch Gen Psychiat 23:326–336, 1970.

Bender, L.: Childhood schizophrenia. Psychiat Quart 27:663–681, 1953.

Benjamin, J.D.: Some considerations in biological research in schizophrenia. Psychosom Med 20:427–445, 1958.

Bishop, M.P., & others: Ultracentrifugal serum proteins in schizophrenia. Arch Gen Psychiat 15:337–340, 1966.

Burch, P.R.J.: Schizophrenia: Some new aetiological considerations. Brit J Psychiat 110:818–824, 1964.

Cancro, R.: Prospective prediction of hospital stay in schizophrenia. Arch Gen Psychiat 20:541–546, 1969.

Dunham, H.W.: Sociocultural studies of schizophrenia. Arch Gen Psychiat 24:206–214, 1971.

Epstein, S., & M. Coleman: Drive theories of schizophrenia. Psychosom Med 32:113–140, 1970.

Fessel, W.J.: Interaction of multiple determinants of schizophrenia. Arch Gen Psychiat 11:1–18, 1964.

Fish, B.: The detection of schizophrenia in infancy. J Nerv Ment Dis 125:1–24, 1957.

Fromm-Reichmann, F.: Psychotherapy of schizophrenia. Am J Psychiat 111:410–419, 1954.

Gottlieb, J.S., Frohman, C.E., & P.G.S. Beckett: A theory of neuronal malfunction in schizophrenia. Am J Psychiat 126:149–156, 1969.

Greenbaum, G.H.C.: An evaluation of niacinamide in the treatment of childhood schizophrenia. Am J Psychiat 127:89–93, 1970.

Grinker, R.R., Sr.: An essay on schizophrenia and science. Arch Gen Psychiat 20:1–24, 1969.

Grinspoon, L., Ewalt, J.R., & R. Shader: Psychotherapy and pharmacotherapy in chronic schizophrenia. Am J Psychiat 124:1645–1652, 1968.

Heath, R.G., & others: Schizophrenia as an immunologic disorder. Arch Gen Psychiat 16:1–33, 1967.

Hedberg, D.L., Houch, J.H., & B.C. Glueck, Jr.: Tranylcypromine-trifluoperazine combination in the treatment of schizophrenia. Am J Psychiat 127:1141–1146, 1971.

Hoch, P., & P. Polatin: Pseudoneurotic forms of schizophrenia. Psychiat Quart 23:248–276, 1949.

Kallmann, F.J.: The genetic theory of schizophrenia: An analysis of 691 twin index families. Am J Psychiat 103:309, 1946.

Kety, S.: Current biochemical approaches to schizophrenia. New England J Med 276:325–330, 1967.

Mahler, M.S.: On early infantile psychosis: The symbiotic and autistic syndromes. J Am Acad Child Psychiat 4:554–568, 1965.

Mishler, E., & N. Waxler: Family interaction process and schizophrenia. Internat J Psychiat 2:375–428, 1966.

Noreik, K., & others: Reexamination of acute schizophrenic and schizophreniform psychoses. Acta psychiat scandinav (Suppl 203):41–42, 1968.

Pollin, W., & others: Psychopathology in 15,909 pairs of veteran twins: Evidence for a genetic factor in the pathogenesis of schizophrenia and its relative absence in psychoneurosis. Am J Psychiat 126:597–610, 1969.

Rosenthal, D.: The offspring of schizophrenic couples. J Psychiat Res 4:169–188, 1967.

Sachar, E.J., & others: Psychoendocrine aspects of acute schizophrenic reactions. Psychosom Med 25:510–537, 1963.

Shakow, D.: On doing research in schizophrenia. Arch Gen Psychiat 20:618–642, 1969.

Singer, M.T., & L.C. Wynn: Thought disorder and family relations of schizophrenics. Arch Gen Psychiat 12:187–200, 1965.

Vaillant, G.E.: The prediction of recovery in schizophrenia. Internat J Psychiat 2:617–627, 1966.

Welch, J.P., Clower, C.G., & R.N. Schimke: The "pink spot" in schizophrenics and its absence in homocytinurics. Brit J Psychiat 115:163–168, 1969.

14 . . .

Manic-Depressive Psychosis

Manic-depressive psychosis is a mental disease of unknown cause. It is likely that there is genetic transmission of some as yet unidentified biochemical or physiologic factor. Attacks may be depressed, manic or hypomanic (mild manic), or mixed. They may alternate or always be the same. In mania there is elation, pressure of speech, and increased motor activity; in depression there is sadness and diminution of the major appetites—food, sleep, sex, and activity. In neither is there any clear precipitating psychologic event.

Rule out depression associated with somatic illness, psychotic depressive reaction (clear-cut precipitating event, no previous attacks), depressive neurosis (less intense, more related to life situation), schizo-affective type of schizophrenia (prominent thought disorder, delusions, or hallucinations), and involutional melancholia.

Troublesome manics and suicidal depressed patients must be hospitalized. Mania usually responds to phenothiazines in large doses or lithium carbonate; depression to the antidepressant drugs. Lithium in maintenance doses may prevent further attacks of either mania or depression. Electroshock may be used in urgent cases. Psychotherapy and enlisting the help of the family are advisable.

The manic-depressive psychoses are a group of "major affective disorders" characterized by severe disturbances of mood—elation or depression, far beyond the range of normal mood swings—that dominate the mental life of the patient. They are classified as manic type, depressed type, or circular type.

ETIOLOGY AND INCIDENCE

The cause is unknown, but at present the dominant view is that the manic-depressive psychoses are due to some as yet unidentified biochemical or physiologic alteration (eg, of catecholamine or serotonin biosynthesis). Various constitutional factors have been proposed, but the evidence presented by different investigators is inconclusive and at times contradictory. The evidence for genetic transmission is strong (see Chapter 8).

Psychodynamic explanations of the development of manic-depressive psychoses stress unsatisfied oral cravings (Abraham), self-hatred (Freud), and loss of self-esteem (Bibring). Klein and others have noted depressions occurring in the first year of life, and Engel has likened the depressive phase of manic-depressive psychosis to the hibernation observed in lower animals. Kraepelin observes that the development of manic or depressive episodes is a reflection of basic personality type and is only minimally related to external events.

The incidence of the manic-depressive psychoses is apparently declining (from 12% of first admissions to psychiatric hospitals in 1933 to 1–5% in 1968). Current estimates of their worldwide incidence are in the range of 3–4/1000 population. Most authorities agree that they are more common among people in the higher social classes. The male/female incidence is about 3:2.

Manic forms of these disorders occur principally in younger people; depressed forms predominate in the older age groups.

Most first attacks occur before age 35.

CLINICAL DESCRIPTION

The patient with manic-depressive psychosis is usually in either a well defined manic or depressive phase, a transitional phase, or a recovered phase. During one episode, there may be an attack of mania or depression followed by the converse phase. There may, however, be recurrences of just one of the phases without the other (eg, recovered mania without depression, or vice versa). Typically, the patient suffers from recurrent psychotic episodes which may be separated by months to years of remission. There have been instances of patients with continuous, repetitive, 24-hour severe mood swings for prolonged periods, and rarely there may be mixed types (eg, agitation and depression). Symptoms such as delusions, hallucinations, and illusions may be part of the clinical syndrome. Paranoid hypersensitivity and projections are often present. The onset of the mood disorder is usually not related to a precipitating life experience.

The diagnosis of manic-depressive psychosis is based on the following: (1) a distinct and marked phasic disturbance of affect, in which thinking is consonant with mood; (2) no intellectual or personality deterioration; (3) well defined attacks; (4) a history of manic-depressive illness in family members; and (5) precipitating psychologic factors inconspicuous or insufficient to account for the degree of illness.

Manic type. The disturbances seen in mania are the mirror image of those seen in depression. The classical triad of mania consists of (1) elated, unstable mood, (2) pressure of speech, and (3) increased motor activity. The mood is one of excess gaiety, euphoria, geniality, disinhibition, and at times ecstasy. Transitory, brief moments of depression may occur. There may be boisterous joking and unrestrained good humor until the patient is frustrated, whereupon the humor may become caustic, insulting, and sarcastic and the patient himself irritable, abusive, or violent. He behaves in a grandiose manner and is invulnerable to reason and logic. He alludes frequently to his outstanding personal achievements, and bends every circumstance to the service of self-aggrandizement. His thinking demonstrates flights of ideas, easy distractibility, absence of self-criticism, little true self-awareness, a tendency to blame others, and at times extremely poor judgment. Paranoid thinking may be present.

The manic patient is usually involved in many schemes and projects and is often able to engage others in fully planned, extravagant enterprises. The excess of activity may ultimately lead to a state of exhaustion. He may at times be exhibitionistic or seductive. Excessive speech causes the hoarseness which is so characteristic of manic patients.

Appetite may be voracious but is usually diminished. There seems to be little increase in sexual drive or potency. The patient is so wound up in his expansive feelings, thoughts, and activities that he has difficulty falling asleep and, when asleep, awakens early. The insomnia is similar to that seen in the depressed state but usually is more severe.

Hypomania may arise almost imperceptibly in a person who is known to be energetic, buoyant, and a central figure in many groups. It may persist for many months before it is recognized as pathologic. Symptoms resemble mania but are milder, and some may be absent. Many of these patients cause great embarrassment, frustration, and chagrin in those who try to help them (wives, lawyers, business advisers, physicians) because they refuse to acknowledge illness. If their behavior is sufficiently aberrant, they can be legally committed or have a conservator appointed by the court, but often this is impossible and they must be permitted to career along until they do something outlandish enough to convince the authorities. If they can be persuaded to cooperate in treatment (as for mania), there is hope for them.

Delirious mania, the severest form of mania, is rare. The patient is out of contact, and his speech is incoherent (often a "word salad"). He is constantly and purposelessly active. He may be hallucinating, delusional, and extremely dangerous. Without treatment, he may die of exhaustion.

Depressed type. In depression, the classical triad is (1) depressed mood, (2) slowed thinking, and (3) psychomotor retardation. The predominant emotions are despondency, gloom, agitation, perplexity, hopelessness, and helplessness. The patient feels extremely inadequate, has no confidence, and may feel that he is a worthless person. All of life's endeavors seem meaningless and without value. There may be sullen bitterness and anger.

The patient's retarded thought processes make it difficult for him to concentrate. Physical tension and anxiety produce a variety of bodily sensations which at times become the major focus of the patient's attention ("somatic equivalents"). There may be excessive preoccupation with a particular, personally meaningful life event. A sense of dread or fear of dying may be present. He loses interest in his usual activities, friends, and family as his attention is completely turned inward.

Memory and orientation are intact. Physical activity is retarded, although there may be marked agitation. There is a paralysis of the will. Even such simple activities as getting out of bed and dressing are markedly slowed. At times the patient can be mobilized only with intensive supervision or aggressive prodding. If he is agitated, he may wring his hands, move about restlessly, cling to others for comfort, or constantly pace the floor.

The patient may appear chronically ill and complain of dryness of the mouth, lack of appetite, constipation, marked fatigue (particularly in the early morning), and coldness of the extremities. Insomnia, characterized by early morning rising with light sleep ("matutinal wakefulness") may be present. There is a loss of sexual interest and drive. Women may complain of dysmenorrhea, amenorrhea, or hot flashes.

One of the major clinical problems of the depressive phase of manic-depressive psychosis is the possibility of *suicide.** It is estimated that 1—5% of depressive patients commit suicide, but these figures are probably high if one includes the huge number of mild or subclinical depressions. The best clue to the possibility of a suicidal attempt is the patient's own testimony. About half of successful suicides have said they would kill themselves. Women make more attempts, but men are more frequently successful. There are approximately 9 attempts for every successful suicide. The major mode of suicide for women is drugs; for men, firearms. The danger of suicide seems to be greatest when the deep, retarded depression lightens so that an active, self-destructive solution is possible. The risk is high during leaves of absence from the hospital and within 1 month after discharge from the hospital. The sense of hopelessness and pessimism is strongly related to suicide wishes and attempts. A previous unsuccessful suicide attempt increases the probability of a subsequent successful attempt.

Circular type. The circular type is characterized by an alternation of manic and depressed phases, with occasional progression to delirious mania or depressive stupor.

Onset and Course

The first attack of manic-depressive psychosis may occur at any time between adolescence and age 45. Manic episodes are more frequent between ages 20—35, and depressive episodes between ages 35—50. The premorbid personality usually is cyclothymic, hypomanic, or depressive.

Attacks may be mild and attenuated, moderate, or severe. The same patient may have recurrent episodes of the various clinical types, with variable durations, severity, and periods of remission. For example, the first episode may be entirely manic, the second circular, and the third depressive. About 75% of episodes begin acutely. In a few cases, the onset may be insidious over a period of 8 months to 10 years. Many first attacks of depression occur in college, cause the student to "drop out," and are unrecognized. Most episodes terminate in improvement or a return to the premorbid state.

In general, the more confused the patient, the shorter the duration of illness. Fifty to 75% of patients have relapses, and about half undergo 3 or

*See further discussion in Chapter 22 and Psychiatric Emergency Routine.

more recurrences. Relapse may occur after many years of reasonably stable functioning. With each successive episode, the symptom-free interval tends to be shorter. The highest probability of recurrence is within 6 years after the first attack. Some patients ultimately develop frank schizophrenia. The more rigid the criteria for diagnosis of manic-depressive psychosis, the more likely the probability of an eventual diagnosis of chronic schizophrenia.

DIFFERENTIAL DIAGNOSIS

Depression Associated With Somatic Illness
Subclinical or clearly established physical disease may be accompanied by marked depressive symptoms. Depressed mood, apathy, or irritability are especially prominent in hypertensive cardiovascular disease, uremia, hepatitis, various intracranial lesions (including cerebral arteriosclerosis and brain tumor), psychomotor epilepsy, drug intoxications, drug withdrawal states, and after severe infectious diseases. On the other hand, there are patients who undergo repeated surgical and somatic treatments when they actually are suffering from a depressive state characterized primarily by somatic complaints.

Psychotic Depressive Reaction
Psychotic depressive reaction is characterized by the same clinical depression as in manic-depressive psychosis, but the life history does not reveal a cyclothymic temperament or a history of manic-depressive attacks. The psychotic depression seems to follow directly upon a clear-cut precipitating event, usually a great loss.

Depressive Neurosis
These episodes are usually specifically related to external precipitating events, and there tend to be many of them in the patient's life. The depressions are labile and less intense, and improve rapidly. Reality testing and functioning are minimally impaired, but other neurotic symptoms are usually present.

Schizophrenia, Schizo-Affective Type
This condition is characterized by a psychotic episode, usually in a young adult. The patient will show a dominant affective disorder, such as depression or mania. In addition, however, there may be a prominent thought disorder, distortions of reality, marked delusions, paranoid ideation, and hallucinations. The patient does not usually have the direct and engaging personality of the manic-depressive. The premorbid personality has usually been more reserved, remote, and ruminative. The symptoms are not reported in a direct manner, The experiences are usually more personalized, bizarre, and less comprehensible.

Involutional Melancholia

This disorder, which usually involves agitation as well as depression, occurs later, during the involutional period, and there is no history of previous episodes. The personality is usually compulsive rather than cyclothymic.

An endocrine factor in this condition has never been demonstrated, and treatment with male or female hormone preparations, while it may help concomitant somatic symptoms, does not affect the depression or agitation. Psychologic factors, however, may be prominent ("empty nest syndrome," loss of vigor, youth, beauty, etc).

TREATMENT

The aims of treatment are (1) to prevent suicide, homicide, or other destructive behavior; (2) to relieve suffering; (3) to shorten the course of the illness; and (4) to prevent or attenuate future episodes.

In both the depressed and the manic phases of the illness, careful attention should be paid to the sleep disorder. The use of hypnotics such as chloral hydrate is advisable. For the illness itself, drug therapy seems to be almost as effective as ECT (about a 75% recovery rate for individual attacks).

Hospitalization

If the patient is in a state of acute mania with impaired judgment, overactivity, and poor planning with regard to his business and financial affairs, hospitalization is advisable. In hypomanic patients, outpatient or day care treatment may be attempted, with medication and frequent examinations. For patients in a state of acute depression, with progressive weight loss, insomnia, agitation, inability to function, a sense of hopeless resignation, and progressive withdrawal with suicidal ideation, hospitalization is mandatory.

If the patient sought help for himself, this is a good sign. If friends, work associates, supervisors, or family made the referral, it may be difficult to persuade the patient to accept hospitalization.

Pharmacotherapy*

A. Manic States:

1. Lithium carbonate—This drug, although still in its early developmental stage, has been demonstrated to give dramatic results in 2—10 days in most manic patients. Maintenance therapy with lithium also seems to be remarkably successful in preventing recurrences of both manic and depressive phases.

2. Phenothiazines—This group of drugs is still the most commonly used form of treatment for manic states. Chlorpromazine (Thorazine), 100—200 mg every 6 hours (or equivalent of another phenothiazine), usually controls excitement.

*See Chapter 24 for further details about the use of these drugs.

3. Haloperidol (Haldol)—This drug, a butyrophenone derivative, has also been used with success.

B. Depressive States: Drug therapy is usually tried first even though ECT (see below) is slightly more effective.

1. Imipramine (Tofranil) and amitriptyline (Elavil)—In moderate to severe depression, the patient usually responds to either of these drugs or other tricyclics, starting with 25 mg 3 times a day and gradually increasing the dosage over a period of 1 week to 150 mg/day. Initial effects are first observed within 5—14 days. The toxicity of these drugs is considerably less than that of the monoamine oxidase inhibitors, and they are also more effective.

2. Chlordiazepoxide (Librium) and diazepam (Valium)—These drugs are useful for anxiety and agitation. The dosage of diazepam is 5—10 mg 4 times a day; the dosage of chlordiazepoxide is twice that much (or more). Neither affects the depression.

Electroconvulsive Therapy

This is the treatment of choice in acutely suicidal patients or where for other urgent reasons (eg, persons with vitally pressing financial, governmental, or other reality stresses that require immediate attention) it is imperative to diminish the depression as fast as possible. It is also used in patients who are refractory to drugs. Antidepressant medication is usually the treatment of first choice for most depressive illnesses (because it does not cause loss of memory or confusion) even though ECT is more effective (see Chapter 25). Transient confusion and memory loss make psychotherapeutic work difficult during and after the period of shock treatment. Six to 8 treatments are usually sufficient to initiate improvement in depressed patients. Several more are often given to ensure maximum and lasting effect. A working rule that some use is to note the number of treatments before improvement first occurs and double this number for the total series.

ECT is at times used as sedative treatment for acutely excited manic patients. Outpatient ECT is at times used on a therapeutic or prophylactic basis, but adequate supervision by responsible friends or relatives must be provided. Patients should not drive themselves home after a treatment and usually should not attempt to work or study on that day.

Psychotherapy

Psychotherapy with the manic-depressive patient can take a variety of forms. Most important is the establishment and maintenance of a sound, trusting doctor-patient relationship. Therapy should be realistic and supportive of the patient's assets. Uncovering therapy is not advisable during the acute illness. Long-term therapy may be indicated later, particularly to help the patient see the unrealistic nature of his self-deprecating attitudes.

The family may be worked with, at first diagnostically, in order to assess the interpersonal relationships and to find the most helpful family members. The family may require education to report early signs of subsequent attacks.

Maintenance pharmacotherapy, with alterations made according to the phase of the illness, is a matter to be decided in each case. See Chapter 24 for the use of maintenance lithium for preventive purposes. Early recognition of an episode of mania or depression, with rapid initiation of treatment, is certainly part of the goal of long-term follow-up.

PROGNOSIS

Studies of the long-term course of manic-depressive illness reveal that almost 90% of patients recover from their attacks. Before treatment with pharmacotherapy and ECT became available, manic attacks lasted, on the average, about 3½ months and depressive attacks about 6½ months. Attacks in patients over age 45 last longer than those in the younger age group. Fifty to 75% of patients have 2–4 attacks. About 5% of cases become chronic.

REFERENCES

Books and Monographs

Abraham, K.: *Notes on the Psychoanalytical Investigations and Treatment of Manic-Depressive Insanity and Allied Conditions: Selected Papers.* Basic Books, 1963.

Beck, A.T.: *Depression: Clinical, Experimental, and Theoretical Aspects.* Harper & Row, 1967.

Grinker, R.R., Sr., & others: *The Phenomena of Depression.* Hoeber, 1961.

Hordern, A.: *Depressive States: A Pharmacotherapeutic Study.* Thomas, 1965.

Kallmann, F.J.: *Heredity in Health and Mental Disorder.* Norton, 1953.

Journal Articles

Beigel, A., & D.L. Murphy: Unipolar and bipolar affective illness. Arch Gen Psychiat 24:215–220, 1971.

Bond, E.: Results of treatment of psychosis. Am J Psychiat 110:881–887, 1954.

Bratfos, O., & J.O. Faug: The course of manic-depressive psychoses. Acta psychiat scandinav (Suppl 203):43–44, 1968.

Brodie, H.K.H., & M.J. Leff: Bipolar depression. Am J Psychiat 127:1086–1090, 1971.

Carroll, B.J., & others: Sodium transfer from plasma to CSF in severe depressive illness. Arch Gen Psychiat 21:77–81, 1969.

Cohen, M.B., & others: An intensive study of twelve cases of manic-depressive psychosis. Psychiatry 17:103–137, 1954.

Dasberg, H., & M. Assabel: Somatic manifestations of psychotic depression. Dis Nerv System 29:399–404, 1968.

Earle, B.V.: Thyroid hormone and tricyclic antidepressants in resistant depressions. Am J Psychiat 126:1667–1669, 1970.

Fieve, R.R., Platman, S.R., & R.R. Plutchik: The use of lithium in affective disorders: Prophylaxis of depression in chronic recurrent affective disorders. Am J Psychiat 125:492–498, 1968.

Gibson, R.W.: The family background and early life experience of the manic-depressive patient: Comparison with the schizophrenic. Psychiatry 21:71–90, 1958.

Gibson, R.W., Cohen, M.B., & R.A. Cohen: On the dynamics of the manic-depressive personality. Am J Psychiat 115:1101–1107, 1959.

Glassman, A.: Indoleamines and affective disorders. Psychosom Med 31:107–114, 1969.

Heller, A., Zahourek, R., & H.G. Whittington: Effectiveness of antidepressant drugs: A triple-blind study comparing imipramine, desipramine, and placebo. Am J Psychiat 127:1095, 1971.

Kerry, R.J., & G. Owen: Lithium in manic-depressive illness. Am J Psychiat 124:1702–1705, 1968.

Leff, M.J., Roatch, J.F., & W.E. Bunney, Jr.: Environmental factors preceding the onset of severe depressions. Psychiatry 33:293–311, 1970.

Rennie, T.A.C.: Prognosis in manic-depressive insanity. Am J Psychiat 98:801–814, 1942.

Reynolds, E.H., Preece, J.M., & A. Coppen: Folate deficiency in depressive illness. Brit J Psychiat 117:267–274, 1970.

Rosenthal, S.H.: Changes in a population of hospitalized patients with affective disorders, 1945–1965. Am J Psychiat 123:671–681, 1966.

Rosenthal, S.H., & G.L. Klerman: Content and consistency in the endogenous depressive pattern. Brit J Psychiat 112:471–484, 1966.

Sachar, E.J., Fukushima, D.K., & T.F. Gallagher: Cortisol production in depressive illness: A clinical and biochemical clarification. Arch Gen Psychiat 23:289–298, 1970.

Slater, E.T.O.: The inheritance of manic-depressive insanity and its relation to mental defect. J Ment Sc 82:626–634, 1936.

Wharton, R.N., & R.R. Fieve: The use of lithium in the affective psychosis. Am J Psychiat 123:706–712, 1966.

Wilson, I.C., & others: Thyroid-hormone enhancement of imipramine in non-retarded depression. New England J Med 282:1063–1067, 1970.

Winokur, G., & V.L. Tanna: Possible role of X-linked dominant factor in manic depressive disease. Dis Nerve System 30:89–93, 1969.

Wolpert, E.A., & P. Mueller: Lithium carbonate in the treatment of manic-depressive disorders. Arch Gen Psychiat 21:155–159, 1969.

15 . . .

Organic Psychosis

Failure to recognize an organic psychosis ranks as one of the major sins in medicine. Differentiation from the "functional psychoses" usually is not difficult.

Psychiatrists as well as other physicians must learn to recognize mental disturbances caused by organic illness. It is tragic to do a routine autopsy on a back ward mental hospital patient and find an operable brain tumor or subdural hematoma—even granted that in some cases the lesion may be unrelated to the mental condition; it is dismaying when a suddenly "psychotic" patient dies in unrecognized diabetic coma, uremia, or of thyrotoxicosis; and it is both a medical disaster and a legal injustice to convict and punish a "criminal" for acts of violence committed as a result of demonstrable brain disease (eg, psychomotor epilepsy or temporal lobe tumor).

The official psychiatric nomenclature attaches the term organic brain syndromes to mental disorders "caused by or associated with impairment of brain tissue function." This is comparable to applying the term "organic lung syndrome" to all pulmonary disease—a gross anatomic localization but not much more than that. The first edition of the *Diagnostic and Statistical Manual of Mental Disorders* (DSM-I), published by the American Psychiatric Association, classified organic brain syndromes into acute and chronic, which had some descriptive and prognostic usefulness; but the current edition (DSM-II) classifies them as psychotic or nonpsychotic, which is like dividing lung diseases into those with fever and those without fever. The DSM approaches were devised in response to administrative and forensic needs. In this chapter (and elsewhere in this book), reference will be made to the corresponding DSM terms; but for the purposes of exposition and practical clinical value, a descriptive and pragmatic nosology will also be employed here.

The organic psychoses divide naturally into delirium and dementia depending upon whether the basic dysfunction is at the lower or the higher mental level. The 2 mental levels and their normal characteristics are presented in Chapter 3. The highlights of the present chapter are summarized in Table 15—1.

TABLE 15–1. The organic psychoses contrasted with the "functional" psychoses.

Type	Mental Level	Chief Involvement	Anatomic Localization	Psychologic Area	Chief Symptoms	Causes
Delirium	Lower	Sensorium, instincts, feelings	Brain stem, limbic lobe, autonomic nervous system, sensory cortex	Id, ego	Clouded consciousness, disorientation, abnormal emotions and mood, confusion, visual hallucinations	Acute trauma, toxic, metabolic, drugs
Dementia	Higher	Intellect, abstraction, judgment, programming, creativity	Temporal, parietal, frontal lobes	Ego, superego	Loss of memory, learning, reasoning, problem solving, personality characteristics, judgment	Residual trauma, structural and degenerative disease
Functional psychosis	Not known; perhaps upper-higher	Self evaluation, interpersonal and social relations	Not known; perhaps frontal lobes	Ego, superego	Loss of reality sense, insight; delusions, depression, mania, hallucinations	Not known

DELIRIUM

Clinical Findings

Dysfunction at the lower (primitive and sensorial) mental level results in the clinical condition known as delirium, which is recognizable by any or all of the following characteristics:

(1) Impaired consciousness: This may vary from slight mental cloudiness to stupor, often changing rapidly from moment to moment. As it fluctuates, so do other mental faculties.

(2) Disorientation.

(3) Abnormal emotions and mood: These correspond not to the reality situation but to disturbed sensory data, including hallucinations (usually visual), illusions, and delusions. A labile mood may swing from apathy or shallow silliness to rage or sudden panic.

(4) Mental confusion: This is manifested by garbled thinking, often dreamlike or nightmarish in content and quality. It occurs in severe cases of delirium because of effects on the higher mental level. Thus, memory, comprehension, factual knowledge, reasoning ability, and judgment are impaired, and insight is usually lacking. These changes are transient and reversible.

(5) Inappropriate, impulsive, irrational, or violent behavior: This often occurs in automaton- or trance-like fashion.

The chief parts of the brain responsible for the delirious state are thought to be the brain stem, autonomic nervous system, limbic system, and sensory cortex and pathways.

The principal causes of delirium are trauma, acute poisoning, metabolic disorders, and drug abuse or overdosage.

Head Trauma

The most common cause of delirious states is head injury. In a typical example, a football player is knocked out during a game. The trainer or a physician runs out onto the field and usually finds that the player has already recovered consciousness. If the player knows where he is, what he is doing, what down it is, etc, no great concern arises and he may even be permitted to remain in the game. If he seems hazy, does not know the score, starts walking toward the wrong sidelines, or talks or acts peculiarly, he will be benched, kept under observation, or even hospitalized.

Head trauma can produce any degree of mental impairment from momentary "concussion" (with brief "blackout" or feeling of being stunned or dazed and nothing more) to increasing degrees of neurotic or psychotic illness. **Posttraumatic neurosis** is usually attributed to the emotional reaction of the individual to the injury; **posttraumatic psychosis** is considered to be a result of physical damage to the brain. In the former, subjective symptoms predominate (eg, anxiety, panic states, insomnia, nightmares, phobias, various somatic complaints); in the latter, some or all of the signs of delirium or dementia (see below) are present.

In posttraumatic psychosis, the period of unconsciousness is usually longer (several hours or days), and there may be concomitant physical and neurologic evidences of damage to the brain (including abnormal x-rays of the skull and abnormal CSF and EEG findings). The psychotic state follows the course of the damage to brain substance, the former improving with the latter. Days, weeks, or even months may pass before recovery is complete, and residuals usually are attributable to irreversible damage at the higher mental levels caused by widespread traumatic encephalopathy. Treatment, other than neurosurgical procedures that may be indicated, is purely symptomatic, and optimism is generally warranted.

Fever

Febrile delirium is common in children, often with the exanthematous diseases, and usually only if the fever is high (over 104° F). The child is restless, irritable, and "talks out of his head." He may not recognize his parents or be able to cooperate in his care. Panicky behavior and wild visual hallucinations may dominate the clinical picture. Treatment is largely medical: lowering the temperature, sedation, antibiotics and other specific measures, fluid and electrolyte replacement, and restraints as needed. The presence of a reassuring adult and adequate sensory stimulation (day and night lighting, and background music) are important.

Metabolic, Toxic, and Other Causes

In adults delirium may be seen under a variety of other conditions as follows:

Drug intoxication or overdosage (alcohol, corticotropin, bromides, hallucinogens, belladonna alkaloids).

Drug withdrawal (eg, narcotics, alcohol, barbiturates).

The postoperative state.

Infectious (especially febrile and debilitating) diseases such as pneumonia, typhoid, tuberculosis, emphysema.

Metabolic disorders (vitamin B deficiencies, uremia, liver disease, diabetic acidosis, porphyria).

Circulatory disturbances (congestive heart failure, cardiac arrhythmias, cerebral emboli, strokes, hypertensive encephalopathy).

Epilepsy (postictal, psychomotor attacks, petit mal status).

Endocrine disturbances (hyperthyroidism, hyperadrenocorticism, hypoadrenocorticism).

Cerebral neoplasms.

Sensory deprivation (see below).

Lupus erythematosus.

Respiratory insufficiency (mountain sickness, bends, Pickwickian syndrome).

Episodes of pathologic violence, wife-beating, child-battering, rape and other sexual offenses, and some homicides may occur as part of the delirious state, especially in certain cases of psychomotor epilepsy and temporal lobe disease.

Often multiple causes coexist. For example, in a postoperative patient who suddenly becomes psychotic, one should think of one or more of the following: drug reaction (including anesthetic), infection, fluid and electro-lyte imbalance, cerebrovascular accident (especially embolic), and sensory deprivation (see below). The effect of the emotional situation on the pre-existing personality must also be considered. A history of mental distur-bances or an unstable personality makeup, or a history of extreme preopera-tive dread or tension may be diagnostically significant.

Sensory Deprivation

In rare cases, sensory deprivation or isolation can cause a mild delirious, psychotic-like state, usually quickly reversible when the deprivation or isola-tion ends. This has occurred in shipwrecked sailors, military men on lonely watches, long-distance truck drivers, pilots flying high and out of sight of the horizon ("gray-out"), Arctic explorers ("white-out"), deep-sea divers ("rapture of the deep"), postoperative cataract patients ("black patch psychosis"), overly isolated cardiac patients ("cardiac psychosis"), and numerous other clinical situations.

DEMENTIA

Clinical Findings

Dysfunction at the upper mental level (intellectual and judgmental) produces impairment of the intellectual processes (dementia), recognized largely by loss of any or all of the following:

(1) **Memory:** Recent events are most affected, causing absentminded-ness and carelessness at first. Later, recognition, retention, and recall may all be involved, and serious blunders may occur, eg, overdosing oneself with pills, getting lost in a familiar dwelling or neighborhood, forgetting impor-tant business matters, and being unable to remember well known informa-tion. If the patient attempts to fill the memory gaps, confabulation results. Memory of remote events may persist even in severe dementia. (*Example:* In a patient with advanced Alzheimer's disease, ability to speak Yiddish, the first language learned as a child, continued long after the ability to speak and understand English had been lost.)

(2) **Learning, comprehension, calculation, reasoning, problem solving, and other cognitive powers:** Many of these functions are complex and over-lap with one another, with memory, and with the lower mental functions. Clinically, one at first sees increasing difficulty in adjusting to new situa-tions, learning people's names, performing unfamiliar duties in a new job or home situation, and getting around in a hospital; later, there may be loss of business acumen, of ability to read or understand printed matter or spoken instructions, or even to care for oneself in eating, getting dressed, or going to the bathroom. The condition can usually be differentiated from the aphasias of more localized neurologic origin by the widespread nature of the mental loss. At times, however, aphasia may coexist with dementia.

(3) **Personality characteristics:** The last acquired are the first to go. Habits of refinement, culture, polish, and sophistication slowly peel away,

followed by good manners, dignity, polite behavior, and consideration for others. "Second childhood" becomes second infancy as the demented patient is reduced to a kind of vegetative existence.

(4) Judgmental and creative functions: These high level mental functions depend on the ability to think abstractly, and thus to think about oneself, judge, evaluate, plan, idealize, create, and imagine. They are intimately personal characteristics, difficult for an outside observer to observe, thus rarely available for clinical use. For artists, research workers, or creative leaders in responsible and sensitive positions, losses in this category can be critical and may become manifest in the nature and quantity of their work output. Thus, one's spouse, close relatives, or work associates may be the first to notice the "slipping" that may herald the onset of dementia. The patient often deludes himself for some time into believing that nothing is wrong—largely through using the mental mechanisms of repression, denial, displacement, and projection.

The higher level mental functions are thought to be widely distributed anatomically in the brain, with some degree of interchangeability, overlap, and redundancy among the parts. The temporal, parietal, and frontal lobes predominate, the last holding sovereignty over the very highest functions. There is reason to believe that the quantity of brain loss as well as distribution determines the degree of dementia.

Etiology

The dementias are usually brought on by chronic, progressive, structural, or degenerative conditions that are not reversible.

Cerebral arteriosclerosis and other **cerebrovascular diseases** are the commonest causes of dementia. The etiologic factors are unknown, but heredity, hypercholesterolemia, hypertension, and diabetes have been implicated. The onset may follow a stroke or several "little strokes," and the course, though variable, is usually downhill. Clinical improvement can be expected only in symptoms due to acute aspects of the disorder (eg, localized edema around a thrombotic area may subside and thus diminish the size of the disabled brain substance). If the progress of the organic disease is arrested, however, the dementia may proceed no further, in which case what seems to be improvement can take place as both the patient and his caretakers learn to adjust better to his impairments.

Senile dementia is a more steadily progressive disease, also of unknown cause. The pathology is cellular rather than vascular and results in widespread atrophy of the brain and gross mental loss. Many comparable **degenerative disorders** have been described, eg, Alzheimer's disease and Pick's disease, but clinically they all share the same dementia, the same lack of response to therapy, and the same fate.

Prolonged **toxic** conditions brought on either by drugs or by metabolic disturbance can sometimes lead to dementia. Years of alcoholism, drug abuse, vitamin deficiency (beriberi, pellagra, Korsakoff's or Wernicke's disease, vitamin B_{12} deficiency), or the **residuals** of acute insults to the brain (severe head injury, carbon monoxide poisoning, heavy metal poisoning, prolonged anoxia, etc) may also cause dementia. In recent years, many enzymatic metabolic deficiencies have been found to be responsible for mental retardation in children (much as hypothyroidism produces cretinism).

Various other **neurologic conditions** can be associated with dementia, eg, brain tumors (especially metastatic or slow-growing and infiltrative gliomas or tumors associated with prolonged internal hydrocephalus), subdural hematoma, syphilis of the CNS (general paresis), severe encephalitis, last stages of multiple sclerosis, Huntington's chorea, repeated head traumas ("punch drunk" boxers), hydrocephalus, and "occult hydrocephalus."

It may be noted that some organic conditions can produce delirium, dementia, or no mental disturbance at all (trauma, tumor, encephalitis, drug abuse, alcoholism).

General Management

Although a history of a steady, downhill course in an elderly, mentally declining individual gives one little reason to be clinically optimistic, the physician must avoid being too pessimistic. Emotional elements that are reversible may be playing an important role in early cases. Depression, for example, is a severe problem in elderly people, and this may exaggerate the abnormalities in the patient's mental outlook considerably. Poor nutrition and neglect of other elements in good physical hygiene and unsuspected chronic drug abuse or alcoholism may also be complicating the picture. Good management and an air of hopefulness on the part of the physician may bring about improvement which, even if minimal, will be greatly appreciated by the patient and his family.

DIFFERENTIAL DIAGNOSIS OF DELIRIUM AND DEMENTIA

Full-blown cases of delirium or dementia are unmistakable, but difficulties sometimes arise in diagnosing early or mild cases. The most common error is a misdiagnosis of "functional psychoses" (schizophrenia, manic-depressive psychosis, or a mixture of the 2—ie, schizo-affective disorder).

In delirium, the break with reality differs from that in the functional psychoses. The delirious patient is disoriented, and the break is at the primitive, sensorial level, usually fluctuating from time to time as the underlying organic condition waxes or wanes. The schizophrenic's break with reality occupies a more abstract level, having to do with his thoughts about himself and his status in the world. He tends to harbor delusions of his special significance in a universe that is no longer impartial. The manic patient and the depressed one also see the world in a distorted way, either in overly rosy or blue hues.

The delirious patient's hallucinations resemble kaleidoscopic embellishments of his true sensory impressions, often misinterpreting actual perceptions (illusions). Eg, "The bugs are crawling all over me! Get them off, they're killing me!" (There are a few bread crumbs on his skin.) He usually sees things that stir up great emotion in him, either frantic fear or, less commonly, ecstatic joy. They come and go and follow no connected plot. However, the schizophrenic hears voices verbalizing his own deluded concepts of himself—voices that persist with unswerving monotony and deadly accusation. ("You have committed the Unpardonable Sin. You are forever doomed.") Manic and depressed patients rarely hallucinate.

The demented patient's mental status is characterized by loss; the schizophrenic's by distortion; the manic-depressive's by mood exaggeration. In early dementia, patients may blame others or distort the reality situation in attempts to explain away their mistakes, and unreasonable emotions may crop up. ("Somebody has deliberately been hiding my glasses on me again!" "He's lying. I never told him he could cancel the order!") The grumpy patient's foibles are usually superficial and transparent. The schizophrenic may be devious, subtle, and convincingly misleading. ("Look at these newspaper clippings and this log I have been keeping. No one can deny the facts.") The manic is ebullient. ("I tell you I made a fantastic investment! My money will be tripled by next week!")

Occasionally, a schizophrenic with an acute and violent psychotic outbreak (as in catatonic frenzy) may resemble a patient with severe delirium (as in alcohol withdrawal). He may refuse to answer questions, so that his orientation remains in doubt and he may guilefully feign quiescence and compliance to dupe the "enemy," thus resembling the fluctuating delirious patient. However, the course of the illness will soon distinguish the acute organic situation from the protracted delusionary state.

Occasionally, a severely depressed patient or a mute schizophrenic may seem to be demented. The history usually clarifies the diagnosis, or the reaction of the patient to continued intensive efforts to induce him to respond may do so. Substantial improvement will rule out dementia. The patient's own explanation for his silence (eg, dejection or hostility) may rule in depression or schizophrenia.

REFERENCES

Books and Monographs

APA Committee on Nomenclature and Statistics: *Diagnostic and Statistical Manual of Mental Disorders,* 2nd ed. American Psychiatric Association, 1968.

Brain, W.R.: *Clinical Neurology,* 2nd ed. Oxford Univ Press, 1964.

Chusid, J.G.: *Correlative Neuroanatomy & Functional Neurology,* 14th ed. Lange, 1970.

Dreisbach, R.H.: *Handbook of Poisoning: Diagnosis & Treatment,* 6th ed. Lange, 1969.

Lennox, G.W., & M.A. Lennox: *Epilepsy and Related Disorders.* Vols 1 & 2. Little, Brown, 1960.

Mark, H., & R. Ervin: *Violence and the Brain.* Brunner/Mazel, 1970.

Journal Articles

Adams, R.D., & others: Symptomatic occult hydrocephalus with "normal" cerebrospinal fluid pressure. New England J Med 273:117–125, 1965.

Beach, G.O., & others: Hazards to health: Scopolamine poisoning. New England J Med 270:1354–1355, 1964.

Chynoweth, R., & J. Foley: Pre-senile dementia responding to steroid therapy. Brit J Psychiat 115:703–708, 1969.

Dalal, P.M., & others: Cerebral embolism. Lancet 1:61–64, 1965.

DeJong, R.N.: Psychomotor or temporal lobe epilepsy. Neurology 7:1–14, 1957.

Dewhurst, K.: The neurosyphilitic psychoses today: A survey of 91 cases. Brit J Psychiat 115:31–38, 1969.

Fine, E.W., & D. Lewis: The effect of cyclandelate on mental function in patients with arteriosclerotic brain disease. Brit J Psychiat 117:157–161, 1970.

Gottfries, C.G., & B.E. Roos: Homovanillic acid and 5-hydroxyindoleacetic acid in cerebrospinal fluid related to rated mental and motor impairment in senile and presenile dementia. Acta psychiat scandinav 46:99–105, 1970.

Heiser, J.F., & J.C. Gillin: The reversal of anticholinergic drug-induced delirium and coma with physostigmine. Am J Psychiat 127:1050–1054, 1971.

Henderson, L.W., & P.J. Merrill: Diagnosis and treatment: Treatment of barbiturate intoxication. Ann Int Med 64:876–891, 1966.

Johnson, J.: Organic psychosyndromes due to boxing. Brit J Psychiat 115:45–54, 1969.

Korolenko, C.P., Yevseyeva, T.A., & P.P. Volkov: Data for a comparative account of toxic psychoses of various aetiologies. Brit J Psychiat 115:273–280, 1969.

Mark, V.H., & others: Brain disease and violent behavior. Neuro-ophthalmol 4:282–287, 1968.

McDonald, C.: Clinical heterogeneity in senile dementia. Brit J Psychiat 115:267–272, 1969.

Victor, M.: Treatment of alcoholic intoxication and the withdrawal syndrome. Psychosom Med 28:636–650, 1966.

Wooster, A.G., Dunlop, N., & R.A. Joske: Use of an oral diuretic in treatment of bromide intoxication. Am J M Sc 253:23–26, 1967.

16...

Neurosis

Neuroses are exaggerations of what we all feel at times—symptoms due to emotions instead of organic disease. Causes involve conflicts, often unconscious, deep-seated, and rooted in childhood. Varieties are largely descriptive: anxiety, hysterical, phobic, obsessive compulsive, depressive, etc. Treatment may be supportive (symptomatic) or uncovering. The former may include medication, reassurance, reeducation, and perhaps technics such as group therapy or behavior therapy; the latter requires bringing unconscious conflicts to consciousness.

Before Sigmund Freud's discoveries about the neuroses became generally accepted, the term signified a number of diseases thought to be referable to the nervous system and implied a long, slowly progressive downhill course. They included anxiety neurosis or anxiety hysteria, phobias, obsessions, compulsions, and neurasthenia; this latter is now part of a larger group of syndromes described as depressive neurosis.

Since no physical cause could be found for the neuroses, they were usually thought to be due to degenerative processes that were either idiopathic or hereditary. Although numerous palliative methods of treatment were advocated, neurotics could expect little relief from their symptoms. Rest cures were advocated in the USA for neurasthenia; various types of electrical stimulation treatments for hysterical symptoms enjoyed brief vogues on the continent; and hypnosis was widely used in an effort to give symptomatic relief. In France, the neurologist Charcot gave particular attention to the hysteria syndromes, and Janet is best known for his description of the obsessive compulsive neuroses.

Our understanding of the emotional basis of the neuroses dates from 1893 with the publication of Freud and Breuer's *Preliminary Communication on the Psychical Mechanism of Hysterical Phenomena*, where for the first time it is stated that memories of a trauma can be responsible for hysterical symptoms. A key passage reads as follows: "We must, however, mention another remarkable fact, which we shall later be able to turn to account, namely, that these memories, unlike other memories of their past lives, are not at the patient's disposal. On the contrary, these experiences are completely absent from the patient's memory when they are in a normal psychical state or are only present in a highly summary form." The concept of the *unconscious* is herewith set forth.

Breuer and Freud later outlined the series of events leading to neurosis that have now become common knowledge among educated people: A psychologic trauma takes place, and is not reacted to but is repressed into the unconscious. The affect persists in the unconscious along with the memory, and may return to awareness in distorted form as a neurotic symptom. The cure lies in once again making accessible to consciousness that which has been repressed so that affective abreaction (release of previously bound emotion) can take place.

Although this simplified scheme of the mental processes involved in neuroses needed a number of elaborations and modifications, the concept of the unconscious remains central to the psychodynamic explanation of neurotic illness. Of equal importance is the now widely accepted view that the neuroses are psychologically determined in the life history of the individual.* The technic of psychoanalysis evolved originally from the concept of making the unconscious conscious. The principal tools of psychoanalysis from the earliest days were the understanding of free associations and the interpretation of dreams.

The psychologic exploration of the emotional traumas that lead to repression of painful memories, which was the first aim of psychoanalysis, led to the discovery of what since has come to be known as psychosexual development. A vast body of knowledge accumulated about physical and emotional development from early childhood into adult life and the specific tasks that the growing child must master at every stage of development. The original theories focused on libido and its discharge at various stages of development. (See Chapter 31.)

The discovery of *infantile sexuality* proved particularly fertile since it led to the formulation of the so-called Oedipus complex. At ages 4–6, the child becomes infatuated with the parent of the opposite sex. The little boy wishes to displace his father in his mother's favor, and the little girl wishes to take mother's place with father. In exploratory therapy with adults, it is often possible to reconstruct the events of this period. Deviations from the normal such as the absence of one or both parents, emotional coldness on the part of the beloved parent, parental abusiveness or excessive seductiveness—all may lead to neurotic symptoms in later life. The success with which the so-called oedipal conflict (in the male, the wish for the mother but fear of retaliation from the father) is resolved is an important factor in determining the character of the individual. Resolution of the oedipal conflict normally occurs through identification with the father, "internalizing" him to form the "superego." In effect, the little boy settles the issue through the unconscious maneuver: "I don't have to envy or compete with father—I am like father." Thereafter, he has his conscience to contend with. Reconstruction of the so-called infantile neurosis, ie, the events around the oedipal phase and their impact on later life, constitutes the core of therapeutic psychoanalysis.

*Freud, however, maintained throughout his life that organic factors might also be operative in the neuroses.

Conflict. In the treatment of the neuroses it is important to remember that conflict in one form or another is always at the root of the presenting symptom. Successful treatment depends upon clearly identifying the conflict and upon helping the patient to recognize and live with his conflicts and find better solutions for them than neurotic symptom formation. The therapist's task consists principally of identifying the pertinent psychic issues. Supportive treatment without insight is insufficient. Insight alone may also be insufficient.

In Freud's early work it was assumed that painful memories were forced out of awareness into the unconscious because of reality considerations—eg, social convention or personal pride. Freud later developed a more sophisticated structural model of the personality which consisted of the *id,* the repository of the instinctual drives always striving for expression; the *ego,* a sort of central coordinating (executive) branch of the personality; and the *superego,* part of which is analogous to the conscience, ie, the body of demands and prohibitions derived originally from parental authority and later self-imposed, and part the *ego-ideal,* the individual's concept of how he would like to be. Neurosis occurs when there is conflict between the ego and the id, and the so-called defense mechanisms are the ego's way of thwarting the demands of unacceptable instinctual drives. In psychoanalytic theory, conflict is considered as always involving the ego. If it is between the ego and the id, the result may be neurosis; if it is between the ego and the superego, the result may be depression; if it is between the ego and an unassimilated or threatening outside world, the result may be various behavioral or psychosomatic illnesses. Psychosis may result if any conflict becomes too great or long-lasting.

ANXIETY NEUROSIS

Anxiety is the term used to describe the subjective experience of unpleasant tension, uneasiness, and distress that accompanies psychic threat or conflict. It is often attended by physical reactions such as increased pulse and respiratory rate and elevated blood pressure. It may be said to be "unconscious anxiety" if the subjective awareness is absent but sufficient causes and clear effects can be identified, and especially if the anxiety later becomes conscious. Anxiety in various forms plays a prominent role in most psychiatric disorders.

(1) Signal anxiety: Freud originally conceived of anxiety as frustrated (and consequently repressed) libido. Later he developed a more useful concept of anxiety as having a *signal function* against danger approaching the ego from the instinctual drives. If the course of action required for the satisfaction of id-based drives is unacceptable to the ego, anxiety arises and leads to the establishment of the so-called defense mechanisms. When anxiety is very great, the individual may be assumed to be under severe pressure from his instincts without having as yet worked out a means of either providing satisfactory outlets or establishing successful defenses. Characteristically, he is aware of his anxiety but is unaware of a reasonable cause for it. He may overreact to annoying trivia in his daily life, may have nightmares, or may be generally irritable, upset, or "nervous."

Example: A woman in her 30's complained about "nervousness" and showed many symptoms of anxiety such as restlessness and inability to sleep at night. She also had physical symptoms such as "heart beats" and digestive disturbances. She had a history of dysmenorrhea as a younger woman. During interviews with her psychologically oriented family doctor, she related her anxieties to her daily life with her husband and gave long recitals of her "miseries" with him. Time and again, the physician led her away from the present and into her past. As a girl she had had frequent angry interchanges with her mother, whom she described as cool and rejecting, and a secret but powerful love for her alcoholic father, who was neglectful of her and her mother but nevertheless radiated affection. She recognized that her husband was a better man than her father and had none of his vices. As her daughter entered the same stage of life (about age 7), the patient's feelings about her own childhood led to a revival of her desire for an affectionate relationship with her devalued father. Her husband, with his impeccable habits and morality, did not suffice as a father substitute, so she attacked him. It is significant that he once cried out, "You're going to drive me to drink!"

In this case the patient's anxiety is a signal of danger, that of reactivating her childhood oedipal conflict when her positive feelings for her father had run counter to her mother's quite reasonable objections. When the patient was able to understand her need for affection from her father, her anxiety subsided.

(2) Separation anxiety: Separation anxiety is the anxiety connected with impending or feared abandonment or loss of a person whom one needs. It is common among young people who are dependent on parents, immature people at any age, and psychotics. Separation anxiety may be the cause for the so-called "school phobia" syndrome, which often keeps young children away from school and with their mothers. It is not a phobia in the true sense, and most often is not expressed as, "I am afraid to go to school," but by often-repeated physical complaints such as stomach aches or headaches which make school attendance impossible. The issue is not school but separation from the mother.

Separation anxiety should be distinguished from a deep and almost indescribable horror spoken of mostly by psychotics and associated with thoughts and feelings of annihilation or extinction or ceasing to be (not simply death).

(3) Castration anxiety: Anxiety in the male may often be due to the fear of castration which is part of the Oedipus complex.

Example: A student complained of inability to sleep, nightmares, difficulty in concentration, and general fearfulness. He was involved in a neurotic relationship with an older divorced woman. When the relationship came to an end, his anxiety subsided; but not until he realized that the affair had raised earlier problems connected with his desire for his mother, who had been rather seductive toward him when he was a young and sickly boy. With this insight, he became free of anxiety and regained his former efficiency in pursuing his career objectives.

Although when Freud introduced the concept of castration anxiety and stressed its importance in the Oedipus complex he meant castration literally, later workers have extended the meaning of the term to include symbolic castration and punishment or injury generally.

Treatment

The treatment of anxiety neurosis begins with exploration, particularly of the instinctual drives that may be temporarily causing alarm in the ego. The patient should not be allowed to continue to complain about his present problems but should be urged to seek their antecedents in his past life. Supportive treatment alone is rarely effective, and drugs* give only temporary relief. Exploratory therapy is usually successful within weeks or months.

<h2 style="text-align:center">HYSTERICAL NEUROSIS</h2>

The word hysteria has passed through a great many variations of meaning since it was first employed to express the belief that nervous conditions arose from abnormalities of the womb. It is still used loosely today to mean anything from wild "hysterics" (temporary emotional loss of control) to any neurotic (or even psychotic) condition whatever.

Correct usage now confines the term to a specific form of neurosis characterized by loss of function in either the physical or mental spheres. Physical loss (*conversion*) may be of motor function ("paralysis" or inability to speak) or sensation ("anesthesia," "blindness"); mental loss (*dissociation*) may be in consciousness ("faints," trances, fugues), memory (amnesia), or total integration (spells, "split personality"). Familiar accompaniments are *emotional indifference* (*la belle indifférence*), and *secondary gain* (indirect benefit from the symptom). A "lump in the throat" (*globus hystericus*) is not unusual, presumably a psychosomatic emotional concomitant. (See Chapter 18.)

Psychodynamically, it is presumed that the buried conflict (oedipal) does not just leak out from its repression, as in anxiety neurosis, but threatens complete disruption, so that major defenses are resorted to. The symptom chosen depends on unknown organ fallibility (*locus minoris resistentiae*) and the previous psychologic background. The *meaning* and *symbolic value* of the body part or function determines the clinical picture, eg, paralysis of the legs means inability to "stand up to" one's problem; blindness signifies unwillingness to "see" the true situation; muteness stands for protective silence. Characteristically, the single symptom represents both indirect gratification of the forbidden impulse (to run away, devour or ravish

---

*Antianxiety agents are discussed in Chapter 24.

visually, destroy verbally) and punishment. The paralyzed soldier has left the fight but can no longer walk; being safe, he blandly accepts his crippled state.

Major hysteria seems to be disappearing from modern civilized communities. One sees it now primarily in primitive societies or in young adolescents of limited intelligence. When it is associated with bizarre phenomena (peculiarities of identity or intellectual functioning) or hallucinations, the possibility of schizophrenia arises. Some authorities believe that the severe ego pathology in hysteria warrants the diagnosis of psychosis in every case.

The treatment of hysteria involves the management of the presenting symptoms and the rehabilitation of the background personality. Various tricks have been employed for the "cure" of the conversion symptom—hypnosis, static electricity, Amytal interviews, sleep therapy. These seem to reach behind the patient's wall of resistance and pull up enough hidden data to force abandonment of the symptom. But the resistance remains intact, and emergency defenses, largely depression, are then evoked to support it. Better strategy is to permit the patient to retain his symptom and let it serve as a barometer during prolonged psychotherapy for deep-going self-understanding and change.

PHOBIAS

The principal symptom of the phobic reaction is anxiety. However, diffuse anxiety may attach itself to any external, interpersonal, or physical issue, whereas in the phobias the patient fixes his anxiety on a given object or situation which he then can avoid. The anxiety of the phobic patient is more properly called *fear* because in its clinical form it presents as such.

Common phobias are *agoraphobia,* fear of open places; *claustrophobia,* fear of being closed in; *acrophobia,* fear of high places; *xenophobia,* fear of strangers; *aquaphobia,* fear of water; and *zoophobia,* fear of animals. Specific syndromes reported in modern times are *subway phobia* and *airplane phobia.*

Phobias share one characteristic feature: The sufferer avoids the object of his fear out of a feeling that otherwise something bad will happen to him although he doesn't know what.

Exploratory therapy will ultimately reveal the reason for the fear, but aggressive interpretations in the early phase of treatment are rarely successful. Even though the therapist may know some of the causes of the phobia, simple reassurance is rarely effective because the symptom serves an important function in promoting emotional comfort. By concentrating all his anxieties on one thing, the patient manages—even at great cost—to avoid the pains of diffuse anxiety.

Separation anxiety frequently underlies the phobic syndromes. Fear of open spaces may represent the fear of separation from a protective home environment. People with claustrophobia may fear the loss of power to make their own decisions (a frequent feature of alcoholism).

A pertinent feature of phobic symptoms is their ambivalence. Like neurotic symptoms in general, a phobia serves 2 purposes: (1) It must help the individual to adapt to his emotional problem in some way, even though it is an unsatisfactory and painful way; and (2) it must serve as a fulfillment, at least in phantasy, of unacceptable repressed wishes, the pain and suffering being the concomitant punishment.

Example: A young woman suffered from fear of trains, especially crowded subway trains. While it was convenient for her to focus all her anxieties on the ride home in the evening, thus permitting her to function responsibly during the day, the subway phobia also was related to a secret wish for a sexual encounter in the traffic and excitement of the rush hour.

The ambivalence of phobic symptoms is well demonstrated in Helene Deutsch's view of the role of the protector in the phobic syndrome. A phobic patient can often overcome his fears when he is protected by someone, usually one particular person. In phobic young girls the mother often assumes the protecting role. Characteristically, the protector is a person for whom the phobic individual harbors ambivalent feelings of hate and love.

What determines the choice of the phobic symptom is as little understood as the choice of psychiatric symptoms in general. Nevertheless, the meaning of the avoided situation in a phobia is often quite evident.

Treatment

The proper treatment of phobic patients became a very difficult matter to the early psychoanalysts who advocated only a passive and interpretative role for the therapist. Sandor Ferenczi was the first to recognize that active intervention by the therapist was required to help the phobic patient face and conquer his terror. Although some phobic patients will eventually decide to do this by themselves, continued avoidance of the feared situation constitutes a therapeutic stalemate that cannot be ignored. Particularly among older patients, long-standing phobic patterns become so firmly established that a phobic character structure develops and the patient considers any attempt to break his symptom's hold a threat and challenge to his entire mode of life.

For this reason, the prognosis for cure of the phobic reactions is often considered poor. Patients are helped by treatment, but many remain partially crippled by their symptom. Still, without treatment, many patients grow steadily worse, their phobic objects increasing until they include almost everything. Some must remain indoors for years, virtual prisoners of their disease.

The newer active methods of treating phobia such as desensitization, operant conditioning, and behavior therapy have shown considerable promise. (See Chapter 28.)

OBSESSIVE COMPULSIVE NEUROSIS

Obsessions are recurrent thoughts that intrude upon consciousness without the individual's being able to do anything about it. Compulsions are repetitive acts that must be performed no matter how irrational and useless they seem. The patient is intensely uncomfortable with his symptoms (usually both kinds), tries unsuccessfully to resist them, and experiences anxiety if he is prevented from performing his rituals. As with the phobic patient, the obsessive compulsive needs his symptoms as a shield against anxiety. Unlike the phobic patient, however, he cannot objectify his fears and then avoid the object or situation but must deal with them in his own characteristic way which resembles magical thinking (expecting that things will happen by wishing rather than by doing or other logical means). It is useless to point out the irrationality of his obsessions or compulsions because he knows this already and suffers from it.

Examples: The patient who fears he may have hit someone with his car without being aware of it and retraces his path to see if anyone is lying on the road; the patient who has an inexplicable urge to kill someone he loves. But the one who fears he will kill continues to have the same fear even when the person involved is out of the country. Similarly, the obsessional fear of syphilis cannot be disarmed by avoiding intercourse or by continually repeating negative serologic tests.

Although obsessional temptations and fears are almost never acted out or realized, they often call for the performance of certain harmless acts that seem to serve as countermeasures. These acts (often called rituals) usually consist of some repetitious and ceremonial elaboration of ordinary daily activities, eg, special routines of washing, dressing, and arranging the room. The meaning of the act may be clear to the patient—eg, keeping the hands tucked into the jacket sleeves, Mandarin style, to guard against choking someone, or continual washing to prevent contamination with germs. At times, however, it is not clear what (if anything) the action means—eg, compulsive touching, counting, or stepping over cracks. Whether the act is meaningful or not, it proceeds from inner necessity, and resisting by an act of will causes anxiety.

Obsessive compulsive symptoms take many forms. The most characteristic feature is the vacillation and doubt that occur as a result of the continuing inner struggle against the symptom. The periodically renewed conviction that an absurd symptom must be resisted always provokes an attitude of doubt and apprehension of the unformulated consequences. Normally, doubt is part of critical thinking; in its obsessional form, it defeats the purpose of thought. Rational conclusions and logical decisions become impossible, and the endless cycles of frustrated resolutions make the mental life of the individual a broken record that never ends. The fuzzy area between doubting as skepticism and doubting as compulsive rumination separates the mental world of the obsessional from that of normal cognitive experience.

Psychodynamically, one may note that the characteristic defense mechanisms of the obsessive compulsive are isolation and reaction formation.

Isolation is a prime factor in obsessive compulsive pathology. Characteristically, the obsessive compulsive remembers innumerable facts, including emotionally loaded ones, but the affect that accompanied the emotionally loaded events is not available to him. In contrast to the anxious person, who seems to be oversupplied with affect for reasons he does not understand, the obsessive compulsive knows the facts but does not feel the anxiety, anger, or depression that ought to be associated with pertinent psychic events in his past life. His characteristic pattern is to remain aloof from emotionally loaded situations, to stand at a distance from people who tend to press their feelings upon him, and to be generally unaware of or helpless with the emotional needs of others.

Reaction formation usually takes place by a process called *undoing.* The obsessive compulsive patient is constantly preoccupied with balancing 2 opposites against each other. If one day is good, the next one necessarily will be bad; if progress is achieved in one area, disaster will strike in another. Elaborate justifications are often devised in an attempt to make these superstitious beliefs acceptable. The obsessive compulsive person is not really superstitious, but he behaves as if he were superstitious against his wishes and better judgment. The young girl in latency age who playfully sings, "Step on a crack, break my mother's back" is demonstrating a highly condensed version of such thinking. She may still wish that some disaster would overcome her mother, but by this time these wishes are thoroughly unacceptable and their fulfillment must be prevented by the magical act of avoiding cracks in the sidewalks.

Diagnosis

Although fleeting experiences with obsessional thinking or compulsive behavior are universal, the neurosis as such is a justified diagnosis in fewer than 5% of neurotic patients. This is in contrast to the character type, which is very common.

An obsessive compulsive reaction is one in which the typical symptoms cause considerable anxiety and significantly interfere with work, personal relationships, or the capacity to enjoy life. The symptoms are often intermittent, or at least wax and wane markedly in severity.

The symptoms themselves are easy to identify. The only difficulty is differentiating the neurotic syndrome from other psychiatric disorders in which obsessional phenomena play a part.

In phobias, the patient's own testimony about his symptom can be taken as diagnostically valid. If he can avoid something outside himself to escape anxiety, he has a phobia; if he is fearful of his own inner thoughts or impulses, he has an obsession. In some cases, however, the distinction is not so clear—eg, a knife phobia may reflect the obsessional thought that one may stab someone with a knife.

Depression often accompanies obsessive symptoms. The principal complaints of the patient who is predominantly depressed involve loss of hope and interest in life and no expectation of help from others, while the obsessive compulsive neurotic tends to be more anxious than depressed. Moreover, neurotic obsessions tend to be less acutely disabling than depression, and obsessive compulsive neurotics rarely commit suicide.

It is common to consider schizophrenia in the diagnostic evaluation of any obsessive compulsive patient because his obsessions or compulsions may have an irrational or bizarre quality. Obsessions occasionally do occur as part of schizophrenic syndromes, but in general—in the absence of other major signs of schizophrenia—one can be confident that the obsessive compulsive is not developing a psychosis. Despite the "magical thinking," there is no real withdrawal from the world of other people. The obsessional may fear he is "going crazy" but he rarely does so. Some reassurance can even be given that a well structured obsessive compulsive neurosis protects against psychosis.

When the obsessive compulsive says he is tempted to perform vicious acts, a decision must be made about whether a real danger exists. In general, the obsessive compulsive will give evidence of overcontrol, without even the normal amount of spontaneity and impulsiveness. The person who is liable to act out violently usually gives a history of difficulty in controlling his rages and of reckless, irresponsible behavior in the past—especially in childhood. The obsessive compulsive usually realizes that it is the idea of his violent action that he fears rather than the action itself. Admittedly, this is a fine point, and any patient who persists in the belief that he may hurt someone should be helped to control his behavior. Fortunately, the obsessive compulsive usually responds to a reassuring discussion about the difference between thoughts and acts. While his neurotic disability may remain unimproved, the issue of violent behavior can usually be quickly resolved.

Treatment

Psychotherapy is generally regarded as the treatment of choice when obsessive compulsive symptoms are severe enough to require medical attention. Most authorities agree, however, that some modifications of classical psychotherapeutic technic are desirable, and some go so far as to advocate drastic new technics such as various forms of behavior therapy. In psychotherapy, it is important to focus on the current realities of the patient's life and the relationship with the therapist. The problems of how to handle anger and the quest for certainty are the most common major issues. In successful therapy, it often is discovered that inability to express positive feelings is a basic issue—more important, even, than anger.

It is customary to consider the dynamic psychotherapy of obsessive compulsive neurosis an arduous, lengthy undertaking of doubtful outcome. This therapeutic pessimism is warranted only if the (unrealistic) goal of therapy is radical reorganization of the personality. Obsessive compulsives go through crises of anxiety and depression which may be severe. However, these patients are usually well protected from impulsive suicidal attempts, and they respond readily to supportive measures. If their crises are properly handled, obsessive compulsive symptoms become less painful and may not seriously interfere with the patient's life.

The patient should be helped to arrange his life so that it causes him less anger and anxiety. In this way, the energy that fuels the symptoms is cut off even though the defenses shaping the symptoms are unaltered.

Somatic therapy is generally of secondary value (phenothiazines and ECT are not usually helpful) but may be useful in 2 instances:

Drugs may be used to combat anxiety and depression during exacerbations. Sedatives (usually barbiturates) and the minor tranquilizers (meprobamate, chlordiazepoxide) are most often used. (See Chapter 24.)

Leukotomy is said to be helpful in the rare case in which obsessive compulsive symptoms are chronically severe, unremitting, and grossly disabling. In such cases, the patient appears to be so overcontrolled that the disinhibiting effect of leukotomy is normalizing.

The prognosis is hard to assess, and traditional accounts of great chronicity apply only to a few patients. As is true of other psychiatric disorders also, a history of good premorbid personality functioning, onset in response to obvious environmental stress, marked affective response, short duration of symptoms, and favorable social and cultural circumstances have favorable prognostic implications. Even in prolonged and severe cases, although progression to obsessive compulsive character may take place, progression to psychosis or antisocial behavior is uncommon.

DEPRESSIVE NEUROSIS

Depression is a common phenomenon variously characterized as gloominess, sadness, retardation of motility, tearfulness, etc. The range of depressive reactions stretches from mild sadness about a concrete disappointment through moderate and long-lasting reactions to severe psychotic depression or melancholia. Although neurotic depressive reactions can be fairly serious and occasionally lead to suicide, the more severe depressions are usually psychotic reactions and are discussed elsewhere (Chapter 14).

Object Loss in the Developmental History

In the depressive syndromes, the element of loss is always of paramount importance. The loss may be obvious, recent, and real, as in normal grief*; or it may have occurred in the past and never have been properly experienced, as in delayed grief and depressive guilt reactions (see below); or the loss may have been not of something concrete but rather of something intangible such as affection or self-esteem. The loss may not even be actual, but something impending or threatening or incipient (eg, failing health, departing youth, fading beauty, a tottering business, waning sexual vigor). What matters is not the facts themselves but what the patient believes to be the facts. Identifying exactly what the depressed patient has lost is usually a major therapeutic goal. After it has become clear what the patient has to be sad about, the work of grief proper can proceed.

*See discussion in Chapter 5.

The "grief work" entails reviewing all the significant life experiences with the lost object and seeing them afresh in a world in which this object is gone. For example, at an Irish wake or Jewish shiva, much of the conversation consists of reminiscences about the departed person.

Object losses at certain phases of development can be related to psychopathology in later life, but this relationship is not simple. Many people who have suffered severe losses at crucial periods in their development have few or no problems, whereas others who have suffered relatively minor losses develop severe disturbances. In working with disturbed persons, establishing the relationship between early object loss and the present illness provides valuable guides for treatment. It is the task of the therapist to determine the life situation of the depressed patient and to help him resolve his depressive feelings and move on toward a new adjustment commensurate with his life stage.

(1) **Object loss during infancy**: In the earliest stage of development, the kind of mothering received is of great importance. Some mothers are naturally confident and loving, whereas others have unending difficulties. A close and supportive relationship with the mother in the first year will enable the child to form relationships with others in his turn. If the infant is denied the early advantage of a close and affectionate relationship with his mother, he may remain aloof later on, unable to form intimate relationships. In so-called borderline patients, there is often a depressed and aloof mother in the family history. From this it follows that a baby with a severely depressed mother should be taken care of by other people at least part of the time, so that it can experience some natural mothering. Institutionalized children must be provided not only with proper physical care but also with adequate emotional mothering (best carried out by the same person).

(2) **Object losses during childhood**: A developmental phase in infancy is that of self-object differentiation. Sooner or later the child discovers that mother is not there all the time and that therefore he is apart both from his mother and, by implication, the outside world. On the basis of a clear differentiation between the self and the world, the child learns to say "I," and self-assertiveness begins. Insufficient self-object differentiation can occur if the child has not received sufficient emotional mothering; he will not let go. It can lead to symbiotic relationships between children and parents, to distorted communications, and a series of developments commonly associated with psychotic disorders (inhibited affect, disturbed appreciation of outer reality, concretism in thinking, and autism).

If the absence of one parent occurs later in the child's development, a number of neuroses or character disturbances may result. Where a normal triangle situation (oedipal) between father, mother, and child does not exist, the remaining parent figure, usually the mother, will become the target of strong ambivalent feelings and the relationship is likely to be conflictual and unsatisfactory. A young girl with only a mother and no father is likely to develop masochistic character traits, since the positive aspects of heterosexuality (care and affection) are not available. A young boy with mother only is more apt to demonstrate passive-aggressive characteristics and may become a delinquency problem as he grows older, particularly if seductive behavior on the mother's part has led to guilt feelings which had to be repressed. Masculine identification then becomes a problem, and overaggressiveness a neurotic solution. In the much rarer occurrence in which a child grows up without a mother or mother substitute but with a care-giving father, a girl will have to assume a mother's role too early in her life. Constriction of emotional functioning may be the result. A boy in that situation may be under pressure to assume a partially feminine role toward his father, with a resulting confusion of sexual identity.

It must be noted that such general statements have no predictive value. They are meant as post facto reconstructions which, when they are applicable, help the adult neurotic tie together some of his puzzling feelings and fantasies. In the context of psychotherapy, they provide understanding of "how it all came about."

(3) **Object loss during adolescence**: At some point in mid-adolescence the individual begins to realize that he must give up some of his ideas about his parents. The depression caused by relinquishing the image of his parents as infallible and supremely powerful beings is often manifested as adolescent rebellion and defiance, but withdrawal and sullen behavior are common symptoms of this essentially depressive constellation. When national leaders (generalized and symbolic parents) are considered fallible and corrupt, the resultant disenchantment may reach violent and mutinous proportions (the national scene, 1971?).

The desirable result, as in earlier developmental stages, is greater individuation. Through the process of separation from the parents, a new self-object differentiation is possible and a personal identity is within reach. Erikson has defined the main task of adolescence as the attainment of a personal identity.

(4) **Object loss in adulthood**: Depression in adult life may also be viewed as crises which, if optimally resolved, could lead to a creative new adjustment to life tasks. Quite often the task is not only to accept the present loss, but also to relive past losses.

Delayed or Incomplete Grief

Grief is a normal response to the loss of a loved one. In many cultures, it is expected that grief will be expressed in prescribed ways, and bereaved persons profit emotionally from conforming to the patterns that tradition has made available. This is less true of American culture, where the work of grieving is often left undone or only partly done so that delayed grief reactions tend to appear later as neurotic symptoms.

Normally, the bereaved person bemoans the loss he has suffered and feels that his world has become empty and meaningless. In contrast to the depressed person, however, he maintains his dignity and makes no exaggerated self-accusations. In time, he accepts his loss, the wound heals, and the beloved deceased remains only a positive memory.

Any interference with this normal process of grieving may result in a number of adverse consequences. For example, proper expression of grief is often not possible in children, adolescents, or affect-inhibited individuals. The grief is borne "with a stiff upper lip," and the realization of the terrible event is partly or wholly suppressed. A frequent consequence of this is constriction of emotional functioning. Suppression of the emotion of loss takes so much psychic energy that little is left for other purposes. For example, a young man whose wife died continued to pursue his professional goals even more ambitiously than before. For 3 years he found himself unable to make meaningful emotional contacts and became increasingly isolated. In therapy he came to realize how much he had *not* felt at the time of his wife's death, and only after a dramatic grief reaction was he able to regain his capacity to form relationships with other people. The diagnosis was one of delayed grief.

Adolescents are often unable to express feelings of grief. Sullen behavior, uncommunicativeness, social isolation, and delinquency may be expressions of improperly experienced grief. In younger children, aggressive behavior may represent a grief equivalent.

Diagnosis

Neurotic depression is a common disease entity. The depression is usually not as severe as that which occurs in psychotic depression. The predominant manifestation may be sadness and a feeling of helplessness in the face of a difficult life situation. These feelings may be related to objective difficulties at home or at work or to a health problem, but the patient is typically aware that his depressive response is not justified by the facts. The patient feels unable to perform up to capacity. Some degree of self-blame may be present, but the most important underlying feature, *guilt* is either not mentioned or not consciously acknowledged.

Example: A 45-year-old man sought psychiatric treatment because he was morose and dissatisfied with his job and his family life. A recent job change had proved not to be as rewarding as he had anticipated; his wife had suffered for years from a debilitating disease; and he had moved to a new part of the country where he had no friends. In the initial interviews, he appeared to be an open and outspoken person, able to express himself clearly and engagingly. After intensive therapy he was able to free himself from repression and express his dissatisfaction with the way he had been brought up in an emotionally cold atmosphere. He had never been able to reach his father, who refused to give him his approval and insisted always on more and more accomplishment. He grew up to be a professional man and appeared to be successful. A crisis in his marriage brought on feelings of anger and guilt toward his wife and, more significantly, his parents. In therapy he was able to relieve his guilt about early anger and delinquent tendencies and his depression disappeared.

A neurotic depressive reaction sometimes manifests itself in a different way than the classical symptoms of feelings of helplessness, sadness, crying, etc. The depressed adolescent in particular, instead of being sad, often resorts to desperate actions to cause grief and hardship for others while he remains apparently unmoved and unconcerned. Older people may adhere rigidly to their daily routines while they so mismanage their affairs that their careers or personal relationships deteriorate; the sad situation that results is not consciously felt as such except by others, and the patient is not aware of his role in bringing it about. This *acting to prevent sadness* must be recognized by the psychiatrist so that he can perceive the real intentions behind the patient's actions and not be side-tracked into exploring only their rational antecedents. For the depressed individual, it is the end result that matters: someone must feel sad; there must be grief and hardship. In *masked depression*, the psychiatrist must make the patient feel his depression, then come to grips with and master its origins.

Example: A 17-year-old boy had recently moved from a rural area, which he liked very much, into a suburb of a major city. He was caught trafficking in a relatively harmless drug which he brought from his new residence back to his old friends. He was impassive and apparently unconcerned about the charges against him. His past history demonstrated that the family move had entailed serious losses for him, particularly the loss of a grandfather with whom he had strongly identified. His parents had also lost a great deal by the move and were only marginally aware of the depressive family environment that had resulted.

In the fourth interview, the patient confirmed the depressive origin of his delinquent act by explaining that the effects of the drugs were such that it was a pleasure to supply them to his friends. The therapist said, "It must have felt good to be close with them again." The patient burst into tears and blurted out his misery and loneliness. Therapy then proceeded rapidly, and the patient was able to make a good adjustment.

Another form of masked depression is seen in *overcompensation.* People in a depressive situation may appear unconcerned and relatively happy ("smiling depression"). Such patients are at times dismissed as having nothing wrong with them, whereas in fact they are under serious pressure. Eventually they may commit suicide. The psychiatrist may see such people because of chronic pain, alcoholism, or other symptoms on a neurotic basis. If the patient's life situation is one in which it would seem he ought to be depressed, the psychiatrist should probe cautiously to see if he can unmask the depression. If he can do so readily, he can then proceed to treat it (with psychotherapy and drugs, as before); if it comes too hard, he had better desist, even if he is sure there is depression there. Some sleeping dogs should be allowed to lie undisturbed (eg, repressed feelings about a bad limp or other deformity, or having a feeble-minded child) since there are worse things than chronic pain or alcoholism (eg, psychosis, suicide), and some reality problems defy psychologic solution.

Treatment

The definitive treatment of depressive neurosis is psychotherapy, intensive and usually prolonged (many months). Neurotically depressed patients are often ideally suited for deep-going, interpretive technics based upon psychodynamic principles. Psychoanalysis or psychoanalytically oriented psychotherapy may be the treatment of choice if it is available.

Although the gratification that is inherent in supportive psychotherapy must be avoided in uncovering interpretive therapy, neurotically depressed patients must sometimes be supported. The psychic pain and anxiety of facing up to deeply buried material may be so great as to make the possibility of suicide very real. (See Chapter 22.) At such times, the frequency of visits may be increased, even to the point of more than one a day if necessary. Some matter-of-fact reassurance may be given that when the patient has been depressed long enough it will pass. Antidepressant or sedative drugs may be prescribed. Amitriptyline (Elavil) and imipramine (Tofranil) and their derivatives usually give symptomatic relief for depression without interfering greatly with therapy. Meprobamate or small doses of phenobarbital may be helpful for intense anxiety.

The prognosis of neurotic depressive reactions is favorable, but the pain experienced by the patient may be severe, particularly that related to guilt and aggression. A depressive syndrome may become rigid and remain chronic, with the patient underperforming for the rest of his life in an internal environment of private misery which he is unable to share. The psychiatrist should attempt as soon as possible to determine how rigid the depressive syndrome has become. If the patient is willing and able to share his painful feelings, he will show this by improving noticeably in the early interviews. If there is no change early in therapy, the prognosis is less optimistic.

ADDITIONAL TYPES OF NEUROSIS

Neurasthenic Neurosis (Neurasthenia)

This is an old descriptive term for patients who complain of chronic fatigue and little else. In many of them, organic disease is later found to be responsible. Some of them are simply depressed, and some have various other forms of psychiatric disorder.

Depersonalization Neurosis

Depersonalization refers to a peculiar feeling of unreality or detachment that can occur occasionally in normal people when they are physically ill, greatly fatigued, or very drowsy. It occurs frequently in other psychiatric disorders, especially in schizoid or schizophrenic conditions. It probably does not warrant the status of a diagnostic entity.

Hypochondriacal Neurosis

Patients who complain constantly of bodily aches and pains and discomforts (in the absence of organic disease) are frequently tagged with this diagnosis. If the complaints are intense and circumscribed, they may represent somatic delusions and indicate psychosis. Frequently they are associated features of a depression, perhaps partially masked, or of an anxiety neurosis.

REFERENCES

Books and Monographs

Bibring, E.: The mechanism of depression. Pages 13–48 in: *Affective Disorders.* Greenacre, P. (editor). Internat Univ Press, 1953.

Blos, P.: *On Adolescence. A Psychoanalytic Interpretation.* Free Press, 1962.

Deutsch, H.: Agoraphobia. Pages 97–116 in: *Neuroses and Character Types.* Internat Univ Press, 1965.

Deutsch, H.: Absence of grief. Pages 226–36 in: *Neuroses and Character Types.* Internat Univ Press, 1965.

Erikson, E.H.: *Childhood and Society,* 2nd ed. Norton, 1963.

Fenichel, O.: Anxiety as neurotic symptom: Anxiety hysteria. Pages 293–315 in: *The Psychoanalytic Theory of Neuroses.* Norton, 1945.

Freud, A.: *The Ego and the Mechanisms of Defense.* Internat Univ Press, 1946.

Spitz, R.A.: Hospitalism. An inquiry into the genesis of psychiatric conditions in early childhood. Pages 53–74 in: *The Psychoanalytic Study of the Child,* Vol 1. Internat Univ Press, 1945.

Spitz, R.A.: Pathology of object relations. Pages 197–300 in: *The First Year of Life.* Part III. Internat Univ Press, 1965.

Stone, A.A.: Neurosis: The symptoms of anxiety. Pages 7–20 in: *The Abnormal Personality Through Literature.* Stone, A.A. (editor). Prentice-Hall, 1963.

Wolpe, J.: *Psychotherapy by Reciprocal Inhibition.* Stanford Univ Press, 1958.

Zilboorg, G.: The discovery of neurosis. Pages 361–78 in: *A History of Medical Psychology.* Norton, 1941.

Journal Articles

Erikson, E.H.: Identity and the life cycle. Psychol Issues 1:1, 1959.

Goodwin, D.W., & others: Follow-up studies in obsessional neurosis. Arch Gen Psychiat 20:182–187, 1969.

Hollender, M.H.: Perfectionism. Comprehensive Psychiat 6:94–103, 1965.

Ingram, I.M.: Obsessional illness in mental hospital patients. J Ment Sc 107:382–402, 1961.

Lindemann, E.: Symptomatology and management of acute grief. Am J Psychiat 101:141–148, 1944.

Michael, R.P.: Treatment of a case of compulsive swearing. Brit MJ 1:1506–1508, 1957.

Pollitt, J.: Natural history of obsessional states. Brit MJ 1:194–198, 1957.

Rickels, K., & others: Hydroxyzine and chlordiazepoxide in anxious neurotic outpatients: A collaborative controlled study. Compr Psychiat 11:457–474, 1970.

Salzman, L.: Therapy of obsessional states. Am J Psychiat 122:1139–1146, 1966.

Stern, R.: Treatment of a case of obsessional neurosis using thought stopping techniques. Brit J Psychiat 117:441–442, 1970.

Woodruff, R.A., Jr., Clayton, P.J., & S.B. Guze: Hysteria. JAMA 215:425–428, 1971.

17 . . .

Character Disorders*

Character (personality) disorders are lifelong patterns of behavior, largely acceptable to the individual but productive of conflict with others. Causes may be in part genetic or constitutional and in part developmental or emotional. Types are descriptive: schizoid, obsessive compulsive, hysterical, antisocial, passive-aggressive, masochistic, etc. Treatment may consist of counseling and reeducation or of deep-going psychotherapy.

In psychoanalytic terminology, patients with character disorders have "character neuroses" as opposed to "symptom neuroses." They usually come to therapy with complaints about how they get along in the world. These complaints are usually about other people who are not behaving properly toward them or about specific unfavorable situations in their lives. Their own makeup is acceptable to themselves. In rare cases a patient may offer an insightful complaint that he knows he has not been doing business with the world in the most suitable way. Patients with symptom neuroses, on the other hand, have complaints within themselves that are unacceptable and undesired (eg, headaches, phobias, fatigue, insomnia, impotence).

It should not be assumed without question that character defects are always present when difficulties in social relationships are brought up in therapy. Problems of communication may actually exist and may be solved by helping the principal parties understand each other better. Furthermore, many of the troubles people have in getting along in the world have more to do with the social derangements and stresses of our time than with diseases of character. Even when character disorders are validly assumed to be present, faults in the environment cannot be ruled out since people who do have character problems are also likely to get into difficult social situations and then complain about them.

Both explanations, therefore—character problems and social problems—must always be sought, even with patients who give a history of prolonged maladaptation to their environment. In this chapter we will first discuss the commonly recognized character disorders assumed to result from develop-

*The terms character and personality are here used interchangeably.

mental processes and then outline some of the social processes, such as
deprivation or alienation, that cause or contribute to the kind of personal
difficulty that impels some patients to seek psychiatric help.

DEVELOPMENT AND CHARACTER

In *Psychoanalysis of the Neuroses,* Otto Fenichel, following classical
Freudian theory, explains abnormal character development as the perpetua-
tion of some inappropriate means of solving problems during the oedipal
period. It is at this time that solutions must be found to the instinctual
problems arising from the attraction of the young child to the parent of the
opposite sex. In general, these solutions involve renouncing the too-
possessive desire for the parent of the opposite sex and identifying with the
parent of the same sex. Although some believe that the sexual drives are
relatively unimportant, the solutions that the child finds to the interpersonal
and family relations will set a pattern for later adult behavior.

As the child grows older, he will continuously seek partial solutions to
residual problems in his relationship to his family. He will look around him,
for example, to discover how problems of aggressiveness or self-assertiveness
are being handled at home. The person who develops a character disorder is
different from the neurotic or normal person in the *rigidity and repetitiveness* with which he applies these partial solutions to his problem-solving tasks
or conflicts. A young child may learn that he can get his way with his
mother by threatening to leave. The solution to his problems then becomes
"threatening to leave." The young man who gets what he wants when he
threatens to leave will continue to expect rewards and live his life according
to this principle. He may easily become an unreliable and aggressive
employee who, after he has actually left a few times, becomes a drifter or an
altogether incompetent person.

The types of solutions to early life problems or to the oedipal conflict
that are brought about in this way determine the type of character difficulty
that develops. Some typical character disorders are the hysterical, compulsive, masochistic, schizoid, passive-aggressive, and passive-dependent. The
principal difference between the symptom neuroses and the character
neuroses is that in the latter the individual makes the resolution of his
childhood problems or his oedipal conflict once and for all and lives his life
according to it. This manner of resolving conflicts becomes built into the life
of the individual, is no longer questioned, and is never recognized as a
symptom to be complained about.

The person with a symptom neurosis suffers a great deal from anxiety.
The person with a character disorder does not overtly experience anxiety
from his built-in neurosis, but if his behavior pattern is questioned he
becomes anxious and uncomfortable. He presents a problem on the surface—
eg, aggressive, provocative, or promiscuous sexual behavior—which
apparently represents a simple drive that has gotten out of hand. Underneath
this manifestation, there is considerable latent anxiety.

Many people with character disorders believe (sometimes unconsciously) in an almost phobic way that their survival depends on continuing to behave as they always have even though this gets them into trouble. Because their ego structure is usually not competent to deal with anxiety or depression, people with character disorders tend either to act or escape, and their instinctual drives are poorly controlled.

SPECIFIC TYPES OF CHARACTER DISORDERS

Schizoid Character

The schizoid character is concerned less with problems of sexuality or aggressiveness than with relationships with others. The presenting complaints are variable. Schizoid persons tend to be suspicious, not easily drawn into social interaction, afraid of people, often overdependent on others, and have difficulties in almost all areas of human intercourse. They may be overcompliant and get hurt; they may be given to temper tantrums or sudden inexplicable rages. Homosexual concerns and frank homosexuality are not uncommon, as well as heterosexual adventures which stem from a need for closeness but always fail because they are ineptly pursued or because the object of attraction is an entirely unsuitable person. A suicide threat or attempt is often what brings the schizoid into therapy.

Affective deprivation is almost always present. The past history regularly reveals gross deficiencies in object relations and loss of the parents or parental aloofness due to their own depressive or compulsive character disorders. Cruel treatment is almost always a part of the history.

The first consideration in treatment is the schizoid's extraordinary hunger for human relationships. For this reason, rapid improvement often occurs as soon as a relationship with the therapist is established.

Another prominent feature of the schizoid personality is the fragility of the defensive structures. The schizoid patient often becomes suicidally depressed over a minor incident in therapy or in his daily life, and this hypersensitivity to minor traumas can be a serious handicap to treatment.

A third characteristic of the schizoid individual is the constant life-or-death exigency of every aspect of their lives, including the therapeutic relationship. For this reason it is advisable to have these patients not only in individual therapy but also in a group setting where alternative relationships are available as others break down. The therapeutic objective is to consolidate whatever ties to reality are in existence and to seek out suitable contacts if the patient has been avoiding meaningful human relationships.

The Obsessive Compulsive Character

The obsessive compulsive character can be described as meticulously concerned with doing things right, insecure about details, persistent, ungiving, scrupulously prompt, parsimonious, and retentive. He may be rigid and unadaptable, but he is persistent and disciplined. He may be boring and narrowly precise, but he is conscientious and predictable. The character type is not abnormal in itself. An optimal number of obsessional character traits is associated with high ethical standards and has practical value in terms of accomplishment and reliability. The character type becomes pathologic only when obsessional traits are markedly overdeveloped.

The obsessive compulsive character's problems may lie in the area of competitiveness, self-assertiveness, or the manifestations of aggression. He may have concerns about status and performance and present manifold complaints: inability to study, undue (but self-generated) pressures at work, and the failure of other people to understand his ways of doing things. Common personality features are procrastination, inability to resolve issues or finish work projects, and isolation from the environment. A pathologic degree of obsessional traits makes him a slave to minor rules and inconsequential details. Devoted to trifles, he may on occasion overlook essentials. His orderliness will be costly and inappropriate. Fiercely committed to his own routines and opinions, he may be a great trial to others whose needs lie outside his imagination. He tends to be so engrossed in the minute details of his life that he is unaware that the main direction of his life is off course.

The relationship between obsessive compulsive symptoms and obsessive compulsive personality is complex. Both may be present in a given patient, but either may occur without the other. Orderliness and perfectionism as character traits appear logically on a continuum with a tendency to compulsive ritual—just as honest doubting borders on obsessional rumination. In each case, morbid symptoms seem to be an exaggeration of normal character traits.

The obsessive compulsive's basic assumption is that in order to avoid disaster he must be very careful, stay aloof from people, and hold fast to everything he has. The past history of such persons often reveals strong authoritarian parents, a rigid upbringing, and similar problems in other members of the family.

The therapeutic aim is principally to allow the patient to understand his fear of closeness with others and his concerns with aggression—both his own and other people's. He will submerge his doctor in limitless detail about his problems without ever making clear what is really wrong. None of the physician's perceptions about him are quite right, but he is unable to say what is right because he is too busy apologizing for not making himself clear. The patient is anxious, and beclouds the interpersonal situation in a smog of words and vaguely irrelevant detail. As a result, treatment is characteristically difficult, prolonged, and rarely more than partially successful.

The Hysterical Character

The hysterical character—usually a woman—is often deeply concerned with sexuality and tends to be emotional, often irresponsible, flamboyant, or theatrical. Frequent complaints in young women suffering from this disorder are difficulty in relationships with men, a general dissatisfaction with themselves, and angry feelings about the world. They resent the feminine role, are competitive with men, have strong wishes to be men, and try to prove that all men fit the same pattern. Men are sought out, found to be inadequate, and then discarded. The basic problem seems to be the castration complex, ie, the young girl's feeling that she has been deprived of a penis. If the young girl adopts the "once and for all" solution that "castration is a lie," ie, that she is in reality the genital equal of the men and boys around her, the foundation of a hysterical personality pattern in later life has been laid down.

Psychotherapy or psychoanalysis fairly regularly will lead the woman first to painful awareness of the reality that she has so long tried to avoid, and then to the gratifying acceptance of the satisfactions of femininity.

The Antisocial Character

Antisocial personality is the official APA term for what was first called moral insanity, then constitutional psychopathic inferiority or psychopathic personality, and then sociopathic personality disturbance with the sub-categories antisocial reaction, dyssocial reaction, sexual deviation, and addiction (drug and alcohol).

The antisocial personality gets into repeated conflict with society. He has no loyalty or concern for others, ignores social codes or values, and acts only in response to his own desires and impulses. Punishment does not touch him, and experience teaches him little. He cannot resist temptation since he cannot tolerate frustration, and he blames others skillfully when he is caught.

Since many people flout the rules of society to satisfy their own desires at one time or another, a diagnosis of antisocial personality depends on both quantitative and qualitative data and on an assessment of a patient's total life style. One must consider *how much* disregard for the ethical standards of society the patient has shown, *how long* he has shown this disregard, and how basically unsocialized and unsocializable he is.

The antisocial personality is usually first manifested in childhood or early adolescence by such behavioral problems as truancy, theft, running away, incorrigibility, associating with "bad companions," impulsiveness, lying, and a poor record of achievement in school or employment. Strangely, enuresis is often part of the history.

It is generally considered that the patient with an antisocial personality is unable to postpone immediate pleasure or gratification of an impulse, lacks the capacity for maintaining a close relationship with another person, and feels no guilt or anxiety over his antisocial acts. Such persons dissipate anxiety by immediate and impulsive actions with essentially no delay between stimulus and response.

The symptoms and signs persist into adult life as poor marital adjustment, bad work history, repeated arrests, impulsiveness, pathologic lying, sexual promiscuity, vagrancy, and social isolation. In women, the history usually includes prostitution, venereal disease, and illegitimacy.

The antisocial person is not a stupid individual who has been unable to learn the rules of society; he may be very bright or even brilliant. Many of these people have great social charm, usually developed over a lifetime of practice in the art of "cunning, conning, and guile"—all directed toward immediate gratification of desires. The "con men" and the "manipulators" are apt to be found in this category along with those who use other people for their own ends with little regard for consequences.

The psychodynamic understanding of this condition is much the same as for the passive-aggressive personality (see below), the pattern arising from grossly faulty mothering, ambivalent parental relationships, and unresolved oedipal conflicts. Behaviorists stress the lack of opportunity to learn the values of society from socially acceptable models. They emphasize that anti-social behavior can be consciously or unconsciously taught to a developing child. The father who lies and cheats to his son's certain knowledge is teaching him that the rules of society are for other people; that it is all right to lie, cheat, and steal; and that one does not need to feel guilty about it. (See also p 235.)

Psychotherapy has had little success in the treatment of these individuals. Classically, the analytic approach is to confront the patient and convince him that his problems are not with the outside world but within himself. Having thus in a sense converted his problem to a neurosis, the usual psychotherapy for the neurosis is instituted.

Since many people with antisocial personality spend time in prison where facilities for individual psychotherapy are limited, it is not surprising that milieu treatment and group therapy have enjoyed some vogue with these patients. Any psychologic approach that offers no rewards for anti-social behavior and definite rewards for social behavior would seem a valid approach based on learning principles. When a social situation is provided, as with milieu or group therapy in prison, from which the patient cannot easily escape, the consequences of his antisocial behavior are forced on him, ie, since he cannot run away impulsively as he would ordinarily do, he is forced to come to grips with some aspects of society. Only limited success has been reported with these types of therapy, but they perhaps represent our best hope for future therapeutic approaches to this treatment-resistant group of patients.

Some antisocial persons, in spite of their lack of ability to learn from experience, nevertheless seem to "burn out" in their middle and late 30's and become respectable citizens.

The Passive-Aggressive Character

In some individuals with a passive-aggressive character disorder, the aggressiveness is concealed and the passivity or dependency is blatant. These individuals are sometimes referred to as "passive-dependent" characters. They are frequent visitors to the outpatient clinic or family service agency, where they present themselves as helpless persons who feel they are not being adequately taken care of by others. The dependent person is susceptible to depressive episodes when he feels his needs are not satisfied. At such times, his reactions are apt to be particularly inept and inadaptable.

The crucial conflict is in the area of *loss* or *fear of loss* and can sometimes be traced back to early affective deprivation such as lack of mothering. However, unlike the schizoid person—who, feeling that he has been utterly renounced, gives up, becomes distrustful, and relies only on himself—the dependent person has not given up hope. He feels that at some time somehow fulfillment of his often childish wishes will come about through some person other than his mother provided he waits long enough or insists long enough on receiving the help he feels he is entitled to.

Treatment must focus not only on identifying the patient's dependent characteristics but (and principally) on uncovering the angry and aggressive component to his constant demands. The helpless and dependent person tends to see himself as good and deserving of the good things that are his due. He has no notion that he harbors negative feelings toward others. There is little or no awareness that some benefits might have to be earned rather than just received. A progressively wider spacing of appointments will often bring home to the patient the realization that he must make his own decisions and become more self-reliant. Group therapy is often the treatment of choice to help the dependent person see the ineffectiveness of his behavior patterns and find more suitable ones.

In contrast to the above type of character, who tends to be depressed, many passive-aggressive characters present themselves as angry, injured parties who have not been treated fairly or been appreciated, whose feelings have been disregarded, and whose self-esteem has been injured. Somewhat like masochistic characters, they subtly provoke others to their own disadvantage, mostly by passive and sullen behavior, and are unaware of the role of their own aggressions in their misery. They characteristically wait in a sulky way for others to come to them, being careful to give them nothing they have not already earned. Conflicts with authority figures are a predictable feature in the life of the passive-aggressive character, starting with difficulties with parents and going on to school officials, employers, and the police. A characteristic family background is an ambivalent relationship with the mother, who is alternatively and inconsistently protective and punitive. In many cases, one parent was either absent or ineffectual during childhood.

In the treatment of this latter type of passive-aggressive personality, the major difficulty is to avoid a repetition of the characteristic fight-or-flight pattern of the patient. The chances are great that he will feel slighted and misunderstood by the therapist whenever he is disagreed with. He will again retreat from the situation, avoid treatment by unannounced absences, and remain emotionally unchanged in his infantile, pouting attitudes.

It is therefore important to deal with the *manifest and actual* interpersonal conflicts first and foremost rather than to wait for a suitable therapeutic relationship which may never materialize. Direct confrontations with significant people in the patient's life (such as the spouse or relevant family members) are most often useful. It is particularly with these elusive and not "treatment-minded" people that the newer conjoint methods of treatment have had success. Examples are marital couple treatment or family therapy, where a passive-aggressive youngster may resolve some of his conflicts with his parents.

The Masochistic Character

The most noteworthy tendency of the masochistic character is the talent for getting hurt. Careful investigation reveals an intricate network of subtle provocation, unconscious aggression, saying exactly the wrong things without realizing it, and, inevitably, receiving conscious and overt suffering as the victim of "injustices" from others. The masochistic character is unaware of his own role in the social and interpersonal disasters that periodically overtake him. He is surprised when people get angry or retaliate against his provocative behavior.

The childhood history regularly reflects a similar pattern. The masochist characteristically sees himself as a passive victim of other people's sadism. The infantile developmental history, when available, often shows that the masochistic character has been exposed to considerable abuse and rejection. In psychodynamic terms, masochism may be explained as the attempt to live up to the expectations of a rejecting parent. If the parent reiterates often enough how bad the child is, he will eventually feel himself to be bad, act accordingly, and spitefully vindicate the parent's view. Usually he also manages to mortify the parent in the process (eg, by appearing all bloody, by being arrested, by dropping out of college)—thus the frequent term, "sadomasochism." A tendency to ingratiate the rejecting person is rarely absent, and bearing this in mind will often lead to an essential clue to this puzzling and refractory character disorder.

Other Types of Character or Personality Disorders

Paranoid: Most of these patients resemble arrested paranoid schizophrenics (residual type).

Cyclothymic: Patients with cyclothymic personality resemble those with mild cases of manic-depressive illness.

Explosive (epileptoid): This is a newly official term used to characterize individuals subject to outbursts of rage or violence with impaired self-control. Many of them have paroxysmal cerebral dysrhythmia (abnormal EEGs) and perhaps should be diagnosed as having psychomotor epilepsy or other organic brain disorders.

Asthenic: This is an old term used to denote emotionally enfeebled persons, anhedonic and unresponsive to their environment. They may be physically ill, depressed, or mildly catatonic.

Inadequate: This frequently used term is more of a moral judgment than a diagnosis. Most patients so characterized are mentally defective, passive-dependent, or schizoid.

Emotionally unstable: This nonspecific descriptive term is sometimes used to denote the hysterical character. Emotional instability may be a feature of any type of personality, including the relatively normal.

GENERAL CONSIDERATIONS IN
TREATMENT OF CHARACTER DISORDERS

Because the problems of the character disorders are perceived by the patients as largely outside themselves and because their distorted ways of relating to their families and associates cause more trouble for others than for themselves, it is difficult to engage them in the necessary therapeutic alliance. Before any kind of treatment can begin, the person with a character disorder must be *confronted* in one way or another with what might be the matter with him, even if he feels he is perfectly justified in the actions and responses that get him into trouble. The therapist starts at a disadvantage as an ally of unfriendly society and a potential enemy in his patient's eyes. The patient may eventually come to see the therapist as a helper but may not acknowledge this change of attitude. The upsurge of anxiety that regularly follows a confrontation may become a major problem if it leads to unwise actions ("acting out") designed to relieve the anxiety engendered by the relationship with the therapist. Patients with character disorders have such a low tolerance for anxiety or pain that they may break off therapy before anything has been accomplished.

Group therapy has gained increasing acceptance for the treatment of character disorders. Since the patient's problem is his way of relating to others, the interactional setting of group therapy would seem to be ideally calculated to force the necessary confrontation and to provide a sheltered opportunity for working out more adaptive solutions to problems of relationship. The group setting also provides much more support for the patient than he can find in individual therapy. The feeling of being included in events and participating in a group endeavor means a great deal to these people, particularly the schizoid personalities who have difficulties with object relations. The opportunity to relate to a variety of people also offers greater resources for testing action patterns than the one-to-one relationship with the therapist. If the patient fears too much closeness with one person, there are others to whom he can turn. If he fears losing people, a one-and-only relationship with the therapist is more vulnerable than a group situation where other people are available as the need arises. Of course, individual and group therapy combined may be the treatment of choice for some patients.

For severely handicapped people with social difficulties—particularly those who are unable to earn a living—day care facilities are becoming more widely available. In most such settings, the elements of peer support and participation in communal activities offer important therapeutic benefits.

Unfortunately, a great many people with character disorders—sometimes quite severe—never come to psychiatric treatment. These people continue to inflict misery on others and on themselves without self-awareness.

For descriptions of particularly colorful or interesting character disorders, one may turn to the great novelists such as Balzac and Dostoevski.

CONSIDERATION OF CHARACTER DISORDERS
FROM THE POINT OF VIEW OF SOCIAL INTERACTION

The character disorders can be profitably examined as derangements of social or cultural interaction in specific relationship settings. An example is the sadomasochistic marriage where the wife complains of a withdrawn husband and the husband complains of a nagging wife. Taking each of these people individually, a diagnosis of character disorder would be justified in each case. The wife may be a hysterical character who complains loudly to various professionals or agencies about her depression and misery. The husband may be a schizoid character who chooses to withdraw to his basement workshop rather than participate in the life of the family. These diagnoses, however, do little to solve the problem of the marriage, whereas taking the marriage itself as the "patient" has the immediate advantage of addressing the therapist's attention to the chief complaint. The problem may be a breakdown of communication between the 2 partners. Each one is "at fault" in his own way, but identifying these mechanisms of alienation is less productive of good therapeutic results than confronting the situation as a whole. A useful technic is to see the couple jointly and trace the history of their marriage and their interactions with each other rather than their individual development.

Disorders of the parent-child relationship can be approached in the same way. Many adolescent difficulties reflect not only past developmental problems but current intrafamilial malfunctioning as well. Delinquency, withdrawal, and sullen or stubborn behavior may yield more easily to a family-centered approach than to individual treatment of the adolescent and his parents. The developing field of family therapy has clearly shown the value of this interactional approach.

Some character disorders such as the passive-dependent, passive-aggressive, and antisocial character may be due not only to family stress but also to widespread social problems during the patient's developing years or current life. If there are urgent practical necessities for welfare assistance or if a barely adequate adjustment to society depends upon job openings for unskilled workers, the problem of dependency as a character disorder fades before the much larger problem of social imbalances which require individual adjustments and compromise just to remain alive and fed.

Some societies seem to have evolved in such a way as to provoke passive-aggressive or antisocial individual adjustments. For the deprived or oppressed person or for entire groups of people subjected to racial or religious discrimination, a passive-aggressive or antisocial attitude may seem to be the only practical solution to the problem of survival.

REFERENCES

Books and Monographs

Berne, E.: *Games People Play*. Grove, 1964.

Boszormenyi-Nagy, I., & J.L. Framo (editors): *Intensive Family Therapy*. Hoeber, 1965.

Deutsch, H.: Hysterical fate neurosis. Pages 14–28 in: *Neuroses and Character Types*. Internat Univ Press, 1965.

Fenichel, O.: Character disorders. Pages 463–540 in: *The Psychoanalytic Theory of Neuroses*. Norton, 1945.

Glueck, S., & E. Glueck: *Toward a Typology of Juvenile Offenders*. Grune & Stratton, 1970.

Jones, M.: *The Therapeutic Community*. Basic Books, 1953.

Reiner, B.S., & I. Kaufman: *Character Disorders in Parents of Delinquents*. Family Service Association of America, 1959.

Robins, L.H.: *Deviant Children Grown Up: A Sociological and Psychiatric Study of Sociopathic Personality*. Williams & Wilkins, 1966.

Salzman, L.: *The Obsessive Personality*. Science House, 1968.

Stock, W.D., & A.M. Lieberman: *Psychotherapy Through the Group Process*. Atherton, 1964.

Stone, A.A. (editor): Character disorder. Pages 21–32 in: *The Abnormal Personality Through Literature*. Prentice-Hall, 1966.

Journal Articles

Grunebaum, H., Christ, J., & N. Nieberg: Diagnosis and treatment planning for couples. Internat J Group Psychother 19:185–202, 1969.

Jenkins, R.L.: The psychopathic or antisocial personality. J Nerv Ment Dis 131:318–334, 1960.

MacDonald, J.M.: The prompt diagnosis of psychopathic personality. Am J Psychiat 122 (Suppl 12):45–50, 1966.

Maddocks, P.D.: Five-year follow-up of untreated psychopaths. Brit J Psychiat 116:511–515, 1970.

O'Neal, P., & others: Parental deviance and the genesis of sociopathic personality. Am J Psychiat 118:1114–1124, 1962.

18 . . .

Psychophysiologic Disorders

Emotions may play a part in originating or intensifying certain diseases (especially of joints and of the stomach, colon, bronchi, and vascular system, with their smooth muscle and autonomic nerves). Do not overlook organic disease, which may be hidden or incipient in these conditions. And do not overlook emotional factors in acute and chronic illness, hospitalization, intensive care and coronary care units, medical life support measures, and surgery. Psychotherapy, usually supportive and not "uncovering," should accompany medical management and should consider the patient's "need" for the disease and his reactions to it.

Psychophysiologic (psychosomatic) disorders are organic dysfunctions in which emotional disturbances presumably play an important etiologic or contributory role. The autonomic nervous system is most frequently involved. The organic symptoms are actually produced or aggravated by emotional disorders and not symbolic substitutes for them, as in the neuroses. Ultimately, pathologic changes may result. *Neurotic (conversion) symptoms* are produced by the transformation of an anxiety state into a bodily dysfunction, usually with partial or complete relief of the anxiety. The voluntary motor and sensory systems are frequently involved, and the particular organ or body part in the symptom is often a symbolic expression of the emotional conflict. *Psychogenic (functional)* is a general term referring to clinical manifestations of psychic origin of any sort. A functional disorder is one in which there is no morphologic change and for which no known organic cause exists. There is widespread agreement that, in general practice as well as in most specialties in medicine, over 50% of cases (and perhaps 75% of physical complaints) are functional in origin.

The distinction between psychophysiologic and neurotic disorders can be illustrated by the following examples: Patient A is unable to walk because of severe arthritic changes in her knees and ankles (psychophysiologic). Patient B is unable to walk because of "paralysis" of his legs (neurotic). Patient A is reacting to a tyrannical husband with tension and rage expressed unconsciously in muscular spasm around the joints, with resultant circulatory and other organic changes. She is in pain and may feel anger, depression, or despair over her affliction. Patient B is a soldier reacting to a conflict between panic at possible death or mutilation and fear of showing cowardice by running away. His paralysis solves the problem that he could not "stand up" to. In hospital he feels blameless and evinces the disarming complacency *(la belle indifférence)* of the hysteric.

Psychophysiologic disorders, therefore, are emotional involvements of organs and viscera, frequently under autonomic nervous system control, and the symptoms are primarily physiologic (peptic ulcer, asthma, etc); anxiety is not relieved and in severe cases life may be threatened. Neurotic (conversion) disorders usually involve the voluntary motor and sensory systems, do relieve anxiety through the symbolic "solution" of the conflict, and the symptoms generally do not threaten life. There is overlap at times, particularly when psychophysiologic symptoms also have symbolic significance (diarrhea as defiling, bronchospasm as "suppressed cry for the mother").

HISTORICAL DEVELOPMENT OF THE CONCEPT OF PSYCHOPHYSIOLOGIC DISEASES

In the study of psychophysiologic disease (less than a century old), the concept of specific (single) causation has gradually given way to the modern view that a variety of factors are usually operative. Early workers did not distinguish between hysterical conversion reactions and psychophysiologic reactions. The leading figures in the field of psychophysiologic medicine have been Cannon, Deutsch, Selye, Dunbar, Alexander, Mirsky, and Wolf. Cannon presented excellent physiologic evidence of his "fight or flight" hypothesis, expounding the role of epinephrine secretion. Deutsch felt that a specific organ was sensitized in early life by trauma and by its accompanying emotional reaction ("organ neurosis"). The "psychosomatic unit" thus created was available later to respond to various psychic conflicts. Selye's concept of "diseases of adaptation" emphasized the role of the adrenal-pituitary axis in its reaction to stress as being responsible for various disease states. Dunbar's specific personality profile ("hypertensive character," "ulcer personality") described statistical correlations between diseases and personality types, eg, coronary thrombosis and striving, goal-oriented, confident, and aggressive individuals. Many later studies, however, failed to corroborate Dunbar's work.

Franz Alexander introduced the concept of the common underlying psychodynamic conflict ("conflict specificity"), where overt personalities differed but there was a specific relationship between certain emotional constellations and certain physiologic responses, eg, the wish to receive love (dependency conflict) and peptic ulcer, or the fear of maternal separation and asthma. Conflicts thus could change in the same patient over the years. In this manner one could explain 2 psychophysiologic disorders in one patient (rheumatoid arthritis and peptic ulcer, bronchial asthma and coronary artery disease).

In addition to emotional trauma, personality profiles, and emotional conflict, constitutional factors have also been implicated. Mirsky's studies of individual variability of peptic acid secretion are noteworthy contributions in this area.

Stewart Wolf was largely responsible for a new approach: multiple forces to the final common pathway—"in *this patient* at *this time*"—including biologic, psychologic, social, economic, hereditary, familial, environmental, and others. Current beliefs emphasize multifactorial etiologic components that interact and produce changes through complex neurophysiologic and neurochemical pathways.

PRINCIPLES OF MANAGEMENT

The major psychophysiologic disorders are discussed briefly below. The physician must bear in mind that there is no scientific proof of emotional involvement in any of them, and that the mechanisms by which emotions trigger physiologic changes are not well understood. Similar disorders may be the result of different combinations of a variety of factors (constitutional, genetic, physical, environmental, emotional), and dissimilar disorders may be the result of apparently similar factors.

Complete Examination

Each patient must be considered individually and a complete medical, psychiatric, and social history obtained, including occupational, educational, and cultural history, domestic factors, and financial status. *Do not overlook organic disease.* A patient may have both organic disease and psychophysiologic disorders. Psychologic evaluation should include a psychiatric diagnostic formulation, identification of current underlying conflicts, and an estimate of emotional maturity and strength. Note particularly (1) any environmental or intrapsychic changes that might help to explain the clinically manifested disease; and (2) loss of important people or serious loss of self-esteem—actual, threatened, or imagined. Anxiety and depression are among the most frequent emotional triggers of somatic distress.

Psychotherapy

Psychotherapy should usually be supportive but may be partly depth-oriented if the patient has sufficient flexibility to change without further disruption of the personality (neurotic or psychotic illness). What is required is the ability to accept and forgive the self and others, to sublimate primitive drives, to pursue long-term instead of short-term goals, and to conform to the demands of reality.

Anaclitic Therapy

Anaclitic therapy ("leaning" on the doctor) may be valuable, particularly in critically ill patients. The patient is permitted to be dependent and infantile. He is dressed, fed, and cared for, and allowed to regress as far as he wishes. Hospitalization is essential, not only for the critical physical problems but also because when severely ill the patient is unable to cope psychologically with his environment. Separation from the family may be an important factor. As improvement occurs, the need for eventual weaning from intense dependency on the therapist must be faced. It is necessary to remind the patient from time to time that one day his present need for doctors will diminish and he will become increasingly mature and independent.

Medical Treatment

Medical treatment, in addition to specific therapy for the disease, may include sedatives, other antianxiety agents, antidepressants, electroconvulsive therapy, sleep therapy, and supportive measures.

Patient's "Need" for the Disease

Consider that the patient may "need" his disease and try to provide something in its place, such as a richer social life, broader vocational interest, or religious involvement. If the psychophysiologic disturbance is serving as a substitute for unacceptable repressed impulses, it may be a better "solution" for his deep feelings than simple conscious realization of the impulses and a resultant psychosis.

The following should be determined: What is the "meaning" of the disease to the patient? Has he had previous contacts with it? Are there rational or irrational fears? Does the illness serve to help him identify with an important person, such as his father? Does the necessary medical therapy have a special significance to the patient, eg, oral or anal gratifications? What does the illness do for the patient? Does it make it possible for him to avoid obligation, responsibility, conflict, or possible failure (emotionally, domestically, occupationally)? Does the illness make dependency and increasing incapacity more tolerable?

MAJOR PSYCHOPHYSIOLOGIC DISORDERS

PEPTIC ULCER

Peptic ulcer has been described as a disease in which the "hungry" stomach eats itself. The longed-for food is equated with love or mother's milk. The "typical" ulcer patient has been epitomized as the tough, hard-driving executive who will not acknowledge his passive-dependent yearnings and thus falls into unconscious conflict and resultant illness. Although this characterization is applicable to many peptic ulcer patients, it certainly does not describe a large number of others.

It is difficult for some individuals to acknowledge their dependency needs. Appropriate dependency needs are just as natural as the need for independence. Dependency is desirable in the patient being treated, in the student being educated, in the learner being trained; interdependency is essential in team sports, orchestras, government, war, sex, and marriage. The denial of dependency in men is often associated with an unconscious fear of homosexuality and the submissiveness connected with it. In women, the denial of dependency may be part of the rejection of the feminine role. Thus, pseudomasculinity in men and masculinity in women have been considered by some to be characteristic of the "ulcer picture."

Also said to be characteristic of the ulcer patient is the "oral" personality. Fixation is considered to have taken place at the early oral stage of development, with unabated emphasis on frequent and regular passive "feedings" ("ego supplies"), not only of food but of affection, money, rewards, satisfaction, and success generally. Note that ulcer pain is relieved by food and increased by hunger.

Organic factors are certainly involved in some cases of peptic ulcer. Cushing's ulcer may occur in brain damage due to trauma, vascular disease, or surgery, especially if the hypothalamic region is involved. Curling's ulcer may follow severe burns or other unusually prolonged stress. The Zollinger-Ellison syndrome produces ulcer as the result of pancreatic disease. Ulcer may be the first manifestation of parathyroid adenoma. Alcoholics are especially prone to ulcer. Finally, many ulcers may be brought about by any of a variety of drugs, eg, corticosteroids, aspirin, phenylbutazone (Butazolidin), or indomethacin (Indocin).

The physician should recognize that in the patient with peptic ulcer he may find relevant data in the psychologic or organic sphere, in both, or in neither. He should investigate both and build his treatment around the positive findings in the individual case. If, as is often the case, there are no findings other than the ulcer, the wise physician will supplement good medical management with special attention to the patient's dependency needs. No attempt should be made to undertake deep-going or interpretative psychotherapy.

ULCERATIVE COLITIS

Tension and emotional stress are known to cause bowel disturbances in many individuals. In ulcerative colitis, the onset or relapse is often clearly and repeatedly associated with emotional duress.

The overactive colon is thought by some to be a means of expressing unconscious defiling hostility. Associated reactions may include enormous guilt and severe infantile dependency. Many patients with ulcerative colitis are considered to be fixated at the anal-expulsive stage of development and to obtain major libidinal satisfaction (on an unconscious level) from anal activity. The anal personality in these patients may also demonstrate the genetically earlier anal-retentive aspects of character (eg, parsimony, compulsiveness, meticulousness, scrupulous promptness, excessive cleanliness, zealous honesty). They are often unable to express aggressive or hostile feelings in a direct manner, but make their relatives suffer secondarily as a result of their illness.

Colitis may, of course, be due to many organic disorders. Gastrointestinal infection must always be considered, as well as Whipple's disease, granulomatous conditions, auto-immune phenomena, and many drugs, especially antibiotics. The *irritable bowel syndrome (mucous colitis)* and functional colonic disturbances may occur in patients with the same personality problems as those with ulcerative colitis but presumably with a more immune colon lining. They have milder symptoms and do not have the structural organic changes (ulcerations of the gut).

In the management of ulcerative colitis, it is important to consider that the patient's ego may be as friable as his bowel mucosa. Treatment should be gentle and considerate, with no attempts at deep-going or interpretative psychotherapy. These patients need strong emotional support. If surgery is required, thorough preoperative psychologic preparation is essential. If colostomy is to be performed, the patient must be informed of its significance in his postoperative way of life. If a major way of dealing with the environment (diarrhea) is taken from certain of these patients, they must be given some alternative or the resultant depression may lead to suicide.

BRONCHIAL ASTHMA

Psychic factors are felt to play a large role in either causing or aggravating bronchial asthma. The wheeze of asthma has been likened to the cry for the mother, and it is true that asthmatics often give a history of a poor mother-child relationship. Attacks are said to be precipitated by threats of loss or separation from the mother or mother substitute. The asthma personality has been described as "pre-oral" or "respiratory," where the fixation upon the mother antedates all other relationships and is of such vital and immediate nature that even brief separation, if threatened as permanent, is reacted to as though potentially fatal.

Organic factors are important in some cases of asthma some of the time. Repeated or chronic pulmonary infections or allergic reactions may be present. Other much less common conditions that produce wheezing are carcinoid syndrome and obstruction (tumor, foreign body). Precipitating factors, besides emotional stress, are exposure to cold and wet, fatigue, and debilitation. To the old medical axiom that, "Not all that wheezes is asthma," one could add, "Nor is all that wheezes a repressed cry for the mother."

In the management of an acute attack proper medical care is vital. Between attacks, attention should be focused on the often severely neurotic or latent psychotic personality of the patient. If the attacks are clearly precipitated by emotional factors or if the patient achieves secondary gains, prolonged psychotherapy may be attempted. If it is suspected that the attacks are psychotic equivalents (substitutes for depression or overt psychosis), antidepressant or tranquilizing drugs may be given in some instances, but with extreme caution because of their anticholinergic effects.

HYPERTENSION

When the popular "raising your blood pressure" occurs without apparent emotional provocation or organic explanation, hypertensive disease is considered to have an underlying psychologic basis. Overly controlled, suppressed rage can act like a pressure cooker with the lid screwed on tight. The distinction between "essential" and "malignant" hypertension is still uncertain despite great advances in the pathophysiologic understanding of hypertension. It is not known whether emotional factors are initial causes of hypertension. However, it has recently been demonstrated that complex cycles involving the secretion of hormones such as renin and angiotensin once set into action will further perpetuate the existing hypertension. The diagnosis of adrenal and renovascular diseases has assumed utmost importance in view of the possibility in these conditions of correction and reversibility of the hypertension by modern therapeutic methods.

Hypertension may be associated with arteriosclerosis, other structural vascular disease, CNS disease (especially in the hypothalamic area), and certain endocrine disorders (eg, Cushing's disease, pheochromocytoma). Various drugs, notably the corticosteroids and the MAO inhibitors, may cause hypertension.

Medical treatment should be supplemented by opportunities for emotional ventilation and better self-understanding. Psychotherapy, though considered potentially dangerous in some psychophysiologic conditions (ulcerative colitis, peptic ulcer), may be undertaken with relative impunity here.

ARTHRITIS

It has been said that the arthritis patient is "able to get his hostility out only as far as his fists," where chronic tension and muscular contractions cause impaired circulation and articular changes. The rheumatoid personality has been described as extroverted, athletic, hyperactive, jovial, and over-ambitious.

Organic factors to be considered are repeated trauma (perhaps partly due to unconscious volition), metabolic disturbances (gout, collagen disease, auto-immune disorders), infections (gonorrhea, Reiter's syndrome), psoriasis, and associated systemic disease.

In addition to giving medical treatment, the physician may wish to explore the possibilities of providing ample opportunities for verbal expression of suppressed resentments and bitterness. Harsh words may be healthier than clenched fists. Muscular activity of various sorts can be encouraged. A well-earned fatigue may be preferable to taut muscles and pent-up feelings.

MIGRAINE

In the patient with migraine the hostility is so deeply repressed that it cannot even be thought of. The typical migraine patient is a hardworking intellectual, with high standards for himself and others and uncompromising with the world.

Migraine must be differentiated from other types of recurrent severe headache, including **anxiety tension headache** and headache associated with brain tumor, hypertensive encephalopathy, renal disease, histamine headache, vascular headache, neuralgia, and toxic and infectious states.

There is an old German saying, "A murder a day keeps the migraine away." Migraine patients often do well in prolonged intensive psychotherapy which permits them to bring unconscious resentments to the surface. A medical therapeutic regimen should be instituted at the same time.

OTHER DISEASES TO WHICH PSYCHOPHYSIOLOGIC FACTORS ARE ATTRIBUTED

NEUROMUSCULAR

Low back syndrome and **coccygodynia** are common complaints among neurotic, dependent, infantile individuals. In industrial and medicolegal cases, these syndromes must be differentiated from malingering. Orthopedic and neurologic factors must be identified.

Epilepsy and **multiple sclerosis** have been erroneously attributed to psychophysiologic causes. In the former, attacks may be precipitated by emotional factors. In the latter, organic brain disease may cause the frequently described hysterical euphoria.

Causalgia and **phantom limb** are phenomena that occur during the healing of severed major peripheral nerves. The pain and discomfort are autonomic in nature and are sometimes attributed to exaggerated emotional stress.

CARDIOVASCULAR

Coronary artery disease. It is felt by many that stress is an important factor in the pathogenesis of this disease. There is a relatively high incidence of coronary disease in driving, ambitious, aggressive, perfectionistic individuals who are always rushing to meet deadlines. Emotional upsets—especially anger—are a well recognized precipitant of attacks of **angina pectoris**.

Raynaud's disease has been attributed to prolonged repressed hostility.

Arrhythmias and **thrombophlebitis** have been attributed by some to psychophysiologic factors.

Syncope, may be vagal or cardiovascular in origin, but sometimes it is induced cortically in high-strung, hyperreactive individuals. A generation or two ago it was not uncommon for delicate and "well bred" girls to "swoon" readily at the sight or sound of emotionally shocking events.

RESPIRATORY

Hyperventilation syndrome due to respiratory alkalosis is not an uncommon disorder. The patient may be observed to have sighing respirations and complains of light-headedness and numbness. In severe cases, symptoms may include tetany and seizures with electrolyte abnormalities. It is seen in anxious and neurasthenic individuals.

Rhinitis. The psychologic factors may be closely related to those seen in asthma (theoretically, a "naso-oral rejection" of the environment).

Laryngitis is frequently seen in manics because of their excessive talking. It may also be associated with anxiety and tension in public speakers and singers.

GASTROINTESTINAL

Aerophagia has psychodynamic factors similar to those observed in hyperventilation.

Cardiospasm is frequently considered to be psychogenic in origin, but severe cases must be treated mechanically.

Psychogenic vomiting may be seen in various forms of severe neurosis or psychosis. Certain cases of **hyperemesis gravidarum** have been attributed to psychologic disturbances (eg, "oral rejection of the fetus").

Constipation may be part of the syndrome of obsessive compulsive neurosis.

Regional enteritis may have emotional components in some patients.

SKIN

Neurodermatitis. Individuals with this disorder are thought to have been subjected to maternal rejection and to have developed subsequent repressed hostility. They are described as driving, ambitious, perfectionistic, wanting to "clean everything up," never able to express enough of their hostility and guilt. The relentless scratching serves as self-punishment through self-mutilation. Others have described repressed erotic needs that are served by the scratching. The location of the pruritus is often thought to be significant psychologically, eg, **anal or vulval pruritus** in sexual pathology.

Eczema in children may begin as a manifestation of atopic disease. Chronic forms are seen in insecure children and those with disturbed mother-child relationships. Hostility, exhibitionism, and shame are often linked to **urticaria.**

Psoriasis has often been suspected of having elements of nonspecific anxiety and tension closely related to it.

Alopecia, primary, or secondary to **trichotillomania** may be associated with severe neurotic disturbances. Masochism is often an element.

In the treatment of all of the above supportive psychotherapy with ventilation and mild sedation are indicated.

ENDOCRINE

Hyperthyroidism is thought to be precipitated by emotional stress when an individual (female) who is closely dependent on the mother tries to function independently. It is thus more frequent at critical times such as leaving home, being involved in demanding jobs, marriage, and childbearing. In young men, the disorder has been linked with emotional immaturity and excessive ambition.

Diabetes mellitus. The onset of the disease and episodes of ketoacidosis are thought to be frequently precipitated by emotional problems. Diabetics (often juveniles) use their disease and its therapy in a manipulative and often sadomasochistic fashion.

Sterility and **repeated spontaneous abortions** are frequently found in women who are consciously or unconsciously rejecting their feminine role and expressing hostility to men.

OBESITY

For years there has been controversy whether nature or nurture is responsible for obesity. The condition of being obese and the process of overeating must be considered separately in order to understand the underlying drives and needs. Being obese may serve as a means of escape from sexuality, social interaction, maturity, responsibility, reality, or life itself. The layers of fat may be insulating in multiple fashion. Overeating in response to a need for love, security, and pleasure occurs in infantile, dependent, passive individuals with poor ego strength who are unable to obtain their gratification and sustenance in more mature ways. Elements of hostility and aggression may be involved.

ANOREXIA NERVOSA

Anorexia nervosa is a serious disease with a substantial mortality rate (40%) seen frequently in adolescent girls but also in women in their 20's and 30's. Occasionally there is a preexisting obesity, and the onset of the anorexia nervosa may be associated with (but not caused by) extreme and overconscientious dieting. Secondary amenorrhea is a constant feature. These patients are immature and narcissistic; often they are obsessive or hysterical in personality makeup, and many of them are preclinically psychotic. They center their lives around a totally irrational approach to food (often "oral impregnation"). No known organic cause exists. The differential diagnosis must include primary disorders of many systems such as the gastrointestinal, gynecologic, and endocrine (eg, hypopituitary or adrenal).

Treatment is largely psychotherapy. Patients should be seen several times a week, often for many months or years. Psychotropic medication may be helpful. Hospitalization, tube feeding, and EST may have to be considered.

UROLOGIC AND GYNECOLOGIC

Dysmenorrhea, amenorrhea, and other abnormalities of the menstrual cycle occur frequently in maladjusted women who are intensely rejecting of their femininity and suffer from deeply repressed hostility.

Pseudocyesis, with many of the signs and symptoms of pregnancy, may mislead the physician.

Impotence, premature ejaculation, frigidity, and **dyspareunia** are discussed in Chapter 19. **Enuresis** is discussed in Chapter 32.

MISCELLANEOUS DISORDERS

Accident proneness may serve both hostile and masochistic needs. It may be easier to be hurt and cared for than to exert oneself to be mature and responsible.

Visual disturbances may occur on a hysterical conversion basis. The organ chosen is unconsciously symbolically significant ("seeing" is equivalent to "understanding"). Impaired motivation may be an element in some cases of poor vision.

Tinnitus, though of organic origin, may be exaggerated and incapacitating on an emotional basis. The same may be said for **vertigo.**

Munchausen's syndrome—repetitive hospitalization with simulation of serious illness, involving pain, bleeding, etc, often for the purpose of obtaining shelter and drugs—has been described in extremely clever, medically well-informed individuals who go from city to city taking advantage of state- and city-supported clinical facilities. They are often successful in obtaining the medical treatment of their choice, thus presenting a compound picture of iatrogenic and self-contrived disease. Patients have been described who can voluntarily alter their blood pressure and cardiac rate.

Polysurgical patients are those who live on the dividends of repetitive surgical care and complications, sacrificing removable parts. The elements of accident proneness are present here.

PSYCHOLOGIC FACTORS IN MEDICAL AND SURGICAL CONDITIONS

The first part of this chapter deals with diseases thought to be caused in whole or in part by psychologic factors (asthma, ulcerative colitis, peptic ulcer, etc). In this section we will discuss the importance of psychologic factors in the management of many medical and surgical conditions of clearly organic origin. With increasing psychologic sophistication on the part of recent medical graduates and of the lay public generally, abundant evidence has demonstrated the critical value of psychologic factors in many health situations.

This chapter will discuss some of the psychologic factors that operate in acute illness, chronic illness, terminal illness, hospitalization, intensive care units, life support measures, and surgery. It will conclude with suggestions for psychotherapeutic management in these areas.

ACUTE ILLNESS AND INJURY

A frequent response to illness is regression toward a childhood dependency state. This can be beneficial, since being taken care of by others allows the body to apply all of its resources to the tasks of defense against the illness and of recuperation. However, some sick people become overly dependent to an unhealthy degree, and some make the opposite mistake of denying legitimate dependency needs and thus either worsen the clinical illness or prolong its recovery.

For example, a busy surgeon who often boasted that he had not missed a day of work because of illness since medical school collapsed one day in the corridor of the hospital after several hours of chest pain. It was assumed he had suffered a heart attack, but in fact he had pneumonia. He had had a sore throat and cough for over a week, and 3 of his patients had developed wound infections postoperatively. Hard work was important to this man because his father and older brother were brilliant surgeons, whereas he had had trouble getting through medical school and felt he had to make up with unremitting effort what he lacked in facility.

Others actually relish the dependency status that their illness confers and tend to languish in it. An example is the young housewife who broke her wrist. Her mother came from a distant city to help the woman's husband take care of the house and children. When the cast was removed, her arm was so weak that she had to continue wearing the sling. After 2 months, the orthopedist called for a neurologic consultation, and all findings were negative except for atrophy of disuse. The family doctor had some long talks with the patient and allowed her to ventilate a number of grievances against her husband and her mother. The arm then gradually recovered.

In the sick room, the physician should pay appropriate respect to the patient's misery, fear, and wish to be taken care of. He should provide reassurance and comfort by maintaining an attitude of understanding, confidence, and matter-of-fact management, making it clear all the while that the patient will soon be expected to cooperate actively in the therapy. "Don't mind if they do everything for you right now. Lie back and enjoy it as much as you can. Soon we will be getting you out of bed and putting you to work at the recovery business."

Most acute illnesses and injuries occur in younger people, and the physician's chief problems in psychologic management are to enlist the patient's cooperation—enough passive acceptance of others' attention in the most acute stages and enough active following of directions in the recovery period. For further discussions of patients' attitudes and the doctor-patient relationship, see Chapter 2 and the concluding section of this chapter.

CHRONIC ILLNESS

Most chronic illnesses occur in older people, and the physician's chief problem in psychologic management is to prevent or to combat depression. Older people yield to depression more easily, since life and hope no longer seem to extend endlessly out into the future. Furthermore, the chronically ill person often has a good deal to be realistically depressed about: pain and other forms of physical suffering; invalidism, with partial or complete loss of ability to walk, work, dress himself, take care of his toilet needs, or even feed himself; relentless progress of the disease, with loss of youth, strength, and appearance; financial ruin, with dependence on relatives, welfare assistance, or charity; and death.

Even so, many chronically ill persons become more depressed than their circumstances warrant, since depression results not only from real losses but also from fantasied, imagined, or feared losses. The physician must explore the patient's dreads about the future and correct any misconceptions and exaggerations he may be harboring. In most cases the physician can honestly reassure his patient about the amount of suffering he should expect. He can almost always suggest constructive, practical possibilities that the patient had not considered. With the help of a social worker, he can enlist the cooperation of community agencies and relevant organizations. The advice of a lawyer, insurance agent, accountant, or investment counselor may be important, and the patient may profit spiritually from a visit from his minister, priest, or rabbi. With the patient's permission, the physician may engage in frank discussions about the patient's predicament with his sometimes reluctant relatives. (For example, the patient himself may be hesitant to mention his plight to a prosperous, aloof son.)

Antidepressant medications are relatively ineffective in depression associated with chronic illness (reactive depression), but they may be useful if the depression is of a mixed type. Mild sedation may be helpful, and many patients respond well to alcoholic beverages in moderation.

The suicide rate increases steeply with age and peaks in sick elderly people (particularly men) who live alone. The physician must beware of the contagion of depression and refuse to side with a patient's desire for death as a means of relief from suffering. An attitude of qualified hope is almost always warranted. The physician should discuss the facts of the illness with the patient with as much frankness as the patient can tolerate and give him every opportunity to ventilate his misgivings. He should be a source of strength, understanding, and help to his patient and should see him as often as necessary—even every day or more than once a day when things are desperate—and he should be available on the telephone at any hour of the day or night.

TERMINAL ILLNESS

Terminal illness differs from other acute or chronic illnesses by the presumed imminence and unavoidability of death. The classic psychologic dilemma of the physician is whether or not to tell the patient that he will soon die. Much has been written about the subject, and strong stands have been taken from moral, ethical, religious, compassionate, and pragmatic points of view. A reasonable working rule judges each case on its merits and applies to each patient the same criterion one applies to a child in deciding how much new responsibility he should carry: "How much is this person under these circumstances able to tolerate and manage well?"

One judges the child's capacity for assuming new responsibilities by considering not only his chronologic age but also his record of past performance and other indications of maturity. In the case of the dying patient, the same general rule can be applied.

Two extreme examples will help to illustrate:

A 40-year-old woman developed unmistakable metastases in the lungs and spine 2 years after radical surgery for breast cancer. She had been a poor mother and wife, taking to her bed with neurotic complaints whenever any serious problem developed in the family, as her own mother had done before her. She had never shown much interest in her breast operation and was content with the explanation that, "It had to be done to prevent anything serious from happening." She accepted radiation without question and marveled at "the wonderful machines." Her husband urgently requested that she not be told of her prognosis. The doctor agreed, and the woman enjoyed her last period of invalidism quite as much as she had her former ones.

A 45-year-old man had had trouble with peptic ulcer for many years. An apparent recurrence progressed to obstruction, and at operation a malignancy and widespread metastases were found. The physician knew that the patient had started a new business a few years before and that he was contemplating a large-scale expansion of it. The patient was a strong, athletic man who had served with distinction as a captain in the Army, and he and his wife had done a good job of rearing 3 children. The physician told him at once of his predicament and later helped him with extra medication before business conferences.

In cases that are not so clear-cut, the physician may obtain clues from the patient. The patient who never asks what is wrong with him or whether his illness will be cured does not want to know. The one who inquires about the significance of every symptom and type of treatment has a right to substantial answers. In doubtful cases, a discussion with the relatives may be illuminating. In many cases the patient already knows he is going to die soon and does not wish to talk about it even to his doctor. Sometimes an elaborate charade goes on in which everybody pretends, although everybody knows, and yet everybody stays as happy as possible under the circumstances.

The patient may fear dying far more than he fears death. The physician may be able to assure him that he will not suffer more than he has already proved he can tolerate; that he will not be alone; that his needs will be taken care of; and that his dignity as an individual will be preserved.

HOSPITALIZATION

Hospitalization becomes a psychologic problem in patient management not because of what a hospital is but because of what it symbolizes. A hospital actually is an efficient place to treat large numbers of sick people with all available skills and technics through the use of a minimum number of doctors and helpers. It represents what schools do for teachers and churches for clergymen. But to primitive people—and to the primitive part of all of us—the hospital is a fearful place where only the hopelessly sick are taken, where horrible things are done to people and their insides, and where people go to die.

Those who cannot control their fear of the hospital may refuse to go when they should. Even today, when many conditions formerly thought to require hospitalization are treated in the home (pneumonia, strokes, mononucleosis), a host of other conditions benefit from hospitalization more than ever (surgical emergencies, diabetic coma, myocardial infarction). Recalcitrant patients should be talked to calmly, unhurriedly, and understandingly. They should not be scolded, badgered, or shamed. They must be told the facts over and over, as simply, reassuringly, and patiently as possible. If necessary, someone the patient trusts (a relative, clergyman, schoolteacher, business associate, or friend) should be brought in to support the physician and help reassure the patient. The physician should give the patient as much time as he can and control his own feelings. The entire hospital stay may go not only for the medical help he received but for the forbearance and kindness he received at a difficult time.

A fearful patient in the hospital may refuse to permit diagnostic tests, especially those he is unfamiliar with (lumbar puncture, electroencephalogram, bronchogram, etc). He should be spoken with patiently and at length and offered reasonably full explanations of what the procedure is, how it is done, and why it is necessary. If he continues to balk, other doctors should talk with him, including, if necessary, a consulting psychiatrist.

A few people like to be in the hospital and will submit to hospitalization on the most minor indications. They regard the hospital as a haven from a troubled home or work situation, and they relish the attention they get and the security they feel. Such patients, once identified, should be gently interrupted in their flight toward dependency. If they are already in the hospital, they should politely but firmly be eased out as soon as their clinical illness is sufficiently improved. The psychodynamics must be remembered and utilized for the patient's benefit later on. These patients also need to be protected against unnecessary investigative procedures and exploratory operations.

INTENSIVE CARE UNIT

The intensive care unit is a kind of hospital within a hospital. It collects in one place those patients who have suffered acute and critical damage either through disease (eg, chronic obstructive lung disease), extensive surgery (eg, organ transplant), or trauma. These patients require constant attention and monitoring by complicated instruments which themselves require constant attention.

When patients are first brought to this unit they are usually too sick to be affected psychologically by the significance of the place. Later they will be bothered by the frequent attentions they and others receive (turning, intubations, intravenous therapy), machine noises, and lack of privacy. Staff people are busily concerned with the myriad details of patient care.

As a result, emotional stress is superimposed on the stress of illness or injury; psychotic breaks occur, and neurotic symptoms are common. The psychoses are variations of delirium, often referred to as "toxic psychosis"; abnormalities of the lower level mental functions predominate (clouded consciousness; disorientation; confusion; visual hallucinations or illusions; restlessness, excitement, and panic), but delusions, frequently paranoid in type, are not unusual. Neurotic symptoms usually consist of anxiety or exaggerations of preexisting neuroses. Complaints may center on convenient reality factors, such as the rough sheets or too cold air conditioning.

The staff share the strains of work in an intensive care unit. If they were to allow themselves to become emotionally involved with their patients, they could not tolerate the daily stress of suffering and death. They may blame themselves for trivial or imagined lapses in technic, and frequently develop a defensive, cold, and detached attitude toward the patients. Many doctors cope with their feelings by focusing exclusively on the technologic aspects of the work; others simply avoid the place.

The implications for improving the psychologic care of patients in the intensive care unit are obvious. Nurses should be briefed in advance about the unavoidable stresses they will be under. They should have regular meetings with experienced supervising staff for discussion of problems, including their patients' and their own emotional reactions.

THE CORONARY CARE UNIT

Coronary care units are much like intensive care units. There are the same dramatic cathode ray lights, red alarm signals, and bells for emergencies, and the same air of impending doom. There is intense preoccupation with the heart. Patients and staff often must face the critical and dramatic attempt to resuscitate a patient with cardiac arrest. Not all attempts succeed, and patients are left to wonder who will be next. When the staff hover excitedly around a machine, the patient often thinks it is his heart that is involved. "Cardiac psychosis"—not clinically to be distinguished from "toxic psychosis"—occurs more commonly in coronary care units than elsewhere.

MEDICAL LIFE SUPPORT MEASURES

Technologic advances in medicine and surgery have provided new ways for the physician to support failing homeostatic mechanisms. The patient's emotional reactions to serious illness are intensified when one of his physiologic systems becomes dependent upon the continuous or intermittent support of a technical device.

Renal Dialysis

The purpose of the dialysis apparatus is to wash the blood when one's kidneys break down so that life can go on. Years of experience have demonstrated the success of the method and have minimized the demands on the patient. Nevertheless, unless he can afford his own dialysis apparatus at home, the patient must visit the hospital twice a week to be hooked up to a noisy machine that cleans his blood for 12–16 hours. He must follow a rigid diet, have his blood chemistry checked frequently, take various medications, and receive intermittent blood transfusions.

Not everyone with hopelessly failing kidneys can be given the benefit of chronic dialysis. The number of apparatuses and supporting funds is limited, and selection of patients becomes a difficult problem. Who shall live and who shall die? How does a desperate candidate feel while awaiting the verdict? Can his family afford the financial and other sacrifices to make the lifesaving program possible? What about their emotional reactions—willingness with resentment, unwillingness with guilt? How do the members of the decision-making committee feel?

The availability of home dialysis machines has greatly increased the number of patients who can be served. However, this places a great responsibility on the family and may be a source of anxiety, fearfulness, and sometimes anger and bitterness.

Cardiac Pacemaker

Although the possibility that life can continue without the apparatus is not always ruled out completely and although the apparatus requires comparatively little attention, the idea of being so critically at the mercy of a battery or of electrical contacts arouses anxiety in every patient.

Respirator

A number of conditions require the use of a respirator for a short time or for longer periods to preserve life. Some of these are neurologic disorders (bulbar poliomyelitis, amyotrophic lateral sclerosis, etc); others are forms of chronic respiratory disease. Sensory deprivation is a regular feature of life in a tank-type respirator, and some patients suffer from psychotic-like states.

Diabetes and Insulin

Since the discovery of insulin, dependence on daily injections has become a regular feature of most diabetic regimens. The diabetic patient may be grateful that regular insulin permits him to eat a fairly normal diet and live a normal life, but he may also resent the necessity. Moreover, since his handicap does not show, he receives no compensatory attention, consideration, or pity from others.

Other Critically Drug-Dependent Conditions

Many other medical conditions have been found to be controllable through the regular administration of certain key substances, usually as a way of supplementing or replacing faulty biochemical systems in the body. A few of these are hypothyroidism (thyroxine), pernicious anemia (vitamin B_{12}), Addison's disease (corticosteroids), diabetes insipidus (vasopressin), familial periodic paralysis (potassium), and even a prospective one in psychiatry—manic-depressive disorder (lithium).

SURGERY

Fears of surgery may be based on realistic threats (complications, death, pain, hospitalization, incapacity, expense) or fantasied threats, often unconscious (annihilation, smothering, loss of control, mutilation, punishment for one's sins). Reasonably normal people react appropriately to the realistic factors, showing concern and apprehension, and may seek a consultant's opinion before agreeing to make plans. Neurotic or psychotic patients respond in an exaggerated way to irrational fantasies and may either overreact or underreact. Some may adamantly refuse a necessary operation or suffer a psychotic break if they are facing one; those who underreact seem to deny that any threat exists and proceed through the operation in automaton fashion. Many of the latter are then unable to resume their former contact with reality and experience a "postoperative psychosis" which is clinically comparable to other psychoses mentioned in this chapter.

In any life-threatening situation, most people want guidance and help from a trusted authority figure. The family physician should have an unhurried talk with the patient and discuss the operation thoroughly. The patient should be given every opportunity to ventilate his doubts and misgivings. Perhaps a talk should also be arranged between the patient and the surgeon. Such interviews help not only realistically but unconsciously; they allow the patient to feel that, "He will do these things to me, but only because they will help me. He likes me and will not let me suffer needlessly."

Special kinds of reassurances are occasionally necessary. The patient may harbor exaggerated fears about the removal of a body part. For some organs, the loss of one (kidney, adrenal, testicle) can be minimized. ("Neither you nor anyone else will ever know the difference.") For others, the technologic advances in prosthetic management can be emphasized (eye, breast, limb). Some specific fears can be dispelled by honestly emphatic denial, eg, that loss of the ovaries causes frigidity; that loss of one eye will cause blindness in the other; or that removal of the prostate invariably causes impotence.

Heart Surgery

Impending cardiac surgery causes extreme foreboding because of the high mortality rate and the symbolic importance of the heart. The high incidence of delirium following open heart surgery has been well documented. Ischemic brain damage and, perhaps, cerebral emboli from the associated procedures are partly responsible for the delirium, but the patient's personality, his emotional state prior to surgery, and the postoperative environment are important contributory factors. Poor prognostic factors are a history of mental or emotional breakdown, somatic preoccupation or withdrawal, and a high level of preoperative anxiety, depression, or denial. Postoperative amnesia is not infrequent, partly on a hysterical basis. Preoperative optimism qualified by a realistic degree of concern implies the best prognosis, and preparatory psychotherapy can improve the patient's chances of uneventful recovery.

Cardiac Transplant

The replacement of a diseased heart with a good one from a cadaver is probably the most dramatic of all surgical procedures. Although there are not yet many long-term survivors, the publicity attending the operation and the implications for the future success of other kinds of transplant have been exciting.

The incidence of psychologic complications of cardiac transplants is high. The preoperative stresses are especially great since candidates for the operation must be on a hopelessly downhill and rapidly fatal course and the certain knowledge of this is itself a heavy burden even for an emotionally strong person. They must then undergo a complicated selection process and, if chosen, wait days, weeks, or months for a suitable donor. Alcoholism and suicide attempts have been reported during this period.

Those who survive the operation are likely to develop a postoperative psychosis. Contributory factors are the high doses of prednisone and other drugs that are administered, ischemic effects on the brain, and excessive sensory deprivation postoperatively. Patients sometimes feel they have acquired the characteristics of their donors (eg, their age) and behave accordingly. Families of the donors frequently take a personal interest in the still-living heart of their relative, eg, if the recipient dies, they grieve again.

Kidney Transplant

Kidney transplants have been more frequent and more successful, if less dramatic, than cardiac transplants. Psychologic problems—especially depressions—have occurred in recipients, donors, unaccepted donors, and unwilling donors.

Hopeful recipients—with failing kidneys, perhaps unsatisfactory dialysis, and a real deadline to meet—may be understandably disappointed and depressed when none of their close relatives can bring themselves to offer a kidney to save their lives. Donors who feel they have been heroic as well as generous learn with bitterness that their sacrifice may be soon forgotten in a busy world. Unaccepted donors worry about what was wrong with them. Unwilling donors may have a difficult time contending with their guilt, especially after the sick person—perhaps a son, daughter, brother, or sister—dies.

Plastic Surgery

Advances in modern surgical and medical technics have made it possible to survive after extensive burns that before would have been fatal and after radical excision of malignant, life-threatening lesions that formerly were considered inoperable. The resulting deformities and disfigurements are sometimes so painful for others to look at that life may seem worse than the death the patient has been saved from. Plastic surgery then becomes the only hope. Patients must understand that there are realistic limits on what to expect from plastic surgery; if they set their goals too high, disappointment and depression will inevitably follow.

Especially when the face is involved, severe emotional problems may be encountered. The face represents the self; we "face" the world, and the face we see in the mirror each morning is important to our body image. Plastic surgery on the face may be obligatory (after trauma, burns, excisions) or optional (cosmetic). Cosmetic surgery is often requested by individuals who blame their unhappiness in life on the way they look and think that if their nose were straightened, ears pinned back, or jaw brought forward they would look so much better that their lives would be different. This may be true, but more often it is wishful thinking; and the patient is doomed to disappointment and mental disturbance if he persuades a surgeon to operate on him. Much the same can be said about women who are getting on in years and think that "face-lifting" will help them retain their youthful appearance. These women are notoriously hard to please, and reality never seems to match their fantasies. Their basic problem is far deeper than the skin.

PSYCHOTHERAPY IN THIS AREA

The attitude of the physician is more important in preventing and managing the problems discussed in this section than in any other field of medicine. He must aim at moderation and avoid extremes. An excessive show of sympathy, warmth, pity, tenderness, or any positive feeling may boomerang, causing the patient to react with distrust and fear. ("Why is the doctor behaving like that? Is he faking? If he is sincere, then I must be sicker than I thought!") The opposite extreme is no better. The completely business-like physician, devoid of emotion and totally objective, appears cold and rejecting. The patient might well respond with resentment and despair. ("How could he help me? He doesn't care a bit! I must be hopeless!")

The successful therapist takes a middle course: kind, pleasant, matter-of-fact, and interested. He is neither overly optimistic nor pessimistic, but realistic. He must maintain his affability and equanimity in the face of emotional outbursts and not respond to stress by imposing further stress. He may laugh with his patient but never cry or fight with him.

The doctor's job is to draw the patient out about his feelings and help modify those that are unrealistic, painful, or potentially destructive. Troublesome emotional symptoms must be studied thoroughly, their origins reviewed, and similar symptoms explored. Critical events in early childhood may be responsible for the tendency to react unrealistically in adult life crises.

In a crisis, the patient faces both danger and opportunity. The danger is that he will be so paralyzed with fear that he will regress to immature or even childish behavior and damage himself (by decision or indecision) irrevocably. The opportunity is that under the great stress of the emergency he may be able to exercise inner controls that he has never used before, "rise above himself," take a giant step toward greater emotional maturity, and make of the crisis a turning point in his life. This can often be suggested to the patient in such a way that he gains perspective and objectivity about his problems, and finds it easier in the future to make a decision on rational instead of emotional grounds.

The person who has the best chance to do this psychotherapy is the family physician, who functions as the first line of defense in all matters of physical or mental health. He has a tremendous head start since he knows the patient's background and has his trust. If the family physician needs help, he can turn to the patient's relatives, clergyman, lawyer, and friends or enlist the aid of a psychiatrist.

REFERENCES

Books and Monographs

Alexander, F.: *Psychosomatic Medicine.* Norton, 1950.

Balint, M.: *The Doctor, His Patient, and the Illness.* Internat Univ Press, 1957.

Cannon, W.B.: *Bodily Changes in Pain, Hunger, Fear, and Rage,* 2nd ed. Appleton-Century-Crofts, 1929.

Dunbar, F.: *Emotion and Bodily Changes.* Columbia Univ Press, 1954.

French, T.M., & F. Alexander: *Psychogenic Factors in Bronchial Asthma.* Psychosomatic Medicine Monograph No. 4. National Research Council, 1941.

Geist, H.: *The Psychological Aspects of Diabetes.* Thomas, 1964.

Levine, M. (editor): *Endocrines and the Central Nervous System.* Proceedings of the Association for Research in Nervous and Mental Disorders. Williams & Wilkins, 1966.

Selye, H.: *The Stress of Life.* McGraw-Hill, 1956.

Sifneos, P.E.: *Ascent From Chaos: A Psychosomatic Case Study.* Harvard Univ Press, 1964.

Journal Articles

Bastiaans, J.: Psychosomatic investigations on the psychic aspects of acute myocardial infarction. Psychother Psychosom 16:202–209, 1968.

Brown, E., & P. Barglow: Pseudocyesis. Arch Gen Psychiat 24:221–229, 1971.

Bruch, H.: The insignificant difference: Discordant incidence of anorexia nervosa in monozygotic twins. Am J Psychiat 126:85–90, 1969.

Bruhn, J.G., & others: Patients' reactions to death in a coronary care unit. J Psychosom Res 14:65–70, March 1970.

Cleveland, S.E., & D.L. Johnson: Motivation and readiness of potential human tissue donors and nondonors. Psychosom Med 32:225–231, 1970.

Freeman, E.H., & others: Psychological variables in allergic disorders: A review. Psychosom Med 26:543–575, 1964.

Glassman, B.M., & A. Siegel: Personality correlates of survival in long-term hemodialysis program. Arch Gen Psychiat 22:566–574, 1970.

Liljefors, I., & R.H. Rahe: An identical twin study of psychosocial factors in coronary heart disease in Sweden. Psychosom Med 32:523–542, 1970.

Luparello, T., & others: Influences of suggestion on airway reactivity in asthmatic subjects. Psychosom Med 30:819–825, 1968.

Luther, I.G., Heistad, G.T., & S.B. Sparber: Influence of pregnancy upon gastric ulcers induced by restraint. Psychosom Med 31:45–56, 1969.

McFadden, E.R., Jr., & others: The mechanism of action of suggestion in the induction of acute asthma attacks. Psychosom Med 31:134–143, 1969.

Mendelson, M.: Psychological aspects of obesity. Internat J Psychiat 2:599, 1966.

Minc, S.: Psychological factors in coronary heart disease. Geriatrics 20:747–755, 1965.

Mirsky, I.A.: The psychosomatic approach to the etiology of clinical disorder. Psychosom Med 19:424, 1957.

Moos, R.H.: Personality factors associated with rheumatoid arthritis: A review. J Chronic Dis 17:41, 1964.

Muslin, H.: On acquiring a kidney. Am J Psychiat 127:1185–1188, 1971.

O'Connor, J.F., & others: An evaluation of the effectiveness of psychotherapy in the treatment of ulcerative colitis. Ann Int Med 60:587, 1964.

Schwab, J.J., & others: Psychosomatic medicine and the contemporary social scene. Am J Psychiat 126:1632–1642, 1970.

Seward, G.H., & others: The questions of psychophysiologic infertility: Some negative answers. Psychosom Med 27:533–545, 1965.

Simmons, R.G., & others: Family tension in the search for a kidney donor. JAMA 215:909–912, 1971.

Steiner, J., & others: Psychiatric sequelae to gynaecological operations. Israel Ann Psychiat 8:186–192, 1970.

Wolf, S.: Stress and heart disease. Mod Concepts Cardiovas Dis 29:599, 1960.

Note: The editors and the author of this chapter wish to acknowledge the valuable assistance of Albert S. Norris, MD, who suggested several of the topics that have been added to the chapter since the first edition.

19 . . .

Normal & Abnormal Sexual Behavior

There are enormous individual variations in healthy sexual endowment, appetite, sensitivity, aptitude, and preferred objects and technics of sexual expression. Impotence, premature ejaculation, and frigidity are common, usually transient expressions of emotional disturbance. If prolonged and severe (and organic disease is excluded), an underlying neurosis may be postulated and psychotherapy instituted.

Homosexuality is a way of life, a phase in the normal development of many, a chosen course by some, a perversion in others. Treatment is of doubtful value unless intensive psychotherapy is begun very early; it is usually not wanted by the patient.

Few subjects in medicine or psychiatry are more important or have been subject to more misconceptions than sexual behavior. The scientific investigation and discussion of sex and sexual problems by well trained workers is a late and welcome development in American medicine. The comprehensive statistical analysis by Kinsey and his coworkers of the sexual behavior of men and women—published in 1948 and 1953, respectively—encouraged a more enlightened attitude toward this field and led to the pioneering work by Masters & Johnson in 1966 in which the detailed patterns of human sexual response are documented.

Sexual behavior should always be considered in the context of the whole personality. Pathologic sexual behavior may be a presenting symptom of an existing disorder or transient manifestation of an emotional or personality disorder or of organic disease. A sudden change in sexual behavior is of particular diagnostic importance. Abnormal sexual behavior becomes especially important when legal proceedings are contemplated, since the final legal disposition of the case may be influenced by psychiatric testimony about its causes, treatment, and prognosis.

THE MEDICAL PRACTITIONER'S ROLE IN THE DIAGNOSIS AND TREATMENT OF SEXUAL DISORDERS

Traditionally, the medical practitioner has been the main source of help and guidance to people with a variety of personal, emotional, and physical problems. Because of his training and background, the physician should be uniquely qualified to provide education and information about all aspects of bodily functions, including sexual functions. Unfortunately, many physicians receive inadequate training about the sexual functions and are unable to serve their patients as well as they should.

The patient may state his or her sexual problem directly, or may complain of nervousness, vague pains, headache, etc as a means of establishing the contact in the hope that the problem will be uncovered. Only if the physician is alert to this possibility will he be able to offer maximum pertinent help to his patient.

A sexual problem that appears trivial may be a cause of great torment. For example, a man may wonder if he is a homosexual because at age 16 he engaged in mutual homosexual activity on one occasion; or he may wonder if his symptoms of depression are a consequence of masturbation. In most cases, all that is necessary, after eliciting additional relevant data, is to give reassurance and explain the facts.

At times the physician will be confronted by more serious sexual difficulties in his patients. If a patient complains of recent onset of impotence, the physician will wonder—knowing that a large proportion of these cases are of psychogenic origin—whether he should refer the patient to a psychiatrist or attempt to offer counseling himself. After excluding organic causes, he should take a more thorough psychosexual history. In the light of what he knows about the patient, his socioeconomic circumstances, his relationship with his wife, etc, it may become evident that recent and apparently unconnected events may account for the symptoms. Brief supportive counseling may be sufficient to give relief without recourse to psychiatric referral. If the physician feels that he is ill qualified, either by training or inclination, to offer this help—or if his efforts are unsuccessful—referral to other professionals should be considered.

If the presenting sexual problem is such that brief educational or supportive interviews would be of no avail (eg, most of the sexual deviations), the physician should inform the patient that more extensive psychiatric evaluation and treatment are indicated and should offer to make the necessary referral. It is important, however, whenever a patient is referred elsewhere, that he be told of the nature and reason for the referral.

NORMAL SEXUAL BEHAVIOR

Normal sexual behavior has a wide range and it is difficult to say where it merges into abnormal behavior. This section will attempt to deal mainly with the biologic aspects of sex behavior, especially as it affects the emotional lives of the individuals.

Much depends upon moral, social, and legal norms in a given culture or community, and although these are constantly being reevaluated they may still be contradictory. For example, in most modern societies premarital sexual intercourse is said to be morally wrong, but it is often considered socially acceptable and may or may not be legal depending upon local statutes. Ideas about what constitutes normal sexual activity are gradually becoming less restrictive under the influence of education. However, some individuals still need to be reassured that there is nothing degrading or unhealthy about indulging in certain sexual practices, often as foreplay, in promoting a more harmonious sexual adjustment between sexual partners. Without this reassurance they may be tormented by thoughts of being "perverts" or "sick."

The chief aims of sexual behavior are procreation, demonstration of love for the partner, pleasure, and relief from sexual tension. A sequence of fairly constant physiologic processes culminating in orgasm is involved.

Foreplay

Just as the surroundings, setting, and service of a good meal are important in its enjoyment (and digestion), the circumstances and conduct of the partners in preparation for a sex act may be crucial to the fullest attainment of its goals. Haste, fear of interruption, anger or other negative feelings toward the partner, unsatisfactory physical conditions, severe fatigue, and fear of pregnancy are common unfavorable factors. Music, dancing, and pleasant conversation are desirable preludes leading to lovemaking with warmth, tenderness, and increasing physical intimacies (kisses, caresses, fondling). These preliminaries never seem to last long enough for most women, but men often become importunate and try to proceed faster too soon. Ten to 30 minutes represents a good investment of time. Actual genital contact (mutual digital-genital stimulation and lingual-genital also for those who like it) should precede sexual intercourse. A myriad of variations and embellishments—timing, different places, improvised technics, and imaginative, creative, playful efforts—can add immeasurably to the delights of sex and to the depth of the relationship.

Orgasm

The frequency of orgasm in males varies widely, from one or more daily to one a month; but for mature men the average is 2—3 times a week. The greatest sexual drive in men is reached in late adolescence, after which it usually declines slowly. In women, the period of greatest sexual desire is reached in the 30s, often after the birth of one or more children.

Orgasm may be defined as the physiologic changes and the paroxysmal emotive sensations experienced at the culmination of a sexual act. The work of Masters & Johnson has resulted in further elucidation of this phenomenon. They recognize 4 stages:

A. Excitement Stage: In men, the initial physiologic change is penile erection, which can occur within a few seconds following an adequate erotic stimulus. In women, the initial response can occur within 30 seconds and consists of a sweating transudate of the vaginal walls, although the latter contain no glands and the cervix produces no secretions. Breast enlargement, nipple erection, and areolar engorgement also occur.

This stage may last from a few minutes to 2—3 hours in both sexes.

B. Plateau Stage: This is characterized by an increase in intensity of the above changes and lasts a variable time depending upon the sexual stimuli and drive. At the end of this stage in women, a "sexual flush" is present over the breasts, anterior chest wall, and neck, signifying marked sexual tension.

C. Orgastic Stage: The climactic stage in both men and women is reached suddenly like a sneeze and lasts only a few seconds.

1. In men, orgasm is manifested by ejaculation of semen followed by relief from muscular tension and venous congestion.

2. In women, the duration and intensity of orgasm varies widely and is associated with definite anatomic and physiologic changes: There is no distinct "clitoral" and "vaginal" orgasm, as described in the old texts. Orgasm is accompanied by rhythmic contractions of the outer third of the vaginal barrel with subsidence of venous congestion of the outer third of the vagina. The clitoral sensations are more important for orgasm than the vaginal, and at the height of the sexual tension the clitoris and labia minora retract.

Other widespread physiologic changes occur that affect the whole body, eg, variations in blood pressure, pulse rate and respiratory rate, and myotonia.

D. Resolution Stage: Immediately after orgasm, resolution of the above changes proceeds in reverse order. In women, if no orgasm is achieved, the resolution changes occur slowly and the clitoris may remain engorged for up to 3 hours. In men, there is a refractory period before further excitation can occur, but some women are capable of having many orgasms during the same coitus.

Contraception and Sterilization

Contraception may be defined as the prevention of impregnation in normal fertile partners while engaging in coitus. Abstinence, abortion, sterilization, and castration are not usually classified in the same category.

There are many technics to prevent contraception, some applying to females and some to males. The reliability of the various methods depends on the effectiveness of the contraceptive technic, its acceptability to the user, and the user's motivation for contraception. Impregnation most often results because of difficulties with the second and third factors.

For the male, coitus interruptus (withdrawal) and the condom are the most common methods of contraception. The female uses douches, chemical foams, vaginal diaphragms, cervical caps, intrauterine devices, oral contraceptives, and the "safe period," especially the last two. The most reliable methods have been shown to be the condom for the male and the oral (hormonal) contraceptives for the female.

The psychologic implications of using contraceptives may be profound. If fear of pregnancy has been great in one or both partners so that secondary manifestations of anxiety—eg, frigidity and dyspareunia in the female and premature ejaculation or decreased sexual vigor in the male—have resulted, effective contraception may significantly improve sexual harmony and performance. On the other hand, the use of contraceptives by members of certain religious groups may result in much anxiety and guilt, so that the end result may be of dubious benefit.

Today, however, with widespread concern about overpopulation and greater emphasis on family planning, many marriage partners resort to some method of birth control in their search for social and psychologic harmony. Sterilization may be defined as the act which makes a male or female incapable of reproduction. It should be distinguished from impotence and castration. In impotence, a man is usually fertile but has difficulty in obtaining an erection and hence in impregnating a female. Removal of the testes invariably results in sterility but also in other evidence of hormonal imbalance.

Sterilization may be performed on the male or on the female. In the female, a major operation is required, usually excision and ligation of the fallopian tubes (salpingectomy); rarely, removal of the ovaries (oophorectomy) and hysterectomy may be performed. In the male, sterilization is a relatively minor surgical procedure and entails ligation and excision of part of the vas deferens (vasectomy). In both male and female, sterilization is almost always permanent, although restoration operations may be performed (eg, vasovasotomy in the male) with up to 90% success claimed.

Indications for sterilization are never absolute. They fall into 3 main categories: (1) eugenic (usually if a dominant gene is involved, eg, Huntington's chorea); (2) therapeutic, if the life of the woman is threatened with further pregnancies; and (3) socioeconomic, to prevent further anguish due to unwanted pregnancies. Sterilization is most often performed for the third reason; indeed, in certain parts of the world it is the principal means of population control, the operation usually being performed on the male.

Before sterilization is contemplated, it is imperative that the partners involved understand the nature and implications of the procedure. Poorer and less well educated couples often request it, but the permanency of the procedure may not be fully appreciated. Even when the procedure is consented to with full knowledge, difficulties may arise if the couple gets divorced and the man remarries and wishes to raise a new family.

The psychologic aspects are similar to those involved in contraception. If fear of pregnancy is great, release from this fear may result in a much happier, less tense, and more satisfactory sexual performance. However, men often worry about loss of sexual vigor or bodily change such as feminization. These never occur on an organic basis, but worry about them can lead to impotence and other neurotic symptoms. Feminization may result from castration.

Some individuals may suffer from anxiety about their "change in identity," ie, a man about his masculinity and a woman about her femininity, the latter especially after "physiologic sterility" (the menopause). Adequate reassurance is all that is usually needed. In some cases, deep-going psychotherapy is necessary.

Masturbation (Onanism, Auto-Erotism)

Masturbation is defined as sexual gratification through noncoital stimulation of the sexual organs.

Masturbation has been a subject of discussion for ages. Misinterpretation of Onan's behavior in the Old Testament led to its condemnation by religious authority, and it became the subject of many myths, being blamed for such disabilities as "weakness," "impotence," and "insanity." These attitudes persist, and several orthodox religions continue to regard masturbation as a sin. However, the only harm that can result from masturbation comes from the feelings of guilt and shame that may be present.

A. Incidence and Frequency: Most reports confirm Kinsey's findings that over 90% of males and 70% of females have masturbated at some time in their lives. The frequency of masturbation in adolescence averages 2–3 times a week in boys and 2–3 times a month in girls. After adolescence, this frequency decreases gradually in men but increases in women, reaching a peak around middle life, when it is more common among women than among men. Women often reach orgasm sooner by masturbation than by normal coitus. (Rich fantasies can easily outstrip meager reality.)

The incidence of masturbation also varies according to education. The single college-level man in the 20–30 age group masturbates more frequently than single men of the same age in the lower socioeconomic groups.

Masturbation may continue into married life and even into old age, especially if other sexual outlets are limited or temporarily unavailable (menstrual periods, pregnancy, illness of the partner, long trips away from the partner, or jail sentences).

B. Psychopathology: In infancy and early childhood, masturbation is considered part of an instinctive search for pleasurable sensations similar to those resulting from exploration of other parts of the body such as the fingers and toes.

At puberty and during adolescence, however, masturbation is a manifestation of emerging sexuality and is almost universally practiced before opportunities for mature sexual outlets appear. Nocturnal emissions ("wet dreams") are also common in boys during this period or in any later period of prolonged abstinence. Orgastic dreams in girls are uncommon.

The main stimuli to masturbation are the pleasure derived and the desire for relief from sexual tension. (Sexual tension probably arises from multiple sources, but the chief physical one is distention of the seminal vesicles. These little sex bladders, like the urinary bladder, produce their unique sensation when filled. If not emptied through sexual intercourse, masturbation, or nocturnal emission, and if the overflow—unfelt—at the end of urination is insufficient, considerable tension and restlessness can result.) Masturbation may be accompanied by sexual fantasies, and props (nude pictures, etc) may be used. The fantasies are often of psychologic interest; they may represent gratification of forbidden or infantile wishes and thus may serve a protective function. Gradually, however, adult heterosexual coital fantasies take their place.

C. Methods: The male usually manipulates the penis and the woman the clitoris with the hand and fingers. Rarely, males may masturbate by rubbing the penis against clothing, sheets, etc, and females may perform masturbation with suitably shaped objects. Some females gain pleasurable sensations by rubbing the thighs together.

D. Varieties of Masturbation:
1. Compulsive masturbation—Masturbation performed in a compulsive manner up to several times a day for long periods may be a manifestation of excessive anxiety resulting from neurosis, psychosis, or a borderline state. Treatment must be directed at the underlying disorder.
2. In association with abnormal sexual behavior—Masturbation is often the means of achieving orgasm with some types of sexual deviations.
3. Mutual masturbation—Simultaneous manual masturbation by 2 individuals may be part of normal heterosexual relations or a homosexual act. It may or may not be a prelude to other sexual activities.
4. Group masturbation may occur at puberty among 3 or more youngsters of the same sex, often as part of normal sexual experimentation and inquisitiveness. In older individuals, group masturbation may be a manifestation of psychopathology or delinquent tendencies.
5. Urethral masturbation (rare) is done by inserting objects into the urethra. It is more common in females.
6. Psychic masturbation (rare) is the ability to achieve orgasm purely by concentrating on sexual fantasies.
7. Anal masturbation (rare) consists of achieving a pleasurable sensation by caressing or manipulating the anus.
8. Oral masturbation (extremely rare)—The ability of some flexible males to insert their own penis into the mouth is called "auto-fellatio."
E. Treatment: Treatment is unnecessary except for the anxiety that may be associated with the act. The guilt and shame that may be reported can be relieved by assuring the patient that masturbation is a normal biologic tendency. The answer to the question, "How often may one do it?" is, "As often as one enjoys it."

Oral Sexual Intercourse (Oralism)

Oralism is defined as obtaining sexual pleasure from mouth-genital contact. Oral contact with the penis is called fellatio; oral contact with the female genitalia is called cunnilingus.

Oralism may be homosexual or heterosexual. When it is performed as part of the foreplay, preceding normal heterosexual intercourse or occasionally even leading to orgasm in the recipient, it is not a perversion. It is considered a perversion only when it replaces normal intercourse completely, frequently, or compulsively.

In some states there are laws (rarely enforced) against these practices, even when performed by married couples.

Anal Intercourse (Sodomy, Buggery)

Sexual pleasure obtained by intercourse per anum is not a perversion if indulged in as an occasional variation among heterosexuals, although it is against the law in many jurisdictions. It is not uncommon among male homosexuals, although experience is sometimes required before it becomes pleasurable. Orgasm can occur in the passive as well as in the active partner.

Extravaginal Orgasms

Sexual pleasure obtained from phallic contact with the partner's axillas, breasts, or interfemoral region is not considered abnormal. The passive partner rarely gets much pleasure.

ABNORMAL SEXUALITY

Sexual disturbances are common in both sexes and at all ages, and often result in much anguish. Normal sexual functioning is a sensitive indicator of emotional and physical health; therefore, illness in extragenital areas may cause transient or prolonged alterations in sexual function. Accurate diagnosis depends upon both psychiatric and physical examination.

The following abnormalities in sexuality are arranged approximately in the order of their frequency in the general population.

IMPOTENCE

Impotence occurs only in males, and may be defined as weak, unsustained, or complete lack of erection resulting in impaired sexual performance. Transient impotence is fairly common at all ages and occurs in most men at one time or another. It is most disturbing in the young.

The following stages of sexual activity occur in the normally potent man: libido, or desire for coitus; sufficient libido for erection; erection sufficient for penetration; ejaculation with orgasm after penetration; and relaxation.

Impairment can occur on different occasions at each of these stages, resulting in complete absence of erection, poor or unsustained erection, delayed ejaculation, or lack of orgasm.

Etiology

Although the most common cause of impotence is psychologic, organic and toxic causes are also recognized.

A. Organic Causes:

1. Systemic—Any general condition producing weakness or lethargy may interfere with sex drive. Examples are anemia, malnutrition, severe infections, neoplastic disease, uncontrolled diabetes mellitus, and hypothyroidism.

2. Neurologic (rare)—Impotence due to diseases of the sacral segment of the spinal cord, cauda equina, and parasympathetic plexuses is often associated with bladder disturbances and loss of the anal reflex. Nerve damage may be produced by trauma, syphilis (tabes dorsalis), and multiple sclerosis. Prostatectomy may (but usually does not) result in impotence.

3. Physiologic conditions—Exhaustion and aging may cause impotence. It has been found, however, that sexual potency in older men is more often a function of the availability of a suitable sexual partner than of age. Men who have intercourse regularly remain potent to a later age. After age 60, 50% of men are potent; after age 70, 30%; after age 80, 20%.

4. Anatomic defects—Hypospadias and phimosis are rare anatomic causes of impotence. Traumatic or surgical loss of the testes before puberty sometimes results in impotence.

B. Toxic Factors:

1. Hormones—Excessive use of estrogens, eg, in the treatment of carcinoma of the prostate, may diminish sexual desire with resulting impotence.

2. Sedative and hypnotic drugs—Alcohol in moderation may produce an initial increase in sexual desire, but impotence may result during periods of inebriation as well as after prolonged use. Certain sedatives, tranquilizers, and opiates in excess (eg, morphinism and chronic barbiturate intoxication) frequently produce impotence. Phenothiazines and antidepressants, eg, thioridazine (Mellaril) and imipramine (Tofranil), often result in delay or inhibition of ejaculation. Marihuana decreases sexual desire in many and produces impotence in some.

C. Psychologic Factors: Psychogenic impotence is rarely absolute. It is almost always caused by anxiety, shame, guilt, fear, or anger, and may be due to external realistic situations or internal moral prohibitions.

It is essential to obtain a detailed sexual history, inquiring into factors such as the strength of the initial sexual urge, circumstances of the first failure, the presence or absence of any subsequent erection, the occurrence of morning erections and wet dreams, and the timing of ejaculation. The background, details of sexual development, moral attitudes, attitudes toward contraceptives if used, attitudes toward the partner, sexual fantasies, current mental status, and the patient's own theories about his problem all have to be considered. For example, the impotence may be "facultative," ie, the patient may be impotent with his wife but not with his mistress, or impotent with his girl friend but not with a prostitute (or vice versa), or impotent with women but not with men, or impotent with both men and women but able to masturbate successfully.

Impotence may be mild and transient, or severe and prolonged.

1. Usually transient—The patient often knows the cause. A rigidly moralistic upbringing is often an aggravating factor.

a. Honeymoon impotence, or sudden impotence in the young man about to perform his first act of sexual intercourse, may be due to fear of failure, fear of impregnating or hurting the partner, fear of discovery, etc. With increasing confidence, potency is gradually restored.

b. Unsustained potency or rapid detumescence prior to penetration may be associated with fear of discovery, impairment of sensation by a condom, or anger at the partner, eg, if she is unresponsive or uninterested. It is possible for a woman to make a man impotent by derogatory remarks or by manifesting excess anxiety at crucial moments.

c. Impotence with specific individuals, usually the wife, is often an expression of hostility if of recent onset; or it may be due to an underlying neurotic conflict in which "love" and "sexual passion" have become mutually exclusive emotions that cannot be directed toward the same woman.

d. Specific fears may cause impotence, eg, fear of venereal disease. Another example is the patient with pulmonary or cardiac disease who becomes impotent because he has been instructed not to exert himself.

e. Specific psychiatric disease—Impotence may be a symptom of a specific psychiatric disorder, eg, depressive reaction or schizophrenia.

2. Usually prolonged—The patient is often unaware of the cause or rationalizes it. Impotence may be an expression of aversion to intercourse or one aspect of a generalized antisexual and antifeminine attitude. The patient with protracted impotence often has a punitive conscience and severe problems with castration anxiety (a relic of the oedipal phase of psychologic development).

a. Castration complex—The "phallic woman" (who wishes she had a penis herself and acts competitively and often hostilely or sarcastically toward men) often causes impotence in her sexual partner. Impotence may be brought on in some men by an overly aggressive woman who attempts to control the sex act by commenting unfavorably on and minimizing her partner's contribution to her pleasure. Impotence may also result from excessive punishment in childhood for sexual "misbehavior"; with repression of the subsequent rage, the symptoms become part of an anxiety or hysterical state. Childhood sex traumas, especially if repeated, may have a similar result.

b. Hypochondriacal ideas concerning physical attributes may lead to feelings of inadequacy. The embarrassment of thinking that one's penis is too small is common, although Masters has reported that the small penis enlarges to a relatively greater extent on erection than the larger penis. Similarly, men with good physiques who are popular with women often have a fear of being sexually inadequate, which would be a blow to their narcissism.

c. Impotence associated with sexual deviations—Men who are latent or overt homosexuals or have other compulsive sexual deviations may be impotent in heterosexual coitus.

d. In rare cases it may not be possible to identify the cause of impotence, the reason presumably being strongly repressed.

Treatment

Treatment depends upon the cause, type, and duration of the disability, with emphasis on the first.

A. Impotence Due to Organic and Toxic Causes: Give medical or surgical treatment as indicated.

B. Impotence Due to Acute Situational Stress: Counseling, reassurance, and education, with attempts to allay guilt and anxiety, will usually result in rapid improvement. If the anxiety is great, the following may help:

1. Intercourse should be discouraged initially to interrupt the vicious cycle which can result from repeated failures.

2. Provide counseling to the female partner and eliminate as many contributing factors as possible. If both partners are available for counseling, the chances for success are improved.

3. Mild tranquilizers before bedtime—or even alcohol in small quantities —may be helpful. So-called aphrodisiacs are of no value, and some, such as tincture of cantharides, are dangerous.

C. Prolonged Psychogenic Impotence: The measures outlined above should be tried, but if no improvement results and the condition is apparently of long standing and there are severe neurotic conflicts or personality problems, the following are indicated:

1. Intensive (often prolonged) psychotherapy—The prognosis is fairly good except in older men in whom the disability has become more fixed.

2. Antidepressant drugs—These are indicated if a clinical depression exists. Imipramine (Tofranil) taken at bedtime may give symptomatic relief even in the absence of depression. Suggestion probably plays a role here.

3. Hormone therapy—This is of benefit only if there is clinical evidence of endocrine malfunction. Testosterone propionate may be used in cases of hypogonadism.

4. Mechanical aids—These are not favored by most psychiatrists or patients, but occasionally a well fitting "penile splint" is greatly appreciated. Similarly, a rubber "penile prosthesis" may be received with gratification by the wife.

PREMATURE EJACULATION

Premature ejaculation may be defined as orgasm occurring before or soon after insertion of the penis into the vagina. The definition is sometimes broadened to include orgasm that occurs before the male wishes it, considered by some to be "partial impotence." This rather common disability results in humiliation for the male and lack of sexual gratification for the female, and is of particular concern for modern sophisticated couples who strive for the supposed ideal of simultaneous climax. (Many couples prefer female-male sequential orgasms.)

Etiology

Normal orgasm and ejaculation result from a reflex action which is triggered when the psychic and tactile stimuli reach a certain threshold. The duration of intercourse before this occurs varies greatly even in long-married couples. Most men want to be able to prolong intercourse until the partner reaches orgasm, or at least for a few minutes. In most cases of premature ejaculation, orgasm takes place after a few seconds of intercourse. Apart from the problem of not satisfying the woman, premature ejaculation is disturbing to the male both quantitatively and qualitatively since the orgasm is apt to be shorter and less pleasurable.

Two divergent points of view have been expressed about underlying constitutional causes of premature ejaculation: (1) In the "athletic" males of Kretschmer, premature ejaculation is considered to be a sign of high sexual tension and superpotency associated with excessive penile sensitivity. It would be more likely to occur, therefore, after a prolonged period of abstinence. (2) In the "asthenic" male and often the older man, premature ejaculation is considered to be an indication of low potency with weak libido and poor erection.

There can be no doubt, however, that neurotic elements, largely unconscious, almost always exist, usually in the form of deep-seated feelings of inadequacy, castration fears, and unresolved oedipal conflicts.

Treatment

A. Physical Methods: The following procedures, though ostensibly based on physical management, contain psychologic features of suggestion.

1. Decreasing psychic stimulation—This involves various technics that can be employed during coitus to delay the climax, eg, occupying the mind with nonsexual fantasies (counting sheep) or tightening the anal sphincter and keeping it tight.

2. Decreasing tactile stimulation—This can be done either by reducing friction from the vaginal walls or by making the glans penis less sensitive, or by both means. The former may be achieved by moderating the extent and thrust of the penis in the vagina, or by inserting it deeply. The latter may be effected by wearing a condom or by the application of 1% dibucaine (Nupercaine) ointment about 30 minutes before intercourse.

3. Alteration of excitability threshold—Deconditioning procedures may increase tolerance to pre-orgastic excitement. The penis is stimulated manually to a stage just prior to orgasm and allowed to subside. This is repeated several times. After several days or weeks of this exercise, coitus may in some instances be markedly prolonged.

B. Psychotherapy: If a neurotic basis for the disorder is present, intensive psychotherapy should be offered. This is especially important in the man with low potency, in whom the various means of decreasing sensory stimuli should not be used.

The prognosis is generally good, but relapses are not uncommon.

FRIGIDITY

Frigidity may be defined as partial or complete lack of sexual enjoyment or gratification in the female. It is a common psychosexual dysfunction but less disabling than impotence since a woman can perform sexually without desire or enjoyment. Severe frigidity, however, may have a far-reaching effect on the life of a marital pair, causing resentment, hostility, and frustration in both husband and wife. The recent trend toward greater sexual freedom with a greater willingness to talk about and engage in sexual experiences aggravates the feeling of personal failure in the female if orgasm is not achieved.

The degree of sexual arousal in any woman will vary on different occasions depending upon many factors, including her emotional state at the time. Different types of frigidity may be distinguished, as follows:

(1) **Negative feelings about coitus:** About 1% of women have an aversion to intercourse. This is the most severe form of frigidity, and the repugnance and resentment felt toward the sexual act are associated with feelings of shame, guilt, and anxiety. Pelvic pain, dyspareunia, and vaginismus may also be present (see below).

(2) **Failure of sexual arousal:** Although the woman is willing to have coitus, little or no sexual arousal results and no enjoyment or orgasm. About 3% of women have this complaint.

(3) **Failure to attain orgasm:** In this type of frigidity the woman has the desire and is able to be aroused but does not reach a climax. Kinsey reported that 25% of women who have been married for 1 year or less are frigid in this way, but the frequency of orgasm gradually increases in later married life. Other authorities report that the percentage of women who never or rarely have orgasm is much higher—up to 40% in some studies.

Masters & Johnson have established that the clitoris is the principal orgastic area and that the physiologic changes associated with "clitoral orgasm" also occur in "vaginal orgasm," thus disproving the existence of a separate and more "mature" entity of vaginal orgasm. Women, like men, have only one kind of orgasm, but in both women and men it can vary enormously in intensity and duration from a mild but pleasurable climax to an overwhelming experience of ecstasy.

Dyspareunia and Vaginismus

Dyspareunia (painful or difficult sexual intercourse) and vaginismus (involuntary spasm of the vaginal wall, preventing insertion of the penis) are sometimes present with severe or chronic frigidity. They may also be present with milder degrees of frigidity in young or inexperienced women.

Vaginismus is always psychogenic in origin. It is a form of neurotic conversion symptom, protecting the woman from the feared act.

Etiology

A. Organic Causes (Rare):

1. Systemic—Frigidity may accompany acute or chronic illnesses, pain, or endocrinopathies, eg, hypothyroidism or hypogonadism.

2. Neurologic—Frigidity can be ascribed to neurologic disorders only when sensory supply to the pudendal (S3–S4) area is destroyed, eg, in tabes dorsalis, multiple sclerosis, or other spinal cord diseases.

3. Physiologic (eg, aging)—Aging is not an important cause of frigidity. Libido may actually increase gradually with age until the menopause. After the menopause, sexual desire may diminish, but it need never be lost completely if a regular sexual partner is available. However, psychologic maladjustments common at the menopause may produce secondary frigidity. Fatigue may cause transient frigidity.

4. Anatomic defects—Many local conditions such as endometritis, cystitis, vulvovaginitis, leukoplakia, etc may produce dyspareunia, which leads to anxiety and frigidity.

B. Drugs and Hormones:

1. Drugs—Impaired libido is a not uncommon side-effect of the major tranquilizers. The minor tranquilizers (including alcohol) may increase sexual desire by relieving anxiety.

2. Hormones—The androgens normally present in the female body help to produce sexual stimulation; if they are deficient, sexual anesthesia may result. Oral contraceptives sometimes interfere with sexual arousal because of their progesterone content. Some improvement may result if sequential contraceptives are used.

C. Psychosocial Factors: These are the commonest causes of frigidity.

1. Frigidity due primarily to sexual inhibition—Sexual inhibition is the most common cause of severe and chronic frigidity. In this group, frigidity causes marital discord and other maladjustments. In group 2 discussed below, marital maladjustment produces the frigidity.

a. Hostility to men is usually learned from a mother who believes that men are "brutes," unreliable and exploitative. Such a mother is often frigid and dominating herself, and the father is either passive and uninvolved or tyrannical. Sometimes these women, who have no wish to be prudish, sincerely desire orgasm consciously. They feel ashamed that they do not achieve it and become excessively concerned with technics of intercourse instead of relaxing during coitus.

b. Attitude toward sex—A prudish or moralistic attitude toward sex acquired from the parents may result in guilt and shame regarding the sexual act. Similarly, fear of rejection and ridicule, fear of impregnation, feelings of inferiority, feelings of dependency, fear of loss of self-control, and intense narcissism may all contribute to frigidity.

c. Unresolved oedipal conflicts—These women may unconsciously view the lover or husband as a father substitute. Their histories show that they were often close to their fathers and in stormy competition with their mothers. Socially, they often prefer men with whom they compete; they are dissatisfied with the feminine role, and are anxious and guilty about sex. Frigidity often gets worse after marriage and pregnancy, as the relationship with the husband becomes more closely identified with the father.

d. Occasionally, a single traumatic sexual incident in childhood may lead to sexual difficulties in later life. Repeated exposures to traumatic situations (violence, incest, squalor) are much more apt to lead to frigidity in adulthood.

e. Severe neurotic or psychotic states may interfere with gratification in heterosexual relations, eg, depressions and schizophrenias, or perversions.

2. Primary fault in partner ("pseudo-frigidity")—The husband may display poor precoital technic; may be physically unattractive to his wife or too demanding; may have other quirks which cause annoyance to the woman, justifiable or otherwise; or coitus may be performed in unsuitable surroundings. During episodes of marital discord, temporary frigidity is not uncom-

mon, and the wife may even withhold sexual relations as a weapon against her husband. The frigidity is often facultative, since the wife may find that she functions quite well with a lover; it is more properly called "pseudo-frigidity" since manipulation of the environment and simple instruction will usually alleviate the problem.

Treatment

A. Medical Treatment: A general medical and gynecologic examination is important. Any organic disorders found should be treated as required. An interview with the husband is desirable.

Drug therapy is occasionally useful, perhaps partly or wholely because of its psychologic effect.

1. Mild tranquilizers or alcohol may be of benefit one-half hour before coitus if extreme apprehension is present.

2. Androgens, eg, methyltestosterone, may be of benefit if the clitoris lacks sensitivity, but side-effects are common and may be unacceptable (hirsutism, voice changes, acne).

3. Aphrodisiacs (eg, cantharides, nux vomica, yohimbine) are of no value.

4. Oral contraceptives may improve sexual adjustment if fear of pregnancy or distaste for other contraceptive measures are factors in the frigidity. However, in some women the pill may produce a slight decrease in libido, in which case a change to another product or withdrawal for a trial period may be of diagnostic help.

B. Psychotherapy: Psychologic treatment will be more acceptable after medical and gynecologic causes have been ruled out. There are several methods:

1. Counseling primarily involves education of the couple. Frank advice on sex technics, especially regarding foreplay, is essential. Coitus should be attempted when both the husband and wife are relaxed, not pressed for time, and have no overbearing worries. Kind words and consideration by the male, together with adequate stimulation of the more sensitive erotic areas, preferably with multiple body contacts, will help to produce sexual arousal; the latter may be further enhanced if the female actively concentrates on erotic fantasies and if coital technics are varied. Mutual oral-genital stimulation may be of benefit to both parties.

Recently, Masters & Johnson have published technics for treating common sexual problems such as premature ejaculation and frigidity. The method involves both marriage partners receiving counseling daily for 2 weeks under supervision of a male-female therapy team, and attempting intercourse each evening as prescribed, in the privacy of their quarters. As much as 80% success has been claimed.

2. Intensive psychotherapy is indicated if the above fails, since a deep-seated neurotic conflict is probably present.

3. Behavior therapy has been advocated by some. The neurotic or maladaptive behavior, especially fear of the sex act, is unlearned by means of deconditioning technics so that sexual acts cease to produce anxiety. The

technic entails graduated exposure (verbal or visual) to the anxiety-provoking situation until the patient feels minimal anxiety at the thought of the previously repugnant act.

The prognosis generally is only fair. Many women remain frigid or obtain only partial gains in spite of prolonged and intensive therapeutic efforts. Some achieve complete success in a short time; others may suddenly obtain it only after several years of psychotherapy.

EJACULATORY DISTURBANCES

Retarded ejaculation, absent ejaculation, ejaculation without orgasm, failure of relaxation after coitus, and postcoital depression may be manifestations of an organic disorder or of a serious neurotic conflict. They should first have urologic investigation and then, if necessary, intensive psychotherapy. Some ejaculatory disturbances occur as side-effects of certain drugs (eg, antidepressants) or as a result of neurologic disorders (eg, multiple sclerosis or spinal cord tumors). Treatment is either obvious or nonexistent.

HYPERSEXUALITY

Excessive desire for or engagement in sexual acts may occur in both men and women. The limits of normal are not clearly defined, but pathologic hypersexuality may be said to be present if sexual preoccupations tend to dominate conscious thought even after the sexual act has been performed or if sex is such a domineering influence that it interferes with other aspects of the individual's daily life. *Satyriasis* in men, with its compulsive characteristics, must be distinguished from *Don Juan behavior* and *philandering,* which imply great variety in sexual partners by choice, and from *priapism,* or prolonged erection with or without sexual desire. Similarly, *nymphomania,* or increased and compulsive desire for sexual experiences in women, must be distinguished from *promiscuity,* which implies deliberate though wayward sexual acts, with or without sexual desire or enjoyment.

Sexual performance, capacity, and drive are biologically and psychologically determined in both men and women, and are modified by many factors.

Etiology

Hypersexuality is usually a manifestation of psychologic problems, but it may occur in certain organic states.

A. Organic Hypersexuality:

1. Lesions in the limbic area of the brain, eg, certain tumors and cerebrovascular accidents, may cause hypersexuality. In monkeys, bilateral extirpation of the temporal lobes—especially the tips, involving the hippocampus, uncus, and amygdala—causes extreme hypersexuality as well as other manifestations (Klüver-Bucy syndrome). Lesions of the limbic sys-

tem and hypothalamus result in marked accentuation of basic emotions; when the amygdala is involved, extreme satyriasis or nymphomania may result.

2. Psychomotor epilepsy—Hypersexuality may be manifested during an episode of temporal lobe seizure via stimulation of the above areas. During such episodes, sexual crimes may be committed in a state of automatism or fugue; afterward, the patient is amnesic for the incidents.

3. Dyscontrol syndrome—Hypersexuality is here seen along with physical brutality, dipsomania, and a tendency to many driving accidents. The cause is neurologic but often unlocalizable.

4. Drugs—Certain drugs (eg, amphetamines, opiates, and androgens) may produce an increase in sexual desire in some individuals some of the time. Aphrodisiacs do not increase desire.

5. Physiologic changes may produce a temporary increase in libido which in rare instances may be quite powerful. For example, at menopause, the physiologic decrease in estrogens results in a relative increase in androgens. Some women have marked increases in sexual desire during their menstrual periods.

B. Psychogenic Hypersexuality:

1. Psychiatric disease—Hypersexuality may be a transient secondary manifestation of some psychiatric diseases, eg, organic brain syndrome, the hypomanic phase of manic-depressive psychosis, and a few schizophrenias. The patients lack full responsibility for the sexual acts they commit, although they may be fully aware of what they are doing.

2. Personality disorders—The borderline personality, the sociopathic personality, and the hysterical personality disorders may be associated with hypersexuality which is psychoneurotic in origin and may more precisely be termed "pseudosexual" behavior.

The *Don Juan* male acts as he does not because of true sexual need, since a normal person loses his desire when satisfied, but because of a narcissistic need to mask unconscious feelings of inadequacy. In these individuals, self-esteem is elevated by erotic conquests, which "prove" that they are potent and desirable. They are in a constant search for new partners, since after each conquest they begin to have doubts about their ability to arouse other women. These men characteristically suffer from an unresolved Oedipus complex. Unconsciously, they seek a maternal figure whom they never find; hence they are never satisfied.

Similarly, *nymphomania* may be an obsession with analogous dynamics. The constant threat here is not being loved. Frigidity and castration conflicts ("penis envy") commonly coexist. The woman searches for satisfaction from multiple partners with whom she often has an ambivalent relationship, using dependent, sadistic, or coercive means.

In both men and women, if excessive inhibition coexists with hypersexuality, compulsive masturbation may occur.

Clinical Manifestations

Hypersexuality is usually manifested by a compulsive (neurotic) desire to have sexual intercourse. The sexual act is often devoid of real satisfaction, so that, although appearing vigorous, the male may be "orgastically impotent" and the female frigid. One male patient said, "It's like urinating"; a woman reported, "I have to do it, but I don't feel a thing." Thus, they have to pursue their relentless, repetitive, promiscuous course, looking vainly for satisfaction and "true love." The relationships formed are usually superficial and include little interest in the personalities of the partners. In the sex act, foreplay often assumes an inordinate role. Vague neurotic symptoms are commonly present, such as restlessness, impaired concentration, and general dissatisfaction with life.

Treatment

A. Organic Causes: Treatment of the specific cause should be offered.

B. Psychogenic Causes: Long-term psychotherapy is indicated to cope with the deep personality problem.

The prognosis is generally good. Time, physiology, and society work with the therapist.

SEXUAL DEVIATIONS

A sexual deviation, perversion, or paraphilia is defined as a pattern of sexual behavior in which the *predominant source* of sexual gratification is by means other than normal heterosexual intercourse. Hence, some "perverse acts" may be within the normal range if indulged in sporadically or as foreplay preceding normal coitus.

Sexually deviant acts are usually impulsive and compulsive in character. Individuals who practice them may seem outwardly as normal as anyone else; indeed, a man's wife may be ignorant of his sexually deviant tendencies for years. The legal status of sexually deviant acts is often culturally influenced—eg, homosexuality between consenting adults is no longer a crime in England, but it is in most of the USA. From a legal standpoint, homosexuality in the female is more tolerated or acceptable than in the male in the USA.

Understanding of the psychodynamics of sexual deviation began in 1905 with Freud's *Three Essays on the Theory of Sexuality.* Freud speculated that sexual energy or libido is present from birth in an unorganized form. This pregenital, "polymorphous perverse" stage is characterized by satisfaction derived from nongenital, auto-erotic sources, eg, sucking, eating, defecating, smearing, and, later, looking and exhibiting. Each of these is a "partial instinct." These partial instincts gradually become integrated, leading to genital dominance in the adult, but they never disappear completely and many of them persist in the forms of kissing, fondling, and exhibiting, often used in foreplay.

If, because of fixation at (or regression to) the pregenital stage, one of these partial instincts remains the dominant source of sexual gratification in an adult, an infantile form of sexuality or deviation results but with the difference that the potential for genital orgasm is present.

Tendencies toward perversion exist in everyone in latent form; the factors that make it overt are debatable. Castration anxiety, oedipal conflicts, and other abnormalities of the family environment during childhood are the most common causes.

Because the mental mechanisms involved in sexual deviations are similar to those involved in the neuroses, deviations have been viewed by some as a form of neurosis. However, Freud called them "the negative of neurosis," since they involve the expression and exaggeration of instincts rather than their repression.

Punishment under the law has been the usual method of management of persons apprehended for deviant sex practices. More enlightened attitudes are now beginning to penetrate the legal system (punishment largely for the use of force or for the involvement of minors—as in illegal normal heterosexual acts), and sexual perverts are being referred for psychiatric treatment rather than sent to jail. The prognosis, however, is in most cases poor since these individuals often have little motivation for change.

HOMOSEXUALITY

Homosexuality is defined as desire for sexual contact with persons of one's own sex. However, a history of isolated homosexual experiences, usually in adolescence, does not constitute homosexuality. Homosexual behavior between women is termed *lesbianism.* Men or women who enjoy sexual contact with both sexes are termed bisexual. It is generally considered that most bisexuals are primarily homosexual, although they can bring themselves to perform heterosexually, and even enjoy it somewhat.

Homosexuality is the most common of sexual deviations. Its prevalence is not precisely known and varies in different societies. In Kinsey's survey, 4% of Caucasian males in the USA were found to be exclusively homosexual and 37% reported some homosexual contact with or without orgasm during their lives. In females, corresponding figures showed one-third of this prevalence in all categories. However, Kinsey defined homosexuality very broadly by rating homosexual activity on a 7-point scale. A zero score meant exclusive heterosexual desires and experiences; a 3 point score implied a mixture of heterosexual and homosexual activity; and a rating of 6–7 was given to exclusive homosexuals.

Homosexuals congregate largely in urban areas. Most homosexual pickups are made at certain locally known sections of town ("gay bars," Turkish baths) or by cruising the streets. Homosexual prostitution is not unusual. Some individuals live open, exclusively homosexual lives, whereas others are more discreet and live (and "pass") in the predominantly heterosexual world. Certain occupations are overrepresented by homosexuals. In men, these include acting, interior decorating, dancing, and hairdressing; in women, aggressive, masculine occupations are more apt to attract homosexuals, eg, truckdriving, machinist work, and engineering.

Some homosexuals attempt to emulate heterosexual relationships and may even be "married"; after a passionate start these relationships almost always break up.

The homosexual may be of any socioeconomic class. He (or she) usually hunts alone and constantly seeks sexual satisfaction through repetitive, often emotionally shallow relationships which are sometimes anonymous and almost never completely gratifying.

Occasionally, episodes of compulsive homosexual outburst may occur in married bisexuals under stress or when intoxicated; these men are often sexually inadequate as husbands.

Homosexuals are constantly exposed to the risks of arrest, blackmail, robbery, venereal disease, and violent assault by gangs of roving adolescents. In a more enlightened society, homosexuals will be treated with more understanding, acceptance, and decency. The opinion has recently been expressed that, in view of the overpopulation threat in the world, a certain percentage of homosexuals is desirable.

Etiology

There are many theories to account for homosexuality. None have attracted universal support.

A. Constitutional Factors: All persons have homosexual and heterosexual components in their sexual drives. Overt homosexual behavior depends upon the degree of control and the ability to sublimate one component or the other. (Heterosexual men can sublimate their homosexual component in friendship with other men and in music, art, etc; similarly, women can sublimate in friendship with other women, and in sports, politics, etc.) The ascendancy of the homosexual drive is sometimes attributed to biologic factors such as biochemical, genetic, or physical abnormalities. The support for this "bisexual theory" stems mainly from Kallman's study of homosexual male twins. He found that in monozygotic twins the concordance rate of homosexuality was 100%, and that it was no higher in dizygotic twins than in the normal male population. However, the interpretation of these figures has been challenged, since psychic and social factors were not adequately controlled.

B. Psychoanalytic Theories: These are based on the concepts of castration anxiety and the Oedipus complex. By castration anxiety is meant the feelings engendered in the little boy during the oedipal phase when he believes that his erotic attraction to his mother and his desire to possess her exclusively are threatened by retaliation from his rival, the father. More specifically, the boy suffers from severe anxiety as he believes that his penis will be cut off if he continues to show his interest in his mother. Satisfactory resolution of this dilemma—the oedipal complex—results when the boy renounces his oedipal love of his mother and begins to identify with his father and incorporate his father's ideals into his own personality.

Freud speculated that regression to or fixation at a pregenital oral or anal psychosexual phase occurred after prolonged frustration (usually by the mother), with identification with the frustrating object.

1. In male homosexuals, identification with the mother is usually present. Because he has unresolved oedipal strivings, he attempts to find a substitute for his mother and, in a narcissistic manner, bestows on effeminate men or adolescent boys the tenderness he received or would like to have received from his mother. He may be attracted to women, but he refuses sexual contact with them. As a result of identification with the mother, love for the powerful father may develop, and with it the wish to enjoy sexual gratification as the mother did, ie, by passively submitting to the father. These individuals may have obvious feminine traits, and the choice of love object is often an older man. Occasionally, a person who has been brought up by his father in the absence of his mother may react to frustration by regressing, with loss of interest in women and a preference for men as his primary love object.

2. In female homosexuals, analogous mechanisms operate. Persisting castration anxiety due to the unresolved oedipal complex (strictly speaking, *Electra complex,* a term now rarely used) results in identification with the father. This is manifested by a masculine love of a person resembling the feminine mother. Also analogous to the psychodynamics in the male, a narcissistic type of love may result from fixation on the homosexual first love, the mother, and a sexual orientation toward women.

C. Environmental Theories:

1. Male homosexuality—Bieber described recurring adverse influences in the intrafamilial (especially parental) relationships in male homosexuals, and suggested that these were of paramount importance. The mother was often overprotective, overintimate, possessive, seductive, and domineering, and minimized the boy's masculine interests, especially during adolescence. She was often frigid herself and sought an alliance with the son against the father. The son admired the mother (although he may have feared her) and would turn to her for protection. The father was usually detached, unaffectionate, absent, or hostile and minimized the son's value as a person; the son thus either lacked respect for or felt nothing but fear or anger toward his father. The father, in turn, never had a close and warm relationship with his son.

2. Female homosexuality—The mother's role is also an important etiologic factor. The mother was hostile, competitive, and defeminizing and favored the sons. In some cases a "female companion" type of relationship existed with the daughter. The father was often submissive to the mother and distant with the daughter.

D. Cultural Theories: Because of its widespread occurrence in past and present cultures, homosexuality is viewed by some as being within the range of biologic normality, only the social and legal taboos making it appear deviant. Clinically, homosexuals often have discernible psychopathology, but so do heterosexuals. Interestingly, there are certain isolated American Indian cultures where homosexuality is completely unknown.

Situations may produce transient homosexuality, eg, fear of sexual inadequacy, experimentation during adolescence, disorganized psychotic states, and circumstances in which heterosexual partners are not available (in prison). It may also occur as a form of antisocial behavior (simply to defy the conventions or the rules of society).

Clinical Features

Homosexual tendencies and behavior may occur at any age. Awareness of sexuality usually appears earlier in homosexuals than in heterosexuals, often with homosexual fantasies. A preoccupation with sex frequently dominates their lives.

A. Male Homosexuality: Some male homosexuals may be effeminate in appearance, manners, gestures, or speech, but most are normal and masculine in appearance. Appearance has no relationship to the type of activity preferred, ie, active or passive. Although certain physical qualities are popular—eg, a large penis and a handsome masculine figure—some homosexuals prefer partners with feminine traits or transvestites. Many have some interest in women, and a significant number (including some "happily married" men) have attempted heterosexual intercourse, sometimes with success. Sexual behavior with other homosexuals varies but usually includes fondling and kissing, interfemoral intercourse, mutual masturbation, fellatio, and, less commonly, anal intercourse. Strong preferences and dislikes are often present, and active and passive roles may be interchanged. Other perversions may be associated with homosexuality.

B. Female Homosexuality: The female homosexual has analogous relationships, varying from the aggressive, and dominant, "butch" to the submissive, and dependent, "femme." There is a greater stability in "couple" relationships among lesbians. Their activities may include passionate kissing and fondling, manual and oral stimulation of the breasts and genitals, and simulated heterosexual intercourse, sometimes with an artificial phallus or "dildo."

C. Latent Homosexuality: This rather loose term refers to the repressed infantile homosexuality which is sublimated in normal males. It may be considered that the degree of latency varies inversely with the adequacy of the repression: If the repression is only slight the latent homosexuality will be great and vice versa. Homosexual trends (latency) may sometimes be revealed by passive and feminine traits and interests; fears of being a homosexual or of homosexual fantasies; excessive disgust with homosexuality; a regular preference for the passive role in sexual intercourse; desiring intercourse in the presence of other men, or with promiscuous women (ways of sexual "sharing" with other men); and, in females, having aggressive interests in male activities. In both male and female latent homosexuals there is no conscious erotic interest in members of the same sex.

Latent male homosexuals have a basic dread of competition and attack, and this may become manifested in any threatening or intimate association with other males. This may lead either to a pathologically dependent relationship with a male (a kind of symbolic yielding) or, if the repression of the latent homosexuality is threatened even more severely, to a state of acute anxiety known as "homosexual panic." They may sometimes project their conflicts onto others, resulting in a paranoid state.

Treatment

Distinction should be made between treating the basic sexual orientation of homosexuals and treating the various other neurotic or personality problems that they may have. The latter are treated much as in heterosexuals, with the result that a maladjusted homosexual may succeed in becoming a better adjusted homosexual. The former should not be treated in individuals who wish to remain homosexuals.

The pessimistic attitude of the past toward the possibility of redirecting the basic sexual orientation of homosexuals is now slowly giving way to more optimism as successes in treatment are being reported with increasing frequency. Favorable prognostic signs are a genuine desire for change, spontaneously expressed; early treatment before complete commitment to a homosexual way of life has occurred; previous attempts at heterosexual intercourse; an admiration for the father; dreams with heterosexual content; and the absence of overly effeminate attitudes and mannerisms.

A. Psychoanalysis: Psychoanalysis, or intensive analytically oriented psychotherapy of long duration, gives the best hope of effecting a significant change in sexual orientation.

Superficial treatment is of no avail. Insight into the origin and irrationality of prevailing fears and resolution of underlying conflicts is the goal of therapy. Treatment, however, is usually requested because of depression and anxiety and not because of the sexual orientation; with treatment, a better interpersonal adjustment usually results. Success rates of 30% in changing the sexual orientation have been claimed. Others are skeptical of such high rates and feel that genuine and permanent changes are rare, but Hatterer's recently published work using intensive psychotherapy and the "tape-capsule" innovation, indicates that this long-held skepticism should be reexamined.

B. Behavior Therapy: Negative conditioning consists of showing pictures with erotic homosexual content to produce sexual arousal, at the same time injecting apomorphine or giving a painful electric shock to produce an "aversion" to the homosexual stimulus. Variable success has been reported with this technic.

C. Drug Therapy: Apart from tranquilizers and other drugs for coincidental psychologic symptoms, drugs are of no use. Androgens are contraindicated, since they produce an increase in sexual drive without altering its direction.

D. Group Therapy: Beneficial results with group psychotherapy have recently been reported, the homosexuals usually being in heterogeneous groups. However, some experienced group psychotherapists would specifically exclude these individuals from group therapy.

EXHIBITIONISM

Exhibitionism is a common deviation which is defined as deliberate and compulsive exposure of the genitals in public, almost always by a male, as a means of achieving sexual gratification. Females usually derive more pleasure than males in displaying other parts of the body.

Psychoanalytic theory holds that exhibitionism serves as a denial of castration anxiety. The male seeks reassurance from the reaction of the female audience, often made up of little girls, that he has a penis, and that they fear him because of it.

Exhibitionistic play is common in preadolescence and is not a perversion. In the pervert, exposure leads to sexual excitement which culminates in orgasm, either spontaneously or, more commonly, by masturbation. Exhibitionistic behavior is often a compulsive and repetitive act, committed usually around strangers and in busy streets or in street cars or theaters, with much guilt after the act. Exhibitionists usually have inadequate personalities and sadistic and masochistic tendencies. They tend to return to the scene of the incident, and hence are often apprehended. The frequency of exposure varies and there are wide fluctuations. There is no regular progression or diminution over the years, although cessation eventually occurs with aging.

Ideally, psychoanalysis or intensive psychotherapy is indicated, but the prognosis is poor as help is rarely sought voluntarily. Exhibitionists are usually referred to psychiatrists by the courts. The voluntary, cooperative patient, however, has a good chance for substantial improvement and a fair chance for recovery.

VOYEURISM
(Scopophilia)

Voyeurism is obtaining sexual gratification through observing sexual organs and sexual activities of others, usually women. It is common in preadolescence purely as sexual excitement seeking. In adults, voyeuristic traits may be normal, as in foreplay prior to intercourse and the arousal caused by occasionally viewing pornographic films or reading pornographic literature. The deviant, however, obtains his major satisfaction by compulsively and repetitively observing others, often at great risk. His methods vary from Peeping Tom activities to prearranged observations of elaborate sexual performances. Masturbation may or may not be required to achieve orgasm.

TRANSVESTISM

Transvestism is obtaining sexual arousal and gratification by wearing clothes appropriate to the opposite sex. It must be distinguished from transsexuality (see below). Orgasm usually occurs by masturbating in contact with this clothing, and the transvestite may have a complete wardrobe of feminine attire which he wears in secret. Some transvestites also have fetishistic, homosexual, or masochistic traits. Masochistic activity during sexual excitement may be severe enough to cause death (eg, through hanging which was intended to last only to the point of heightened sexual excitement).

FETISHISM

Fetishism, defined as obtaining sexual arousal and gratification from inanimate objects—eg, shoes or lingerie—or from parts of the body—eg, the feet or hair of persons of the opposite sex—is predominantly a male form of sexual deviation. Orgasm can be spontaneous upon contact with the fetish, or by masturbation or coitus in the presence of the fetish.

Fetishism is an exaggeration of the normal sexual overvaluation of certain articles associated with the love object. In males, the main source of erotic gratification often occurs in the presence of objects such as women's shoes or undergarments and even hair cuttings. Excessive attention to certain parts of the female body—eg, breasts, buttocks, legs—is called *partialism.*

The female fetishist sometimes engages in compulsive kleptomania, which may have unconscious sexual significance.

SADISM AND MASOCHISM

Sadism consists of obtaining sexual arousal or gratification by inflicting pain or humiliation on the partner; masochism is sexual pleasure derived from suffering pain or humiliation. The 2 are always present together (although one or the other is apt to be dominant) and are referred to as sadomasochism. The terms are derived from the Marquis de Sade, a French writer, and Leopold von Sacher-Masoch, an Austrian novelist who wrote on this subject.

A certain amount of mild sadistic behavior is common during normal sexual activity in males, and some masochistic elements are common in females; both are present to some extent in all normal men and women. The dominant deviation may vary in different circumstances, eg, sadistic social relationships may coexist with masochistic sexual needs in the same person.

Clinically, as a prelude to coitus, the sadist may bite the partner, perform flagellation or other physical assault—even to the point of causing bleeding—or insist on other humiliations. Extreme sadistic acts are forcible rape, which may end in murder to prevent discovery; and lust murder, the ultimate sadistic perversion which involves killing and then mutilating the corpse for sexual gratification—usually without sexual intercourse, gratification being obtained by masturbation. Extreme sadism is usually (perhaps always) indicative of psychosis, but can be the result of organic brain disease ("dyscontrol syndrome," psychomotor epilepsy, temporal lobe epilepsy).

Sadism also refers to cruel acts unassociated or minimally associated with sexuality—beating children, some forms of game hunting, fanatical persecutions, etc. Men who indulge in excessive cruelty often have potency problems.

Masochism, on the other hand, involves suffering, usually to allay guilt and feelings of worthlessness. In extreme forms, regressive acts such as coprolalia, coprophilia, and coprophagia (see below) may be necessary for sexual arousal.

In "moral masochism," the sexual component is in abeyance and the guilt is experienced through self-induced psychologic suffering, humiliation, and failure.

TRANSSEXUALITY

Transsexuality is the conscious, compelling desire to change one's sex. A male transsexual is a person who thinks, feels, and acts like a female, but is biologically male. In contrast, the hermaphrodite has biologic abnormalities of intersex (both sexes) but, usually, the sex-role orientation appropriate to his predominant external sexual characteristics.

Transsexuality is often confused with transvestism and homosexuality. Most transvestites are not transsexual, but most transsexuals wear the clothes of the opposite sex, as transvestites do at times. Similarly, passive feminine homosexuality in the male transsexual is usual, but most homosexuals have a normal gender role although the object choice is reversed. Occasionally, an individual becomes convinced he is actually changing sex, usually against his will; such an individual is psychotic and not a transsexual.

In recent years, male transsexuals have become increasingly successful in inducing legitimate surgeons to perform plastic operations upon them, with castration and the provision of a vagina-like organ. Female transsexuals resort to mastectomy and prostheses.

PEDOPHILIA

Pedophilia is defined as sexual arousal and gratification through sexual contact with a child or a sexually immature person of either sex. The pervert, usually male, can be either a heterosexual or (more commonly) a homosexual.

Partial impotence is usual; hence, gratification is limited to fondling, masturbation, and exhibitionistic activities. Rarely, anal intercourse with a child may be attempted, sometimes with physical harm to the victim. Although secretive, the pedophile is often caught because of ineptness brought about by unconscious guilt. Some, however, murder their victims to avoid detection.

Occasionally, adolescent "victims" may be actively seductive, and, since they may also appear older than their true age, the act may not strictly be a deviation. Maladjusted adolescent girls have been known to get many relatively normal men (sometimes their own fathers or brothers) into serious sexual and legal trouble.

GERONTOPHILIA

Gerontophilia is defined as obtaining sexual gratification with an elderly person of either sex. Gerontosexuality is difficult to detect as it is not uncommon for a young woman to marry an old man for love or a young man an old woman for love, or in either case for conscious materialistic reasons. However, if a young person compulsively and exclusively prefers a succession of elderly mates, it is a perversion.

BESTIALITY

Bestiality consists of obtaining sexual gratification with living subhuman animals. The term usually denotes actual sexual intercourse with animals and not sexual arousal through observing sexual activities of animals nor a form of fetishism in which animal objects (eg, fur) may be the sexual object. Zoophilia denotes sexual excitement through stroking or fondling animals and mild forms of this may occur transiently in normal persons.

Bestiality occurs most commonly in individuals who live in rural areas, are socially isolated, have a schizoid personality, or are overtly psychotic or mentally retarded. However, intelligent and educated people may also practice this deviation, sometimes only when intoxicated. The activity occurs mostly at adolescence and then declines rapidly. Household pets are the most common animals involved, but farm animals have been used.

NECROPHILIA

Necrophilia is defined as obtaining sexual gratification from corpses, usually by intercourse, with or without subsequent mutilation. It is rare.

If the victim is first killed and then sexually assaulted, the act is an extreme form of sadism, with the sexual object being a fetish, ie, lust murder. If the corpse is directly violated, a very deep personality disorder, usually a psychosis is present.

Considerable risks may be taken by necrophiliacs in removing corpses from graves. They often obtain jobs in morgues and funeral parlors. Although they have little sexual interest in live women, some are able to perform coitus if the woman lies absolutely still (as though dead).

COPROPHILIA, COPROPHAGIA, AND COPROLALIA

Coprophilia is an abnormal sexual interest in excretions; coprophagia, a desire to eat secretions or excretions; and coprolalia, compulsive utterances of obscene words (Gilles de la Tourette syndrome).

These disorders are often associated with other perversions. For example, a prerequisite for sexual arousal may be sadistic, through urinating on the partner; or masochistic, by being urinated upon; or voyeuristic, by observing excretory functions. Orgasm is usually achieved by masturbation.

FROTTAGE

Frottage means sexual pleasure obtained by rubbing or pressing against the object, usually the buttocks of a fully clothed woman. It commonly takes place in subways or other crowded situations, and may pass unnoticed by the victim. Frotteurs are perverts only if this is their sole mode of obtaining orgasm.

GROUP PERVERSION

Group perversion (apparently on the increase) implies sexual arousal and gratification by participating in sexual activity with 2 or more persons simultaneously. Usually one member, a pervert, initiates others, who are not true perverts but who compliantly indulge in these activities. Although they seek gratification through excitement, novelty, and variety, they often fail to get it. Group sex acts usually turn out more disturbing than exciting.

The activities can take the form of an "orgy"—an occasion for relaxation of inhibitions and permission for sexual excesses; group rape, in which one woman is raped by several men; group voyeurism, sexual arousal achieved through watching mutual sexual participation by several individuals; and *ménage à trois,* or a triangular sex situation involving, for example, a husband, his wife, and her lover. The last-mentioned situation implies a strong latent homosexual component in the husband under a heterosexual guise. The same may be said for "swapping wives." (The 2 men "meet" sexually in their respective wives.)

BONDAGE

This is a rare perversion in men in which the individual insists on tying up the woman as a prelude to sexual gratification. The crucial element is the helplessness of the partner and not, as in sadism, her suffering.

CAUSES OF SEXUAL DEVIATIONS

The causes of sexual deviations are unknown. The psychoanalytic view, which is plausible and of practical therapeutic value in many cases, stresses the defense against castration anxiety in deeply buried oedipal conflicts. The specific deviation seems to be determined by the pathologic experiences of childhood, reinforced by parental rejection, hostility, or ambivalence.

The perverse act is usually impulsive, with a compulsive element. Schizophrenia or a borderline state may coexist, and the deviation may be one manifestation of personality difficulty. Perverse acts may also result from organic brain disease, as in the senile, or from episodes of temporal lobe epilepsy. Hence, a neurologic examination and an EEG is important for diagnosis.

TREATMENT OF SEXUAL DEVIATIONS

Psychoanalysis or intensive psychoanalytically oriented psychotherapy offers the main hope in those persons with adequate ego strength and with no other serious concomitant disorder. Behavior therapists claim fair success for their methods in the treatment of perversions, but their data are not convincing. Many patients can be helped to live more comfortably with themselves as they are by achieving better conscious control and self-discipline through counseling and supportive psychotherapy.

OTHER SEXUAL PROBLEMS WITH SOCIAL & LEGAL RAMIFICATIONS

INCEST

Incest refers to sexual activity or coitus between members of the same family. It usually refers to coitus between father and daughter, mother and son, or between siblings, but it may involve other close relatives such as stepchildren or uncles. The ban against incest is one of the most stringent of sexual prohibitions in all cultures.

Normally, oedipal incestuous strivings of childhood are gradually resolved and replaced by adult sexuality. If they remain dominant in adulthood, neurotic conflicts manifested by psychosexual disturbances and deviations may result. Owing to the social taboo against incest, an individual who actually carries out the incestuous wish is usually suffering from an ego defect and is often psychotic.

Father-daughter sex relationships are not uncommonly uncovered in clinical practice. The eldest daughter is usually the victim, but younger daughters may be drawn into an incestuous relationship as the eldest moves away. The father may be an alcoholic or have sociopathic traits, or he may appear remarkably competent though he has doubts about his masculinity. The mother often is strangely accepting of the situation.

Mild incestuous behavior in siblings is common in preadolescence as sex play, and is harmless; if it occurs later, it may be an indication of serious neurotic conflict. Mother-son relationships are the rarest form of incest, and usually one or both partners are psychotic.

The future of the son or daughter in these cases is variable, but severe psychopathology is not as frequent as used to be thought.

If possible, the son or daughter should be removed from the home. The prognosis for the parent is usually poor because of the degree of psychopathology involved. Prison sentences do no good, but often cannot be avoided when the authorities have been involved.

RAPE

Rape is defined legally as sexual intercourse between a man and a woman (who is not his wife) against her will or without lawful consent, either by force or threat of force, or by deceit.

The definition, laws, and penalties governing rape are remarkably inconsistent and severe in different jurisdictions. Thus, in some states of the USA, sexual intercourse is said to occur if the penis brushes against the vulva without penetration or emission. In others, a woman who is mentally retarded, psychotic, or under the influence of drugs or alcohol cannot give lawful consent to intercourse. The same applies if she is a minor, which is defined as being under 16 or 18 years depending on the state, and intercourse with her is regarded as statutory or second degree rape. Hence, a 17-year-old boy who has intercourse with a 17-year-old girl with her full consent may be committing a felony if the age of legal consent is 18 years, and he may be subject to several years' imprisonment.

In forcible or first degree rape, damage to the female genitalia may occur. Rape is usually committed under strong emotions, and often under the influence of alcohol. Sadism is not usually the prime motive, as the pain involved is incidental, but the rape may be unconsciously incestuous (with a fantasied resisting "mother"). Rape may lead to murder out of fear of apprehension.

Rapists often have underlying inferiority feelings, and a sense of dominance is compulsively important to them.

The legal penalties for rape are severe, and include even the death penalty.

Some rapists have organic brain disease ("dyscontrol syndrome"), and all should therefore be studied neurologically. Underlying neurosis or sociopathy should be treated in the usual ways. The prognosis is good, with time and the law on the therapist's side.

SEDUCTION

In seduction the woman is induced to consent to sexual intercourse by enticements, bribes, or deceit but not force or the threat of force. In some states of the USA it is grounds for a civil "breach of promise" suit to make a promise of marriage to a woman to obtain sexual favors and then break the promise. Seduction of men by women is usually not considered pathologic (but see below).

In psychiatry, seduction as a trait—as in a parent's sexual advances to a child or a patient's sexual advances to a physician—can be of considerable significance. In the former, the overpermissive, seductive, and excessively caressing attitude of a father for his daughter may hinder the satisfactory resolution of the Oedipus complex in the child, producing psychosexual difficulties, eg, frigidity or nymphomania, later in life. Similarly, the overprotective, smothering, and immodest attitude of the mother toward her son may lead to deviations such as homosexuality. Seductive attitudes may be unconscious with no malicious intent.

Seductive patients are often encountered by the physician. Usually they can be classified as hysterical personalities, their histrionic behavior and provocative attitudes being characteristic of their neurosis. However, these women do not usually become involved in actual sexuality, as may women with sociopathic personalities whose seductive behavior may have a definite hedonistic aim. The psychotic patient may suddenly begin to distort and misinterpret the physician's behavior and make him the object of her sexual attention. Mildly neurotic women may occasionally become seductive as a consequence of the transference process, perhaps complementary to the countertransference of the physician.

Seductive behavior by children toward grown men is seen also, but more rarely.

NUDITY

Problems with regard to nudity (other than in exhibitionism, noted above) occur in 2 situations: social, in nudist colonies or camps; and domestic, among family members.

Serious psychologic or sociologic investigation of either of these has been scanty, which is perhaps an indication of disapproval of it even by professionals. The organization of social nudism in the early decades of this century coincided with the rebellion against the excessively moralistic attitudes then prevailing. The aim was a democratization of man and desexualization of genital sex. This "back to nature" movement was accompanied by high sexual mores in the camps, the nudists maintaining that naturalism fostered emotional health and that for this purpose it was necessary to adopt uninhibited and realistic views of sexuality. Despite the continuing obstacles to social nudity (it is outlawed in several states of the USA, and many nudist publications have been declared obscene), the custom is gathering strength and nudist camps continue to flourish, especially in Europe, California, and Florida. Recently, nude group therapy has made headlines, to the consternation of most psychiatrists.

Domestic nudism, however, remains a controversial issue. Psychoanalysts state that the castration anxieties of young male children are kindled by the sight of the penisless mother or sister, while the sight of a well developed male penis in the father or big brother traumatizes the little boy with his small penis. Analogously, the penis envy or trauma evoked when the little girl sees her father's genitals may lead to deviant sequels. For these reasons, some psychoanalysts advise that children should not be exposed to parental nudity; if exposure is unavoidable because of living conditions, an attitude of casualness should be maintained.

Nudists, on the other hand, state that attempting to conceal the sex differences from children is futile, since children have a great propensity to fantasize about the unknown; and that allurement by concealment is more likely to lead to tensions and misconceptions.

It is not known if children exposed to excessive domestic nudism suffer from psychosexual disturbances to a greater degree than others.

PROSTITUTION

Prostitution signifies the giving of sexual favors—usually promiscuously, anonymously, and without affection—for a fee. Prostitution usually refers to female heterosexual acts, but female homosexual prostitution, male homosexual prostitution, and male heterosexual prostitution (the female paying the male "gigolo" for sexual services) all exist. The distinction between prostitution and amateur fornication is vague at times, as when a woman gives sexual favors for personal gain (eg, in procuring employment) or when she receives gifts from regular male consorts.

Because of the almost universal illegality of their trade, prostitutes are gradually decreasing in number and are being replaced by "amateur prostitutes." These women may have full-time jobs or may be housewives, divorcees, or students; they work at prostitution part time, often temporarily, to supplement their incomes.

The lures of prostitution for women are money, adventure, sex itself (although most prostitutes are frigid), a neurotic need for punishment, revenge against the parents, family, or society, or the promise of a job to a woman with no other qualifications. Prostitution is justified by some women as analogous to using female sexuality for nonsexual purposes, eg, in jobs where feminine attractiveness is used as a bait for customers; hence, they have fewer scruples in offering sexual services temporarily—eg, to tide them over a financial crisis.

Men may be attracted to prostitutes out of a need for variety, an unwillingness to accept the obligations involved in marriage, an unwillingness to pursue women, advancing age, and physical or other handicaps that make it difficult to succeed with women in socially acceptable ways. Despite police vice squads and civic clean-up campaigns, the male's biologic need for such sexual outlets remains; hence, commercial sex continues to meet the demand, and it probably never will be suppressed completely. There is evidence that attempts at suppression of prostitution have been followed by an increase in sex crimes.

The dangers of prostitution are considerable for both the prostitute and the client because of the legal and social taboos against it. She is a social outcast, open to exploitation and arrest, and may be led toward drug addiction and alcoholism, especially after she has passed her peak earning capacity. The client is open to blackmail, robbery, and scandal. Both may be infected with venereal disease, but this is now more widely spread by free love, homosexuality, and adultery than by prostitution. In one European country the serious suggestion has been made that prostitution and brothels should be made legal as a means of controlling the spiralling venereal disease rate.

PORNOGRAPHY

Pornography may be defined as writings or pictorial arts whose sole aim is to arouse the reader or viewer sexually, ie, act as a psychologic aphrodisiac. The terms obscene, lewd, lascivious, and "hard core" relate to the work itself and not to the reaction of an individual.

Controversy over pornography continues to rage. Because of the permissiveness associated with the changing cultural climate, censorship has gradually weakened and pornography has become increasingly difficult to define. In legal battles, eminent persons testify on the socially redeeming nature of works of literature previously considered obscene or pornographic. However, pornography, together with the increase of permissiveness, disregard for authority, violence, and crime, has also been labeled a sign of the decay of society. The principal "consumers" of pornography are the over-40 members of the middle and lower classes, usually the more conservative members of society.

Psychologically, pornography is related to voyeurism, and those persons habitually using pornographic material as a means of stimulation to achieve orgasm (usually by masturbation) are sometimes considered to be scopophilic perverts. However, Fenichel has written that masturbation with the help of pornographic materials (eg, by men isolated from heterosexual opportunity) is nearer to normal sexuality than is masturbation by itself, the literature being a medium between sexual fantasy and sexual reality.

Pornographic writings frequently have recurring themes. These involve seduction, defloration, incest, profanity, hypersexuality, flagellation, contact with animals, etc, with emphasis on the physical aspects of the acts and not the emotional content. These themes may have psychologic significance in that they involve the most primitive and universal instincts which are taboo in all cultures, and therefore "exciting" to transgress. However, most persons soon find pornography joyless, repetitious, depersonalized, and boring.

The psychologic effects of pornography continue to be debatable. Evidence is now accumulating—most recently by the United States Congressional Commission on Pornography (1970)—that pornography per se does not result in an increase in frequency of sex crimes or antisocial behavior; it may, in fact, reduce the incidence of sex crimes by acting as a safety valve. Denmark, the first country in the world to remove all forms of censorship, noted an initial increase in interest in pornographic literature, followed by a waning to preexisting levels and no increase in the sex crime rate. Studies with sex deviates and offenders show that they had *less* exposure to erotically stimulating material in childhood and adolescence than did the average person. They more often suffered from a family background which was excessively repressive and punitive toward sex.

The effects of prolonged contact with pornographic material and the effects on minors remain unknown. Perhaps the sadism and violence depicted with sex may be damaging. Perhaps pornography is nothing more than educational for the normal curious person.

REFERENCES

Books and Monographs

Allen, C.: *A Textbook of Psychosexual Abnormalities.* Oxford Univ Press, 1962.

Bieber, I., & others: *Homosexuality: A Psychoanalytic Study.* Basic Books, 1962.

Caprio, F.S.: *Female Homosexuality.* Grove Press, 1964.

Deutsch, H.: *The Psychology of Women.* Vols 1 & 2. Grune & Stratton, 1944.

Ellis, A., & H. Ababanel (editors): *The Encyclopedia of Sexual Behavior.* Hawthorn Books, 1961.

Hastings, D.W.: *Impotence and Frigidity.* Little, Brown, 1963.

Hatterer, L.: *Changing Homosexuality in the Male.* McGraw-Hill, 1970.

Karpman, B.: *The Sexual Offender and His Offenses.* Julian, 1954.

Kinsey, A.C., Pomeroy, W.B., & C.E. Martin: *Sexual Behavior in the Human Male.* Saunders, 1948.

Kinsey, A.C., & others: *Sexual Behavior in the Human Female.* Saunders, 1953.

Kronhausen, P., & E. Kronhausen: *Erotic Art.* Grove, 1968.

Lorand, S., & M. Balint (editors): *Psychodynamics and Therapy.* Random House, 1956.

Marmor, J. (editor): *Sexual Inversion.* Basic Books, 1965.

Masters, W.H., & V.E. Johnson: *Human Sexual Response.* Little, Brown, 1966.

Masters, W.H., & V.E. Johnson: *Human Sexual Inadequacy.* Little, Brown, 1970.

Reuben, D.: *Everything You Always Wanted to Know About Sex But Were Afraid to Ask.* McKay, 1969.

Rosen, I. (editor): *The Pathology and Treatment of Sexual Deviation.* Oxford Univ Press, 1964.

Stoller, R.J.: *Sex and Gender: On the Development of Masculinity and Femininity.* Science House, 1968.

United States Congressional Commission on Obscenity and Pornography: *Report.* Washington, DC, 1970.

Wahl, C.W. (editor): *Sexual Problems: Diagnosis and Treatment in Medical Practice.* The Free Press, 1967.

Wolfendon, J. (chairman): *The Wolfendon Report: Report of the Committee on Homosexual Offenses and Prostitution.* Stein & Day, 1963.

Journal Articles

Bene, E.: Genesis of female homosexuality. Brit J Psychiat 111:815–821, 1965.

Benjamin, H.: Transsexualism and transvestism as psychosomatic and somato-psychic syndromes. Am J Psychotherapy 8:219–230, 1954.

Bieber, I.: The married male homosexual. Med Aspects Human Sexuality 3:76–85, May 1969.

Brady, J.P.: Frigidity. Med Aspects Human Sexuality 1:42–48, March 1967.

Brunstetter, R.W.: Some psychiatric comments on the current move toward sex education programs in the school. California Med 112:7-12, May 1970.

Cartwright, R.D., & others: Effect of an erotic movie on the sleep and dreams of young men. Arch Gen Psychiat 20:262–271, 1969.

Cooper, A.J.: An innovation in the "behavioural" treatment of a case of non-consummation due to vaginismus. Brit J Psychiat 115:721–722, 1969.

Cooper, A.J.: Disorders of sexual potency in the male: A clinical and statistical study of some factors related to short-term prognosis. Brit J Psychiat 115:709–720, 1969.

Ellis, A.: Why married men visit prostitutes. Sexology 25:344–347, 1959.

Erikson, E.H.: The theory of infantile sexuality; eight ages of man. Childhood and Society 2:48–108, 247–274, 1963.

Farnsworth, D.L.: Sexual morality and the dilemma of the colleges. Am J Orthopsychiat 35:676–681, 1965.

Finkel, A.L., & others: Sexual potency in aging males. JAMA 170:1391, 1959.

Green, R.: Persons seeking sex change: Psychiatric management of special problems. Am J Psychiat 126:1596–1603, 1970.

Greenson, R.R.: On sexual apathy in the male. California Med 108:275–279, 1968.

Heersema, P.H.: Homosexuality and the physician. JAMA 193:815–817, 1965.

Hoenig, J., Kenna, J., & A. Youd: Follow-up study of transsexualists: Social and economic aspects. Psychiat Clin 3:85–100, 1970.

Hollender, M.H.: The prostitute's two identities. Med Aspects Human Sexuality 2:45–51, Feb 1968.

Irving, B.: Survey on incest. Excerpta Criminol 4:137–155, 1964.

Kallmann, F.J.: A comparative twin study on the genetic aspects of male homosexuality. J Nerv Ment Dis 115:283–298, 1952.

Levine, S.: Sexual differentiation: The development of maleness and femaleness. California Med 114:12–17, Jan 1971.

McConaghy, N.: Subjective and penile plethysmograph response following aversion-relief and apomorphine aversion therapy for homosexual impulses. Brit J Psychiat 115:723, 1969.

Pauly, I.B.: The current status of the change of sex operation. J Nerv Ment Dis 147:460–471, 1968.

Pfeiffer, E., & others: Sexual behavior in aged men and women. Arch Gen Psychiat 19:753–758, 1968.

Raybin, J.B.: Homosexual incest. J Nerv Ment Dis 148:105–110, 1969.

Saghir, M.T., & E. Robins: Homosexuality: Sexual behavior of the female homosexual. Arch Gen Psychiat 20:192–201, 1969.

Sex, censoring and society's psyche. Med World News, Oct 2, 1970.

Solomon, P.: Love: A clinical definition. New England J Med 352:345–351, 1955.

Stoller, R.J.: The term "transvestism." Arch Gen Psychiat 24:230–237, 1971.

Waggoner, R.W., & others: Viewpoints: What questions on sex are asked most frequently by your patients? Med Aspects Human Sexuality 3:8–13, May 1969.

Ziegler, F.J., Rodgers, D.A., & R.J. Prentiss: Psychosocial response to vasectomy. Arch Gen Psychiat 21:48–54, 1969.

20 . . .

Chronic Alcoholism

The physician should consider alcoholism a symptom and search for causes—social, neurotic, and psychotic. The social alcoholic drinks to conform with his peer group or his family, and his treatment involves reeducation. The neurotic alcoholic has a deep-seated emotional conflict, uses drinking as an escape, solace, ego bolster, etc, and needs psychotherapy. The psychotic alcoholic uses a drinking spree in lieu of (or as a symptom of) a psychotic breakthrough, schizoid, paranoid, or manic-depressive. These patients usually require phenothiazines, antidepressants, lithium, or EST. General measures for all alcoholics include patience and tolerance, continuous attention to physical and mental hygiene, and imaginative utilization of friends and relatives, AA, and social, religious, vocational, recreational, and other organizations.

Overindulgence in the pleasures and comforts that society makes available is a natural human tendency that most people manage to resist most of the time. Abuse of alcohol, tobacco, and other drugs, overeating, and sexual promiscuity are some of the ways in which individuals may pursue momentary pleasure and relief from tension and anxiety at the expense of great danger to their lives.

It makes no more sense to search for *the* cause of excessive drinking than for the cause of overeating, inappropriate sexual behavior, extreme religiosity, or fanatical preoccupation with baseball statistics. The frequent, persistent, or uncontrollable drinker has found that a numbed consciousness is often preferable to sobriety, and the resulting syndrome of physical and social consequences is one that probably serves a unique function in each individual.

Alcoholism is too complex a problem to be considered solely as a criminal or spiritual offense, a bad habit, an addiction, a toxic state, or a disease. It is also an affliction of society itself, and a problem of concern and interest not only to the physician and pharmacologist but also to the anthropologist, sociologist, legislator, jurist, criminologist, penologist, lawyer, welfare worker, and economist.

General Considerations

Even though the treatment of alcoholism involves the understanding and manipulation of the psychic life of the victim, it should not be considered as a problem that only a psychiatrist can manage. In most cases it is the general practitioner who should treat the alcoholic patient—just as it is the general practitioner who should treat the obese patient. He may find these patients either by direct referral by themselves or (more often) by family members, or he may identify them through a careful history and examination which he conducts for other presenting conditions. In the discussion that follows we will classify alcoholism as social, neurotic, and psychotic. The nonpsychiatrist physician can and should care for the first 2 categories of patients, with psychiatric consultation as required. Psychotic alcoholism should be managed by a psychiatrist.

The degree of specificity in treatment depends upon the accuracy of diagnosis, which in turn depends upon an understanding of the patient as a human being. There is no such entity as "the alcoholic personality." Some alcoholics are orally neurotic, submissive, dependent, and latently homosexual and some are none of those things.

However, certain nonspecific considerations apply to all types of alcoholism. One general rule is that the alcoholic should avoid the first drink, ie, he should strive for complete abstinence. Unfortunately, this is not always possible, and accepting an alcoholic for treatment means that the physician must be prepared to accept therapeutic setbacks ("falling off the wagon") in a therapeutically realistic way—ie, by continuing to be judgmental and disapproving about the act of drinking but not about the patient himself. This distinction is important, for the patient must be convinced that he himself is accepted by the therapist no matter what he does—even though what he does might be condemned.

This can be most difficult for the physician because the alcoholic often gets into trouble and needs help. Much will depend on the patient's age and social circumstances, the strength and integrity of his personality, and the loyalty of his family. The skill and sincerity of the therapist will be constantly tested. The success rate is directly related to the therapist's tenacity and his ability both to help the patient and to hold him in therapy. This is an important first step, since something must be substituted that is better than alcohol before alcohol can be safely interdicted. There are some things that are worse than alcoholism—eg, psychosis or suicide.

The more specific considerations of therapy relate to the type of alcoholism, and the treatment of each type is different.

TYPES OF ALCOHOLISM

A logical approach to the problem may be constructed if one considers 3 possible diagnostic entities: (1) social alcoholism, (2) neurotic alcoholism, and (3) psychotic alcoholism. These categories are not mutually exclusive, and are in fact rarely seen in pure form. A patient who begins in one category may later assume the characteristics of another or even of all 3. However, one form usually predominates and will dictate the therapeutic approach.

SOCIAL ALCOHOLISM

"Conforming to the group" is often the basis of early drinking. In some subcultures, being able to "hold your liquor" is part of the definition of manhood. This is no different from other forms of behavior acquired in the same way—eg, drug abuse, gambling, or delinquency. At times it is not the peer group but significant family members who serve as the model for drinking behavior.

A careful history will often reveal a characteristic pattern of development of alcoholism, and the diagnosis can be made with confidence.

Treatment

The treatment of social alcoholism differs from the treatment of other forms of social delinquency (which involves the establishment of a strong positive transference and transformation of the delinquency into a neurosis which can then be handled by uncovering technics). The relationship of the social alcoholic patient to the therapist, although it may seem warm and friendly, is often capricious and opportunistic. The patient does not find it easy to trust anyone fully because he has been hurt too often—usually by the people closest to him—and it takes a great deal to convince him that anyone is really interested in his ultimate welfare. Relentless optimism and tenacity are the physician's most essential tools in proving over and over again his desire to be of real help. Instead of engaging the patient in interpretive discussions about his unconscious need for mothering, he simply mothers the patient without comment and helps in all ways possible to extricate him from whatever trouble he gets into—eg, jail, lawsuits, absenteeism at work, rejection by his wife, and financial distress.

A thorough physical examination, including a neurologic work-up, is a good starting point. Advice should be given about how to improve general health; this may involve diet, exercise, sleep, posture, or correction of such problems as refractive errors, tooth decay, skin diseases, hemorrhoids, varicosities, and corns or bunions. Most patients are grateful for this kind of concern and respect their physicians for offering it. This puts the physician in a good position to exert a favorable influence as the relationship develops.

Environmental changes are important since the environment is the primary problem in social alcoholism. In most cases, however, the damage has already been done and the most reasonable therapeutic objective is to help the patient stop drinking where he is. The use of organizations such as Alcoholics Anonymous (AA) is in some cases the single most important factor in encouraging the patient to stay sober. They often provide a new outlook on life and a new set of sympathetic friends who can understand the problem because they have "been there" themselves. AA groups vary in their effectiveness with the quality of the people in them, and if the patient finds himself in an ineffective group the therapist should attempt to direct him to a new group if that can be done. Other useful organizations are the churches, YMCA and YWCA, Salvation Army, and some fraternal orders. With national losses due to alcoholism approaching 7.5 billion dollars a year, many business organizations are wisely attempting to offer treatment programs for alcoholics in order to save their investments in employees with drinking problems.

The therapist himself must usually supply the initiative for utilizing these resources, and any physician who is likely to have to deal with alcoholic patients should familiarize himself with what is available in his community.

Disulfiram (Antabuse) is often useful, but it is probably best not to urge its use against the patient's reservations. If he wants a "built-in policeman," particularly in the early phase of treatment, the drug may help him resist temptation. However, the alcoholic receiving disulfiram can stop taking the drug and some can drink right through it, accepting the resulting sickness as a just punishment for failure to remain sober.

NEUROTIC ALCOHOLISM

In neurotic alcoholism, drinking (like any other neurotic symptom) is based mostly on unconscious motivation and serves as a means of maintaining psychodynamic equilibrium. People who are not alcoholics may take a few drinks now and then or even (rarely) get drunk, but they usually remain in control even though alcohol serves some function for them. In the life of the neurotic alcoholic, loss of control is a regular occurrence. Some of the common functions of alcohol in these patients are the following:

(1) **Build confidence:** With alcohol, the patient is able to overcome his feelings of inferiority. These feelings are often conscious, but their underlying causes are not.

(2) **Relieve anxiety:** Alcohol allows the patient to function in situations where he would otherwise be paralyzed.

(3) **Escape from responsibility:** Alcohol can be used to help suppress guilt, anger, and grief.

(4) **Substitute for hostility:** Getting drunk can be used as a substitute for direct expression of aggressive feelings.

(5) **Substitute for sex:** Persons of the same sex are able to use alcohol and maudlin behavior as an unconscious substitute for heterosexual or latent homosexual behavior.

(6) **Regress:** Alcoholism may facilitate unconscious regression to early childhood behavior patterns which at one time elicited mothering responses from others.

The history and careful attention to patterns of behavior and neurotic needs establish the diagnosis of neurotic alcoholism.

Treatment

The treatment of neurotic alcoholism consists of treatment of the neurosis itself. As in all forms of psychotherapy, the most important element is the proper use of the personality of the physician. Authoritarian, pessimistic, cynical, and moralistic attitudes have no place in this relationship, but neither do softheartedness, hearty overoptimism, naivety, nor sanctimonious and "do-gooder" attitudes. The therapist should be realistic, friendly, accepting, and fair. Complete and permanent sobriety is the goal of therapy, but lapses and imperfection must be tolerated.

The response to the physician's attention—particularly if the patient has been "down and out"—will be rapid and most rewarding. The patient's dignity and self-esteem must be reestablished as a foundation on which to rebuild a shattered life. A strong positive relationship with the therapist is the major ongoing stimulus to change, and this can be strengthened at the outset by attention to the patient's total needs—including a physical examination as outlined in the previous section, with correction of organic disorders, even minor ones such as bad teeth, improper glasses, skin problems, varicose veins, hemorrhoids, etc.

The frequency and duration of visits must be individualized according to feasibility and need. At first, most severe cases are best handled by admission to a general hospital; this can always be justified by the need for "a complete work-up and tests." Interviews may last anywhere from 10 to 50 minutes, but the time must be set aside exclusively for the patient without interruption. The patient should do most of the talking, with the therapist responding according to the style he has found to be most comfortable. The therapist should emphasize positive features of the content of the patient's reflections and underplay negative features such as tears and self-recrimination.

The patient should be helped to realize that there are psychologic reasons for his drinking and that not all alcoholics have the same reasons. He must accept the idea that he is in therapy for his nervous trouble and that he and the therapist must work together to understand all of the important things that have ever happened to him. These include his early life, family, school, friends, sexual experience, jobs, hobbies and social interests, religion, successes and failures, children, illnesses, accidents, and everything about his drinking.

At the same time, the patient's immediate life situation with all of its problems at home, at work, and in society must be handled satisfactorily. This merges with the future and involves helping the patient widen his life with satisfying involvements and activities, increasing his skills and effectiveness so that he can afford to abandon the use of alcohol to fulfill his unmet needs.

It is often useful to bring significant people in the patient's life (often wife or husband) into therapy. The wife of an alcoholic husband may have unrealized needs that are being satisfied by her husband's drinking; if so, she may develop (or cause) problems as the husband begins to achieve sobriety. When domestic strife is the major consideration, conjoint family therapy—in which the patient is seen at the same time as other key members of the family (see Chapter 27)—is often desirable. Group therapy, usually with carefully matched alcoholics in a group of about 8, may be useful, particularly in clinics where individual therapy is not feasible.

Medication is often helpful, particularly in the early phases of treatment. There is a symbolic relationship between medication, mothering, giving love, and magical cures. The patient must understand that the medication is only temporary until the therapeutic process enables him to understand his drinking and give it up. Tranquilizers, particularly the benzodiazepine group (chlordiazepoxide [Librium] or diazepam [Valium]), or phenobarbital several times a day in small doses are the drugs of first choice. If sedation is desired, particularly in the evening, give phenothiazines (eg, chlorpromazine [Thorazine]) in small amounts. Further sedation may be obtained with chloral hydrate if necessary.

Watch for and avoid habituation.

Most physicians are capable of undertaking the psychotherapy of the neurotic alcoholic patient. Some will wish to have occasional or regular supervision by a psychiatrist. Others will prefer to have a psychiatric consultation and perhaps turn the case over to the psychiatrist altogether.

PSYCHOTIC ALCOHOLISM

This type of alcoholism includes 2 subtypes: schizophrenic alcoholism and manic-depressive alcoholism. In either type, assistance is often sought at the end of a spree when the patient is experiencing delirium tremens or some other form of withdrawal symptomatology. The morbidity and mortality rates are high in these cases. Hospitalization is usually indicated, and adequate treatment has lowered the mortality rate in recent years from 15% to 5% or less.

Psychotic alcoholism is an indication of severe underlying psychopathology. The drinking bout may represent a desperate attempt to stave off a psychotic break, or it may be part of the early stage of an actual break.

These patients should always be handled by a psychiatrist.

1. SCHIZOPHRENIC ALCOHOLISM

Schizophrenic alcoholism is characterized by impulsive heavy drinking accompanied by signs of mental dissociation that greatly exceed those observed in ordinary alcoholic intoxication, eg, amnesia, fugue states, bizarre behavior, sex orgies, wild rages, and violent behavior even to the extent of mayhem and murder. Between drinking bouts, some of these patients may appear normal, with a minimum of schizoid personality traits; at the other extreme, patients may be clearly schizophrenic but retain barely enough control to continue to function in the community. Patients in this category are often described by their associates as "high strung," "unstable," or "different." Psychiatric investigation will usually disclose delusional or hallucinatory content. The psychotic core of the personality is often paranoid and includes persecutory ideas or irrational jealousy centered on the spouse or a close relative. The family history often includes other instances of serious mental illness such as "nervous breakdowns," suicides, severe alcoholism, and mental hospital admissions. The patient himself will often have a history of trouble with the police and the courts and interrupted relationships with other psychiatrists.

Treatment

Treatment is primarily psychopharmacologic. The phenothiazines (chlorpromazine [Thorazine], trifluoperazine [Stelazine]) and butyrophenones (haloperidol [Haldol]) are the drugs of choice and should be continued indefinitely. They should be prescribed as outlined in Chapter 13 for the schizophrenic patient. If medical control can be established, the frequency of alcoholic sprees will decrease. When they occur, hospitalization is both a safety and disciplinary measure.

It is realistic to expect lapses, and the physician's attitude should not be condemnatory. Prodromal signs of a spree can often be detected if the physician knows his patient well. The family and the patient himself often become quite astute about recognizing these signs and should be urged to alert the physician when they appear. The patient usually becomes listless, disinterested in daily activities, apathetic, and seclusive. Anxiety, restlessness, and irritability increase. Craving for alcohol may or may not be present.

At this point all of the available resources should be mobilized. The patient's friends and relatives should be alerted to help him utilize his assets and control himself. If he is a member of AA, other members should be enlisted in his aid. He should not be alone or idle. His time should be filled with heavy work, exercise, and absorbing activities. Each day should be full and tiring, so that sleep will come easily. Drugs should be given in increased dosage as needed, and appropriate medications used for particular symptoms. The primary consideration during this crucial period is to get the patient through the crisis without drinking. If this can be done, the result is a tremendous boost to the patient's self-confidence, one that makes the next crisis easier to handle. "Crisis intervention" is never more effectively used than in this situation.

Long-term psychotherapy with these patients involves many risks and should not be undertaken lightly. The physician's major role is supportive. Formal uncovering technics should be reserved for selected patients with the means and motivation to stay in therapy, and should be attempted only by an experienced therapist.

Without treatment, the schizophrenic alcoholic usually goes progressively downhill to more frequent and more prolonged bouts of drinking until he dies of either an overdose of alcohol, intercurrent infection, suicide, or violent accident. With vigorous treatment, many of these people can be helped to live longer and more satisfactory lives.

2. MANIC-DEPRESSIVE ALCOHOLISM

Manic-depressive alcoholism is also characterized by serious drinking bouts—often less impulsive than in schizophrenic alcoholism and often alternating with severe depression. There may be a history of hypomanic episodes. The mood is often mercurial, swinging from silly, hilarious behavior to combative belligerence. In some cases the alcoholic spree terminates with a period of prolonged depression from which the patient is unable to extricate himself. The patient may isolate himself for long periods and may commit suicide or die accidentally. Between attacks he may be a pleasant, even ebullient person who is quite objective and disapproving of his drinking, insisting that he abhors alcohol even when he is drinking heavily. The genetic components of manic-depressive disease are well documented, and the family history usually reveals instances of severe depression, suicide, and serious emotional problems.

Treatment

The tricyclic antidepressants (amitriptyline [Elavil], imipramine [Tofranil]) are effective in most cases (see Chapter 24). The butyrophenones and phenothiazines (chlorpromazine [Thorazine]) are useful in the manic phase. ECT is indicated if the suicide risk is judged to be great or if medications are ineffective. In spite of the patient's assurances that "it will never happen again," maintenance doses of drugs should be given indefinitely. In occasional cases it is necessary to give prophylactic ECT—eg, once a month. Lithium carbonate (Lithonate, etc) has shown promise in the treatment and prophylactic follow-up care of these patients, and will be a valuable drug if current studies corroborate the early reports. This drug is discussed further in Chapter 24.

Psychotherapy should be used sparingly with these patients. Adequate supportive and somatic measures are usually sufficient to help manic-depressive alcoholics maintain a productive existence.

UNSOLVED PROBLEMS

In spite of the increased tempo of research in the problems of alcoholism, many aspects of this condition remain as baffling today as they were centuries ago. *Craving* is not well understood; it may be independent of addiction and due to organic factors in one patient and psychologic in another. It is hard to explain, for example, why an apparently healthy, well-adjusted man, dry for many months, may suddenly, on his way to church with his family, have such a powerful urge to drink that he leaves abruptly and gets drunk on all the liquor he can lay his hands on.

Loss of control is another puzzling feature. Some alcoholics drink slowly and steadily, apparently titrating their blood alcohol level with exquisite care. Others, after one drink, seem compelled to drink everything in sight until there is no liquor or money left or until a rebellious stomach can hold nothing more.

Addiction seems to be easily established in some alcoholics but never develops in others. Perhaps anyone can become addicted if he is able to drink enough for a long enough period of time. Recent claims have been made that in some individuals alcohol (as well as other sedative drugs) inhibits aldehyde dehydrogenase in the normal metabolism of dopamine, thus augmenting an alternate condensation of the aldehyde intermediate of dopamine to tetrahydropapaveroline. Alkaloids of this type are known to produce analgesia and addiction, presumably through the endogenous formation of morphine-like substances in the nervous system.

In the complications of chronic alcoholism, *organ specificity* has never been adequately explained. Why do some alcoholics develop cirrhosis of the liver, others Korsakoff's psychosis or Wernicke's disease or peripheral neuritis or myositis or myocarditis? Nutritional deficiencies seem to be only partial answers. Why is there such individual variability in the appearance of *delirium tremens* and other withdrawal phenomena?

REFERENCES

Books and Monographs

Alcoholics Anonymous: *The Story of How Many Thousands Have Recovered From Alcoholism.* Alcoholics Anonymous Publishing, Inc, 1955.

Blum, E.M., & R.H. Blum: *Alcoholism: Modern Psychological Approaches to Treatment.* Jossey-Bass, 1967.

Catanzaro, R.J.: *Alcoholism: The Total Treatment Approach.* Thomas, 1968.

Cole, J.O.: *Clinical Research in Alcoholism.* Psychiatric Research Report No. 24. American Psychiatric Association, 1968.

Jellinek, E.M.: *The Disease Concept of Alcoholism.* Hillhouse Press, 1960.

Ludwig, A.M., Levine, J., & L.H. Stark: *LSD and Alcoholism: A Clinical Study of Treatment Efficacy.* Thomas, 1970.

Mendelson, J.H., & P. Solomon: Alcoholism. In: *Current Therapy, 1964.* Conn, H.F., Clohecy, R.J., & R.B. Conn, Jr. (editors). Saunders, 1964.

Mendelson, J.H., Mello, N.K., & P. Solomon: Small group drinking behavior: An experimental study of chronic alcoholics. In: *The Addictive States.* Proceedings of the Association for Research in Nervous & Mental Disorders, Vol 46. Williams & Wilkins, 1968.

Plaut, T.F.A.: *Alcohol Problems: A Report to the Nation.* Oxford Univ Press, 1967.

Scott, E.M.: *Struggles in an Alcoholic Family.* Thomas, 1970.

Solomon, P.: A new look in alcoholism. Pages 76–86, 96–112 in: *Practical Lectures in Psychiatry for the Medical Practitioner.* Usdin, G. (editor). Thomas, 1966.

Solomon, P.: *Psychiatric Treatment of the Alcoholic Patient.* International Psychiatric Clinics (No. 2), 1966.

Journal Articles

Childs, A.W.: Metabolic basis for recommending how to use alcohol. California Med 113:7−11, Aug 1970.

Davidson, E.A., & P. Solomon: The differentiation of delirium tremens from impending hepatic coma. J Ment Sc 104:326−333, 1968.

DeVito, R.A., Flaherty, L.A., & G.J. Mozdzierz: Toward a psychodynamic theory of alcoholism. Dis Nerv System 31:43−49, 1970.

Ditman, D.S., & G.G. Crawford: The use of court probation in the management of the alcohol addict. Am J Psychiat 122:757−761, 1966.

Goodwin, D.W., Crane, B.J., & S.B. Guze: Alcoholic "blackouts": A review and clinical study of 100 alcoholics. Am J Psychiat 126:191−198, 1969.

Hayman, M.: Methods of therapy in alcoholism. California Med 105:117−123, 1966.

Johnson, L.C., Burdick, J.A., & J. Smith: Sleep during alcohol intake and withdrawal in the chronic alcoholic. Arch Gen Psychiat 22:406−418, 1970.

Kaim, S.C., Klett, C.J., & B. Rothfeld: Treatment of the acute alcohol withdrawal state: A comparison of four drugs. Am J Psychiat 125:1640−1652, 1969.

Keehn, J.D., Bloomfield, F.F., & M.A. Hug: Use of the reinforcement survey schedule with alcoholics. Quart J Stud Alcohol 31:602−615, 1970.

Linsky, A.S.: The changing public views of alcoholism. Quart J Stud Alcohol 31:692−704, 1970.

Ludwig, A., & others: A clinical study of LSD treatment in alcoholism. Am J Psychiat 126:59, 1969.

Nathan, P.E., & others: Behavioral analysis of chronic alcoholism. Arch Gen Psychiat 22:419−430, 1970.

Papas, A.N.: An Air Force alcoholic rehabilitation program. Mil Med 136:277−281, 1971.

Pattison, E.M., Coe, R., & R.J. Rhodes: Evaluation of alcoholism treatment. Arch Gen Psychiat 20:478−488, 1969.

Rosenberg, C.M.: Young alcoholics. Brit J Psychiat 115:181−188, 1969.

Schuckit, M., & others: Alcoholism. Arch Gen Psychiat 20:301−306, 1969.

Selzer, M.L.: Alcoholism, mental illness, and stress in 96 drivers causing fatal accidents. Behav Sc 14:1-10, 1969.

Wanberg, K.W., & J. Knapp: Differences in drinking symptoms and behavior of men and women alcoholics. Brit J Addiction 64:347−355, 1970.

Winokur, G., & others: Alcoholism. Arch Gen Psychiat 23:104−111, 1970.

21...

Drug Dependence

Most drug abuse today is social, based on peer group acceptance, curiosity, alienation, defiance, and the like. Management rests with law enforcement, legislative, civic, educational, and social leaders. Drug addiction may be neurotic, an expression of deep-seated emotional conflict requiring psychotherapy. Psychotic *drug dependence may be an expression of schizoid, paranoid, or manic-depressive disease requiring appropriate psychiatric attention.*

Methadone maintenance or withdrawal should be considered for heroin addicts. Barbiturate dependence may require a dose-response trial before gradual withdrawal. Treatment of dependence on stimulants and hallucinogens is symptomatic, followed by consideration of the total patient. Watch for mixed drug abuse.

The problem of drug use, abuse, misuse, habituation, and addiction has expanded with explosive force in recent years. Drug taking, previously considered a deviant, dangerous, and "out" thing to do, has become accepted by much of the younger generation as a proof of courage, self-realization, defiance of the "establishment," and definitely "in." The practice has spread through the colleges, high schools, and even the elementary schools.

Although marihuana is the drug most extensively resorted to, the stimulants and hallucinogens are widely abused, and addiction to the "hard" narcotics has increased considerably. The general public as well as government and professional authorities have become increasingly alarmed at the evidences of a "drug culture" that seems to have taken root in this country and many others throughout the world.

The variety of drug effects and the constant introduction of new drugs and agents and rediscovery of old ones have led to some confusion in the terminology of inappropriate or inadvisable drug use. *Misuse* implies overzealous or indiscreet administration of drugs by physicians. *Abuse* implies the use of drugs for other than legitimate medical purposes. *Habituation* and *addiction* imply dependence with the absence (habituation) or presence (addiction) of physical withdrawal phenomena—a distinction made explicit by the WHO Expert Committee on Addiction-Producing Drugs in 1957.

In 1964 the Committee recommended that the general term *drug dependence* be accompanied by a qualifying phrase specifying the drug or class of drugs involved, eg, "drug dependence of the morphine type." The Committee's position is that drug dependence is a state of psychologic and, in many cases, physical dependence, and that dependence as such says nothing about the degree of risk to the individual or about the public health problem and need for control.

Psychologic dependence means that there is a compulsion to continue taking a drug despite untoward consequences. *Physical dependence* causes a specific and characteristic syndrome of physical symptoms upon abrupt withdrawal. *Tolerance* is a declining effect upon administration of a given dose, so that the dose must be increased in order to achieve the initial effect. *Cross-tolerance* occurs when the use of one drug induces tolerance to another drug of the same class. Finally, the psychophysiologic aspects of drug intoxication and the social consequences of drug abuse are essential parts of the description of the type of dependence characteristic of any given drug.

The subject of this chapter will be drug dependence due to the use of opiates, sedatives, marihuana, amphetamines, cocaine, and the psychedelic drugs. Inhalants that are used to produce acute intoxication will be mentioned briefly.

Medical Practitioner's Involvement in Problems of Drug Abuse

Problems related to drug dependence come to the medical practitioner's attention in several ways. Cases of acute or chronic toxicity usually come to medical attention if the individual himself or someone close to him decides he is sick or out of control. The chronic sequels of drug abuse may lead to medical consultation even when the cause is not obvious. Drug withdrawal syndromes may lead to medical contact in response to social pressures (family, friends, employees, law officers), or the individual may himself decide that he must interrupt a cyclic pattern of dependence and abstinence.

A patient may seek psychiatric contact for difficulties associated directly or indirectly with drug use. In many such cases, drug use may be overlooked in the initial psychiatric work-up. In others, the patient may be suffering from obvious toxic or withdrawal effects of the drug at the first interview.

Finally, problems of drug dependence may come up unexpectedly in the course of medical management of other conditions, especially accidents, hepatitis, malnutrition, venereal disease, pneumonia, tuberculosis, skin infections, and pregnancy.

General Considerations

A provisional diagnosis of drug dependence and an initial estimation of the level of tolerance are based on the history taken from the individual, although the history cannot always be relied upon with certainty. People dependent upon opiates often overestimate the amount they have been using, whereas those dependent upon barbiturates frequently underestimate it. Corroboration is important in the initial as well as after-care stage. Clues include a history of withdrawal symptomatology (especially convulsions) and broken social relationships, the patient's general physical state, and specific signs of drug administration (eg, needle marks, scars, and nasal ulcerations).

A wide range of diagnostic categories and socioeconomic backgrounds are represented by the total group of people who become dependent upon drugs. Although it is not possible to isolate an addiction-prone personality, a few generalizations are feasible about patients who become dependent upon different types of drugs. Dependence of the opiate type is more frequently found in patients with socially deprived (ghetto) backgrounds and is found relatively more frequently among various minority groups. Psychodynamically, they have been described as of oral character and narcissistic, operating on a level of immediate gratification of needs. Dependence on barbiturates is often seen in chronically neurotic adults, particularly women, who use the drug as a haven. Amphetamine dependence occurs more frequently among teenagers with borderline social and psychologic adjustment. The "thrill" that frequently motivates the dependence is of a more volatile and aggressive character than that seen with opiate dependence. Patients with dependence of the marihuana or psychedelic type are more frequently young adults of middle class background with some college experience. The motivation more frequently arises from a desire for personal psychologic insights or for group acceptance.

The use of combinations of drugs of different classes is a frequent phenomenon. Usually one drug predominates, but problems of withdrawal from more than one drug are not rare. The most prevalent combinations are opiate-barbiturate, opiate-marihuana, barbiturate-amphetamine, marihuana-amphetamine-psychedelics, and opiate-cocaine. Alcohol may also be combined with any of these, but frequently is combined with barbiturates.

Because of the screening effect of the sometimes dramatic symptoms of toxicity or withdrawal, the physician must be alert for intercurrent medical problems. In addition to those mentioned earlier, cardiac disease and coincident infections should also be considered.

In most cases, hospitalization is indicated for the management of drug withdrawal or intoxication. Unfortunately, with the recent enormous increase in such cases, it is available for only a tiny fraction of those who should have it. Moreover, problems arise when young people avoid recognized clinics or hospitals for fear of being "busted" (arrested) or having their parents notified. Preventable serious illness and deaths have thus resulted. Many organizations have sprung up in urban areas all over the country, and the laws have been modified in several states to permit help and immunity to youngsters with drug problems. "Emancipated minors" (not living at home) are widely treated with confidentiality. Nevertheless, the great bulk of youngsters who abuse drugs will not trust members of the "establishment" and turn instead to those who look and talk like themselves in special groups set up to help them.

Definitive treatment begins only after the presenting disorders have been treated successfully. It is important to attempt to identify the psychologic disturbances and social drives that have led to drug dependence. After-care and continued contact with the individual are essential to long-term success. In most cases, supportive psychotherapy is indicated with attention to the social, interpersonal, and psychologic problems.

A great deal of time and effort are required to assist the patient in dealing with his particular constellation of psychologic and social needs. Active therapeutic involvement with problems of social adjustment, vocational training, counseling, or placement may be required, as well as medical care, conventional psychiatric management, and insight therapy.

DRUG DEPENDENCE OF THE MORPHINE TYPE

The drugs involved in opiate dependence constitute a group of analgesic compounds for which morphine serves as a convenient reference. These include opiate derivatives, synthetic opiates, and synthetic compounds with morphine-like properties, even though the last may bear little resemblance to morphine in chemical structure. In addition to morphine, the drugs most frequently involved are heroin, oxymorphone (Numorphan), meperidine (Demerol), dihydromorphinone (Dilaudid), omnopon (Pantopon), levorphanol (Levo-Dromoran), methadone (Dolophine), codeine, and paregoric. Although heroin is the drug most frequently involved, patterns of multiple opiate use are not rare. These arise either because the preferred drug is difficult to obtain or out of preference for a mixed effect. Multiple use often involves other drugs, particularly barbiturates and, less often, marihuana, alcohol, and cocaine.

The Evolution of Drug Dependence

Except for methadone, the properties of the opiates differ little, and continued administration of any of them results in tolerance. They can produce physical dependence and self-limited abstinence syndromes which, though varying between drugs and somewhat between individuals, have many features in common. The time required for drugs to produce physical dependence also varies somewhat, but generally it takes at least 2 weeks of continuous administration at moderate therapeutic dosage to produce a definite though mild abstinence syndrome upon abrupt cessation. In addition, drugs of this class produce a syndrome of intoxication which is generally characterized by sedation, decreased physiologic and psychologic "drive," and a sense of inner pleasure or well-being (the "high"). Clinically, this presents as an increasing drowsiness (the "nod"), flushing, itching, constricted pupils, decreased rate and depth of respiration, decreased blood pressure and temperature, and slow pulse.

From the point of view of opiate-dependent persons, the initial motivation for drug use is frequently the "high" derived from the drug. In only a few cases does dependence develop initially from medical use. Motivation for the "high" experience extends beyond the pharmacologic effects of the drug to psychosocial factors, such as the desire to emulate drug-dependent peers and the excitement that goes along with acquisition of the drug ("being in the life").

Heroin dependence frequently begins by snuffing or subcutaneous injection, progressing to intravenous injection. Once physical dependence is established, the motivation shifts from the search for pleasure to a flight from the suffering of abstinence. The "life" then becomes a relentless pattern of decreasing highs, as tolerance develops, and increasing lows, as physical dependency hardens. All this is made more frustrating and unsatisfactory by the difficulties of obtaining illicit drugs.

The appearance of abstinence phenomena follows a predictable time course for any given drug, although there are considerable variations with different drugs. For example, meperidine, dihydromorphinone, heroin, morphine, and codeine range (in that order) from 4–48 hours for the time from last drug intake to onset of spontaneous withdrawal symptoms. It is possible to group the signs and symptoms of withdrawal in increasing levels of severity: (1) restlessness, anxiety, and a craving for the drug; (2) yawning, lacrimation, rhinorrhea, perspiration, and light, restless sleep (the "yen"); (3) dilated pupils with decreasing reactivity to light, gooseflesh, anorexia, hot and cold flashes, muscular twitches, and muscle and joint pains; (4) insomnia, elevated temperature, increased rate and depth of respiration, increased pulse and blood pressure, marked restlessness, nausea, vomiting, diarrhea, weight loss, and spontaneous, unenjoyable orgasm.

Treatment

Experimental treatment programs, some of which use an outpatient model with or without some form of substitution or maintenance therapy, have yielded encouraging though limited results. For most cases, however, the most feasible treatment begins with substitution therapy in a hospital setting. Estimation of the patient's degree of physical dependence may be gained in part by historical items: length of time of current drug use, frequency and amount of daily use, and the interval since the last dose. Withdrawal signs and symptoms at the time of examination give more concrete clues.

If signs are not in evidence, there should be a 24-hour observation period, with provision made to begin substitution at the first appearance of pupillary dilatation and gooseflesh, the most consistent and reliable withdrawal signs.

Because methadone (Dolophine) has a 12-hour action, it is the preferred drug for substitution (*"methadone withdrawal treatment"*). Oral administration of 5, 10, or 15 mg (depending on the extent of dependence) twice daily is in most cases sufficient to delay the discomfort of withdrawal. After 1–2 days of stabilization at one of these levels, methadone may be withdrawn in decrements of 5 or 10 mg/day depending upon the patient's medical status as well as the severity of withdrawal phenomena. If withdrawal is characterized by protracted vomiting, methadone may be administered intramuscularly at equivalent oral dose levels.

In some centers, addicts are kept on methadone indefinitely (like diabetics on insulin), with a daily dose that not only eliminates the craving for opiates but would block the action of ordinary doses of opiates if they were taken. This *methadone maintenance therapy* has become increasingly available in the major cities of the USA. Thousands of narcotic addicts have become rehabilitated through its use, and the laws of many states have been modified to permit the treatment to be given legally. Methadone is inexpensive (about 10 cents a day), is taken orally, does not produce tolerance, and has little or no untoward or chronic adverse effects. There are indications that newer similar drugs may soon be available that will have to be taken only 2 or 3 times a week for the same effectiveness. Objections that this kind of therapy condones drug addiction are varied and sanctimonious. The success rate of the treatment has been reported to be 70–90%.

Special problems:

(1) The physician should keep in mind that certain secondary or concomitant medical problems occur more frequently among addicts under treatment than in the general population: hepatitis, tuberculosis, pneumonia, cardiac disease, and severe diarrheas.

(2) Simultaneous withdrawal from opiates and barbiturates may necessitate more gradual withdrawal. In these cases the degree of barbiturate dependence largely determines the time course of withdrawal.

(3) Concurrent medical conditions—in particular, infections and fevers of any origin—may transiently increase tolerance and the severity of withdrawal phenomena; depending upon the individual circumstances, withdrawal should be either slowed or stopped during this period.

(4) Seizures of the grand mal type may result from meperidine intoxication at levels of 1.2–2 gm/day. The seizures are self-limiting and disappear after a few hours of abstinence. These seizures must be differentiated from those arising from barbiturate abstinence or other causes.

DRUG DEPENDENCE OF THE SEDATIVE TYPE

It has been said that the overall problem of sedative dependence is second only to that of alcohol dependence, and indeed the 2 have many features in common. Dependence of this type involves most of the barbiturates, particularly the short- and intermediate-acting barbiturates—pentobarbital, secobarbital, and amobarbital.

In recent years a number of drugs—mostly chemically unrelated—have been introduced which are variously identified as nonbarbiturate sedatives, relaxants, psychotropic agents, and minor tranquilizers. All produce sedation, intoxication, and psychologic and physical dependence similar to (but milder than) that observed with the barbiturates. The drugs which most frequently produce a barbiturate type dependence are glutethimide (Doriden), methyprylon (Noludar), ethchlorvynol (Placidyl), ethinamate (Valmid), meprobamate (Miltown, Equanil), chlordiazepoxide (Librium), and diazepam (Valium).

The Evolution of Drug Dependence

Barbiturates produce an intoxication syndrome characterized by feelings of relaxation and euphoria, increasing nystagmus (present first as fine lateral gaze nystagmus and proceeding to coarser nystagmus on forward gaze), increasing dysarthria and ataxia, and decreasing mental alertness (with a corresponding increase in confusion, memory disruption, disorientation, and emotional instability). At higher levels of intoxication, the following may result (in more or less progressive order): semicoma with constricted pupils, respiratory depression, shock with dilated pupils, and death. Excessive doses of drugs of the sedative-tranquilizer group have been reported to cause decreasing mental alertness (with confusion, memory impairment, and emotional instability), slurred speech, ataxia, coma, and, in some cases, death.

Continued exposure to the barbiturates and other sedative drugs results in variable degrees of tolerance. It may result in physical dependence. Unlike morphine-type drugs, these drugs produce the withdrawal syndrome at levels considerably above therapeutic levels of the drug, as indicated by studies of barbiturates and meprobamate in man and clinical reports of other drugs. For example, in one study abrupt cessation after administration of 400 mg of pentobarbital daily for 6 weeks produced only minor transient effects. Furthermore, although the administration of 1200–1600 mg of meprobamate daily for 8 weeks resulted in no discernible withdrawal phenomena after abrupt cessation, 3200 mg/day regularly generated withdrawal syndrome on abrupt withdrawal. Numerous case reports concerning other drugs would indicate that greater than therapeutic levels for extended periods of time are necessary to produce physical dependence. Cross-tolerance among the barbiturates is striking, and probably exists also to a considerable degree between the barbiturates and other sedative drugs.

The first exposure is usually on medical indication, but for a variety of psychologic reasons the individual finds the development of tolerance increasingly more difficult to handle. It has been suggested that chronic barbiturate use represents an "adjustive" mechanism for coping with a variety of adverse psychologic states: anxiety, guilt, depression, inadequacy, unacceptable sexual urges, and dependency. Dosage increases gradually to the point where many individuals fluctuate between intoxication and the severe stress of withdrawal. Because of the nature of chronic intoxication, these people are prone to accidents and overdosage. Satisfactory social functioning is obviously impaired in such a situation.

Abrupt discontinuance of barbiturates or other sedatives in a physically dependent individual results in a characteristic withdrawal syndrome that appears usually within 24 hours after cessation. In moderately severe untreated cases, withdrawal phenomena last approximately 1 week. The withdrawal syndrome presents (in progressive order) as weakness, restlessness, and tremulousness; anxiety, insomnia, blepharoclonus, and elevated blood pressure at rest but postural hypotension if the patient stands up suddenly (these latter 3 are the most dependable criteria); and hyperthermia, generalized convulsions, and psychotic behavior. The psychotic behavior is characterized by paranoia, visual and auditory hallucinations, and grossly disturbed emotional balance and intellectual functioning. If convulsions occur, they usually do so on the second or third day, whereas psychotic behavior usually appears in the 4th–7th day. Psychotic behavior, once begun, may continue for several weeks and then gradually decrease.

Treatment

The life-threatening nature of withdrawal demands a close estimate of the degree of dependence. A specific dose-response trial is indicated, and is of particular value in mixed patterns of dependence where barbiturate abuse may only be suspected. Administer 200 mg of pentobarbital orally (debilitated or elderly patients may require less), and evaluate the sensorium after 1 hour. A nontolerant person will usually be somnolent though arousable. A person tolerant to 500–600 mg/day will show nystagmus and mild dysarthria and ataxia; one tolerant to 700–800 mg/day will show some nystagmus; and one tolerant to 900 mg or more per day will show no signs of intoxication. If the level of tolerance is still uncertain, 200 mg may be given every 2 hours until a mild state of intoxication is achieved. Once 24-hour tolerance is estimated, the individual should be stabilized at that level (in divided doses) for 1–2 days. Reduction by 100 mg/day may then be started and continued until withdrawal is complete.

The principle of barbiturate treatment is applicable to the treatment of withdrawal syndromes of the other sedatives. Barbiturate substitution has been used with the same degree of success in the treatment of meprobamate and glutethimide withdrawal.

Special problems:

(1) Prompt attention to barbiturate withdrawal is imperative because of the life-threatening nature of abrupt abstinence.

(2) The convulsions that occur in barbiturate withdrawal respond readily to barbiturate treatment but not to diphenylhydantoin (Dilantin) or other nonbarbiturate anticonvulsants.

(3) Anxiety and agitation are best managed with barbiturates; the phenothiazines add to the danger of seizures.

(4) Psychotic behavior does not usually respond readily to barbiturate treatment and may persist for weeks.

(5) Intercurrent medical problems, particularly infections and cardiac disease, may necessitate prolonging or delaying withdrawal because of increased difficulties in nursing care and possibly a transient increase in tolerance.

(6) The general medical management must include standard procedures for the care of extremely agitated, accident-prone, confused, and potentially convulsive patients, including maintenance of electrolyte and water balance and dietary supplementation.

DRUG DEPENDENCE
OF THE CANNABIS (MARIHUANA) TYPE

Cannabis—the flowering tops and leaves of the hemp plant—produces a resinous exudate that in antiquity was valued for its medicinal properties. In recent times it has been valued for its intoxicating properties. It is used almost all over the world, presumably because of the plant's wild growth and easy cultivation in a variety of climates. Varying with its geographic distribution, the method of preparation, and the route of consumption, its names include *hashish, bhang, ganja, charas, dagga,* and *marihuana.* The active principle of the exudate is a tetrahydrocannabinol.

The Evolution of Drug Dependence

Cannabis has enjoyed a long history of varied social, cultural, and medicinal uses. Although it has no known medicinal value now and there is virtually a worldwide ban on its use, it continues to be used because of its psychic effects. In most areas the dried preparation is combined with tobacco and smoked, most commonly in cigarettes.

There is no evidence that tolerance or physical dependence develops when cannabis is used either on a few occasions or repeatedly. The development of psychologic dependence is variable.

The behavioral effects depend upon the quantity consumed, which in turn is dependent upon the substance used, the strength of the preparation, and the route of consumption. If not reinforced, the effect of a usual dose persists for about 2—4 hours. The most common effect is a "dreamy" state, often characterized by euphoria, hilarity, and an intense, excited inner feeling of well-being. Speech is rapid and voluble, and at times disjointed. This leads to impairment of memory and judgment. Thoughts may take on new or special meanings. If he is alone, the individual may be drowsy or moody; in the company of others, he may become restless, gregarious, and garrulous. Behavior may be impulsive and emotional responses eccentric. Perception of space and time seems distorted and extendable. Higher doses may cause a subjective experience of lowered sensory threshold, diminished sexual desire and potency, hallucinations, and delusions—or may simply produce drowsiness and coma.

Casual or brief use of cannabis appears to be widespread, particularly in the teen-age and young adult population. Its use is motivated in part by curiosity and in part by the desire for social or "in-group" acceptance, and may be related to a questioning of social norms and values in the process of growth and search for maturity and "identity." Its use often represents part of the younger generation's defiance to government action or inaction in such matters as poverty, racial discrimination, environmental pollution, and undeclared wars.

Although the personal and social hazards of cannabis use must not be minimized or overlooked, there is no clear evidence that it leads to psychic dependence except in a small percentage of users or that lasting mental changes result. It is almost impossible to estimate reliably the number of users who progress from marihuana to narcotic use ("escalation"), but reports from informed observers suggest that the percentage is low but increasing. Chronic use is much less common than brief or occasional use.

It appears likely that persons using marihuana on a chronic basis represent a wide spectrum of psychiatric syndromes. It is useful to consider them under the broad classification of social, neurotic, and psychotic, a division that may be applied to users of other drugs as well.

Social drug takers are usually motivated by curiosity or thrill seeking. They may be going along with the gang, expressing "independence," or searching for "identity." Very few of these take the drug regularly or become habituated.

Neurotic drug takers are those in whom drug taking serves the purpose of any other neurotic symptom—an attempt to relieve anxiety and reestablish psychic equilibrium in the face of deepseated conflict and emotional turmoil. It succeeds no better than other neurotic symptoms, and the additional reality problems that usually supervene add to the individual's already overfull pool of misery.

Psychotic drug takers are not necessarily psychotic all the time. Some are, and may by virtue of that fact be led easily by unscrupulous individuals into troubles of various sorts—delinquency, crime, promiscuity, alcoholism, or drug taking. Others learn to reach for alcohol, marihuana, or other drugs when they sense an attack of psychosis coming on. The attempt, often on an unconscious basis, is to ward off the attack (depressive mostly, but sometimes manic or schizo-affective) and escape from it.

The dangers of marihuana are the following: (1) It produces social problems in that its use is illegal. (2) It is intoxicating. Accidents (some of them fatal) have occurred for this reason. (3) Some individuals ("potheads") tend to use it on a chronic basis to the detriment of school work, family relationships, and other reality factors.

American insurance companies, on the basis of their own research, have begun to deny life insurance to users of marihuana.

Research on the action and chronic effects of marihuana is urgently needed. Many projects are actually in progress, largely sponsored and supported by NIMH. Now that the problem of standardizing the active marihuana dosage has been solved, it may be anticipated that the widespread theorizing and speculation about this controversial drug will soon be replaced by solid knowledge. When this occurs, it is likely that the present ill-advised agitation to legalize marihuana (because it is "no worse than alcohol") will subside.

Treatment

Treatment is aimed at one of 2 problems: acute toxic psychosis and chronic use. The acute episodes are characterized by marked anxiety or depressive affect; delusional ideation, often of a persecutory nature; and hallucinatory behavior. These are the symptoms, usually, which cause the patient to seek medical attention. These episodes are evidence of intoxication rather than withdrawal and usually subside within hours. They may persist for longer periods, but the role of the drug in precipitation of longer episodes is not clear.

The acute episodes are best managed with a protective environment and firm, calm, friendly reassurance. Isolation aggravates the anxiety and panic that frequently accompany these reactions and should be avoided.

The treatment of chronic marihuana use, with or without acute toxic episodes, requires much time and effort. Where the causes are largely social, environmental approaches and educational efforts are indicated. In many school systems, efforts are being made (1) to teach children about the decision-making process, (2) to provide alternatives to drugs (sports, spiritual values, opportunities for involvement in relevant community activities), and (3) to encourage "rap" sessions—open discussions with parents and other adults. In neurotic drug taking, the treatment, as for any other neurosis, is psychotherapeutic, with the emphasis on the resolution of underlying intrapsychic conflicts. In psychotic drug taking, the treatment should be largely organic, ie, antidepressant or antipsychotic medication (see Chapter 24) or ECT (see Chapter 25).

Attention must also be directed toward the management of concurrent disease, usually the sequel of malnutrition.

DRUG DEPENDENCE OF THE AMPHETAMINE TYPE

In the past 25 years, the amphetamines and related sympathomimetic amines have had wide medical use as mood elevators in depression and as appetite depressants for weight reduction. They have had equally wide non-medical use by truck drivers and students in combating drowsiness and simple fatigue. This background of use, the relative ease of acquisition, the tendency for development of tolerance, and the sense of well-being induced by these drugs have contributed to a high incidence of psychologic dependence. In some areas of the USA, informed estimates have placed amphetamine dependence at a higher level than opiate dependence. These drugs are usually taken orally but may be taken intravenously ("speed"). Drugs frequently encountered are amphetamine (Benzedrine), dextroamphetamine (Dexedrine), methamphetamine (Desoxyn, Methedrine), and phenmetrazine (Preludin). Methylphenidate (Ritalin) may also be mentioned here, although it is not an amphetamine derivative, since its action is similar and it is frequently abused. Other drugs of this type are listed in Chapter 24.

Recently, the FDA has ordered drug manufacturers to limit their production of amphetamines sharply and voluntarily and to label these drugs as approved only for use in (1) narcolepsy, (2) certain behavior problems in children ("minimal brain damage"), and (3) the early and limited adjunctive treatment of obesity.

The Evolution of Drug Dependence

Psychologic dependence may develop even on therapeutic doses, presumably because the user needs to maintain the experience of well-being the drugs provide. The fatigue, lassitude, and mild depression that occur after the effect has dissipated serve to promote continued use and psychologic dependence.

With continued use, tolerance develops rapidly and the daily dose may gradually be raised to several hundred times the therapeutic level. Physical dependence does not develop, although a characteristic syndrome of psychologic responses upon withdrawal does occur. (See below.)

The psychologic effects, which depend for their intensity upon the amount and route of administration, are characterized by euphoria, an exhilarated sense of well-being, an impression of increased mental and physical prowess, and decreased appetite (variable). These may be accompanied by the appearance of restlessness, excitability, and irritability.

As tolerance develops with higher doses, the lassitude and depression between doses increase. The sense of well-being is increasingly blurred by apprehension and by an increasing emotional lability characterized by hostile impulsiveness. Judgment becomes faulty, and memory is sporadically impaired. Eventually, frightening persecutory delusional ideas may develop, together with visual, auditory, and tactile hallucinations. The syndrome may be indistinguishable from paranoid schizophrenia, although some patients retain perception of the delusional character of their thoughts.

In increasing order of drug effect, the physical signs are increased pulse and blood pressure, fine tremors of the extremities, headache, anorexia, nausea, bruxism, dilated pupils with decreasing reactivity to light, and delay of orgasm in sexual activity.

Abrupt cessation of drug intake results in a variable syndrome often characterized by lethargy, somnolence, and depression—in some cases, serious suicidal preoccupation or actual suicide. A seriously disabling series of events may persist for weeks. There is no characteristic syndrome of physical symptoms even though a high degree of tolerance may have developed.

Amphetamine dependence occurs in individuals representing a wide spectrum of socioeconomic backgrounds. In some areas of the USA the use of these drugs by adolescents appears to be high. Peer relationships partly determine the amount and frequency of use. Amphetamine dependence can be categorized according to (1) medical or nonmedical introduction and (2) the amount and frequency of use. If dependence originates in medical use, the dose tends to remain low although use is continuous. Nonmedical use, particularly that which is determined by the emulation of peers, may be periodic (eg, weekends only) or continuous. Continuous users may progress to intravenous administration in order to intensify the effect. High intake, oral or intravenous, often evolves into a spree pattern in which a constant level of intoxication is maintained by repeating the dose every 2 hours for several days. Exhaustion, mental confusion, paranoia, and somnolence eventually terminate the cycle.

Mixed drug use is of 2 types: (1) alternation and combination with psychedelic drugs, which seems to arise out of preference for the effects of these drugs; and (2) alternation or combination with opiates or barbiturates, usually for the purpose of controlling the intensity and less desirable aspects of amphetamine intoxication.

Treatment

Periodic or continuous high intake and the resulting toxic disturbance produces a toxic syndrome usually lasting a few days to a week; during this time, protective hospitalization is recommended. Psychosis, particularly if accompanied by marked agitation, may be treated with phenothiazines, and insomnia with barbiturates. The possibility of barbiturate tolerance must be kept in mind. Attention should be given to associated medical problems, usually sequels of poor nutrition and the self-administration of the drugs (eg, hepatitis). When the toxic syndrome subsides, an effort should be made, as with other drug-dependency syndromes, to explore the psychosocial reasons for drug use. After discharge from the hospital, continued follow-up with regular contacts is essential.

DRUG DEPENDENCE OF THE COCAINE TYPE

Cocaine is the prototype of stimulant drugs that, in sufficient quantity, induce euphoric excitement and hallucinatory experiences. It is derived from the leaves of the coca tree indigenous to the northern Andes, and has for centuries been used by Indians native to that area to increase physical endurance. It has had wide medical use as a topical anesthetic.

The Evolution of Drug Dependence

The effects sought by the chronic cocaine user are an ecstatic euphoria and a feeling of enhanced mental and physical prowess. These lead to an overestimation of abilities and frequent accidents. Pronounced persecutory delusions develop in conjunction with anxiety, illusions, and visual, auditory, and tactile hallucinations, resulting at times in a dangerous potential for antisocial activity. Formication, diarrhea, nausea, appetite loss, and insomnia are common. Depressive symptoms and delusional ideation may continue for some time after cessation of intake. Acute poisoning can occur, with dilated pupils, exophthalmos, nausea, vomiting, delirium, and, in the terminal state, convulsions, coma, respiratory arrest, and death.

The use of cocaine alone is now rare; in recent years cocaine users have combined it with other drugs, particularly opiates, to intensify the initial effect. Administration is either by snuffing or intravenously. A strong psychologic dependence develops, but physical dependence and withdrawal phenomena do not occur. Tolerance does not develop, presumably because the drug is rapidly destroyed in the body. This allows relatively large doses to be taken in a 24-hour period by repeated administration. In extreme cases the drug may be administered as often as every 10 minutes.

Treatment

In acute poisoning, treatment consists of a protective environment and barbiturates for the control of delirium. The management may be made difficult in some cases by an extremely rapid progression of toxicity. Short-acting barbiturates and artificial respiration may be necessary. These procedures are aided by the rapid in vivo destruction of the drug.

As with other drug-dependent syndromes, continued after-care and exploration of the disturbed psychosocial relationships that underlie drug use are required.

DRUG DEPENDENCE OF THE PSYCHEDELIC TYPE

Of the various labels for the drugs of this group, the most prevalent are *psychotomimetics, psychotogens, hallucinogens,* and *psychedelics.* The drugs most frequently used and most widely studied are LSD, mescaline, and psilocybin. LSD (lysergic acid diethylamide), a semisynthetic derivative from the ergot fungus, was at first thought to cause a "model psychosis" that could be studied profitably by mental health investigators. Mescaline (*mescal* or *peyote*) is an alkaloid contained in the buttons of certain cactuses indigenous to Mexico and the southwest USA. Psilocybin and its analogue psilocin are isolated from the "sacred" mushroom (*Psilocybe mexicana*) found in various parts of Mexico. In the past, the cactus buttons and mushrooms have played significant roles in the religious rites of some Indian groups in Mexico and the USA. Other agents of this class are bufotenine and harmine. In addition, morning glory seeds provide an active principle similar in chemical structure and effect to LSD.

The Evolution of Drug Dependence

Studies have demonstrated that tolerance to LSD and psilocybin comes and goes rapidly and that tolerance to mescaline develops more slowly. All 3 drugs exhibit a high degree of cross-tolerance. There is no evidence of physical or psychologic dependence.

These drugs are almost always taken orally, usually on 1 or 2 occasions or periodically. Sometimes one to several doses are taken over a 4- or 5-day period. Chronic intake occurs but is infrequent.

The psychologic effects run a course, as a rule, of 8–12 hours, and some of them have had a great deal of publicity in the lay press. The most dramatic effects are kaleidoscopic visual hallucinations of vivid colors and forms. Auditory and tactile hallucinations, illusions, and distortions of perception and body image also occur. The individual is often preoccupied with his own thoughts and perceptions. Mood may be ecstatic but may alternate with uncertain, anxious, and depressive feelings. A feeling of estrangement and depersonalization is common. Long-term periodic or chronic use tends to cause looseness of associative processes, vagueness of formulations, and difficulty with coherent communication.

Users of these drugs represent a broad range of socioeconomic backgrounds, but their use is most common among white middle-class college students. Motivation arises from a desire for "kicks," for the changing moods, for alternating perceptual patterns, for the induction of reveries, and for the relief of anxiety and a desire to gain psychologic insights into personal problems. There is a widespread belief among users that the "consciousness expanding" properties of these drugs lead to beneficial personality changes.

Adverse reactions occur most often in people who have made borderline or conflicting adjustments to life and who are ill prepared to control the unconscious impulses, thoughts, and feelings induced by the experience.

A few psychiatrists have claimed beneficial effects through the use of LSD in the treatment of chronic alcoholism. Others, in controlled studies, have been unable to verify these claims.

Adverse Reactions to Psychedelic Drugs
The overall incidence of adverse consequences of single or repeated use of the psychedelic drugs is not known, but it is probably low. Studies suggest that the incidence is lower in controlled, supervised settings than in unsupervised settings. Physical disturbances are reported to be rare.

The characteristics of a "bad trip" (as judged by the individual) vary considerably, although some are reported more often than others. Extreme anxiety may develop, bordering on panic and characterized by overwhelming fears of loss of control and of physical and psychologic disintegration.

A little understood but not uncommon sequel is the periodic recurrence ("flashback") of features of the drug experience during abstinent periods for as long as 3 years afterward. The most frequent is recurrence of hallucinations that are similar, at least in form, to those that occurred during the drug experience and accompanied by varying degrees of anxiety and fears of losing control. At times this appears as an impending psychotic reaction. (Of course, similar experiences are reported by patients who have never taken psychedelic drugs.)

A psychotic reaction may develop after the drug experience. Individuals in whom this has occurred most probably were at a marginal level of adjustment prior to the drug experience and were unduly stressed by the necessity for accommodating the insights they derived from the drug with the realities of their nondrug existence.

Other sequels are depressive and paranoid reactions and the accentuation of preexisting sociopathic tendencies. Serious accidents have reportedly resulted from the apparently drug-induced belief that superhuman powers had been acquired. This happens most often in emotionally labile persons, in those with hysterical and paranoid personalities, and in those who have shown prior evidence of psychologic difficulties.

There is conflicting evidence both in animal experiments and in humans that LSD produces chromosomal damage to the cells of the body and thus poses a serious genetic threat to users. A higher incidence of malformations in infants born to mothers who used the drug during pregnancy has been reported. This kind of evidence has become a telling argument against the use of LSD by young people.

Treatment
Treatment involves both the management of the undesirable sequels and the concurrent psychiatric problems. Most panic reactions respond to supportive management in a friendly, protective environment and are resolved within a few days. Isolation aggravates the panic. Phenothiazines have proved effective in terminating the drug experience induced by LSD. Most patients manifesting anxiety (with or without hallucinations) or depressive, paranoid, and psychotic reactions respond to conventional medical and

psychiatric management. Some remain sick and require hospitalization for many months or indefinitely.

DEPENDENCE ON INTOXICATING INHALANTS

A number of gaseous substances have been used to produce an intoxicating or exhilarating effect. Among these are ether, carbon tetrachloride and other cleaning fluids, gasoline, kerosene, ethylene oxide (used in glass frosters), and glue vapor (especially model airplane cement). Various aerosols, hair sprays, spray paints, shellacs and varnishes, and insecticides have also been so used, but rarely.

Children and adolescents have been the chief offenders in the abuse of inhalants, and several deaths have occurred. The inhalants are extremely toxic; some can cause immediate death through mechanical airway obstruction or a noxious effect upon the lungs; others can cause death later through destruction of the liver, kidneys, or bone marrow.

Prevention is clearly by education and better supervision on the part of parents, educators, and others responsible for the behavior of children. Treatment consists of immediate hospitalization and supportive therapy as needed.

REFERENCES

Books and Monographs

Brill, L., & others: *Rehabilitation in Drug Addiction.* Publication No. 1013. US Public Health Service, 1963.

Glaser, E.M.: *Psychological Basis of Habituation.* Oxford Univ Press, 1966.

Maurer, D.W., & V.H. Vogel: *Narcotics and Narcotic Addiction,* 3rd ed. Thomas, 1970.

Solomon, D. (editor): *The Marihuana Papers.* Bobbs-Merrill, 1966.

Wilner, D.M., & G.G. Kasselbaum (editors): *Narcotics.* McGraw-Hill, 1965.

Journal Articles

AMA Committee on Alcoholism and Addiction: Drug dependence and other sedative drugs. JAMA 193:673–677, 1965.

AMA Committee on Alcoholism and Addiction: Dependence on Cannabis (marihuana). JAMA 201:368–371, 1967.

AMA Committee on Alcoholism and Addiction: Dependence on LSD and other hallucinogenic drugs. JAMA 202:47-50, 1967.

AMA Committee on Alcoholism and Addiction: Dependence on amphetamines and other stimulant drugs. JAMA 197:1023–1027, 1966.

Bialos, D.S.: Adverse marijuana reactions: A critical examination of the literature with selected case material. Am J Psychiat 127:819–823, 1970.

Black, S., Owens, K.L., & R.P. Wolff: Patterns of drug use: A study of 5482 subjects. Am J Psychiat 127:420–423, 1970.

Brill, N.Q., & others: The marijuana problem. Ann Int Med 73:449–465, 1970.

Cherkas, M.S.: Synanon Foundation: A radical approach to the problem of addiction. Am J Psychiat 121:1065–1068, 1965.

Cole, J.O., & M.M. Katz: The psychotomimetic drugs. JAMA 187:758–761, 1964.

Connell, P.H.: Clinical manifestations and treatment of amphetamine type of dependence. JAMA 196:718–723, 1966.

Crane, G.E., Johnson, A.W., & W.J. Buffaloe: Long-term treatment with neuroleptic drugs and eye opacities. Am J Psychiat 127:1045–1049, 1971.

Dole, V.P., & M. Nyswander: A medical treatment for diacetylmorphine (heroin) addiction. JAMA 193:646–650, 1965.

Eddy, N.B., & others: Drug dependence: Its significance and characteristics. Bull World Health Organ 32:721–733, 1965.

Ellinwood, E.H., Jr.: Assault and homicide associated with amphetamine abuse. Am J Psychiat 127:1170–1175, 1971.

Essig, C.F.: Clinical and experimental aspects of barbiturate withdrawal convulsions. Epilepsia 8:21–30, 1967.

Essig, C.F.: Addiction to nonbarbiturate sedative and tranquilizing drugs. Clin Pharmacol Therap 5:334–343, 1964.

Fink, M., & others: Prolonged adverse reactions to LSD in psychotic subjects. Arch Gen Psychiat 15:450–454, 1966.

Fischmann, V.S.: Drug addicts in a therapeutic community. Psychother Psychosom 16:109–118, 1968.

Freedman, A.M., & R.L. Sharoff: Crucial factors in the treatment of narcotic addiction. Am J Psychother 19:397–407, 1965.

Graff, H.: Marihuana and scopolamine "high." Am J Psychiat 125:1258–1259, 1969.

Houston, B.K.: Review of the evidence and qualifications regarding the effects of hallucinogenic drugs on chromosomes and embryos. Am J Psychiat 126:251–253, 1969.

Kramer, J.C.: Methadone maintenance for opiate dependence. California Med 113:6–11, Dec 1970.

Mirin, S.M., & others: Casual versus heavy use of marihuana: A redefinition of the marijuana problem. Am J Psychiat 127:1134–1140, 1971.

Pearson, M.M., & R.B. Little: The addictive process in unusual addictions: A further elaboration of etiology. Am J Psychiat 125:1166–1171, 1969.

Pillard, R.C.: Marihuana. New England J Med 283:294–302, 1970.

Ramer, B.S., Zaslove, M.O., & J. Langan: Is methadone enough? The use of ancillary treatment during methadone maintenance. Am J Psychiat 127:1040–1044, 1971.

Robbins, E.S., & others: College student drug use. Am J Psychiat 126:1743–1751, 1970.

Schremly, J.A., & P. Solomon: Drug abuse and addiction. JAMA 189:512–514, 1964.

Solomon, P.: Medical management of drug dependence. JAMA 206:1521–1526, 1968.

Ungerleider, T.J., & H.L. Bowen: Drug abuse and the schools. Am J Psychiat 125:1691–1696, 1969.

Weil, A.T.: Adverse reaction to marihuana: Classification and suggested treatment. New England J Med 282:997–1000, 1970.

Wikler, A.: On the nature of addiction and habituation. Brit J Addiction 57:73–79, 1961.

22...

Suicide

Suspect the possibility in association with depression or psychosis, present or past. Inquire frankly about death wishes and suicidal ideas or impulses, specifically about actual plans or attempts. Share the responsibility and hospitalize when necessary. In treating a suicidal risk, scrupulously maintain continuous contact with the patient and enlist the help of all possible interested persons.

Suicide is the 10th leading cause of death in the USA. The suicide rate is 12 per 100,000 population, accounting for over 24,000 deaths annually. One suicide occurs about every 20 minutes, and there are 10 unsuccessful attempts to every fatal one. Elsewhere in the world, the suicide rate seems to be increasing, with over 500,000 fatal cases being reported annually.

Suicide is neither a "sign of insanity" nor a "mark of genius." The high incidence of suicide is not due to the "jet age" or the "tensions of civilization." The rate now is not substantially different from what it was in 1900.

Suicide is uniquely a human problem. Most animals can kill, but only man can decide to kill himself.

It is not true that people who threaten to commit suicide never do so. Most people who attempt suicide actually warn someone—often their doctors—beforehand. Potential suicides can usually be recognized before they act.

In the past, suicide was regarded as a heinous offense, a crime against the state, and one that called for retaliation and vengeance by society. The Common Law in England confiscated the suicide's property in the name of the Crown. (It was said that you could not commit suicide "on pain of being regarded as a criminal if you failed and a lunatic if you succeeded.") Other penalties for attempted or successful suicide were social banishment and religious excommunication, and the sacrament of last rites (and burial in hallowed ground) was denied.

Toward the end of the last century, many suicides were believed to be caused by reading trashy novels or romantic sentimental stories such as Goethe's *Sorrows of Werther*. After 1900, suicides (and most social ills) were attributed to a faulty educational system. During the 1930s, a blues ballad

("Gloomy Sunday") was banned from the radio because it was said that a rash of suicides always occurred after it was played. After World War I and through the depression years, constitutional and hereditary factors were held responsible; since then, with the upsurge of psychoanalytic influence, deeper underlying motivation has been sought.

PSYCHOLOGIC THEORIES OF THE CAUSES OF SUICIDE

Freud believed that the loss of someone on whom an individual is ambivalently dependent results in pathologic depression. During the period of mourning, the individual takes into himself (incorporates) the image of the departed person and begins to have the same feelings toward himself that he had toward the departed person. The unconscious hostility originally directed toward the lost person then becomes directed against the self and may culminate in the ultimate act of self-hostility, self-destruction. Suicide can thus be regarded as "murder in the 180th degree." Freud linked suicide also with "the death instinct," a concept that explains nothing and is essentially a tautology.

According to Menninger, suicide is an act of self-murder. The person involved must have the wish to kill, the wish to be killed, and the wish to be dead.

Schneidman and Farberow classify people who commit suicide into 4 general types: (1) Those whose beliefs induce them to view suicide as a transition to a better life or as a means of saving reputation (eg, hara-kiri); (2) those who are old, bereaved, or in physical pain, who regard suicide as a release; (3) those who are psychotic and kill themselves in response to hallucinations or delusions; and (4) those who kill themselves out of spite, with the belief that people will mourn and that they themselves will somehow still be around to witness their sorrow.

Others have stressed numerous additional psychologic factors. Friendless children or those with a history of poor impulse control may commit suicide in the apparent absence of depression following some trivial frustration such as a minor injury or accident (often after running away from home). In adults, the escape from an intolerable real life situation is often stressed. If there have been suicides in the family, identification is considered a factor of importance, the suicide often occurring as an "anniversary phenomenon" (eg, a woman committing suicide at age 40, the age at which her mother committed suicide). Suggestion may also be a factor, especially in determining the method used, eg, after seeing suicide portrayed on TV or in a movie, or following the suicide of a celebrity (eg, Marilyn Monroe). However, recent attempts to evaluate the influence of newspaper articles on suicides (by studying the suicide rates before, during, and after prolonged newspaper strikes in certain cities) have been inconclusive.

In the psychodynamics of suicide, serious losses (or threats of loss) take high priority. These include loss of health, loved ones, money, earning power, job, pride, beauty, honor, status ("success"), independence, and friends, and the "empty nest syndrome" (when the children have grown and moved away). Chronic or terminal illness often contributes to loneliness, emptiness, and "existential dread" that presages suicide. Suicide is readily understandable in prisoners facing execution or spies anticipating capture or torture.

Suicide has been called "a litany of the dire consequences of alienation, disfranchisement, ostracism, and disparagement"—also an act "designed to put an end to all future competition by the final play of an unbeatable trump in a winner-take-all competition," paradoxically seeking to convert a total loss to a gain (in the unconscious).

Most authorities agree that there is rarely a single precipitating cause of suicide and that several are usually operative in an additive way. Some take a neurophysiologic approach and feel that the final decision to commit suicide may depend on weakening of the higher cerebrocortical functions, with sleeplessness, barbiturates, and alcohol often playing a contributory part. Anxiety may serve as a protective mechanism by means of the cerebral excitation it causes. Grinker confesses, "I do not know—despite lengthy clinical experience—what the dynamics are that push the patient from thought to action."

Suicide may be considered the final common pathway and outcome of a progressive failure of adaptation, with isolation and alienation from the usual network of human relations that support us all and give meaning to our lives, and with waning of that vital and mysterious force that makes every living creature want to stay alive.

SOCIOLOGIC THEORIES OF THE CAUSES OF SUICIDE

Suicide and the Intensity of the Relational System

The more intimately one is involved with others, the less the wish for suicide. The suicide rate is higher in cities (where apartment dwellers often do not know one another) than in rural areas; higher in the centers of cities than in residential areas; and higher among the divorced and widowed than among the married. Interestingly, both the married state and the state of war are associated with a low suicide rate and a high homicide rate.

Suicide and Business Cycle

A downward trend in the business cycle is associated with an increase in suicide, especially in the upper socioeconomic classes where the losses are greatest.

The Relationship to Social Status

There is a direct relationship between suicide and social status. In the American army, the suicide rate is higher among officers than enlisted men, and in society at large blacks are less susceptible to suicide than whites. Professional workers are more susceptible than laborers. The higher one is on the social scale, the more susceptible one becomes to suicide.

Sex Incidence

In 1960, the suicide rate for white males was 16.6 per 100,000; for white women, 4.7 per 100,000. On the West Coast of the USA, however, there have been more successful suicides in women than in men. The rate for Negro men in 1960 was 6.8 per 100,000 and for Negro women 1.4 per 100,000. Conversely, the rates for "attempted" suicide are reversed, women "attempting" suicide at least 5 times as frequently as men. Possible explanations for the sex discrepancy are that women are more protected in our society and mental health care is more available to them, whereas men are not supposed to "cry for help."

Influence of Culture and Religion

Catholic countries generally have lower suicide rates than non-Catholic countries. Ireland has a suicide rate of 2.5 per 100,000, whereas Sweden's rate is 20.1 per 100,000. In the USA, the rate is higher among Protestants than among any other religious group. (Paradoxically, Austria, a Catholic country, has a high suicide rate.)

The prevalent cultural attitude toward suicide is important in the incidence. In the USA, where suicide is condemned, the incidence of suicide is relatively low; in Japan, where it is praised, it is high. However, incidence figures are suspect because of the widely disparate and often inaccurate methods of reporting.

Age Incidence

In the USA, the most significant pattern in the incidence of suicide is the increase with advancing age. Suicide is rare among the young; between the ages of 5–14 years, the rate in 1960 was 0.3 per 100,000. In adolescents from 15–19, there is a marked rise, and suicide is the third ranking cause of death in this age group. In college students it is the second ranking cause of death (after accidents), and men are twice as apt to commit suicide as women. The rate increases with age, so that for the population 85 years of age and older the overall incidence is 26 per 100,000. For white males over age 85, the incidence is almost 70 per 100,000.

ASSESSMENT OF SUICIDAL RISK AND SUICIDE ATTEMPT

Attempted suicide is a common medical emergency, and all such cases should be evaluated by a psychiatrist (see Chapter 23 and the Psychiatric Emergency Routine at the end of this book). A common pitfall for the physician is to regard a suicidal attempt as "only a gesture," to discover later that the patient has successfully committed suicide.

Self-destructive behavior can take many forms, ranging from the consistently reckless "accident prone," self-mutilative person to the protest demonstrator who lies down in front of a car and to the chronic alcoholic whose life may be regarded as a chronic suicide attempt. In assessing the patient who has attempted suicide, a decision must be made about the seriousness of his intent to kill himself.

Grave Risk

A. The Wish to Die: Repeated statements by the patient that he would be better off dead should be treated with the utmost gravity.

B. Presence of Psychosis: The psychotic patient who is impulsive and suspicious, inappropriately fearful, or subject to states of panic should be regarded as potentially suicidal. The risk is greatly increased if, in addition, the patient hears voices commanding him to kill himself.

C. Depression: Depression is the most common precursor of suicide, and the depressed patient who exhibits the following symptoms in severe form should be regarded as a serious risk:

1. Guilt, especially over a dead relative.
2. Feelings of worthlessness and despondency.
3. Intense wish for punishment.
4. Withdrawal and hopelessness.
5. Extreme agitation and anxiety.
6. Loss of the 4 appetites—food, sex, sleep, and activity.

Danger Signs

Any of the following indicates a definite risk of suicide:

A. Previous Attempts: Over half of those who commit suicide have a history of a previous attempt. The setting of the attempt is also an important indication of the seriousness of suicidal intent. If the attempt is made with no one present and the chance of interruption is slight, the wish for death is great. If it takes place in the company of others or in circumstances where it is anticipated that others will intervene, the wish for death is slight.

B. Previous Psychosis: A history of any previous psychiatric episode suggests the possibility of a recurrence, with increased danger of suicide.

C. Suicide Note: Any suicide note must be considered a dangerous sign.

D. Violent Method: In general, the more violent and painful the method chosen, the greater the risk of suicide.

E. Chronic Disease: Patients with severe chronic illnesses may commit suicide at the height of a depressive response to illness.

F. Recent Surgery or Childbirth: The birth of a baby may cause a pathologic depressive reaction in some women. Major surgery, especially mutilative or subtractive surgery, may entail similar risk.

G. Alcoholism and Drug Dependence: Alcohol and other drugs, because of their effect in weakening controls, may contribute materially to the suicidal impulse.

H. Hypochondriasis: Constant and varied physical complaints without organic cause may conceal an underlying dangerous depression.

I. Advancing Age: Particularly in men, advancing age, with its concomitants of failing and "not having made it" or of "life having passed me by," may induce the feeling that life is not worth living. In some women, the menopause, with attendant feelings of depression and loss of worth as a woman, is a time of suicidal risk.

J. Homosexuality: Homosexuals are unusually subject to emotional maladjustment and depression, and their suicide rate is high.

K. Social Isolation: This frequently indicates that other people can no longer help and signifies that the depression is serious.

L. Chronic Maladjustment: The patient with a long history of turbulent or unsatisfactory interpersonal relationships is a poor risk.

M. Bankrupt Resources: The patient without money, job, friends, or future prospects has less to live for than the financially and socially successful patient. Freud was once reported to have said, in a jocular mood, "It is better to be rich and healthy than sick and poor."

N. No Apparent Secondary Gains: If the patient's suicidal threat was directed at some person in the environment, perhaps in an attempt to manipulate or to appeal for help, the risk is decreased. When there is no obvious secondary gain and the threat and urge are truly directed against the patient himself, the risk is greater.

PREVENTION OF SUICIDE

Many organizations ("Rescue," "Save a Life," etc) are available to help individuals with suicidal impulses. In many large cities, one can telephone for help at any hour of the day or night.

Experience has taught many practical tips: Neurotic patients in therapy may frequently speak of suicide, but—unlike others who speak of suicide—they almost never become serious risks.

Beware of sudden well-being in a previously depressed patient. He may be feeling relief at having made the decision to die.

If you decide to hospitalize a suicidal patient, do not let him go home alone to get ready.

Do not discontinue antidepressant medication abruptly.

Accidental overdosage with barbiturates does occur and can be fatal. The mentally befogged patient forgets how much he has taken. Suicide with barbiturates is 5 times as frequent as with tranquilizer drugs. Avoid giving lethal amounts in one prescription.

In appealing to a man on a ledge threatening to jump, use anything he seems to respond to—religion, listening, simple attention, warmth, or bringing in relatives, friends, or a priest. He is usually psychotic, feels friendless and bereft, and should be hospitalized. Patients in therapy who rationally threaten suicide often have temporary "tunnel vision," and their perspective has to be broadened. If they have children or other close relatives, emphasize the right of everyone to lead a life unstigmatized by the suicide of a near relation.

Do not hesitate to bring up the subject of suicide in a patient who has not mentioned it if he is depressed or if you have other reason to suspect he may be considering it. Studies have shown that bringing up the subject has never harmed anyone and has helped a great many.

In talking about how to tell a "gesture" from a genuine suicidal attempt, Grinker points out that the only honest answer is, "Guess." Informed clinical judgment is the only diagnostic tool available in most such cases.

TREATMENT

When the patient is seriously suicidal, the first course of action should be hospitalization. The patient should be placed on suicidal precautions, and every care should be taken to protect him against his impulses. During hospitalization, one or all of the following treatments may be instituted: (1) electroconvulsive treatment; (2) drugs, particularly the antidepressants; and (3) psychotherapy, to help the patient find some solution to his problems other than self-destruction.

Overhospitalization should be avoided. The doctor's trust may be an extremely valuable treatment measure if the physician can control his own anxiety. In any case a patient really intent on suicide can often manage to kill himself even in the best psychiatric hospitals. Adolph Meyer once said, "A mental hospital in which suicide doesn't occur cannot be a good hospital." Such a hospital would be too restrictive.

In psychotherapy, the development of a positive transference may be vital. See the patient often, even more than once a day if necessary, during crucial periods. Let him have access to you by telephone at all times of the day or night. If you must be out of town, let him know where you will be and how he can reach you.

PROGNOSIS

The principal factors that influence the outcome are the following:

(1) **The patient**: The better the former adjustment and the greater the immediate stress that precipitated the suicide attempt, the better the prognosis (when the stress is over).

(2) **The environment**: The more supportive the environment, the greater the number of people who care for the patient, and the greater the number of things that give meaning to the patient's existence, the more optimistic the outcome.

REFERENCES

Books and Monographs

Dublin, L.I.: *Suicide: A Sociological and Statistical Study*. Ronald Press, 1963.

Farberow, N.L., E.S. Shneidman: *The Cry for Help*. McGraw-Hill, 1961.

Meerloo, J.A.M.: *Suicide and Mass Suicide*. Grune & Stratton, 1962.

Menninger, K.: *Man Against Himself*. Harcourt Brace, 1938.

Retterstol, N.: *Long-Term Prognosis After Attempted Suicide: A Personal Follow-up Examination*. Thomas, 1970.

Shneidman, E.S., & N.L. Farberow (editors): *Clues to Suicide*. McGraw-Hill, 1957.

Shneidman, E.S., Farberow, N.L., & C.V. Leonard: *Some Facts About Suicide.* US Public Health Service, 1961.

Shneidman, E.S., Farberow, N.L., & R.E. Litman: *The Psychology of Suicide.* Science House, 1970.

Shneidman, E.S., & D.D. Swenson (editors): *Suicide Among Youth.* US Government Printing Office, 1969.

Wolff, K.: *Patterns of Self-Destruction: Depression and Suicide.* Thomas, 1970.

Journal Articles

Abram, H.S., Moore, G.L., & F.B. Westervelt, Jr.: Suicidal behavior in chronic dialysis patients. Am J Psychiat 127:1199–1204, 1971.

Blaine, G., Jr.: Causal factors in suicidal attempts by male and female college students. J Am Psychiat 125:834–837, 1968.

Bruhn, J.G.: Broken homes among attempted suicides and psychiatric outpatients: A comparative study. J Ment Sc 108:772–779, 1962.

Diggory, J.C.: Calculation of some costs of suicide prevention using certain predictors of suicidal behavior. Psychol Bull 71:373–386, 1969.

Farberow, N.L.: Training in suicide prevention for professional and community agents. Am J Psychiat 125:1702–1705, 1969.

Fawcett, J., Leff, M., & W.E. Bunney, Jr.: Suicide. Arch Gen Psychiat 21:129–137, 1969.

Haughton, A.B.: Suicide prevention programs: The current scene. Am J Psychiat 124:1692–1696, 1968.

Havens, L.L.: Recognition of suicidal risks through the psychologic examination. New England J Med 276:210–215, 1967.

Hilgard, J.R., & M.F. Newman: Anniversaries in mental illness. Psychiatry 22:113, 1959.

Hirsh, J.: Suicide. Ment Hyg 43:516–524, 1959; 44:3–10, 274–280, 382–388, 1960.

Hoch, P.H.: Psychodynamics and psychotherapy of depressions. Canad Psychiat AJ 4(Suppl):24, 1959.

Kreitman, N., Smith, P., & E.S. Tan: Attempted suicide as language: Empiric study. Brit J Psychiat 116:465–473, 1970.

Lester, D., & G.W. Brockopp: Chronic callers to a suicide prevention center. Commun Ment Health J 6:246–250, 1970.

Lindemann, E.: Symptomatology and management of acute grief. Am J Psychiat 101:141, 1944.

Litman, R.E., & others: Suicide-prevention telephone service. JAMA 192:21–25, 1965.

Lukianowicz, N.: Attempted suicide in children. Acta psychiat scandinav 44:415–435, 1968.

Macdonald, J.M.: Suicide and homicide by automobile. Am J Psychiat 121:366–370, 1964.

Mattsson, A., Seese, L.R., & J.W. Hawkins: Suicidal behavior as a child psychiatric emergency. Arch Gen Psychiat 20:100–109, 1969.

Perr, I.N.: Liability of hospital and psychiatrist in suicide. Am J Psychiat 122:631–637, 1965.

Resnik, H.L.P., & L.H. Dizmang: Observations on suicidal behavior among American Indians. Am J Psychiat 127:882–887, 1971.

Robins, E., & others: Some clinical considerations in the prevention of suicide based on a study of 134 successful suicides. Am J Pub Health 49:888–889, 1959.

Rosen, D.H.: The serious suicide attempt: Epidemiological and follow-up study of 886 patients. Am J Psychiat 127:764–770, 1970.

Ross, M.: Suicide among college students. Am J Psychiat 126:220–225, 1969.

Rubenstein, C.R., Moses, R., & T. Lidz: On attempted suicide. Arch Neurol Psychiat 79:103, 1958.

Shein, H.M., & A.A. Stone: Psychotherapy designed to detect and treat suicidal potential. Am J Psychiat 125:1247–1251, 1969.

Solomon, P.: The burden of responsibility in suicide and homicide. JAMA 199:99–102, 1967.

Stengel, E.: Enquiries into attempted suicide. Proc Roy Soc Med 45:613, 1952.

Stone, A.A.: A syndrome of serious suicidal intent. Arch Gen Psychiat 3:331, 1960.

Tabachnick, N.: The crisis treatment of suicide. California Med 112:1–8, June 1970.

Veith, I.: Reflections on the medical history of suicide. Mod Med 37:116–121, 1969.

Weiss, J.H.A.: Suicide: An epidemiologic analysis. Psychiat Quart 28:225, 1954.

PART III.
PSYCHIATRIC TREATMENT

23...

Psychiatric Emergencies

A condensed Psychiatric Emergency Routine is given following the index.

A psychiatric emergency is a disturbance of behavior, affect, or thought for which immediate treatment is judged to be necessary by (1) the patient, because of his discomfort; (2) his family, friends, or the authorities, because of the manifest signs; or (3) the physician, because of the prognosis if untreated. A psychiatric emergency may be a new illness with an acute onset or an acute exacerbation of a chronic illness.

Emergencies with psychiatric symptomatology fall into 2 large categories: those due to psychogenic and those due to nonpsychogenic causes.

The psychiatric examination (Chapter 4) may be of value in helping to differentiate the two. Patients with emergencies of nonpsychogenic origin are generally delirious and show markedly disordered behavior with an intense degree of any or all of the following: anxiety, excitement, disorientation, helplessness, hopelessness, impaired reality testing, labile affect, poor judgment, and inadequate impulse control. These patients require careful evaluation and diagnosis to determine which ones need immediate specific therapy. Some of the disorders are life-threatening and may require medical consultation if the diagnosis is not clear.

Patients may be seen in their homes, may come to the office or hospital alone, or may be brought in by relatives, friends, or the police. They represent emergencies because they may do harm to themselves or to others or because immediate treatment is necessary to avert a catastrophic or even a fatal outcome.

Emergency psychiatric patients are usually overactive or underactive (and possibly suicidal). Overactive patients may be violent, requiring antipsychotic drugs or, at times, physical restraints; others may be agitated, panicky, and anxious, requiring calming and sedation before the causes of their distress can be investigated. A drunken patient may manifest any of the symptoms of overactivity or may be underactive. Patients in drug withdrawal may have a combination of symptoms, although they are usually overactive.

Underactive, depressed, and suicidal patients will usually need hospitalization and close observation. Attempts at suicide must be anticipated and prevented.

On first contact with the patient, the physician should demonstrate an attitude of kind firmness and confidence. This attitude is likely to be communicated to the patient and will help to calm him. It is well to explain the situation to the patient and to interview him privately, if possible. With disturbed patients it is best to open the interview with neutral topics before exploring conflict-laden issues. If the patient appears hostile or resistant, the physician should question him about his attitude rather than ignore it. The patient should be encouraged to put his thoughts and feelings into words instead of into actions.

In evaluating a psychiatric emergency, it is important to distinguish between the signs and symptoms of the immediate disorder and longstanding characterologic problems which must be considered in total management. A physical examination and psychiatric (mental status) evaluation should be performed when possible. Since the patient may be an unreliable informant, a history should be obtained from relatives, friends, or the police. Particular emphasis should be placed on the following:

(1) Detailed history of the chief complaint.

(2) Recent changes in life situation—physical illness and, particularly, losses (real or imaginary).

(3) Level of adjustment prior to the emergency.

(4) Use of drugs.

(5) Past history of medical illness.

(6) Past history of psychiatric illness and response to treatment.

(7) Family history of medical illness.

(8) Family history of psychiatric illness.

PSYCHOGENIC PSYCHIATRIC EMERGENCIES

ATTEMPTED SUICIDE

A suicide attempt may occur in many psychiatric conditions (see Chapter 22). It is the physician's responsibility to give immediate medical aid and prevent further self-injury. Since many patients are still seriously suicidal when brought to the physician, they must be carefully supervised during and after the initial examination. The physician's primary task is to render medical attention: stop bleeding; assist respiration with oxygen, tracheostomy, and artificial respiration, and keep the airway open; and support the cardiovascular system with appropriate measures. If the suicide attempt was by poison, the stomach should usually be lavaged immediately with large quantities of water since the emptying time of the stomach is prolonged by many drugs. The dangers of aspiration must be guarded against. A corrosive poison requires neutralization before lavage if the patient is seen more than 1 hour after exposure.

Immediately after the patient's physical safety has been assured, the reasons for the suicide attempt and the seriousness of the patient's wish to die should be investigated. If the patient has made a serious attempt—ie, one which would reasonably be expected to have been successful, such as jumping from a window, hanging, gunshot to a vital area, or massive ingestion of medication—he should be hospitalized under psychiatric supervision, preferably on a psychiatric ward if his medical condition will permit. If on a medical ward (preferably on a first floor level), he must have 24-hour special nursing care. The greatest problem in evaluation arises in patients who have made minimal or "benign" suicide attempts, in which case the degree of suicidal intent must be evaluated. If such a patient can be interviewed early (while his psychologic defenses are still disorganized), the physician will be better able to determine the patient's real wishes.

The patient's attitudes toward death and his expectations of the consequences of his act are of importance. The patient may safely be discharged to outpatient care if the suicide attempt was clearly manipulative and not expected to result in death; if the patient called for assistance soon afterward; and if he convincingly expresses repentance for his act and denies any intention of repeating it. However, the severity of suicidal gestures should not be minimized, since many successful suicides result from "gestures" that turn out to be more successful than intended. Once a patient has made a suicidal gesture, the chance of his using this method in the future either to release psychologic tensions or to achieve an effect is increased.

If the patient has made a suicide attempt and expresses no regret over the action and a continuing wish to die, he must be hospitalized for treatment. Patients with feelings of guilt and unworthiness who state that they would be "better off dead" or that the world would be better if they were dead are especially poor risks. This is true also of elderly depressed alcoholics; patients with chronic or progressive organic illnesses; patients in alcoholic hallucinosis; schizophrenic patients responding to hallucinations—especially auditory hallucinations commanding them to kill themselves; and patients with a family history of suicide.

THREATENED SUICIDE

The fear of committing suicide is a frequent chief complaint. If it presents as the obsessive thought, "What if I should kill myself?" and the patient denies any wish to die and has no significant depressive symptomatology, the complaint may be explained to the patient as an obsessive thought and he may be reassured that he will never act on it. This reduces his anxiety, and treatment can then be directed toward the obsessional illness. If the patient expresses a fear of committing suicide, a decision must be made about its probability. The patient's reasons for fearing that he may commit suicide should be investigated as well as his thoughts about what effect his death would have on those around him and his expectations about life after death. If he sees no solution to his difficulties other than suicide, he should probably be hospitalized for his own protection. If, on the basis of the initial evaluation, the patient can be restored to hope and a feeling of mastery of himself and his situation—and if solutions to his problems other than suicide can be arrived at—he may be treated as an outpatient provided that he agrees to be seen frequently and the therapist is readily available.

Common reasons for committing suicide are (1) to escape suffering and despair; (2) to punish oneself for guilt, real or imaginary; and (3) to punish a significant figure in the environment. When the possibility of suicide is substantial, the responsibility for hospitalizing the patient should be shared with the relatives. If the physician believes the patient should be hospitalized but the patient and his relatives refuse to consent, involuntary commitment (with the cooperation of legal authorities) should be considered (see also Chapter 22).

ATTEMPTED HOMICIDE

Homicide or attempted homicide is a police matter, and the psychiatrist may be asked for an opinion about the suspect's degree of criminal responsibility (see Chapters 4 and 37). The sooner after the incident the suspect is interviewed, the more reliable will be the psychiatrist's opinion of his mental status at the time it occurred. Therefore, every effort should be made to interview the suspect immediately.

THREATENED HOMICIDE

Threatened homicide and the fear of committing homicide—particularly a mother's fear that she might harm her children—are not uncommon. If this thought takes the form, "What if I should do such-and-such to hurt my child?" and is associated with a great deal of anxiety, and if the patient's impulse control is good and she denies any conscious wish to harm the child, the patient may be assured that this is an obsessive thought that will never be acted on and treatment may be directed toward the basic illness. If the patient threatens homicide, a judgment must be made about its probability. A patient who threatens homicide in response to hallucinations or delusions must be hospitalized.

In other patients who threaten homicide, the reasons for their threats should be investigated and the consequences of their actions pointed out to them. Most patients who are able to discuss the reasons for homicidal thoughts will be able to see less destructive ways to express their feelings, and these patients rarely commit homicide. The possibility must be considered that the target of such feelings may be serving as a scapegoat for someone else, or that the patient is seeking someone to blame for his own faults and problems.

Since most homicides occur in periods of intense excitement, poor judgment, and impaired impulse control, patients who have concern about homicide should avoid situations that will bring these about—especially situations in which arguments and controversy may be expected. They should above all avoid the use of alcohol or drugs. The companionship of a responsible friend during periods of stress should be recommended.

If the patient has taken any action toward homicide (such as acquiring a gun or a knife) or has made concrete plans or shown indications of overpowering impulsiveness, at least part of the burden of responsibility then falls on the physician. In most cases he must report the matter to relatives and authorities even if the patient objects. If he feels he can carry the responsibility entirely himself, he should at least arrange to see the patient frequently and investigate vigorously any missed appointment.

ASSAULTIVE BEHAVIOR

Assaultive behavior occurs in a variety of psychiatric conditions, and the physician must protect himself and others (and the patient) from injury. It is wise to have an attendant present during examinations and interviews, and one or more attendants should always accompany nurses, occupational therapists, visitors, and other vulnerable persons onto wards where physical assaults are possible. Chlorpromazine (Thorazine), 100 mg IM, is usually sufficient to calm assaultive patients, but more may be given provided it does not sedate the patient so much that he is unable to participate in examinations and ward routines.

In psychotic patients, assaultive behavior arises chiefly out of fear or out of anger due to frustration; less often, it is a direct response to auditory hallucinations or delusions. The examination should be directed toward determining and alleviating the cause of the assaultive behavior. During the examination, although the physician is nonthreatening, he should be aware that the patient may misinterpret his words and deeds. What the physician assumes to be nonthreatening may be perceived as a threat by the patient.

Patients with antisocial reactions and emotionally unstable personalities also may show assaultive behavior. It is desirable to help them institute their own internal controls by pointing out the consequences of their actions and helping them to understand the conscious and unconscious causes of their behavior. However, if this is not possible in acute situations, the patient should be confronted with overwhelming force so that the assaultive behavior will obviously be useless to him. Physical restraints such as straitjackets, locked rooms, cold packs, and padded cells are now rarely necessary. The best sedative is a calm, firm, sympathetic doctor or nurse; proper medication is a close second.

Patients under the influence of alcohol whose repressed impulses erupt may become assaultive. It is important to evaluate these patients after the effects of the alcohol have worn off, since many psychotic patients self-medicate themselves with alcohol.

FUGUE STATES

As a part of a dissociative reaction, the patient may suffer from a fugue, which is a state of altered consciousness resulting in dazed or bewildered behavior. During fugue states, patients may commit acts which their consciences would not ordinarily permit. A patient interviewed during a fugue state usually does not remember his name and has amnesia for previous incidents of his life.

An interview under light intravenous barbiturate anesthesia is useful in obtaining a history and assisting the patient to recall facts for which he is amnesic; in skilled hands, hypnosis may be used. An intense emotional experience, such as the arousal of unacceptable sexual, aggressive, or guilt feelings, is frequently the precipitating event. Most of these patients have hysterical personalities, and the prognosis for recovery from the immediate episode is excellent. Head injuries, temporal lobe epilepsy, and alcoholism must be included in the differential diagnosis. A background of character neurosis is usually present, and this is refractory to all but prolonged treatment.

MANIC-DEPRESSIVE PSYCHOSIS, MANIC TYPE

Manic patients become a management problem because of their grandiosity, boisterousness, poor judgment, overactivity, overtalkativeness, and flights of ideas. They are brought to the attention of a psychiatrist by their families or friends or by the police. It is important to remember that manic patients are sometimes able to control their behavior for brief periods and may present a normal facade to the examiner; however, if the interview is left unstructured and the patient is allowed to talk freely, his psychosis soon becomes evident. A third person history is particularly important in these cases since the patient himself is an unreliable informant.

In caring for these patients the physician must bear in mind that they cannot be relied upon to keep their promises no matter how sincere they may appear to be; if their behavior seems likely to be harmful to them, either financially or socially, they should be hospitalized for treatment with drugs or electroshock. For immediate management, chlorpromazine (Thorazine), 100 mg IM, is usually sufficient, although some patients may require 2–3 times this dose. The use of lithium carbonate in these cases is still in the experimental stage, but this drug promises to become the treatment of choice (see Chapter 24).

DOMESTIC CRISES

Domestic crises are usually caused by a breakdown in communications between marital partners or between parents and children and may be manifested by physical abuse, alcoholism, or arguments with threats of violence and suicide. The patients should be interviewed together briefly to determine what each feels to be the problem, and then interviewed separately in a traditional psychiatric manner to determine whether either is mentally ill. If one is, appropriate treatment should be offered; if not, the parties should be brought together again and interviewed jointly. The goal of this interview is to establish meaningful communication and encourage the patients to express their complaints verbally rather than by acting out. It must be emphasized to them that they must both be willing to negotiate a settlement and accede to the other's reasonable requests. In crisis situations, positive recommendations for their behavior and alternative solutions to their problems should be given immediately if possible. Provocative behavior and the ways in which each sabotages the other's goals should be made clear. The impulsive actions the individuals may use in an attempt to resolve crises should be forbidden. At the termination of the first interview, a second appointment should be scheduled in which the patients will be asked to discuss their efforts to resolve their difficulties.

PANIC REACTION, ANXIETY TYPE

Patients with panic reactions may complain of a general fear of impending disaster about which they are unable to be more specific; may fear loss of control; or may express a specific dread—all accompanied by autonomic nervous system dysfunction. A detailed history of the circumstances surrounding the initial attack should be obtained. The physician's approach should be one of keen interest, assurance, and desire to help. Frequently there will be an obvious precipitating cause of which the patient will be unaware until he is questioned specifically. If the precipitating cause can be established, it should be discussed fully with the patient and an explanation of the cause of his anxiety offered to him, with the expectation that when the cause of his anxiety becomes conscious he will be able to deal with it and that the symptoms of anxiety as a defense will no longer be necessary. The common causes of panic reactions are unconscious aggressive and sexual impulses.

It is often difficult and unnecessary to explore the causes of the panic during the crisis. The physician may postpone delving for causes until he has a more relaxed and cooperative patient. If no cause for the panic reaction can be found, the patient should be reassured that no major mental illness is present and be given an appointment to return for more prolonged investigation into the cause of his anxiety. He should not be given premature and meaningless reassurance. Until the cause is established, the patient should be offered tranquilizers with the explanation that they will not remove the anxiety but will reduce it to a tolerable level. Chlordiazepoxide (Librium), 25 mg orally 4 times a day; diazepam (Valium), 5 mg orally 4 times a day; or trifluoperazine (Stelazine), 2 mg orally 3 times a day, may be given initially and the doses increased until the symptoms are alleviated or the side-effects of the drugs (chiefly drowsiness or extrapyramidal symptoms) become severe. If one drug is not effective, another should be tried. If, as is often the case, a depressive element is present, antidepressant medication such as desipramine (Pertofrane, Norpramin), 25 mg orally 3 times a day, should be considered in addition. The physiologic concomitants of anxiety (palpitations, hyperventilation, muscle tension, vascular changes, etc) should be explained logically as part of the fight-or-flight mechanism.

The prognosis for the individual panic attack is excellent, since it rarely lasts more than a few hours with or without treatment. Unfortunately, recurrences are common, sometimes within a few hours and in some cases not for days or weeks. The determining factor is the elimination or modification of the underlying cause through psychotherapy.

PANIC REACTION, HYPOCHONDRIACAL TYPE

In patients with a fear of dying, whether generalized or with specific complaints, the first step is a thorough medical examination so that the patient can be assured that there is no medical illness. A detailed history of the circumstances surrounding the attack should be taken, with emphasis on the meaning of the symptoms to the patient and on the search for significant persons in the patient's life with similar symptoms—particularly if there has been an anniversary or other circumstance which has brought the idea of death to the patient's attention. If these can be found, the connection between the cause and the effect should be made clear. If not, the patient should be given another appointment and tranquilizers prescribed in the interim.

The physician must make it clear that he accepts the symptoms as real in spite of the negative physical findings, and the patient must not feel that his anxiety is regarded as unreasonable or "imaginary." Pointing out that the patient always fears a fatal rather than a benign disease may help the patient to be more objective, and a past history of similar fears which proved groundless is reassuring.

AGITATED DEPRESSION

Patients with agitated depression may present with insomnia, anorexia, fatigue, crying, hopelessness, loss of self-esteem, and guilt, or these may be partially masked by hypochondriacal complaints. Suicidal ideation is common; if the patient seriously expresses the thought that he would be "better off dead," hospitalization is mandatory. If suicide is not considered likely, the patient may be treated on an outpatient basis with a combination of psychotherapy and drugs, the goal of psychotherapy being to restore the patient's feeling of worthiness, to overcome his disappointment, and to make conscious his feelings of anger. Drug treatment directed toward the agitation and depression should be attempted with antidepressants in conjunction with antianxiety agents. If the patient has not improved in a week, the dosage should be increased to the maximum level. If he is no better after 2 weeks and is still severely ill, electroshock treatment should be considered.

During treatment, it is essential that the therapist be available in case a crisis should occur; that the patient's hope for recovery be maintained; that his self-esteem be raised; that he be encouraged to take an active part in helping himself rather than passively waiting for relief; and that he be given sedation to ensure a good night's rest. If, during the course of treatment, the patient's hopelessness and thoughts of suicide increase, he should be hospitalized for his own protection and electroshock treatments started.

TRANSIENT SITUATIONAL DISTURBANCES

The transient situational disturbances ("worried executive" or "harried housewife" syndrome) present as anxiety, tearfulness, hopelessness, and a sense of inability to cope with the situation in which the patient finds himself. Insomnia and fatigue are severe, and if the insomnia is not relieved it will perpetuate the reaction. This syndrome is common among executives promoted to positions of increased responsibility and in housewives placed under increased stress because of geographic removal from family and friends, illness of a child, absence of the husband's emotional support because of his work, or physical illness that prevents them from functioning efficiently.

Psychologic management consists of clarifying the causes of the symptoms and, if possible, removing them. Daytime sedation should be given. However, it must be kept in mind that the tranquilizers may produce dullness and fatigue, so that dextroamphetamine sulfate (Dexedrine) during the day may be indicated. It is particularly important that the patient sleep well at night; chloral hydrate, 0.5–1 gm at bedtime, may be prescribed. If this is ineffective, barbiturates should be used.

PARANOID SCHIZOPHRENIA

Paranoid schizophrenia is characterized by delusions of persecution, and patients with this disorder often present with a fear of being harmed. In the most malignant form of this illness, the patient has a well systematized delusion in which he specifies the persecutor by name. In such cases the patient must be hospitalized.

If the onset is acute, electroshock treatments are indicated. If the onset is gradual, an initial attempt at drug treatment with phenothiazines is indicated; if the patient does not respond within 2–3 weeks, electroshock treatments should be instituted.

When patients present with vague delusions in which the persecutor is indefinite and the purpose of the persecution is not to injure or kill the patient, hospitalization is not mandatory and usually not indicated. Such patients should be offered psychotherapy in an attempt to evoke insight into their own hostility. Oral phenothiazines, in dosages just below those that produce drowsiness, are useful. The physician should be careful not to become too controlling since he may then be included in the patient's delusional system.

Patients with commanding auditory hallucinations should be hospitalized if obeying the command would be harmful to themselves or others. If the commands are benign, these patients may be treated as outpatients; however, they must be closely supervised, since the character of the command may change.

CATATONIC EXCITEMENT

Catatonic excitement is manifested by extremely unpredictable behavior, frequently assaultive and unrelated to external stimuli. The patient's behavior is bizarre and may be grimacing, manneristic, and posturing. He may refuse or be unable to speak; or, if he talks, his speech may be disorganized and incoherent. His hallucinations may have a grandiose or paranoid character. Because of his excitement, he may be constantly overactive, refusing to eat, sleep, or rest. Treatment consists of large doses of phenothiazines, usually given parenterally; if these are insufficient to control his behavior within a few days and he becomes dehydrated, electroshock treatments should be started to prevent death from dehydration and exhaustion.

NONPSYCHOGENIC PSYCHIATRIC EMERGENCIES

Nonpsychogenic psychiatric emergencies are due to organic disorders affecting brain tissue. Regardless of the specific cause, they are characterized by impairment of orientation, memory, intellectual functions (comprehension, calculation, knowledge, learning, apperception, etc), and judgment, and lability and inappropriateness of affect. The specific nature of the symptoms is a function of both the premorbid personality and the area of the brain affected. (See Chapter 15.)

ACUTE ALCOHOLISM

Acute alcoholism is manifested by poor impulse control, drowsiness, incoordination, slurring of speech, and often grandiosity or belligerence. The odor of alcohol may be detected on the breath, and the blood alcohol concentration is over 150 mg/100 ml.

If the patient is drowsy, the best treatment is to allow him to sleep it off; if he is belligerent, sedation with paraldehyde or chlorpromazine given orally is desirable. If the patient refuses to take the medication orally, chlorpromazine (50 mg) may be given IM. (Observe carefully for respiratory depression if the patient is still drowsy from the effects of alcohol.) It is important to rule out organic diseases—particularly trauma, subdural hematoma, and acute infection (especially pneumonia), which are common in alcoholics—as well as diabetes, hypoglycemia, cardiac decompensation, and uremia.

PATHOLOGIC SENSITIVITY TO ALCOHOL

Dipsomania or pathologic intoxication is an unusual sensitivity to the effects of alcohol in which the patient responds with compulsive, furious, and disorganized behavior to small amounts of alcohol. Treatment is the same as for alcoholism but with the special aim of preventing the patient from harming himself or others (through sedation and restraint if necessary). An EEG should be taken to rule out epilepsy, and the patient should be forbidden to drink.

DELIRIUM TREMENS

Delirium tremens is a toxic state that occurs in response to withdrawal or diminution of alcoholic intake. It is particularly common in patients who are withdrawn from alcohol when admitted to the hospital for treatment of pneumonia or fractures. The symptoms are anxiety, tremulousness, irritability, agitation, and insomnia, followed by visual hallucinations, frequently of small, frightening animals or shapes. Tactile and auditory hallucinations may also occur. The patient is frequently frantic, confused, and disoriented, with poor memory and easy distractibility. There is evidence of gross autonomic overactivity with tachycardia, profuse perspiration, nystagmus, and digital tremor, and the patient is difficult to examine because of his restlessness and desire to move. Peripheral neuritis with tenderness in the calves of the legs may be present.

Treatment consists of sedation, such as chlorpromazine (Thorazine), 100 mg 4 times a day orally, and paraldehyde, 12–16 ml orally, in cold fruit juice or cracked ice. The duration of delirium tremens is 2–7 days. Because of the patient's agitation and restlessness, he is difficult to manage on a general medical ward; placement in a seclusion room is recommended. Mechanical restraints are dangerous and should be avoided if possible. The seclusion room should be kept lighted to reduce the incidence of hallucinations, and the presence of an attendant is useful. The patient is usually dehydrated, and fluids should be given—orally if possible, or dextrose and saline solution intravenously if necessary. Vitamins, especially the B group, should be given immediately, intramuscularly at first and then 3 times daily orally. Because of the frequency of convulsions, diphenylhydantoin (Dilantin), 100 mg 3 times a day orally, should be prescribed. Because of the complications of pneumonia and cardiac failure, careful medical supervision is mandatory.

ALCOHOLIC HALLUCINOSIS

Acute alcoholic hallucinosis (a variant of delirium tremens) is a serious psychiatric emergency because the patient may become homicidal or suicidal in response to his hallucinations. Auditory hallucinations of a threatening nature occur, producing intense fear, although the sensorium remains clear. The delusional system forms rapidly and becomes well systematized, and the patient's hallucinations cause much more anxiety than those of the usual schizophrenic patient. These patients must be hospitalized. In the hospital they must be sedated, observed closely, and treated as for delirium tremens.

Alcoholic hallucinosis may be distinguished from delirium tremens by the presence of a clear sensorium and a lack of amnesia for the hallucinatory episode after recovery has taken place.

BARBITURATE WITHDRAWAL

Because of the large number of barbiturate addicts, barbiturate withdrawal has become a serious psychiatric problem with a small but significant mortality rate. Suicidal attempts with overdoses of barbiturates may occur in barbiturate addicts who, after recovery from coma, may develop symptoms of barbiturate withdrawal which resemble delirium tremens: anxiety, restlessness, tremulousness, and convulsions.

Immediate treatment consists of giving barbiturates intravenously in a dose sufficient to produce drowsiness. The addict's daily dose should then be determined and the patient started on this dose; thereafter, the dosage is very gradually reduced (see Chapter 21).

PHENOTHIAZINE TOXICITY

The phenothiazines have a large number of side-effects which create psychiatric emergencies by virtue of the anxiety aroused in the patient. The most common of these are extrapyramidal, with dystonias manifested by spasm of the neck muscles, extensor rigidity of the back muscles, carpopedal spasms, trismus, difficulty in swallowing, and rolling back of the eyes (oculogyric crises); motor restlessness, with a feeling by the patient that he must pace; and pseudoparkinsonism, with mask-like facies, drooling, tremors, and shuffling gait.

Treatment consists of withdrawing the phenothiazine and giving antiparkinsonism drugs such as benztropine mesylate (Cogentin), 2 mg by mouth or IV if necessary, or, if these are not available, diphenhydramine (Benadryl), 10–25 mg slowly IV, repeated as necessary in a dose not to exceed 100 mg.

OTHER DRUG REACTIONS AND DRUG WITHDRAWAL

Meprobamate (Miltown, Equanil), when taken in large doses for prolonged periods, will result in withdrawal symptoms if stopped abruptly. The symptoms are insomnia, severe anxiety, anorexia, vomiting, ataxia, tremors, muscle twitching, and epileptic seizures. Chlordiazepoxide (Librium) in doses over 300 mg/day can produce a similar response when suddenly withdrawn.

Treatment consists of reinstituting the drug and giving phenobarbital 100 mg 3 times a day orally if there are convulsions.

Toxic delirium may be produced by a variety of other sedatives. In patients presenting with an unexplained delirium, a careful investigation of drug use or recent drug withdrawal is indicated. Many nonprescription sedatives and tranquilizers contain agents which may produce toxic psychosis.

BROMIDE INTOXICATION

Bromide delirium is now rare, since bromides are uncommonly prescribed as sedatives; however, bromide is still present in some patent medicines. Symptoms are due to the effect of the bromide on chloride metabolism and are those of toxic psychosis. The presence of dermatitis in a delirious patient should excite a suspicion of bromide poisoning. The diagnosis may be established by a blood bromide level in excess of 150 mg/100 ml.

Treatment consists of administering chloride in the form of sodium chloride or ammonium chloride.

PSYCHOTOMIMETIC DRUGS

Mescaline and lysergic acid diethylamide (LSD) may produce toxic delirium with severe panic, derealization, and depersonalization. The diagnosis can be made by a history of drug ingestion. Treatment consists of withdrawal of the drug and close supervision of the patient. Chlorpromazine (Thorazine) should be used intramuscularly in severe cases.

EPILEPTIC FUROR

Following an epileptic attack, either grand mal or petit mal, the patient may behave in a strange, automatic way and carry out a series of actions which are apparently conscious but of which he has no memory afterward. During this behavior he may become aggressive or assaultive or behave in an unconventional manner.

Immediate treatment consists of giving a barbiturate intravenously. Treatment should then be directed toward control of the epilepsy.

PSYCHOMOTOR EPILEPSY

Psychomotor epilepsy consists of attacks (sometimes with an aura of strange noises in the ear or hallucinations of an unpleasant taste or smell) of disturbance in body sense, feelings of unreality, or disturbances of memory in which the patient may perform automatic acts of which he has little or no awareness. Attacks may last for minutes or hours and may frequently bring the patient to psychiatric attention because of his unexplained behavior. The diagnosis is based on the history and EEG, with particular attention to temporal lobe leads.

Treatment is directed at the underlying cerebral dysrhythmia. Organic cerebral disease should be sought, particularly in the temporal lobes. If none is found, anticonvulsant therapy should be given.

HYPOGLYCEMIA

Hypoglycemia may be manifested by weakness, faintness, hunger, anxiety, emotional instability, and, when severe, disordered consciousness, bizarre behavior, automatic actions, and, rarely, convulsions.

The diagnosis is confirmed by a blood glucose level below 40 mg/100 ml. Treatment consists of giving glucose intravenously—or, if the patient can cooperate, orange juice by mouth—followed by determination of the cause of the hypoglycemia.

HYPERVENTILATION SYNDROME

The hyperventilation syndrome (see Chapter 18) occurs occasionally during an anxiety reaction and consists of air hunger, panicky fear, numbness and tingling of the hands and feet, carpopedal spasm, dizziness, light-headedness, disturbance of consciousness, palpitations, and, rarely, convulsions. The diagnosis may be established by producing the same symptoms by having the patient hyperventilate for 2 minutes while sitting down.

Treatment consists of rebreathing into a paper bag or, if this is impractical, having him hold his breath. Attention should be directed toward the cause of the underlying anxiety reaction.

Hyperventilation may also be caused by intracranial disease, salicylate poisoning, and fever.

THYROTOXICOSIS, MYXEDEMA, AND PARATHYROID DISEASE

Patients with thyrotoxicosis may present with a delirious picture. The usual signs and symptoms of hyperthyroidism are present, and treatment is directed toward the thyroid disorder.

Patients with myxedema may have acute depression or varied psychotic behavior. The diagnosis is based on the symptoms and signs of hypothyroidism. Treatment with thyroid hormone is indicated.

Parathyroid disease may rarely manifest itself first as psychosis, usually schizo-affective, or as neurosis, with varied symptomatology.

POSTPARTUM PSYCHOSIS

Following childbirth—for unknown reasons but perhaps as a result of hormonal changes or of the new responsibilities of the mother—an acute psychosis, usually of the schizo-affective type, may suddenly occur. The signs and symptoms may be manic, depressive, mixed, or schizophrenic, and pharmacologic treatment should be directed toward the predominant symptomatology. It is particularly important that the patient get adequate rest during the day and a good night's sleep. She should also have assistance with care of her baby and supportive psychotherapy.

BRAIN TUMORS

The signs and symptoms of brain tumor (primary or metastatic) depend upon the area of the brain involved. Frontal and temporal lobe tumors may produce no localizing neurologic signs or symptoms, and the patient may be brought to the psychiatrist's attention because of sudden deterioration of personality, poor judgment, poor impulse control, and flattened affect. The emergency management will be according to the predominant symptoms, as above. Special neurologic studies may be necessary to establish or rule out the diagnosis.

SUBDURAL HEMATOMA

Bleeding into the space between the dura mater and the arachnoid, frequently following trauma in alcoholics, may (weeks or months after the trauma) cause headache, fluctuating impairment of consciousness, reduction of intellectual efficiency, or psychosis. The fluctuation in severity of symptoms is sometimes remarkable. The specific neurologic signs and symptoms are those of a space-occupying lesion and are dependent upon the area of the brain affected.

Treatment consists of surgical removal of the clot, which is frequently bilateral.

INFECTIOUS-EXHAUSTIVE PSYCHOSIS

Following high fever, infection, bleeding into tissues, meningitis, or encephalitis, an acute delirium with clouded sensorium, disorientation, excitement, overactivity, poor impulse control, disordered thinking with hallucinations, delusions and illusions, and intense anxiety may occur. Definitive treatment depends upon the specific cause. Chlorpromazine (Thorazine), 50–100 mg orally 4 times a day, fluids, vitamins, measures to lower the temperature, and other appropriate supportive measures are indicated.

ADDISON'S DISEASE

Adrenocortical insufficiency may present with anorexia, vomiting, diarrhea, anxiety, depression, psychomotor retardation, or floridly paranoid symptoms. The diagnosis is confirmed by failure of the adrenal cortex to respond to intramuscular corticotropin (ACTH). Treatment consists of hormone replacement.

PORPHYRIA

This disorder of porphyrin metabolism sometimes is exacerbated by barbiturates and alcohol and produces a peripheral neuropathy with flaccid paralysis, severe pain (frequently abdominal), and signs of bulbar involvement. Because pain can be present with normal physical findings, the psychiatrist may be asked to see the patient. If the attack of pain subsides within 48 hours, it is unlikely that acute porphyria is the cause. The diagnosis is supported by darkening of the urine on standing and established by the Ehrlich aldehyde reaction with a chloroform-insoluble red residue.

No specific treatment is available. Symptomatically, phenothiazines may be helpful. Alcohol and barbiturates must be forbidden.

HOSPITAL EMERGENCY ROOM PROCEDURES*

Many of the procedures discussed above require special modification when employed in the emergency room of a general hospital. In the past 2 decades, there has been considerable growth in the number of general hospitals that maintain psychiatric units and in the number of requests for psychiatric consultations from their emergency rooms. In one general hospital, it is estimated that there are about 250 such requests per month. (These are in addition to over 2000 requests for psychiatric consultation per year from the various wards of the hospital.)

---

*See also Psychiatric Emergency Routine, following index.

The Consultation Process (See also Chapter 38.)

Emergency room requests are dealt with as a consultation verbally requested by the medical or surgical resident on call. Shurley & Pokorny recommend that the consultant answer 4 questions in order to assess the situation: (1) What is the problem? (2) For whom does it constitute an emergency? (3) Is it what it appears? (4) Is it a problem appropriate for the consultant to deal with here and now?

Interviewing the Patient and the Relatives

Eliciting information about the patient follows no absolutely rigid rules, since every case must be dealt with individually. Interviewing the patient on an emergency basis calls for great flexibility and improvisation in the conduct of the interview. If a comprehensive case history is not available, interviewing the relatives or ambulance driver can serve as a useful means of gathering information. Relatives can sometimes be reached by telephone or contacted by the police and may be very helpful in supplying the missing data in the patient's history, particularly if the patient has been previously hospitalized at a mental institution, has been recently ill, or has been taking drugs.

Communication of the Results

This is an important phase of the consultation process since what the consultant communicates, how he communicates, and to whom he communicates have important bearings on the successful outcome of the consultation. In addition to his written report, the consultant should talk personally with the physician requesting the consultation to discuss the rationale of the recommended disposition and to allow the consultee to express his own feelings about the patient. Many consultees are anxious and threatened by the nature of the problem and may occasionally be reluctant to accept what appears to be an overly permissive disposition, eg, sending a patient home after a suicidal gesture.

It is equally important to communicate the results of the consultation to the relatives. This is especially true if the consultant has recommended temporary commitment to a state hospital, as unnecessary legal problems may be avoided by discussing this disposition with the relatives. The consultant ordinarily does not violate confidentiality in this kind of discussion, but he may have to do so (after notifying the patient) in cases where there are threats of suicide or homicide.

TYPES OF EMERGENCIES

The Joint Committee of the American Hospital Association and the American Psychiatric Association recommends the following classification of mentally ill persons who require psychiatric emergency care: (1) Mentally ill persons who seek help or who will accept it voluntarily. (See Voluntary Patients, below.) (2) Nonresistive persons who may not accept care voluntarily at first but who can be persuaded to do so (such as some senile or depressed persons). (See Persuaded Patients, below.) (3) Resistive persons who will not accept care voluntarily and whose behavior may be or may become actually or potentially dangerous to themselves or others. (See Resistive Patients, below.)

Voluntary Patients

A. Anxiety and Panic: Some people with anxiety develop more and more panic until they "lose control." For a discussion of the diagnosis and treatment of these reactions, see pp 339–340 and Chapter 16.

B. Alcohol Intoxication: One of the commonest causes for the appearance of persons at an emergency room and by far the commonest cause of coma on entry is alcohol intoxication. For a discussion of acute alcoholism and the psychiatric complications of alcoholism, see pp 342–344 and Chapter 20.

C. Drug Addiction: Narcotic addicts should be admitted for inpatient drug withdrawal (see Chapter 21). The physician should be alert to addicts masquerading under other diseases in the attempt to obtain treatment with morphine. For a discussion of the psychiatric aspects of drug toxicity and drug withdrawal, see pp 344–345 and Chapter 21.

D. Depression: Mildly depressed patients may present themselves to the emergency room when they are unable to sleep or are restless and agitated. An unhurried psychiatrist who listens to these patients and offers them an appointment for follow-up at the clinic may make a tremendous impact on them and turn the balance against utter despair and helplessness. However, he should not permit the patient to leave if he feels that the danger of suicide is great (see pp 334–336, 340, and Chapters 14 and 16).

Persuaded Patients

This category comprises the more severely depressed patients and the mildly paranoid and senile patients. Most of them benefit by an emphatic talk, and most can be persuaded to report to the outpatient clinic of the general hospital for follow-up.

Resistive Patients

A. Alcohol Withdrawal: This is manifested by a spectrum of behavior that ranges from tremulousness to hallucinosis, convulsive seizures, and delirium tremens. These patients usually are either resistive to any care or are unaware of their predicament. Because of the seriousness of this condition, most of these patients must be admitted to the medical wards of the general hospital for immediate treatment. See pp 343–344 and Chapter 20.

B. The Suicidal Patient: (See also Chapter 22 and pp 334–336.) This is by far the most threatening emergency for the psychiatrist. It is necessary to determine, in an attempted suicide, whether the patient is likely to repeat the attempt, in which case measures must be taken to protect the patient, or whether the act was a mere "gesture" not really intended to lead to death but to afford some secondary gain.

To judge the severity of the threat, 4 practical categories may be employed: (1) The patient has merely thought about suicide. (2) The patient has considered a particular way of committing suicide, such as buying pills, but has not actually done anything about it. (3) The patient has actively procured the means but has not yet attempted to use it. (4) The patient has tried to use the means to commit suicide but has not been successful.

In the last 2 categories (action), it is the responsibility of the psychiatrist to intervene, eg, by hospitalization of the patient or by informing relatives or the authorities.

A summary of the various factors by which to judge the seriousness of a suicide attempt is given in the Psychiatric Emergency Routine on the inside back cover of this book.

C. The Violent or Disturbed Patient: This is the most common major psychiatric emergency. The category includes patients going into psychosis and patients in a toxic or inebriated state. Such patients become hyperactive and threatening, refusing to calm down. Sometimes they react with belligerence to any restraining effort. The psychiatrist should try to gain control of the situation through persuasive questioning and matter-of-fact discussion with the patient (psychologic restraint). Usually it is necessary to employ medication to calm the patient down before a meaningful conversation can be held (chemical restraint). Hospitalization is often necessary (physical restraint). In severe cases the physician may have to call for assistance from colleagues or the police. (See also p 337.)

D. Competency Determination: The psychiatrist may be called to the emergency room to determine the competency of a patient who is refusing treatment. In interviewing the patient, the psychiatrist must clarify 2 points: (1) Does the patient really understand the nature of his illness? (2) Does he recognize the consequences of his refusing treatment? If these 2 questions are affirmatively answered, then the patient is considered competent to refuse treatment even though he might be making an imprudent decision. If either question is answered negatively, as is usually the case if the patient is psychotic, the treatment may be given against the patient's will. (See also p 48.)

TYPES OF DISPOSITIONS

Discharge Home and Follow-up at the Clinic

This applies to the anxious, mildly depressed, and even the compensated psychotic patients seen in the emergency room. This disposition has to be prepared for by an emphatic talk by the psychiatrist. Such a talk should attempt to calm the frightened and anxious patient, soothe the angry patient, clarify reality for the confused, halt foolish or destructive behavior in the impulsive, and offer hope to the patient who has decided to "give up the struggle."

Admission to the Psychiatric Unit at the General Hospital
or Admission to a State Hospital

Whenever the psychiatrist believes that the patient may harm himself or others in the vicinity, it is his responsibility to arrange for hospitalization. Whether this should be in the psychiatric unit of the general hospital or at a state hospital depends on the nature of the problem as well as on the availability of beds. Usually, the more disturbed patient who cannot be handled in an open ward is sent to the state hospital for commitment.

Admission of Psychiatric Patients to the Medical or Surgical Wards
at the General Hospital

Such a disposition may be open to patients with delirium tremens and some suicidal patients, eg, those who attempt to harm themselves seriously by cutting or shooting or other violent means (surgical ward) and those who take sleeping pills, sedatives, tranquilizers, or other drugs (medical wards). When they recover from the acute crisis, they are seen by the psychiatric consultant on the ward who evaluates the suicidal potential and recommends further management.

REFERENCES

Books and Monographs

Bellak, L., & L. Small: *Emergency Psychotherapy and Brief Psychotherapy.* Grune & Stratton, 1965.

Bridges, P.K.: *Psychiatric Emergencies: Diagnosis and Management.* Thomas, 1970.

Caplan, G.: Emotional crises. In: *Encyclopedia of Mental Health.* Deutsch, A., & H. Fishbein (editors). Franklin Watts, 1963.

Lenzer, A.S. (chairman): *Psychiatric Emergencies and the General Hospital.* American Hospital Association, 1965.

The Psychiatric Emergency. The Joint Information Service of the American Psychiatric Association, Washington, DC, 1966.

Shneidman, E.S., & N.L. Farberow: *Clues to Suicide.* McGraw-Hill, 1957.

Shurley, J.T., & A.D. Pokorny: *Handling the Psychiatric Emergency.* American Medical Association, 1967.

Journal Articles

Baxter, S., Chordorkoff, B., & R. Underhill: Psychiatric emergencies: Dispositional determinants and the validity of the decision to admit. Am J Psychiat 124:1542–1548, 1968.

Bill, A.Z.: The effectiveness of a psychiatric service. Delaware MJ 41:241–249, 1969.

Coleman, M., & M. Rosenbaum: The psychiatric walk-in clinic. Israel Ann Psychiat 1:99, 1963.

Darbonne, A.: Crisis: A review of theory, practice and research. Internat J Psychiat 6:371–379, 1968.

Errera, P., Wyshak, G., & H. Jarecki: Psychiatric care in a general hospital emergency room. Arch Gen Psychiat 9:105, 1963.

Garetz, F.K.: The psychiatric emergency. Med Times 88:1066–1070, 1960.

Gross, H.S., & others: The effect of race and sex on the variation of diagnosis and disposition in a psychiatric emergency room. J Nerv Ment Dis 148:638–642, 1969.

Hadden, J., & others: Acute barbiturate intoxication. JAMA 209:893–900, 1969

Johnson, J.: Psychiatric emergencies in the community. Comp Psychiat 10:275–284, 1969.

Kateryniuk, N.: Alcoholic Emergencies. GP 35:14–15, March 1967.

Lion, J.R., Bach-y-Rita, G., & F.R. Ervin: Violent patients in the emergency room. Am J Psychiat 125:1706–1710, 1969.

Mattsson, A., & others: Suicidal behavior as a child psychiatric emergency. Arch Gen Psychiat 20:100–109, 1969.

Miller, W.B.: A psychiatric emergency service and some treatment concepts. Am J Psychiat 124:924–933, 1968.

Morison, G.C.: Therapeutic intervention in a child psychiatry emergency service. J Am Acad Child Psychiat 8:542–548, 1969.

Nigro, S.A.: A psychiatrist's experiences in general practice in a hospital emergency room. JAMA 214:1657–1660, 1970.

Raphlin, D.L., & J. Lion: Patients with repeated admissions to a psychiatric emergency service. Commun Ment Health J 6:313–318, 1970.

Satloff, A., & C.M. Worby: The psychiatric emergency service: Mirror of change. Am J Psychiat 126:1628–1632, 1970.

Shurley, J.T., & A.D. Pokorny: Handling the psychiatric emergency. M Clin North America 46:417–426, 1962.

Solomon, P.: The burden of responsibility in suicide and homicide. JAMA 199:321–324, 1967.

Trier, T.R., & others: Emergency, urgent, and elective admission. Arch Gen Psychiat 21:423–430, 1969.

Ungerleider, J.T.: The psychiatric emergency analysis of 6 months' experience of a university hospital consultation service. Arch Gen Psychiat 3:593, 1960.

Whitely, J.S., & D.M. Denison: The psychiatric casualty. Brit J Psychiat 109:488, 1963.

24...

Drug Therapy

*Advances in psychiatry and pharmacology during the past 2
decades have made drug therapy and somatic therapy virtually
synonymous. These advances have not only resulted in more
effective treatment for many patients but also have renewed
interest in the study of the organic or biologic basis for abnormal
behavior.*

This chapter discusses the effects and application to therapy of the
sedatives, the antipsychotic tranquilizers and lithium, and the antidepressant
drugs.

The distinctiveness of the effects of the antipsychotic or phenothiazine
tranquilizers from those of the sedatives was first clearly recognized by
French surgeons and psychiatrists in 1951 and 1952. The impact of the
tranquilizers on psychiatric practice has been truly revolutionary, and their
effectiveness has stimulated much research in psychopharmacology.

The related antidepressant drugs have reduced the need for ECT. The
availability of new sedatives, some of them drugs whose sedative action was
not always recognized, and the more permissive attitude toward drug therapy engendered by the success of the tranquilizers have encouraged the use
of drugs in the symptomatic relief of anxiety.

SEDATIVES

The sedative drugs are useful for the induction of sleep and for the
relief of anxiety. These 2 uses represent a great need and market, and the
proliferation of compounds is correspondingly great. Loose application of
the term "tranquilizer" has led to confusion.

It is not necessary or feasible for the physician to evaluate separately
each of the drugs available, since drugs can be placed in groups. The drugs
listed in Table 24–1 can all be considered as sedatives. It is most efficient to
consider that all drugs in this category or drug group will have similar properties and then to look for smaller variations between compounds within the
group. This preliminary suggestion is necessary because it has been difficult

TABLE 24–1. Identification of some sedatives by chemical class.

Monoureides
  Carbromal
  Ectylurea (Nostyn)
Diureides or barbiturates
Piperidinediones or "nonbarbiturates"
  Glutethimide (Doriden)
  Methyprylon (Noludar)
Carbamates
  Emylcamate (Striatran)
  Hydroxyphenamate (Listica)
  Ethinamate (Valmid)
Dicarbamates
  Meprobamate (Miltown, Equanil)
  Mebutamate (Capla)
  Carisoprodol (Rela, Soma)
  Tybamate (Solacen)
	Benzodiazepines and a quinazolone
	  Chlordiazepoxide (Librium)
	  Diazepam (Valium)
	  Oxazepam (Serax)
	  Methaqualone (Quaalude)
	Alcohols
	  Ethanol
	  Chloral hydrate
	  Chlorobutanol (Chloretone)
	  Ethchlorvynol (Placidyl)
	  Phenaglycodol (Ultran)
	Bromides
	Ethers
	Paraldehyde
	Hydrocarbons, halogenated hydrocarbons

to integrate the new antipsychotic tranquilizers into practice and avoid confusion with the large number of recently marketed sedatives.

The sedative class of drugs, exemplified by the barbiturates, has been used for the relief of anxiety and the induction of sleep since about 1903. After the antipsychotic tranquilizers were recognized as a separate class of drugs and their use had revolutionized the institutional practice of psychiatry, the physician in noninstitutional practice, dealing more often with anxious and neurotic patients than with psychotic ones, believed that this important advance should have an impact on his practice also. However, when the tranquilizers were used in the treatment of anxiety, the results were disappointing. At this point, many physicians concluded that a drug of the sedative class rather than of the tranquilizer class was indicated (as in the past) for anxious patients. But a series of sedative drugs were advertised as "tranquilizers," "minor tranquilizers," "successors to the tranquilizers," etc, and this led to confusion. Recognition of the fact that meprobamate was merely an expensive variant of an intermediate-acting sedative required 10 years. The influence of advertising and ambiguities in the use of the term "tranquilizer" continues to be confusing.

What Is a Sedative? What Is a Tranquilizer?

Each of the drugs listed in this section as a sedative will, if given in progressively larger doses, diminish anxiety, lead to sedation, excitement, or disinhibition, ataxia, general anesthesia, and, ultimately, medullary (respiratory and vasomotor) depression and death. With repeated or continuous administration, the sedatives are anticonvulsant, habituating, cause physical dependence and a withdrawal state, and are voluntary muscle relaxants and spinal cord depressants.

In contrast, the tranquilizers (represented by any of the phenothiazine compounds discussed below or by reserpine) do not cause general anesthesia, ie, the patient can be aroused even after huge doses. They are convulsant in their action and not habituating. They may cause extrapyramidal signs of parkinsonism and dystonias as well as autonomic effects (atropine-like, sympathoplegic). Their therapeutic usefulness is in the management of psychotic rather than neurotically anxious patients.

Chemical Classification and Identification

The most useful classification of the sedatives is based on their duration of action. There are, however, advantages to considering a chemical classification such as that suggested by Table 24–1. The most important of these advantages is to be able to predict classification of new drugs in the sedative group as they appear on the market. A new modification of a barbiturate, urethane, or alcohol may, as a first approximation, be expected to act quite similarly to other drugs in its class. The metabolism of a drug and its physical and chemical properties are also more easily understood as characteristics of a chemical class of drugs. (For example, all barbiturates are weak acids; all urethanes are neutral compounds.)

Pharmacologic Actions

A. Mechanism of Action: The barbiturates and the few other sedatives and anesthetics that have been studied are selective depressants of the ascending reticular activating system, and this action can explain the loss of consciousness induced. However, they are also general depressants of the CNS.

B. Effects: Several precautions must be observed if the description of the effects of sedatives is to be accurate and the classification of the drugs valid. The drug must be studied over a wide range of doses if the complete sequence of effects described below is to be observed—or, if different drugs are being compared, equally potent doses must be used before a claim of selectivity of effect for one of the drugs is made. Furthermore, many of the effects to be described are subjective, and some drug effects may therefore seem to vary unpredictably. Actually, the drugs themselves, since they can act only on the organic substrate of behavior, are quite consistent in their effects. However, the content and intensity of the patient's reaction to them are conditioned by individual factors and by the setting in which the drug is given. The varied reactions to alcohol in different individuals and in different situations are common examples of this fact.

1. Gross behavioral changes—

a. Sedation—Sedation results from small doses of drugs of this class. It may be defined as decreased responsiveness to a constant level of stimulation or a decrease in spontaneous activity and ideation. It is not the same thing as drowsiness, but drowsiness may also occur and may progress to sleepiness.

b. Disinhibition may occur following the use of larger amounts of a sedative. This effect is presumed to be due to depression of a higher cortical center and release of a lower or phylogenetically older level from constant inhibitory control. It may be minor in degree, may appear as euphoria, or may be absent. The feeling generally is accompanied by impaired judgment and a loss of self-control, neither of which is common in the euphoria seen after the use of the narcotic analgesics. With larger doses, or in the presence of continuous stimulation such as pain, the disinhibition may result in drunkenness and excitement. This excitement is a manifest behavioral change due to disinhibition and is not equivalent to stimulation in the physiologic sense.

    c. Relief of anxiety is an effect that is probably not physiologically separable from the sedative and euphoriant effect, but is mentioned separately because of its therapeutic importance.

    d. Ataxia and nystagmus appear with high dosage and persist until anesthesia supervenes.

    e. Sleep is induced by all of these drugs if sufficiently large doses are administered. Small doses suffice if the patient is ready for sleep. The dose required will vary with the physiologic and psychologic state of the individual (especially the patient's expectations) and the environmental situation in which the drug is given. The resulting sleep is equivalent to normal or physiologic sleep, but with larger doses it can be deeper, ie, less time is spent in the REM (rapid eye movement, dreaming) phase.

    f. Anesthesia (stage III of general anesthesia) can be induced in animals and in humans. Demonstration of this effect in humans often depends upon a suicidal attempt with the drug, although short- and ultrashort-acting barbiturates are used as anesthetic agents. All of the agents classified as sedatives in this chapter have been used in successful suicide attempts or in unsuccessful attempts that demonstrated anesthesia.

    2. Effect on the EEG—The effect of a graded series of doses of a sedative on the EEG is exactly what would be predicted from similar observations on general anesthetics and from studies on sleep. Small doses of sedatives, producing a state of disinhibition or light sleep, lead to an increase in fast activity, particularly of "sleep spindles." With larger doses or when sleep is induced by smaller doses, the pattern is that of slow wave activity equivalent to the normal sleep pattern. Still larger doses, as with general anesthetics, cause a progressive decrease in amplitude with "burst suppression" or periods of inactivity. Finally, all activity disappears.

    3. Analgesia—The barbiturates are said to be poor general anesthetics because the patient may respond reflexly to pain during surgical anesthesia. Deeply anesthetized patients, however, are totally unresponsive.

    The analgesic activity of the barbiturates has been tested on patients with postoperative (incisional) pain. These drugs were found to be effective, although less so than the narcotic analgesics. However, in the presence of pain, the excitement of the disinhibited (stage II) period may be greatly intensified. This inappropriate response to an intense stimulus appears to be equivalent to that seen during induction with general anesthetics. When the barbiturates are used alone for their analgesic effect, the possibility of a paradoxic excitement should be kept in mind.

    4. Anticonvulsant effect—All of the sedatives are anticonvulsants both in the laboratory and clinically. Phenobarbital and other long-acting drugs such as diazepam are more effective in this regard, and are thus used in the treatment of epilepsy.

5. Withdrawal state—When large doses of any of these drugs are given chronically, continued administration or very gradual withdrawal may be necessary to prevent a withdrawal state—ie, physical dependence is present. The withdrawal reaction, as in delirium tremens, may include hyperexcitability, autonomic stimulation, convulsions, psychosis, and even death.

6. Habituation—The relief of anxiety and the euphoria provided by these drugs has led to the casual or compulsive misuse of every member of this group.

7. Spinal cord depression (voluntary muscle relaxation)—The effect of depressing polysynaptic reflexes or internuncial transmission in the cord is of interest because of the claim that some sedatives, notably meprobamate and chlordiazepoxide, are unusually potent in this effect and are potentially useful in relaxing abnormally contracted voluntary muscle associated with joint disease or tension. This effect on spinal cord function actually is so slight in ordinary dosages as to be of no therapeutic importance. It is mentioned here only to negate false claims and to emphasize that it is a property of all drugs of this class. In fact, if the cord depressant action is assayed in animals by the ability of a drug to antagonize strychnine convulsions (which are due to spinal cord facilitation), phenobarbital is seen to be more active than meprobamate.

Monosynaptic spinal reflexes are depressed by the barbiturates and the other sedatives only by very large doses. Therefore, the simple myotatic reflexes persist until deep anesthesia.

8. Cardiovascular and respiratory effects—In ordinary doses, the cardiovascular, respiratory, and autonomic effects of the sedatives are indirect and are due either to the patient's decreased activity or to the occasional periods of excitement that may appear. It is important to recognize, however, that with larger doses respiration is progressively depressed. The peripheral chemoreceptors are less sensitive to the barbiturates and other sedatives than is the respiratory center, and respiration is therefore maintained by the stimulation of hypoxia rather than by an increase in P_{CO_2}. Later, medullary depression occurs and respiration is further depressed.

In the deeply anesthetized patient, shock may occur as a result of vasomotor depression.

Clinical Uses

A. Induction of Sleep: There are some situations where the physician can anticipate the patient's need for medication at the hour of sleep. It is considerate, for example, to offer sedation to a patient attempting to sleep in a strange hospital or to someone who has undergone an anxiety engendering day. However, the indication for sleep-inducing medication is usually established by the complaint of the patient who is dissatisfied with the pattern of his sleep. The nature of his complaint—ie, the pattern of his insomnia—is the important factor in determining the drug selected for use. Many patients, because of anxiety or other reasons, have trouble going to sleep but once asleep have no further difficulty. For such patients a rapidly acting sedative with a short duration of action is adequate. Other individuals have no difficulty going to sleep but awaken after a few hours to spend a restless night and arise unrefreshed. For these individuals an intermediate-acting drug with its attendant risk of hangover may be used, or a short-acting drug is prescribed at bedtime with instructions to repeat it one time during the early part of the night if necessary.

B. Relief of Anxiety; Sedation:

1. Situational anxiety—Anxiety may be an appropriate reaction to some circumstances. If the situation does not recur too regularly, a barbiturate or other sedative may be used over short periods to minimize anxiety. Many people use alcohol in this way, and the risks associated with the use of other sedatives are similar. Relief of anxiety may occur, but with a corresponding decrease in manual proficiency and judgment. In some situations (eg, a critical school examination), sedation may impair performance even though the subject is deceived by the euphoria into believing that he has performed well. There are, however, situations in which mild sedation may improve both mood and performance.

2. Neurotic anxiety—Neurotic anxiety is anxiety in response to an insufficient environmental stimulus or no apparent adequate stimulus at all. It may be manifested as subjective fear or tension; as any of a variety of psychophysiologic disorders; or as obsessive or phobic behavior. The sedatives often provide partial symptomatic relief of anxiety and decrease the intensity of associated organic symptoms. Drugs should certainly not be used to the exclusion of psychotherapy, and the occasional hazards attending their use must be borne in mind.

Patient reports and evaluations by physicians under carefully controlled conditions have established the effectiveness of each of the drugs classified in this chapter as sedatives. In controlled studies, the placebo effect on anxiety—this most subjective of responses—is not so great as might be supposed. In the noninvestigative situation, however, the nonspecific factors are amplified and merge with psychotherapeutic technics such as reassurance.

The long-acting sedatives—phenobarbital is the reference standard—are preferable to short- or intermediate-acting drugs for the relief of anxiety. If short-acting preparations are used, the effect appears quickly and decays rapidly (as with alcohol). The patient soon associates these cyclic changes (3—4 times each day) with his medication, and may tend to take additional doses or larger doses and escalate his drug-taking. The less intense, more constant effect of the long-acting cumulative sedatives is safer and more satisfactory.

When drugs are used in this way, adequate explanation is always necessary so that the patient will not fix upon his organic symptom and its relief and thus fail to cooperate in helping the therapist and himself understand the real origins of his problem.

Anxiety may also occur as a symptom attending other psychiatric illnesses (psychosis, personality problem, psychosomatic disease, behavioral abnormality). In these also, anxiety may be controlled by sedatives, but effective treatment requires far more than sedation.

TABLE 24–2. Dosages of commonly used sedatives.

	Oral Dose	
	For Sleep (Single Dose)	**Sedative** (3–4 Times a Day)
Short-acting*		
Pentobarbital (Nembutal)†	100–200 mg	30 mg
Secobarbital (Seconal)†	100–200 mg	30 mg
Paraldehyde	12–16 ml	4–8 ml
Hexobarbital (Sombulex, Evipal)	250–500 mg	
Ethinamate (Valmid)	0.5–1 gm	
Methyprylon (Noludar)	200–400 mg	50–100 mg
Ethchlorvynol (Placidyl)	0.5–1 gm	100–200 mg
Chloral hydrate	0.5–1 gm	
Chlorobutanol (Chloretone)	0.5–1 gm	
Flurazepam (Dalmane)	30 mg	
Intermediate-acting*		
Amobarbital†	100–200 mg	15–30 mg
Aprobarbital (Alurate)	120 mg	20–40 mg
Butabarbital (Butisol)	100–200 mg	8–60 mg
Vinbarbital (Delvinal)	100–200 mg	30 mg
Heptabarbital (Medomin)	200–400 mg	50–100 mg
Meprobamate (Miltown, Equanil)		200–400 mg
Glutethimide (Doriden)	500 mg	125–250 mg
Diazepam (Valium)†		5 mg
Long-acting		
Phenobarbital†	100 mg	15–30 mg
Mephobarbital (Mebaral)		30–60 mg
Ectylurea (Nostyn, Levanil)		150–300 mg
Chlordiazepoxide (Librium)†		10–25 mg
Oxazepam (Serax)		10–20 mg
Phenaglycodol (Ultran)		200 mg

Note: The following sedatives are listed for purposes of identification only. They are less commonly used or are present only in mixtures. **Short-acting:** Cyclobarbital (Phanodorn), hexethal (Ortal), talbutal (Lotusate). **Intermediate-acting:** Butethal (Neonal), cyclopentyl allylbarbituric acid (Cyclopal), diallylbarbituric acid, probarbital (Ipral), hydroxyphenamate (Listica), carisoprodol (Rela, Soma), mebutamate (Capla). **Long-acting:** Barbital, carbromal, acetylcarbromal. (The action of methylparafynol [Dormison] is too feeble to permit classification.)

*Short- and intermediate-acting drugs are not recommended for continuous sedation.

†These sedatives are also available for parenteral administration. Parenteral forms of other sedatives are available, but experience with their use is limited.

C. Other Uses: Sedatives may be used to reduce excitement due to drugs or disease; to reduce activity when bed rest must be enforced; as anticonvulsants; and, in diagnostic EEGs, to activate latent EEG abnormalities by inducing sleep.

Preparations, Dosages, and Selection of Drug

In classifying the sedatives in relation to their use, duration of action is the most important property. As indicated above, the long-acting sedatives are preferable to the short- or intermediate-acting drugs in the prolonged treatment of anxiety. For the induction of sleep, the short-acting compounds are usually most useful, although the sleep patterns of some patients may suggest the use of a drug with intermediate properties.

Some of the commonly used sedatives are reviewed below. Of the many drugs available, most physicians select only 1 or 2 from each class for their use. The dosages are listed in Table 24–2. The dose for sleeping is given at bedtime, often with permission to repeat once before 1 a.m. if necessary. For sedation, the longer-acting, cumulative drugs are given 3–4 times a day. The effective and tolerated dose varies with the individual and must be determined for each patient. To some extent it may be increased when the patient becomes accustomed to the effect. For example, phenobarbital, 15 mg 3 times a day, may be the initial dose. If this is ineffective, a 4th dose may be added or one or more doses may be increased to 30 mg. A few patients complain of drowsiness unless the dose is reduced to 8 mg.

A. Short-Acting Sedatives:

1. Pentobarbital is the standard drug of this category. Secobarbital does not differ from it in its properties.

2. Chloral hydrate and equivalents—Chloral hydrate is a very rapidly acting hypnotic. It was for many years available only as a salty solution and was, therefore, largely replaced by the more easily dispensed barbiturates. It is now available in a capsule of 0.5 gm. The usual dose for inducing sleep is 0.5 or 1 gm. It occasionally causes gastric irritation.

Chloral betaine (Beta-Chlor) is a solid complex that liberates chloral hydrate after ingestion. It is easier to dispense than liquid chloral hydrate. Tablets are labeled in terms of their chloral hydrate content.

3. Paraldehyde—Paraldehyde is a liquid with an unpleasant taste and an odor that is more offensive to other people than to the patient himself. Paraldehyde acts rapidly. It is primarily metabolized by the liver, but some appears in the expired air, accounting for the odor and the pulmonary irritation that sometimes occurs. Paraldehyde has been a traditional remedy for the excited or inebriated person, but it has no advantage in this context. Like other drugs dispensed as liquids or solutions, it is more rapidly absorbed than solids in tablets or capsules.

Paraldehyde is a cyclic ether formed by the polymerization of acetaldehyde. The reaction is slowly reversible, and the liberated acetaldehyde may be oxidized to acetic acid. Old supplies of paraldehyde may become strongly acid. As paraldehyde stocks are now only slowly utilized, the chance of encountering a deteriorated solution has increased. Paraldehyde from a previously opened bottle should not be used unless it has been kept in a refrigerator.

B. Intermediate-Acting Sedatives:

1. Amobarbital (Amytal) is the prototype of this class.

2. Meprobamate (Miltown, Equanil)—This carbamate is merely another intermediate-acting sedative without any special attributes. The drug was advertised as a "tranquilizer" and was widely recommended for the treatment of anxiety without much mention of the caution that ought to be exercised in its use, as in the use of amobarbital, its nearest equivalent. As a result, misuse, withdrawal states, and ataxic states have been produced more commonly than with the barbiturates. Direct comparisons in double-blind tests on anxious patients, both institutionalized and ambulatory, have shown that neither the patient nor the physician can distinguish meprobamate from amobarbital. The cost of meprobamate is no longer as high as it once was, but the objection to using an intermediate-acting instead of a long-acting drug for continuous sedation remains.

3. Glutethimide (Doriden)—This drug was widely used because it was an early "nonbarbiturate sedative." When used at bedtime, it causes hangover the next morning in many patients. Like other short- and intermediate-acting sedatives, it has greater potential for misuse than do the long-acting drugs. If it has any distinctiveness, it is in its unfortunately greater toxicity. Patients have had convulsions, sometimes accompanied by a toxic psychosis, not only after withdrawal but during continued administration of the drug, and there have been a number of deaths from accidental overdosage.

4. Diazepam (Valium)—Like chlordiazepoxide (Librium), its chemical relative, this drug is currently in wide use. It offers no advantage over other intermediate-acting sedatives.

C. Long-Acting Sedatives:

1. Phenobarbital—Phenobarbital is still the most widely used and generally most useful drug of this category. Its repute has suffered unjustifiably because it was developed and used long before the period of enthusiasm for psychopharmacology and before the reintroduction of drugs into psychiatry.

2. Chlordiazepoxide (Librium), oxazepam (Serax)—These drugs are currently very widely used. Their only distinctiveness is that they are excreted over a period of several days and have a duration of action somewhat longer than that of phenobarbital. A cumulative effect may be seen, and the appearance of withdrawal effects may be delayed for a week or more after discontinuation of the drug.

Each of these drugs is an effective sedative if given in adequate doses. The claim that anxiety can be relieved without the occurrence of drowsiness as a side-effect is based on experience with small doses and with no deaths yet reported from the use of these long-acting benzodiazepine sedatives by themselves. This may in part reflect their distribution in small doses and the failure of the layman to identify these drugs as "sleeping pills" suitable for suicide.

The cost to the patient of treatment with one of these newer drugs is considerably greater than equivalent treatment with phenobarbital.

Adverse Reactions
The undesirable effects of all of the sedatives listed above are similar. They differ in the rapidity of onset of action and the duration of effect.
A. Side-Effects:
1. Drowsiness—All of the sedatives cause drowsiness if enough is given, and some patients will be made drowsy even by small doses. Whether drowsiness is regarded as an undesirable or a desirable effect depends upon physician and patient expectations.
2. Impaired performance and judgment—A person need not be rendered staggering drunk before his motor performance and, probably more important, his judgment are significantly impaired. The most important offender in this regard is alcohol. However, other sedatives are similar to alcohol in their effects and all are additive in their effects with alcohol and with each other. Some simple psychomotor tests—eg, key tapping, auditory reaction time, and memory for digits—are impaired for as long as 8 hours after a dose of pentobarbital.
3. Hangover—The effect of the sedatives may extend beyond a period judged by the patient to be desirable. After a bedtime dose of even a short-acting sedative, the patient may on the following morning complain of feeling dizzy, lethargic, or exhausted. Long-acting agents cause more complaints of this type.
4. Drug abuse or habituation—No other sedative (or any other drug) is abused so widely and with such great social and individual harm as alcohol. However, every one of the sedatives may, like alcohol, be abused continuously and compulsively. More commonly, they are illicitly used as spree drugs or as a substitute for other drugs when the preferred drug (alcohol, methamphetamine, or heroin) is not available. In some subjects the distinction between therapeutic use and misuse becomes blurred—eg, in the patient whose physician provides a large supply of a sedative to use daily or several times daily to offset anticipated anxiety-inducing situations.
5. Withdrawal state—All of the therapeutic agents listed, including those most recently introduced, have caused a withdrawal state. The changes may be limited to insomnia and prolonged disturbances in the EEG during sleep. After discontinuance of larger doses, there may be a hyperexcitable state with associated weakness, tremor, anxiety, and elevated blood pressure, pulse, and respiratory rate. Following even larger doses, convulsions may occur and a toxic psychosis may appear with agitation, confusion, and hallucinations. If the drug is alcohol, the state is called delirium tremens.

In experiments on humans who have been given pentobarbital or secobarbital for many weeks, it was shown that withdrawal after daily doses of 0.4 gm resulted in only minor symptoms. Withdrawal after doses of 0.5 gm/day caused pronounced tremor and anxiety. Following withdrawal from 0.8 gm/day, 75% of the subjects had at least one convulsion and 60% had a toxic psychosis.

Meprobamate may pose a special hazard in this regard since doses of 800 mg 4 times a day—amounts that are not unusual—may result in pronounced withdrawal signs in patients who have taken the drug for some weeks.

The symptoms of withdrawal following abuse of a short- or intermediate-acting sedative appear in 18–24 hours and increase to a maximum in 2–3 days. When phenobarbital, chlordiazepoxide, or a similar long-acting depressant is withdrawn, symptoms may not appear for a week. A withdrawal state is very rare after the use of these slowly eliminated compounds since they usually accomplish their own slow withdrawal.

Treatment consists of readmininistration of a sedative followed by planned gradual withdrawal. Once a toxic psychosis has developed, it is difficult to shorten the withdrawal syndrome.

B. Chronic Toxicity: Except for the nutritional and direct toxic effects seen in the chronic excessive use of alcohol, none of the commonly used sedatives cause chronic toxicity other than their usual actions of sedation, drunkenness, and the possibility of a withdrawal state.

C. Overdosage Toxicity: In large doses the sedatives produce a state of prolonged, deep anesthesia. Respiration is depressed. If a stage of severe medullary depression is reached, circulatory shock occurs. Tendon reflexes persist until the deepest stages. Nystagmus is seen until the equivalent of plane 2 of stage III anesthesia is reached. Pupillary size is not a consistent sign of intoxication since initial constriction may be replaced by dilatation due to asphyxia.

The diagnosis is usually made on circumstantial evidence: a suicide note, a phone call, or an empty drug container. Simple chemical tests on urine are useful, but treatment must be instituted before the results of blood tests are available.

The lethal dose of a barbiturate or other sedative varies tremendously depending upon the circumstances of ingestion. If the person arranges not to be discovered for some time after ingestion of the drug, as little as 8–10 times the hypnotic dose may be fatal. If he reaches medical care in time, ingestion of many times that amount may be consistent with survival.

The variability in lethal dose reflects the fact that the causes of death differ if death occurs before rather than after hospitalization. Uncared for, the deeply anesthetized patient may die of respiratory depression or obstruction. With appropriate treatment, these usually can be prevented; and if the patient dies, he will probably die from shock, acute renal insufficiency, or pulmonary pathology resulting from immobilization—eg, pneumonia, acute pulmonary edema, atelectasis.

D. Allergic Reactions: Serious allergic reactions to sedatives are uncommon. A morbilliform rash sometimes occurs as an allergic response to barbiturates (especially phenobarbital) and most of the other sedatives. A particularly disturbing pruritic crural rash occurs in a few patients following meprobamate.

Treatment of Acute Sedative Intoxication

A physiologic or conservative plan of treatment derived from a study of the cause of death in many anesthetized patients has reduced mortality to a few percent of cases.

A. Observe Continuously: Treatment is best carried out in an intensive care unit, where observation can be continuous and carefully recorded.

B. Support Respiration: The airway is kept open by an oropharyngeal airway, intubation, or by tracheostomy if necessary. Secretions are aspirated frequently. If necessary, respiration is mechanically assisted. Avoid continuous mechanical respiratory support if possible since it often leads to alkalosis and confusion of the neurologic signs.

C. Prevent or Treat Shock: A fall in blood pressure or narrowing of the pulse pressure should be treated without waiting for the development of overt shock. Blood or plasma substitutes should be given. The same objections to the use of levarterenol (Levophed) and other pressor amines apply here as in shock due to other causes. The use of isoproterenol infusions in patients who do not respond to plasma expansion is now becoming more common.

D. Maintain Renal Function: Whether or not diuresis is induced to hasten elimination of the drug, adequate water (in the form of 5% glucose in water) and saline must be provided. Prevention of prolonged shock protects against acute renal insufficiency.

E. Increase Rate of Excretion of Drug: In profoundly depressed patients, efforts to hasten excretion may be justified—eg, osmotic and alkaline diuresis, peritoneal dialysis, or hemodialysis. Osmotic diuretics—eg, mannitol—are used to increase urine volume to 10 or more liters of urine per day.

If the urine is kept alkaline (pH > 8.0), renal tubular reabsorption of phenobarbital is decreased. The barbiturates are weak acids, and reabsorption is less if they are present in the renal tubular urine in the salt (ionized) form. Phenobarbital has a long half-life in the blood (3 days), is present in high concentration, and its ionization can be easily influenced—ie, it has a favorable pK. Alkalinization of the urine is not useful if intoxication is due to the shorter-acting barbiturates or other sedatives.

Peritoneal dialysis and hemodialysis are both effective in removing practically all of the sedatives but are not often needed since recovery rates are already good, and they add a hazard of their own.

F. Prophylactic Penicillin: Prophylactic penicillin during the treatment of coma due to sedative drug overdose has reduced the incidence of pneumonia.

G. Nursing Care: Nursing service is vital: aspiration of secretions, regular movement of the patient, and packing of pressure points to prevent decubitus ulcers. If the period of anesthesia is prolonged, the eyes should be covered to protect the cornea from dust and drying.

H. Aftercare: Most of these patients will have ingested drugs in a suicidal attempt. Obviously, the need for care does not end when they regain consciousness. Each patient should be considered a psychiatric problem and a challenge.

I. Measures That Should Not Be Used:

1. Gastric lavage—If the patient is reached promptly, gastric aspiration may be advisable. Introduction of additional lavage fluid, however, has repeatedly been shown to hasten gastric emptying and sometimes to lead to bronchial aspiration even in conscious patients. A comatose patient usually should not be aspirated. Some physicians feel that lavage is permissible if a cuffed endotracheal tube is first inserted. Others withhold lavage because it imposes added risks of cardiac arrhythmias and respiratory arrest.

2. Central stimulants—The use of central stimulant drugs such as pentylenetetrazol (Metrazol) and picrotoxin in sedative intoxication is regarded by those who have reported the most favorable survival experience as contraindicated.

ANTIPSYCHOTIC TRANQUILIZERS

All of the drugs classified above as sedatives are useful in the treatment of anxiety. They cannot, however, be expected to alter the course of a psychotic episode and cannot dependably quiet a manic patient without inducing a state of anesthesia. In contrast, the tranquilizers are much less effective against anxiety but are effective "antipsychotic" drugs. Even when huge doses are used, the patient can still be aroused.

The term "tranquilizer" is not precisely defined, and in common usage may be applied to some of the sedatives as well. Confusion can be avoided by using terms such as "antipsychotic tranquilizers" or "phenothiazine-type tranquilizers."

Chemistry and Classification

The tranquilizers most widely used are phenothiazine derivatives. There are, however, 4 general groups:

A. Reserpine and Related Rauwolfia Alkaloids: Reserpine affects behavior as other tranquilizers do, and the drug was used briefly in the treatment of psychotic states. However, it is now regarded as an antihypertensive drug, and the tranquilizing effect is regarded as a side-effect. The effect on amine depletion and storage produced by reserpine does not occur with the phenothiazine tranquilizers.

B. Phenothiazine Tranquilizers: The phenothiazines may be classified according to the nature of the side chain that bears the tertiary amine function. The piperazinylpropyl class causes less sedation and more extrapyramidal side-effects than the other subclasses.

All are bases (some with 2 amine functions) and are dispensed as salts of a variety of acids.

C. Nonphenothiazine Tranquilizers: The phenothiazine part of the tranquilizer molecule is not essential and may be replaced by some other bulky chemical group. Chlorprothixene (Taractan) and haloperidol (Haldol) are quite similar in their effects to chlorpromazine. Others, eg, hydroxyzine (Atarax, Vistaril), are qualitatively similar to the phenothiazine tranquilizers but are less potent in the sense that the greater atropine-like side-effects limit the size of the dose that can be used. Other nonphenothiazine tranquilizers are listed below.

D. Related Drug Groups: The antihistamines, including those used as antiemetics and the parasympatholytic drugs, have CNS effects comparable to those of the tranquilizers. Conversely, the antipsychotic tranquilizers have parasympatholytic and histamine blocking properties.

Pharmacologic Effects

A. Mechanism of Action: The behavioral or manifest effect of the tranquilizers is depression in the sense that activity and attentiveness are reduced, but the neurophysiologic mechanism of action seems—to the extent that it is understood—to be stimulation. As larger and larger doses are given, signs of stimulation appear and may culminate in convulsions. Lower levels of the CNS are depressed, presumably as a result of increased inhibitory influences from above.

Electrographic studies show the limbic system to be the most sensitive electrically. The seizures caused by very large doses begin here and spread to cortical structures.

The diencephalon is inhibited in its function. Hypothalamic control of the anterior pituitary is reduced, temperature regulation is altered, and, in animals, "sham rage" is reduced.

B. Effects:

1. Behavioral—The useful effect of the tranquilizers is a distinctive kind of sedation. Even with the huge doses used in the treatment of psychotic patients, this sedation does not progress to anesthesia. The patient experiences a state of indifference or apathy, with a drowsy feeling and motor retardation, but can be aroused even after large doses by ordinary stimuli. Euphoria is not present, and subjectively the type of sedation is actually unpleasant. Excitement is an unusual effect, but may occur early in the course of treatment. Some tolerance to the sedative effect develops.

This tranquilizing effect can reduce the activity of a grossly disturbed patient without inducing anesthesia. The tranquilizers also act beneficially on the disturbed thinking of schizophrenics who are not excited. Whether this represents a specific antipsychotic effect or is merely an extension of the sedative action is one of the controversial but crucial questions related to this drug group.

2. Autonomic—

a. Parasympatholytic—The synthetic tranquilizers (but not reserpine) have atropine-like properties that become very prominent because of the large doses used. Dry mouth, mydriasis, failure of accommodation for near vision, constipation, and tachycardia are manifestations of this effect.

b. Beta-adrenergic effects—The phenothiazines intensify the vasodilating and other beta-adrenergic effects of epinephrine. Patients may, therefore, show signs of vasodilatation with postural hypotension but nevertheless respond to norepinephrine and other vasoconstricting (alpha-adrenergic) amines.

The degree of postural hypotension may be great enough, especially after parenteral administration of a phenothiazine, to lead to syncope. Even when blood pressure has fallen to very low levels, the skin is warm and dry—demonstrating the difference between shock and hypotension.

3. Temperature regulation—The phenothiazine tranquilizers cause a minor fall in body temperature. Chlorpromazine and its congeners not only cause vasodilatation but suppress shivering as well, and are therefore useful when it is desirable to induce hypothermia by lowering the ambient temperature.

4. Endocrine effects—Hypothalamic influences on the anterior pituitary are reduced. A common side-effect is nonpuerperal lactation, presumably due to decreased production of prolactin-inhibitory factor with resultant increased liberation of lactogenic hormone. Gonadotropin liberation is also decreased, as shown by assays of urinary excretion and by disturbances of the menstrual cycle or even, with large doses, amenorrhea.

5. Extrapyramidal effects—Parkinsonism, dystonias, or akathisia are common adverse effects with large doses. For this reason, antiparkinsonism drugs are often given prophylactically when large doses of antipsychotic tranquilizers are used.

6. Convulsant effect—Huge doses of any tranquilizer may cause convulsions, although this is rare clinically. Epileptics are far more susceptible.

7. Effect on conditioned responses—The distinction between sedatives and tranquilizers can be made in animals by their different effects on operant conditioning. Conditioned avoidance, for example, can be extinguished by reasonable doses of phenothiazine, whereas barbiturates are without effect in this situation until the response is prevented by motor impairment.

8. Effects not present—Habituation to the antipsychotic tranquilizers does not occur, and physical dependence or tolerance does not develop. A withdrawal state does not occur, or is so mild that its existence is debatable. Supposed withdrawal symptoms must be distinguished from exacerbation of the psychosis following discontinuance of the drug.

Absorption, Metabolism, and Excretion

The phenothiazines are absorbed after oral administration, but the maximal effect does not develop for several hours. Response is immediate after intramuscular or intravenous injection. After the large doses used in psychiatry, the effects persist for about 24 hours—ie, the drug need not be given oftener than once or twice daily.

There are important differences in the rate and completeness of absorption between the various preparations. The liquid preparations provide for more complete absorption than the standard tablets (Fig 24–1). Absorption from the "prolonged action" capsules is even less complete.

The principal metabolic pathways involve oxidation to a sulfoxide and hydroxylation of the rings at several sites. The metabolites can be demonstrated in the urine by simple color tests for phenols.

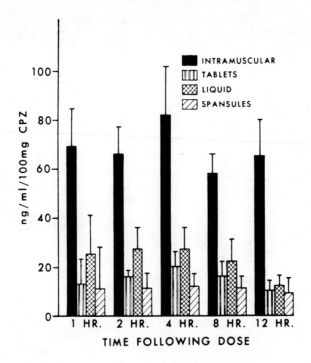

FIG 24-1. **Plasma levels following the administration of chlorpromazine in 4 dosage forms.** Patients had been receiving the same dosage form prior to the test dose but initial plasma levels were low. Levels are adjusted to reflect the difference in dosage between the 13 subjects and the smaller (50–100 mg) IM dose. (Reproduced, with permission, from Hollister, L.E., & others: Studies of delayed action medication. Clin Pharmacol Therap 11:54, 1970.)

Clinical Uses

A. **Treatment of Schizophrenic Reaction:** The phenothiazines can reduce excitement and control hostile and aggressive behavior in psychotic patients. This effect has had a tremendous impact on the institutional practice of psychiatry by reducing the amount of restraint needed.

The tranquilizers also suppress symptoms, particularly psychotic ideation, in a manner that cannot be explained easily by the depressant effect of the drugs. To some observers—especially those who accept the hypothesis that schizophrenia is due to some biochemical abnormality—the normalization of behavior suggests that the phenothiazines exert an antipsychotic effect. Others point out that patients are anything but normal while taking the large doses of phenothiazines required even though they may be able to return to the community on maintenance doses.

TABLE 24—3. Antipsychotic tranquilizers.

	Equivalent Adult Oral Dose (3—4 Times a Day) (mg)	
Chlorpromazine (Thorazine)*	25—50	
Promazine (Sparine)*	50—200	
Triflupromazine (Vesprin)*	10—20	
Thioridazine (Mellaril)	10—25	
Chlorprothixene (Taractan)*	25	
Prochlorperazine (Compazine)*	5—10	
Trifluoperazine (Stelazine)	1	Drugs of this category
Perphenazine (Trilafon)*	2—4	cause less sedation but
Fluphenazine (Permitil,		are more likely to produce
Prolixin)*	1	extrapyramidal side-
Acetophenazine (Tindal)	10	effects.
Butaperazine (Repoise)	5—10	
Piperacetazine (Quide)	10	
Carphenazine (Proketazine)	25—50	
Thiothixene (Navane)	1—2	
Thiopropazate (Dartal)	5—10	
Haloperidol (Haldol)	0.5	
Promethazine (Phenergan)*	25	Produces comparatively greater degree of sedation.

*Parenteral form for intramuscular injection is available. Single maximum parenteral dose equals maximum single oral dose, eg, chlorpromazine, 50 mg IM (maximum); may repeat as necessary.

The phenothiazines have materially decreased the duration of hospitalization for severe psychosis and have prevented hospitalization in many cases. From the starting dosage levels indicated in Table 24—3, the dosage is slowly increased until a therapeutic response occurs or side-effects limit dosage. The patient is kept on smaller maintenance doses after improvement or discharge.

Highly disturbed or otherwise severely psychotic patients may require very large doses of the phenothiazines before they can be controlled. In terms of chlorpromazine, 800 mg/day (by mouth) is not unusual, and amounts from 1000—2000 mg/day may be used. Intramuscular doses of 100 mg may be given every hour if necessary, and a dose of 500 mg IM/day is not unusual. High dosages for the other phenothiazines are comparable.

The potent drugs do not differ in therapeutic effectiveness.

B. Other Psychiatric Problems: Emotional instability and odd behavior in aged patients with "chronic brain syndrome" may be controlled with phenothiazines. Usefulness in other situations cannot be assumed. Disturbed mentally retarded patients, for example, are not improved by phenothiazine treatment.

C. Analgesia: Methotrimeprazine (Levoprome, Nozinan) is a phenothiazine similar in structure and effects to the other tranquilizers. However,
the analgesic properties that are present to a negligible degree in chlorpromazine are greatly increased in this compound. When given by injection,
it is nearly as potent as morphine. Huge doses must be given orally, but this
compound is of great interest because it appears to be the most potent
nonaddicting analgesic so far studied.

D. Other Uses: The tranquilizers are also used for the relief of itching;
for their antiemetic effect; as preanesthetic medication; and to intensify the
effect of the opiates.

Selection of Drug

From controlled clinical trials of the major tranquilizers, the following
conclusions emerge: (1) The true tranquilizers are not effective antianxiety
drugs. (2) In the treatment of schizophrenia, no differences in effectiveness
among the potent drugs have been established. (3) Those phenothiazines
suggested for special application—eg, itching or vomiting—are no different
from the others.

The available tranquilizers, whether phenothiazines or not, can therefore be discussed in 4 classes:

A. Chlorpromazine and Comparable Agents: Chlorpromazine
(Thorazine) no longer causes jaundice with the distressing frequency that it
once did, and the consensus would clearly name it as the standard drug of
the tranquilizer class. In the treatment of psychotics, it is often combined
with one of the piperazinylpropyl compounds such as trifluoperazine
(Stelazine) because of the unquantitated impression that a balance of sedation and stimulation is thus achieved.

Promazine (Sparine) has caused a high incidence of agranulocytosis.
With so many alternative drugs available, there is no need to use it.

Thioridazine (Mellaril) is favored by some physicians because it probably causes less parkinsonism. However, it is also more likely to cause vomiting and retinopathy.

B. "Stimulant" Tranquilizers: There is little basis for differentiating
among the piperazinylpropyl derivatives shown in Table 24–3. Haloperidol
(Haldol) is not a phenothiazine but one of a group of butyrophenones. It
causes many extrapyramidal reactions but little sedation and perhaps fewer
autonomic side-effects. Fluphenazine (Prolixin) is provided in a form slowly
absorbed after injection and can be given in doses of 25 mg every 2 weeks.
The advantages claimed are the saving in nursing time during hospitalization
and less dependence upon patient cooperation after discharge.

C. Tranquilizers That Cause More Somnolence: Promethazine (Phener-
gan) is usually not used in the treatment of psychosis because of the sedation
that it causes.

Propiomazine (Largon) is similar to promethazine and offers no advantage over the more widely used compounds. It is available only in an inject-
able dosage form, and experience has been limited to adjunctive uses in
anesthesia.

D. Less Potent Tranquilizers: Nonphenothiazine compounds may be potent and useful tranquilizers—eg, haloperidol or chlorprothixene. However, the nonphenothiazine tranquilizers listed below are much less useful. They are often called "diphenylmethane derivatives"; but they resemble the antihistamines and synthetic substitutes for atropine, and their dosage and effectiveness are limited by their atropine-like side-effects. They are listed here for identification only and are not suggested for any of the uses discussed above. They should not be used in the treatment of anxiety.

Hydroxyzine (Atarax, Vistaril) is closely related chemically to the familar antihistamines and antinauseants. As Atarax (hydroxyzine hydrochloride), it was not widely used, and the pamoate (oral) and hydrochloride (parenteral) were reintroduced as Vistaril, first as an antiarrhythmia drug and later as a tranquilizer.

Benactyzine is not much used by itself (as Suavitil or Phobex), but is present in Deprol in combination with meprobamate.

Azacyclonol (Frenquel), buclizine (Softran, Vibazine), and pipethanate (Sycotrol) are mentioned only to identify them.

Mepazine (Pacatal) is a phenothiazine but is rarely used today. Its effectiveness is limited by the atropine-like side-effects which appear if the dosage is increased to achieve a therapeutic effect.

Adverse Reactions

In those situations in which a few small doses of a tranquilizer are used, it might be possible to differentiate side-effects and overdosage toxicity. However, because these drugs are most commonly used in large doses for prolonged periods, this differentiation is usually not possible.

A. Side-Effects:

1. Behavioral—Taking an antipsychotic tranquilizer is not a subjectively pleasant experience. The feelings of lassitude and fatigue are unpleasant. With continued administration, patients become somewhat tolerant of or accustomed to this effect.

The incidence of suicide is greater among psychotics receiving drug therapy than in groups receiving only institutional care. It may be that the greater freedom of activity permitted the patient controlled by drugs is a factor. The behavioral depression caused by the tranquilizers may be another, and the selection factor (the more serious cases getting the drugs) is probably a third.

A few patients may experience feelings of excitement and restlessness. These feelings are more common early in treatment and after the administration of those piperazine or piperazinylpropyl derivatives characterized as "stimulant" tranquilizers.

Early in treatment, a rare patient depressed by a tranquilizer may at the same time develop a toxic psychosis with confusion and hallucinations. Such a reaction is more common with those drugs that resemble the antihistamines and atropine substitutes.

2. Extrapyramidal effects—Disturbances of the extrapyramidal motor system appear in 3 general patterns.

a. Parkinsonism equivalent—As the phenothiazines are given to institutionalized schizophrenic patients—ie, to therapeutic response or the maximum tolerated dose—parkinsonism is one of the most frequent side-effects. It consists of muscular rigidity and fine resting tremors and may vary in severity from slight impairment of facial mobility to completely disabling rigidity.

To minimize the development of muscular rigidity, many physicians administer an antiparkinsonism drug prophylactically—eg, benztropine (Cogentin)—when large doses of a phenothiazine tranquilizer are being used. Recent studies to evaluate this practice suggest that it is better to give the antiparkinsonism agents only after the signs appear.

b. Dystonias—Dystonias are most commonly seen in children and young adults either early in treatment or immediately following the injection of a phenothiazine or the accidental ingestion of a single large dose. The muscles of the shoulder girdle and jaws are most likely to be involved. Violent dystonias with movements of the arms and head that can be mistaken for convulsions may occur, or there may be athetoid movements or persistent oculogyric crises. Occurring in a depressed, unresponsive patient, these reactions may be alarming, misdiagnosed, and therefore overtreated.

Dystonias are actually well tolerated and should be treated conservatively. Of the drugs that may relieve the dystonia, diphenhydramine (Benadryl) has been most used in children.

c. Akathisia—Akathisia is a feeling of restlessness or of compelling need for movement. The patient may walk about impatiently ("pacing"), tap his foot incessantly, or complain of "restless legs."

3. Convulsions—Precipitation of convulsions is possible but quite rare during the use of the antipsychotic tranquilizers unless some additional factor is present—eg, if the patient is an epileptic or if another convulsant drug is being used.

4. Atropine-like effects—Parasympatholytic side-effects are often quite prominent. They include dry mouth, blurred vision, and constipation or even paralytic ileus. The expected tachycardia and pupillary dilatation may appear, especially with large doses, but these changes may sometimes be quite small, or bradycardia and pupillary constriction may actually occur. This variability in the response of the heart rate and pupillary size suggests that a central sympatholytic effect may also be present in some cases.

5. Postural hypotension—The intensification of the beta-adrenergic effects (vasodilatation) of the sympathomimetic amines has been described above as the basis for the fall in blood pressure. This side-effect is especially troublesome after injection of the tranquilizer and early in oral treatment. It may be intense enough to cause dizziness or fainting.

6. Metabolic and endocrinologic changes—Weight gain is a common side-effect of prolonged administration of tranquilizers. The increase in caloric intake cannot be explained merely by changes in mood, as is true for the similar effect of the antidepressant drugs.

As discussed above, the endocrinologic side-effects appear to be due to hypothalamic depression and consequent decrease in some of the tropic hormones of the anterior pituitary. Decrease in gonadotropin liberation leads to menstrual irregularities which usually become less with continued treatment. Lactation may occur for the reasons discussed above.

7. Oculocutaneous pigmentation—For some patients, the continued use of large doses of a phenothiazine is the only alternative to grossly disturbed behavior or recurrent hospitalization. In some patients, especially women, the exposed parts of the skin (face, neck, back of hands) take on a mauve or slate color after years of therapy with chlorpromazine. Pigment deposits in the anterior lens capsule and posterior surface of the cornea can be seen by slit lamp examination in one-third to one-half of some groups receiving prolonged chlorpromazine therapy. Some blurring of vision may be reported. At autopsy, the pigment is seen in macrophages throughout the body.

Thus far, chlorpromazine and thioridazine are the only phenothiazines that have caused this state. The daily dosage of chlorpromazine must exceed 500 mg/day. Experimentally, a single large dose followed by exposure to ultraviolet or visible light causes an unusual degree of erythema, but in clinical practice this occurs only after treatment for 3 years or longer. The process is very slowly reversible over a period of several months. Treatment consists of protection from light and substitution of a phenothiazine that requires a smaller absolute dose or of a combination of chlorpromazine with such a phenothiazine.

8. Pigmentary retinopathy—Deposition of pigment in the retina with impaired vision occurs rarely and by a process separate from the more common oculocutaneous pigmentation. Smaller doses and brief periods are involved. Thioridazine (Mellaril) has caused most of the few reported cases.

B. Acute Toxicity: The acute overdosage toxicity of the tranquilizers is very low in adults, and the possibility of a fatal outcome following attempted suicidal or accidental ingestion is negligible unless a second depressant drug is also involved.

These drugs are only slightly more dangerous in children; however, children are especially susceptible to the dystonic state described above, and such states are occasionally seen following accidental ingestion of one of the drugs or its therapeutic use in the treatment of vomiting.

C. Allergic Reactions:

1. Cholestatic jaundice—Chlorpromazine and a few other drugs can cause jaundice or less marked degrees of liver dysfunction by intrahepatic biliary obstruction rather than by direct liver cell damage. The process is benign and completely reversible, although many weeks may be required. The reaction is now only rarely seen, presumably because the impurity responsible for the reaction has been removed. It is assumed, without immunochemical evidence, to have been allergic in origin. Prior sensitization is not a factor since the jaundice appeared in almost every case within the first 6 weeks of treatment.

2. Other allergic reactions—Agranulocytosis occurs rarely and then only with extremely high dosages of the individual drugs except in the case of promazine, which is unusually hazardous in this regard. Contact dermatitis can occur when the situation permits, as in nurses who handle the drug. Other cutaneous reactions also occur, including a photosensitivity reaction that resembles eczema.

LITHIUM

Lithium ion, administered in the form of lithium carbonate, is used as an alternative or supplement to the major tranquilizers in the control of the manic stage of manic-depressive illness. Its mechanism of action is not known, and therapeutic doses do not have gross effects comparable to those of the tranquilizers or the sedatives. The onset of action is delayed for several days after the drug is started and 6—10 days elapse before the peak effect is reached. The drug is well absorbed after oral administration and is excreted by the kidneys.

Clinical Uses

Lithium carbonate is approved for marketing in the USA only for use in the control of mania and the drug has been remarkably successful for this purpose. Its use in any other clinical conditions is still investigative.

A. Control of Manic Episodes: An acute manic state is best controlled by the injection of chlorpromazine or other antipsychotic tranquilizer. The use of an oral preparation of a drug with a long latency of action is less satisfactory, and lithium is therefore not much used by itself. It may be started simultaneously with chlorpromazine or a similar tranquilizer.

B. Prophylaxis Against Affective Illness: Lithium is clearly not effective in the treatment of an established depression, but it has been claimed that it can prevent cyclic changes in mood and thus prevent not only manic attacks but also the development of depression and of the depressed stage of the manic-depressive syndrome. Some of these reports have been quite enthusiastic, and it may be that this use will ultimately be justified by adequately controlled double-blind studies. At present, however, the consensus is that the value of lithium in the prevention of depression is unestablished. If the effect is present, it requires 6—12 months for its appearance.

Adverse Reactions

Toxic effects during chronic administration are predicted by serum levels, which must be determined during treatment with lithium. Side-effects are generally mild if the serum level is kept below 1.5 mEq/liter. Serum levels above 2 mEq/liter are an indication that dosage should be decreased or the drug withheld temporarily. Serum lithium decreases by half every 24 hours.

Toxic effects may be graded as follows:

A. Mild: Nausea passes in a few days. A fine tremor of the hands or jaw may interfere with the patient's function and is not relieved by antiparkinson agents.

B. Moderate: Anorexia, vomiting, diarrhea, thirst and polyuria, coarse tremor, muscle weakness and twitching, sedation, and ataxia.

C. Severe: Chorea, athetosis, confusion, stupor, and convulsions.

D. Terminal: Coma.

Contraindications and Cautions

Lithium should not be used in the presence of impaired renal function or cardiovascular disease or any other situation that involves a restricted diet, diuretic drugs, fluid loss, or inadequate fluid intake. It should not be used during pregnancy or when facilities for the determination of serum lithium levels are not available.

Dosage and Preparations

Dosage is controlled by the regular determination of lithium blood levels.

Manic patients are given initial doses of 600 mg of lithium carbonate 3 times each day, but the serum level should not exceed 1.5 mEq/liter. As excitement subsides, the maintenance dose—usually 300 mg 3 times a day—should give serum levels of 0.5–1 mEq/liter.

Lithium carbonate (Eskalith, Lithonate, Lithane) is available in tablets or capsules of 300 mg.

ANTIDEPRESSANTS AND CNS STIMULANTS

This section defines drugs that are used in the treatment of depressions or are CNS stimulants. There are 3 general groups:

(1) **Antidepressants that resemble tranquilizers:** Drugs of the amitriptyline (Elavil) or imipramine (Tofranil) type are the most widely used antidepressants. Their properties are quite similar to those of the antipsychotic tranquilizers.

(2) **Sympathomimetic amines:** Amphetamine and related drugs are sympathomimetics comparable to ephedrine.

(3) **Monoamine oxidase (MAO) inhibitors:** The monoamine oxidase inhibitors are no longer widely used in the treatment of depression, but great interest in their mechanism of action remains. They have CNS stimulant properties which are qualitatively similar to those of amphetamine.

ANTIDEPRESSANT DRUGS RESEMBLING TRANQUILIZERS

The drugs that are most commonly used in the treatment of severe depression should be classed as a subgroup of the antipsychotic tranquilizers. They are treated as a separate group in this discussion to conform to current (but changing) clinical thought.

When the antipsychotic tranquilizers were first evaluated, a few investigators reported a beneficial effect on patients with severe depressions —especially early in treatment, before the dosage had reached high levels. However, the use of the phenothiazines in depressed patients was generally held to be contraindicated. Imipramine, a compound synthesized as a possible analogue of the phenothiazine tranquilizers, was reported in 1958 to be effective in treating endogenous depression. For a few years, imipramine and related compounds were generally described as a drug class distinct from the tranquilizers. Pharmacologically there was no basis for this distinction, and a few clinicians soon began to substitute mixtures of a phenothiazine tranquilizer and imipramine in treating depressions. It now appears that some of the phenothiazines alone may be preferable to the newer antidepressant drugs. Discussion of these drugs can, therefore, be shortened by reference to the similar properties of the antipsychotic tranquilizers already discussed.

Chemistry

The drugs in this category are identified in Table 24—4. Imipramine and amitriptyline differ from the tranquilizers promazine (Sparine) and chlorprothixene (Taractan) in that a bridge of 2 methylene groups has been substituted for the sulfur of the older drugs and the chlorine present in chlorprothixene is not present in amitriptyline (Fig 24—2).

These drugs are also called imidodibenzyl, dibenzazepine, and tricyclic antidepressants.

Pharmacologic Effects

The section on the pharmacologic effects of the tranquilizers above can be applied without modification to the antidepressants. Some of the effects described for the tranquilizers are much less prominent because the antidepressants are used in smaller doses—ie, a maximum or limit is placed on the dosage.

Treatment of Depression Reaction

A. Problems in Evaluation of Therapy: The usual factors that require a controlled evaluation operate also during the drug treatment of depressions. In addition, the inadequate diagnostic differentiation of depressions can result in confusion if the groups of patients being compared are in fact not really comparable. One cannot assume that all depressions—reactive (situational), neurotic, involutional, endogenous, or psychotic—respond similarly to drugs. Experience with severely ill, institutionalized populations is not interchangeable with experience in office practice, in which much of the depression that is seen is on a neurotic basis.

TABLE 24—4. Antidepressants that resemble tranquilizers.

	Initial Dose 3 Times a Day (mg)	Daily Dose (mg)
Imipramine (Tofranil)	25	200
Desipramine (Pertofrane, Norpramin)	25	200
Amitriptyline (Elavil)	25	150
Nortriptyline (Aventyl)	10	100
Doxepin (Sinequan)	25	300
Protriptyline (Vivactil)	5—10	60

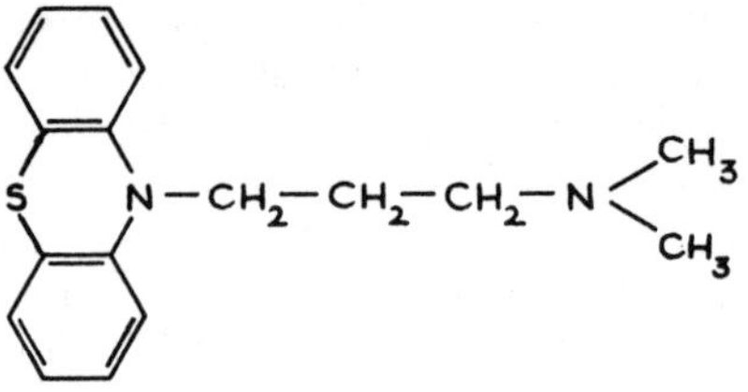

Promazine (Sparine)

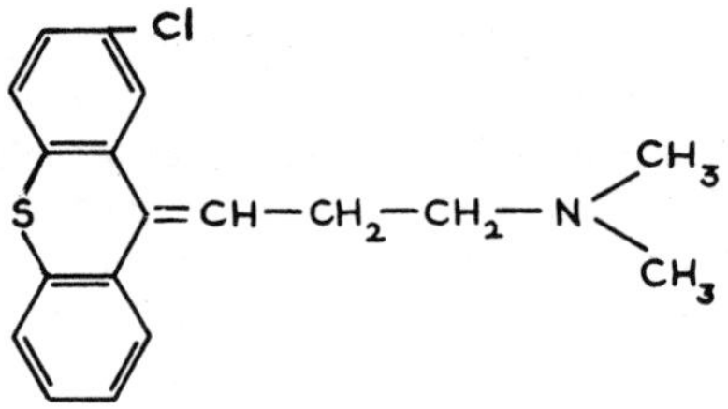

Chlorprothixene (Taractan)

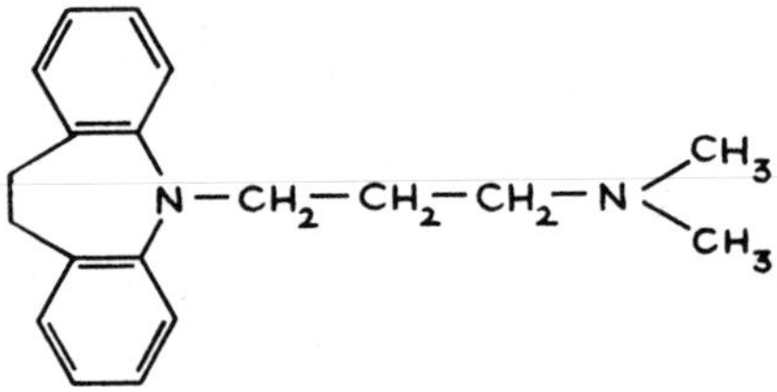

Imipramine (Tofranil)

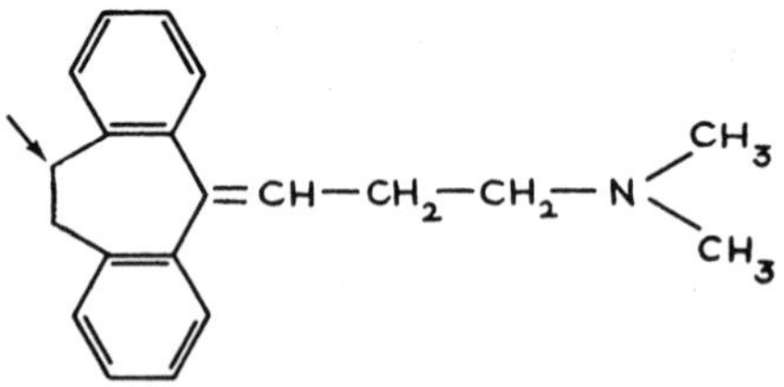

Amitriptyline (Elavil)
Doxepin (Sinequan) has oxygen
at site shown by arrow.

FIG 24–2. Chemical structures of 2 representative antipsychotic tranquilizers (above) and 2 antidepressants (below), illustrating the similarity between the 2 classes.

A precise statement of the results in the treatment of depression is difficult to formulate. Serious depressions are often episodic and self-limiting regardless of treatment. Because of variations in diagnostic criteria, control groups are essential for every new evaluation. The criteria of improvement also vary—eg, duration of hospitalization, a test score, or a subjective estimate of the degree of depression.

B. Alternative Treatments:

1. Antidepressants related to tranquilizers and ECT—The usefulness of the antidepressants as an alternative to electroconvulsive therapy (ECT) is established in the treatment of severe endogenous depressions. ECT is rapid and effective, but it is usually administered only during hospitalization and is an unpleasant experience. Drugs are a less rapid means of combating depression but have the advantages that continued or maintenance treatment is possible and that they are less objectionable to the patient and less expensive. Some psychiatrists start drugs and ECT together.

No important differences among the compounds available have been established. Of greater interest is the suggestion that in some cases phenothiazine tranquilizers are more effective.

2. Amphetamine—Amphetamine and related sympathomimetic amines are generally said to be useful in depressions only if the depression is mild.

3. Sedatives—The older sedatives (eg, phenobarbital) have long been used in the treatment of patients with an agitated depression, or with depressions that are on a neurotic basis. Recently, chlordiazepoxide (Librium), another long-acting sedative, has gained ground as an antidepressant, but its use should be confined to neurotic and situational depressions. In some patients, sedatives increase depression.

4. MAO inhibitors—These agents have been generally replaced by the above-listed classes of drugs.

Preparations and Dosages

Treatment with the antidepressants is started at a usual initial dosage level (Table 24–4). Patients are told that there will be an unavoidable waiting period of 1–3 weeks before the drug can be expected to have a favorable effect. If there is no improvement after 2 weeks, the dosage can be raised to the maximum level. The usual maximum daily dose may be exceeded in hospitalized patients. Aged patients are usually more sensitive to these drugs and thus require a smaller dosage.

When a favorable response is achieved, the same dose is continued for 1–2 months and is then slowly decreased to a maintenance level at or below the usual starting dosage. Treatment is usually continued for at least 3 months after the depression has cleared, and the drug is then gradually withdrawn over the next 3 months.

Adverse Reactions

A. Side-Effects: Side-effects are similar to those seen after the administration of the antipsychotic tranquilizers. After the usual doses, atropine-like effects and postural hypotension are relatively prominent.

1. Behavioral—The distinctive kind of sedation that occurs after the administration of antipsychotic tranquilizers also appears after imipramine and similar antidepressants. The patient may complain of weakness or drowsiness. Increased feelings of tension, tremulousness, visual hallucinations, and agitation are sometimes induced.

2. Autonomic—Dry mouth and constipation are common atropine-like effects; blurred vision and tachycardia are uncommon. Postural hypotension occurs frequently, and is the side-effect that most commonly limits the comfortable dose of these drugs.

3. Other—Extrapyramidal signs are rare with the doses usually employed. Weight gain, an unpleasant taste, edema, and prolonged atrioventricular conduction time occur.

B. Acute Toxicity: The acute toxicity of the antidepressants appears to be greater than that of the phenothiazines in that accidental deaths and suicides have been reported.

C. Allergic Reactions: Isolated reports of bone marrow depression and cholestatic jaundice have appeared.

AMPHETAMINE AND RELATED SYMPATHOMIMETIC STIMULANTS

The drugs in this category are variants of the ephedrine class of sympathomimetics selected because they exhibit relatively more potent central stimulant effects and relatively less potent cardiovascular effects.

All of the compounds of this group (identified in Table 24—5) have a chemical and biologic similarity to ephedrine and amphetamine.

TABLE 24—5. **Amphetamine and related anorexigenic and stimulant amines.**

	Usual Oral Daily Dosage (mg)
Amphetamine (Benzedrine)	5—15
Dextroamphetamine (Dexedrine)	5—15
Methamphetamine (Desoxyn, Methedrine)	5—15
Phentermine (Wilpo; Ionamin, a complex with a resin)	8—40
Chlorphentermine (Pre-Sate)	65
Benzphetamine (Didrex)	25—50
Phenmetrazine (Preludin)	25—75
Phendimetrazine (Plegine)	35
Diethylpropion (Tenuate, Tepanil)	25—75
Methylphenidate (Ritalin)	10—30
Pipradol (Meratran)	2.5—10

Pharmacologic Effects

 A. Sympathomimetic: Blood vessels are constricted. Blood pressure and pulse rate are elevated. The pupils are dilated.

 B. CNS Stimulation: Wakefulness is produced, fatigue is decreased, and euphoria is induced. Tremulousness and anxiety may appear. Larger doses may cause hyperactivity, insomnia, or a toxic psychosis.

Clinical Uses

 In the following clinical situations, an amphetamine such as dextro-amphetamine is given in a dose of 5—15 mg/day (usually prohibited within 8 hours of bedtime).

 A. Obesity: The great interest in the anorexigenic effect of the sympathomimetics is based on more than the vanity of the patient; obesity increases susceptibility to a number of diseases, and life expectancy is reduced by even a minor increase in weight above an ideal based on insurance statistics. In recent years, weight control has become a major concern and interest of a large proportion of the American people.

 The ability of ephedrine, amphetamine, and other phenyliso-propylamines to decrease appetite parallels their potency as CNS stimulants. An intense anorexigenic action can be demonstrated on animals in the laboratory, and a specific CNS effect is therefore assumed to be operating rather than a change in mood, or distraction, or increased activity. The amphetamines act in mentally deficient as well as normal humans.

 When any of the drugs related to amphetamine is tested in obese patients under controlled conditions and is given in adequate dosage, it exerts an anorexigenic effect that is clearly beyond that of the placebo. However, after a few weeks (6—8 weeks maximum), tolerance appears, the weight loss ceases, and the patient usually resumes his previous eating and gaining habits unless other forms of treatment have been more successful. All of the controlled studies utilize a fixed dosage throughout the period of study since a progressive increase in dosage to overcome whatever process is leading to tolerance would presumably add the risk of drug misuse or habituation. Periods of treatment with amphetamines for 2 weeks alternating with equal periods without treatment are more effective than continuous treatment.

 B. As Euphoriant and Antidepressant: Controlled tests show that amphetamines produce euphoria more consistently in normal humans than either morphine or pentobarbital. This action may in part explain the misuse of the amphetamines and their use in mild (usually situational or reactive) depressions. Unfortunately, the amphetamines are essentially impotent in endogenous and psychotic depressions.

 C. To Improve Performance: Amphetamine and its congeners are used, perhaps ill-advisedly but nevertheless effectively, to improve psychomotor performance. The deterioration of performance with fatigue can in part be prevented or reversed and a state of wakefulness maintained. This generalization applies to comparatively simple psychomotor tests; concentration in complex learning situations and judgment are not improved.

Without suggesting that the practice is anything but pernicious, it must be acknowledged that the administration of amphetamine 90 minutes before a test situation improves athletic performance (swimming, running, weight throwing) to a degree that is highly significant in competition. As a result, a strict ban on the use of drugs in athletic competition has become worldwide. The drug has been used in warfare, before battles.

D. Hyperkinetic State in Children: This syndrome (also identified as minimum brain damage or organic behavior problem) is introduced here in order to present the apparently paradoxic effect of the amphetamines in children. The syndrome is defined by the complaints of the parent or teacher rather than of the child—ie, hyperactivity, aggressiveness, perseveration, distractability, poor performance in school. Evaluation of the results of treatment is difficult, but in controlled studies amphetamine (or methylphenidate) does appear to reduce the behavior that is impeding development provided that it is due to organic factors. Adult doses are given each morning (or morning and noon), and the effect is like that of a sedative without stimulation (ie, there is no excitement, wakefulness, etc). Treatment is discontinued after the patient reaches his early teens.

E. Narcolepsy: Narcolepsy is a rare condition characterized by involuntary lapses into normal sleep, especially during periods of monotony or inactivity such as working at some jobs or driving. Amphetamine prevents these lapses. A single morning dose of 10—15 mg may be adequate, or larger doses several times a day may be necessary. *Cataplexy*—ie, sudden generalized loss of muscle tone without loss of consciousness during laughter or at the time of experiencing an intense emotion—is sometimes associated with narcolepsy but is not as readily altered by treatment with amphetamine.

Preparations and Dosages

If the drugs listed in Table 24—5 are given in equipotent doses, they are generally equivalent. A few have not yet been used in doses sufficient to cause toxic psychosis, but other side-effects are similar.

Dextroamphetamine is the standard drug of the group. It is often given in doses of 5 mg 3 times daily before meals. Taking the drug before meals may serve as a reminder to the patient that he must discipline himself, but 15 mg of this long-acting drug as a single morning dose are often equally effective. Some disturbance of sleep habits will be apparent for as long as 24 hours after a single dose—an observation important in interpreting the claims made for sustained release dosage forms.

Racemic DL-amphetamine (Benzedrine) causes more cardiovascular side-effects for the same amount of central stimulation.

Methamphetamine is about twice as potent as dextroamphetamine.

The other available preparations are claimed to have either fewer side-effects or a longer duration of action. The most recently introduced analogue of amphetamine, chlorphentermine (Pre-Sate), causes the same restlessness as amphetamine but also a poorly defined kind of sedation. Amphetamine may cause a similar side-effect, but the sedation is probably a depressive after-effect.

Pemoline (Cylert) is a mild stimulant chemically similar to phenmetrazine. It is an investigative drug publicized for its effect on learning in animals and its possible effect on memory in aged humans. The early enthusiastic reports are being superseded by descriptions that emphasize the similarity of this drug to amphetamine.

Adverse Reactions

This discussion applies to amphetamine, methamphetamine, related anorexigenic drugs, and cocaine.

A. Side-Effects: Common side-effects are tremulousness, anxiety, awareness of heart action, dry mouth, and alteration of sleep habits such as insomnia or increased dreaming. The side-effects are usually not troublesome after a few days of continued use, but some patients are unable to tolerate the stimulation of any amphetamine.

B. Overdosage Toxicity:

1. Acute toxicity—The acute toxicity of the amphetamines is low. Reported fatalities have been due to a complicating coexistent disease or the result of treatment. The lethal dose of dextroamphetamine is probably several grams. Restlessness or toxic psychosis, hypertension, and tachycardia may be prominent. Treatment consists of sedation.

2. Chronic toxicity—The amphetamines may be misused (as described below) but have no other organic toxicity.

3. Toxic psychosis—Behavior is not usually greatly altered by chronic use of these stimulants. The subject complains of depression if he is deprived of the drug but usually does not acknowledge any euphoria when it is supplied. In large and repeated doses the drug becomes a psychotomimetic agent. Intense anxiety, restlessness, feelings of depersonalization, and altered perception may progress to a state similar to paranoid schizophrenia. As in other toxic psychoses, auditory and visual hallucinations may be prominent, but the patient usually continues to recognize the relation between his altered perception and the drug. If paranoia or delirium is prominent, a small dose of chlorpromazine or other antipsychotic tranquilizer may be useful but sedation with a barbiturate is usually adequate treatment.

C. Misuse and Habituation: The amphetamines, like other drugs with a potential for misuse, are abused to different degrees by different users. Amphetamines may be used episodically as "spree" drugs to improve performance, defer fatigue, or prolong an alcoholic binge. They may be used intermittently over a long period but in moderate doses for their euphoriant or antidepressant effect.

A few people become compulsive users of the drug. Some take huge doses by mouth. If the susceptible person is with a drug abusing group in his community, he may use an amphetamine intravenously. In this setting, methamphetamine is the favored agent.

Physical dependence manifested as withdrawal signs is difficult to establish or to distinguish from the exhaustion that follows a period of abuse of the amphetamine group of drugs.

The development of tolerance is commonly seen, and side-effects become less prominent with continued use.

The principal adverse result of amphetamine misuse is the loss of productive activity imposed on the drug-dominated individual by his preoccupation with obtaining the drug. In some individuals, large doses will precipitate the toxic psychosis mentioned above.

AMINE OXIDASE INHIBITORS

Inhibitors of monamine oxidase (MAO) are no longer much used in therapy. The remaining interest in these drugs is based largely on their mechanism of action.

The drugs usually classified as MAO inhibitors are listed in Table 24—6. Iproniazid is no longer available for use in humans because of the liver damage that it caused, but it is still widely used in laboratory investigation because of its potency. Tranylcypromine is closely related to amphetamine. The ephedrine or amphetamine type of sympathomimetic drugs are weak MAO inhibitors.

Pharmacologic Actions

A. Mechanisms of Action: The MAO inhibitors cause a long-lasting inhibition (irreversible or nonequilibrium blockade) of MAO. The action is demonstrable in humans. However, it is not clear which of the pharmacologic effects are due to MAO inhibition and which are independent of enzyme inhibition.

MAO governs the oxidative deamination of many simple primary and secondary amines. The aldehyde formed is converted to an acid. Thus, serotonin is metabolized to hydroxyindoleacetic acid.

During the period of MAO inhibition, the concentration of norepinephrine, dopamine, and serotonin rises in the CNS and heart because destruction is slowed. The activity of the precursors of these amines—dopa and 5-hydroxytryptophan—is greatly augmented. An increased CNS action of the amines themselves cannot be demonstrated since they do not enter the CNS after systemic administration.

TABLE 24—6. Monoamine oxidase (MAO) inhibitors.

	Initial Dose (mg per day)	Maintenance Dose (mg per day)
Iproniazid* (Marsilid)	—	—
Nialamide (Niamid)	100—300	50—150
Isocarboxazid (Marplan)	20—30	10
Phenelzine (Nardil)	30—45	5—20
Pargyline† (Eutonyl)	25—50	10—100
Tranylcypromine (Parnate)	20	10—20

*No longer marketed. Included for identification only.
†Used in treatment of hypertension rather than as stimulant.

B. Effects:

1. CNS stimulation–The MAO inhibitors produce a series of changes similar to those described for amphetamine: wakefulness, euphoria, respiratory stimulation, excitement, and, after large doses, a toxic psychosis. Convulsions are rare, and the drugs are anticonvulsant in the laboratory and clinically. An increase in appetite is much more often seen than anorexia.

2. Sympathoplegic effects–The mechanism by which a decrease in sympathetic influence on the tissues is brought about is not understood, but postural hypotension occurs and cardiac output is reduced.

3. Sympathomimetic effects–Drugs of this class differ in the intensity of their sympathomimetic effects, but after large doses all can produce hypertension, tachycardia, and smooth muscle relaxation.

Absorption, Metabolism, and Excretion

All of the drugs of this group are given by mouth. They are rapidly metabolized and excreted. However, the MAO inhibition persists long after elimination or discontinuation of the medication.

Clinical Uses

The MAO inhibitors have been almost completely superseded by the antidepressants related to the tranquilizers. In retrospect, it is doubtful whether even iproniazid was as effective as ECT. Indeed, there are many studies that question whether the hydrazines have any superiority when compared with placebos.

Preparation and Dosages

If the MAO inhibitors are used, they are given in an initial dosage (see Table 24–6) that is continued for 2–6 weeks or until a response is noted. The dosage is then slowly reduced to the maintenance doses listed.

Excluding pargyline (the hypotensive agent) and tranylcypromine, there is no basis for preferring one or the other of these drugs. Tranylcypromine (Parnate) is a special case. Its return to the market after serious and lethal hypertensive episodes was permitted only with special restrictive labeling. It should be used "only in those depressions that have failed to respond to other [not further defined] therapy." The package insert should be read by anyone contemplating the use of tranylcypromine because it is by law part of the labeling and places the responsibility for any poor result on the physician.

Adverse Reactions

A. CNS Effects. Euphoria or restlessness may progress to excitement or a toxic psychosis. After large single doses, the patient may become stuporous and unresponsive. Convulsions are rare, but fibrillary muscle twitching is common.

B. Sympathomimetic Effects: These are usually limited to constipation, urinary hesitancy, and dry mouth. Hypertension may occur, but is dangerous only in the case of tranylcypromine (Parnate) or when dietary tyramine or other sympathomimetic drugs are ingested concurrently, in which cases a

TABLE 24–7. Toxicity of major groups of psychopharmacologic drugs.*†

★ = Often present ○ = Usually absent	Antipsychotic Tranquilizers	Antidepressants	Sedatives	Sedative Withdrawal	Amphetamines	Narcotics	Narcotic Withdrawal
Autonomic Effects							
Blurred vision	★	★	○	○	★	○	○
Dry mouth	★	★	○	○	★	○	○
Urinary retention	★	★	○	○	★	○	○
Pupillary dilatation	★	★	○	★	★	○	★
Pupillary constriction	★	★	○	○	○	★	○
Paralysis of accommodation	★	★	○	○	○	○	○
Abdominal cramps, diarrhea	○	○	○	○	○	○	★
Constipation	★	★	○	○	○	★	○
Sweating	○	○	○	★	★	○	★
Cardiovascular Effects							
Bradycardia	★	★	○	○	○	★	○
Tachycardia	★	★	○	★	★	○	★
Hypotension, postural	★	★	○	○	○	★	○
Hypertension	○	○	○	★	★	○	★
Edema	★	★	○	○	○	○	○
CNS Effects							
Drowsiness	★	★	★	○	○	★	○
Hyperthermia	○	○	○	★	★	○	★
Insomnia	○	○	○	★	★	○	★
Excitement, hyperactivity, agitation	★	★	○	★	★	○	★
Convulsions	★	★	○	★	○	○	★
Euphoria	○	★	★	○	★	★	○
Depression	★	○	★	○	○	○	○
Ataxia, dysarthria, nystagmus	○	○	★	○	○	○	○
Unconsciousness, coma, anesthesia	★	★	★	○	○	★	○
Respiratory depression	★	★	★	○	○	★	○
Hallucinations	○	○	★	★	★	★	★
Tremors and rigidity	★	★	○	★	○	○	★
Dystonias and akathisia	★	★	○	○	○	○	○
Metabolic and Endocrine Effects							
Menstrual irregularity	★	★	★	○	○	★	○
Galactorrhea	★	★	○	○	○	○	○
Weight increase	★	★	○	○	○	○	○
Anorexia	○	○	○	★	★	○	★

*Courtesy of Carlos E. Climent, MD.
†Variations in effect may be dose-related or may be due to setting or basic personality structure.

serious hypertensive crisis may occur. The most common sources of dietary tyramine, which should be avoided during treatment with MAO inhibitors, are foods prepared by fermentation, ie, some forms of cheese, beer, and wine. The absorbed tyramine is not destroyed at the usual rapid rate and so releases norepinephrine from stores augmented by administration of MAO inhibitors.

The possible hypertensive reactions to dietary tyramine should be explained to the patient, and he should also be cautioned against the use of other sympathomimetic drugs, including over-the-counter cold tablets or capsules. In addition, the MAO inhibitors potentiate the effect of narcotic analgesics, tranquilizers, and sedatives such as alcohol and barbiturates.

. . .

Table 24–7 is a presentation of the toxic signs and symptoms in the major groups of psychopharmacologic drugs and in sedative and narcotic withdrawal. Both side-effects and signs and symptoms of acute and chronic toxicity are included.

REFERENCES

Books and Monographs

Cole, J.O.: *Pharmacotherapy of Depressions.* Thomas, 1966.

Haase, H., & P. Janssen: *The Action of Neuroleptic Drugs.* North Holland Publishing Co., 1965.

Klein, D.F., & J.M. Davis: *Diagnosis and Drug Treatment of Psychiatric Disorders.* Williams & Wilkins, 1969.

Rothlin, E. (editor): *Neuropsychopharmacology.* 2 vols. Elsevier, 1961.

Schildkraut, J.J.: *Neuropsychopharmacology and the Affective Disorders.* Little, Brown, 1970.

Shader, R.I., & A. DiMascio: *Psychotropic Drug Side Effects.* Williams & Wilkins, 1970.

Solomon, P. (editor): *Psychiatric Drugs.* Grune & Stratton, 1966.

Usdin, E., & D. Efron: *Psychotropic Drugs and Related Compounds.* US Department of Health, Education, and Welfare, 1967.

Journal Articles

Ayd, F.J., Jr.: A survey of drug-induced extrapyramidal reactions. JAMA 175:1054–1060, 1961.

Baastrup, P.C., & M. Schou: Lithium as a prophylactic agent: Its effect against recurrent depressions and manic-depressive psychosis. Arch Gen Psychiat 16:162–172, 1967.

Baldessarini, R., & J. Stephens: Lithium carbonate for affective disorders. Arch Gen Psychiat 22:72–77, 1970.

Brophy, J.J.: Single daily doses of neuroleptic drugs. Dis Nerv System 30:120-123, 1969.

Council on Drugs: Evaluation of lithium carbonate for treatment of manic-depressive psychosis. JAMA 215:1486–1488, 1971.

or are

Crane, G.E.: A review of clinical literature on haloperidol. Internat J Neuropsychiat 3 (Suppl 1):111–125, 1967.

Curry, A.S.: Twenty-one uncommon cases of poisoning. Brit MJ 1:687–688, 1962.

Davis, J.M., & others: Overdosage of psychotropic drugs: A review. 1. Major and minor tranquilizers. 2 Antidepressants and other psychotropic agents. Dis Nerv System 29:157–163, 246–256, 1968.

Demers, R., & G. Heninger: Pretibial edema and sodium retention during lithium carbonate treatment. JAMA 214:1845–1848, 1970.

Engelhardt, D.M., & others: Phenothiazines in prevention of psychiatric hospitalization. Arch Gen Psychiat 16:98–101, 1967.

Goldfield, M., & M.R. Weinstein: Lithium in pregnancy: A review with recommendations. Am J Psychiat 127:888–893, 1971.

Hadden, J.: Acute barbiturate intoxication. JAMA 209:893–900, 1969.

Hollister, L.E.: Human pharmacology and antipsychotic and antidepressant drugs. Ann Rev Pharmacol 8:491–516, 1968.

Hollister, L.E., & others: Acetophenazine and diazepam in anxious depressions. Arch Gen Psychiat 24:273–278, 1971.

Hollister, L.E., & others: Withdrawal reactions from chlordiazepoxide (Librium). Psychopharmacologia 2:63–68, 1961.

Lehmann, H.E., Ban, T., & V.A. Kral: Drugs and patients: Evaluating chemicals that change human behavior. Psychopharmacol Bull 6:48–63, April 1970.

Litvak, R., & R. Kaelbling: Agranulocytosis, leukopenia, and psychotropic drugs. Arch Gen Psychiat 24:265–267, 1971.

Lowinger, P., & S. Dobie: What makes the placebo work? Arch Gen Psychiat 20:84–88, 1969.

Lynn, E.J., Satloff, A., & D.C. Tinling: Mania and the use of lithium: A three-year study. Am J Psychiat 127:1176–1180, 1971.

National Institute of Mental Health Collaborative Study Group: Effectiveness of phenothiazine treatment of acute schizophrenic psychoses. Arch Gen Psychiat 10:246–261, 1964.

National Institute of Mental Health Collaborative Study Group: Differences in clinical effects of three phenothiazines in "acute" schizophrenia. Dis Nerv System 28:369–383, 1967.

Overall, J.E., & L.E. Hollister: Psychiatric drug research. Arch Gen Psychiat 16:152–161, 1967.

Powell, L.W., & others: Acute meprobamate poisoning. New England J Med 259:716–718, 1958.

Prien, R.F., & J.O. Cole: High dose chlorpromazine therapy in chronic schizophrenia. Arch Gen Psychiat 18:482–495, 1968.

Rickels, K.: Drug use in outpatient treatment. Am J Psychiat 124:20–31, 1968.

Roth, M., & K. Schapira: Social implications of recent advances in psychopharmacology. Brit M Bull 26:197–202, 1970.

Schildkraut, J.J., & others: Changes in norepinephrine turnover in rat brain during chronic administration of imipramine and protriptyline: A possible explanation for the delay in onset of clinical antidepressant effects. Am J Psychiat 127:1032–1039, 1971.

Schou, M.: Lithium in psychiatric therapy and prophylaxis. J Psychiat Res 6:67–95, 1968.

Schou, M.: Lithium: Elimination rate, dosage, control, poisoning, goiter, mode of action. Acta psychiat scand (Suppl)207:49–53, 1969.

Schou, M., & D. Baastrup: Lithium as a prophylactic agent. Arch Gen Psychiat 16:162–173, 1967.

Van der Velde, C.D.: Toxicity of lithium carbonate in elderly patients. Am J Psychiat 127:1075–1077, 1971.

Weiss, B., & V.G. Laties: Comparative pharmacology of drugs affecting behavior. Fed Proc 26:1146–1156, 1967.

Wheeler, R.H., Bhalerao, V.R., & M.J. Gilkes: Ocular pigmentation, extrapyramidal symptoms and phenothiazine dosage. Brit J Psychiat 115:687–690, 1969.

Zbinden, G., & others: Experimental and clinical toxicology of chlordiazepoxide (Librium). Toxic Appl Pharmacol 3:619–637, 1961.

25...

Electroconvulsive Therapy & Other Somatic Therapies

ECT remains a bulwark of modern psychiatry—safe, easy, and effective. It supersedes medication (or the 2 can be given together) in critical depressions or unresponsive agitations. It has no place in the treatment of neuroses. Lobotomy has become a last resort procedure in various desperate problems.

Physical (somatic) methods of treatment in psychiatry are treatments administered to the patient's body in order to produce changes in his behavior. In the widest sense they include drugs, electroconvulsive therapy, insulin coma therapy, neurosurgery, hydrotherapy, sleep therapy, and body restraints. In common practice, however, the term somatic therapy has come to mean either drug therapy or electroshock therapy since these treatments are in wide use whereas the others are fading into a position of mainly historical interest.

In this chapter, only electroshock therapy will be considered in detail. Drug therapy is covered in Chapter 24. The other physical methods of treatment will be dealt with briefly.

At the outset, it should be stated explicitly that the modes of action of all of the physical methods of treatment are largely unknown. Those who claim that the physical methods of treatment are more "scientific" than psychologic treatment are correct only in the sense that it is easier to apply statistical methods of analysis to their results. One can easily measure and record a drug dosage or the amount of electrical current used for shock treatment, whereas quantitation of the "dose" of psychotherapy is impossible.

Against this claim for the greater scientific validity of the physical therapies, however, is the undeniable fact that there is a psychotherapeutic component inherent in the use of all physical treatments. The physician's enthusiasm for the treatment he is giving undoubtedly influences the response, and the expectations of both the doctor and the patient—as well as the nature of their relationship—can modify the patient's mood and outlook. It is probable that some physical therapies in the hands of an enthusiastic physician have helped some patients as effectively (and for the same reason) as a placebo administered with the same positive, hopeful attitude.

ELECTROCONVULSIVE THERAPY

Electroshock therapy (EST), now usually called electroconvulsive therapy (ECT), is the most widely used of the physical therapies with the exception of drug therapy. Originating with the mistaken observation that epilepsy and schizophrenia never occurred in the same patient and the false conclusion that convulsions might eliminate the symptoms of the illness, efforts were made in the early 1930s to induce convulsions as a form of treatment. Camphor injections, pentylenetetrazol (Metrazol) injections, and, more recently, flurothyl (Indoklon) have been used for this purpose. However, the method of producing convulsions introduced by the Italian psychiatrists Cerletti and Bini in 1938—ie, passing an alternating electrical current through the head and brain—has proved the most reliable, convenient, and effective.

ECT can now be given to patients or selected outpatients with a minimum of preparation. Small, portable ECT apparatuses are available that operate on 110 volts of alternating current and are equipped with a rheostat to deliver 70—130 volts. An electric timer is provided to vary the duration of shock from 0.1—1 second. Current is provided through 2 electrodes which are positioned on the patient's temples. The optimal dosage is the lowest current for the shortest time that will produce a grand mal or generalized tonic and clonic convulsion. It is customary to give 3 treatments a week until substantial improvement occurs and then another 3 or 4 treatments to complete the course. A minimum of 6 treatments, an average of 9 treatments, and a maximum of 25 treatments are considered normal limits for a course of treatment.

Some workers use the rule of thumb of noting the number of treatments before clinical improvement appears and then doubling this number—eg, if the patient first shows improvement after the 6th treatment, 12 will be given in all.

Indications

All depressions other than neurotic depressions tend to respond favorably to ECT. Depressive components of other illnesses are likely to respond as well. Acutely suicidal patients and patients in a state of manic or catatonic excitement may respond at least temporarily. Some psychiatrists feel that ECT is the treatment of choice for acute schizophrenia, but intensive drug therapy with phenothiazine probably should be tried first.

Since effective antidepressant drugs became available, most psychiatrists have preferred to try a course of drug therapy before using shock therapy unless the patient is acutely suicidal, severely retarded or agitated, or unless there is an urgent reason why he must be returned as soon as possible to his role as family breadwinner or other critical position. Antidepressant drugs do not become maximally effective for 3 weeks or more after beginning therapy, whereas the patient is sometimes restored to nearly normal function within 7—10 days after ECT is begun.

Character disorders, neurotic states, and chronic schizophrenias do not themselves respond to shock therapy, but an excited, depressed, or suicidal phase may develop in the course of any of these illnesses and may best be treated with ECT.

Contraindications

The only absolute contraindication to ECT is brain tumor since in this condition the increased intracranial pressure that occurs during the convulsion may have dire consequences. Careful consideration should be given to the underlying disease state in all patients, but shock therapy has been given successfully despite the presence of such serious illnesses as severe myocardial disease or recent coronary thrombosis. With proper care, ECT has a mortality rate of no more than one in 25,000 cases and is one of the safest treatments in medicine.

Preparation of the Patient

When the decision is made to give ECT, the patient must be told even though he is psychotic. Since some patients may equate the term electroshock with electrocution, it is well to use the less frightening term "electroconvulsive therapy." It is also well to tell him that a transient period of impaired memory may persist for nearly a month after treatment. If the patient is told that he will be put to sleep, will receive a treatment, will feel no pain or discomfort, and will wake up before an hour has passed with no recollection of what has happened, it is likely that he will be reassured and cooperative. It is customary to have the patient (if nonpsychotic) or a responsible relative sign a permission form prior to the administration of ECT.

The usual sequence of events is as follows: (1) Give nothing by mouth for at least 4 hours before treatment (to avoid the complications of vomiting). (2) Give 0.8 mg of atropine sulfate subcutaneously 30 minutes before treatment to decrease salivation and bronchial secretions. (3) Give thiopental sodium (Pentothal) intravenously to induce sleep. (4) Just before the shock is delivered, give an intravenous muscle relaxant such as succinylcholine chloride (Anectine), 10–30 mg IV (0.5–5 mg/min), to prevent violent muscle contractions.

Because the muscle relaxant paralyzes the muscles of respiration, it is usually necessary to assist respiration mechanically and through the use of oxygen during a brief period of postconvulsant apnea. *An anesthetist should be in attendance* since prolonged apnea or laryngeal stridor may occur.

During the recovery phase, a qualified person must be present until the patient is awake and able to care for himself. If he is left unattended, he may roll from the recovery bed to the floor or stumble around the recovery room during waking confusion. Because of the period of impaired memory associated with ECT, the patient receiving a course of treatment should be advised against making important business decisions until fully recovered. Also, if he is receiving treatments on an ambulatory or outpatient basis, he should be under someone's supervision while traveling back to his home after treatment. He should not drive his own car, and he should be advised against participating in any activity that could be dangerous to him in his somewhat hazy state until he is fully recovered from the course of treatment.

Before muscle relaxants became part of the ECT routine, violent muscle contractions often produced long bone fractures or thoracic vertebral compression fractures. If the convulsion is not adequately modified, either because the dosage of succinylcholine is inadequate or because of errors in the injection technic, fractures may still occur. An x-ray of the spine is often obtained before beginning treatment to permit evaluation of complications and to avoid malpractice claims.

INSULIN COMA TREATMENT

Insulin coma therapy (ICT) was discovered in 1933 by Manfred Sakel in Berlin. Insulin was used at that time to improve appetite in psychiatric patients and an occasional insulin-sensitive patient became comatose. Sakel observed that some psychotics emerged from coma in an improved mental state. He gradually developed a technic that employed the administration of up to 200 units of insulin to schizophrenic patients. After receiving this large dose of insulin, the patient passed through stages of progressive hypoglycemia manifested by (1) tiredness and perspiration; (2) restlessness, disorientation, dysarthria, hallucinations, and automatic movements with occasional convulsions; and then (3) coma. Periods of coma varying from 15 minutes to 1 hour were induced, and were terminated by administration of glucose.

Because improvement required 40–100 comas, treatment was protracted over a period of several months. The insulin treatment unit required highly competent and experienced personnel to maintain a patient in deep coma for extended periods, yet fatalities were frequent (one in 100 patients).

Although drug therapy and ECT have essentially replaced insulin coma, there are still those who feel that insulin treatment is a valuable therapeutic tool in schizophrenia. However, insulin coma units are rarities in the USA today.

PSYCHOSURGERY

Various neurosurgical procedures have been used in an attempt to improve symptoms in serious and chronic psychiatric disorders by interrupting neural pathways. From the 1930s, when Moniz and Lima in Portugal operated on the frontal lobes of psychotic patients, through the early 1940s, when Freeman and Watts reported some success with relief of depression by cutting the frontal lobes, the neurosurgical approach to psychiatry has held some promise.

Thus far, psychosurgery has been able to offer little more than a last ditch alternative to chronic hospitalization or chronic severe impairment. If improvement is obtained with one of the many surgical technics still utilized on rare occasions, it is apt to be accompanied by undesirable sequelae such

as crude antisocial behavior or emotional flatness. Postoperative deaths
(1–3%) and cortical scarring with subsequent seizure activity (10–30%) are
also reported. Although formal tests of intelligence may show little change
after psychosurgery, higher intellectual functioning such as concept formation and ability to plan for the future is usually affected.

In recent years, Lindstrom has developed a method of ultrasonic
lobotomy (through burr holes in the skull) that eliminates cutting of the
brain and thus the mortality and risk of postoperative seizures. He reports
excellent results in otherwise intractable cases. Other recent developments
have involved stereotaxic procedures (rigid fixation of the skull and highly
accurate localization of deep-lying structures by x-ray) and pinpoint destruction of either the amygdala or the cingulum. Lesions in these areas have been
reported to relieve suffering in cases of intractable pain and in a variety of
unresponsive psychiatric conditions (especially severe agitated, obsessive
compulsive, or anxiety states).

HYDROTHERAPY

Psychiatric illness is no longer treated by means of water baths in the
USA. The technic once used was to place the patient in a large tub filled
with warm water at a carefully maintained temperature. The patient was
then covered with a sheet of canvas so that only his head protruded. "The
tubs" were used for disturbed patients and had the doubtful advantage of
restraining and bathing the patient at the same time. Since careful maintenance of a comfortable temperature was important, it was also necessary
to have someone in close attendance throughout the procedure. In retrospect, it seems clear that this attendant provided some psychotherapy along
with his other duties and perhaps this was the most effective component of
the hydrotherapy regimen.

CONTINUOUS SLEEP THERAPY

Since 1922, when Klaesi, a Swiss psychiatrist, first used drugs to induce
long periods of sleep in psychiatric patients, sleep therapy has enjoyed occasional vogue. Patients have been maintained in deep sleep for over a week at
a time, being awakened only for feeding and elimination of wastes.

The results of sleep therapy seem to be no better than those of ECT.
Consequently, sleep therapy is little used in this country, although it is now
enjoying some popularity in Europe and, particularly, in Russia.

BODY RESTRAINTS

Since Pinel removed the shackles and chains from his patients, physical
restraints of disturbed psychiatric patients have gradually been discarded.
Straitjackets are no longer standard equipment in mental hospitals, although

some police departments still use them to control violent behavior. A patient may be stimulated to even more violent disruptive behavior rather than quieted by the application of restraints. The lesson of the locked ward is that when patients are deprived of their freedom their behavior becomes more regressive and assaultive than when the doors are unlocked and the ward left open. The same seems to be true of physical restraints.

The common practice today is to use drugs as chemical restraints. Physical restraints are now used only for brief periods as a temporary emergency measure to control violent behavior in the absence of other, far more satisfactory measures.

REFERENCES

Books and Monographs

Crue, B.L., Jr.: *Pain and Suffering: Selected Aspects.* Thomas, 1970.

Himwich, H.E., & others: Effect of shock therapies on the brain. Pages 548—567 in: *Biology of Mental Health and Disease: A Symposium.* The 27th Annual Conference of the Milbank Memorial Fund. Hoeber, 1952.

Journal Articles

Ballantine, H.T., & others: Stereotaxic anterior cingulotomy for neuropsychiatric illness and intractable pain. J Neurosurg 26:488—495, 1967.

Bidder, T.G., Strain, J.J., & L. Brunschwig: Bilateral and unilateral ECT: Follow-up study and critique. Am J Psychiat 127:737—745, 1970.

Brown, M.H., & J.A. Lighthill: Selective anterior cingulotomy: A psychosurgical evaluation. J Neurosurg 29:513—519, 1968.

Elithorn, A., & others: Adrenocortical responsiveness during courses of electroconvulsive therapy. Brit J Psychiat 115:575—580, 1969.

Fleminger, J.J., & others: Differential effect of unilateral and bilateral ECT. Am J Psychiat 127:437, 1970.

Foltz, E.L., & L.E. White: Pain "relief" by frontal cingulumotomy. J Neurosurg 19:89—100, 1962.

Impastato, D.J.: The safer administration of succinylcholine without barbiturates: A new technique. Am J Psychiat 113:461, 1956.

Malmquist, C.P., & J.H. Matthews: Electroshock therapy in high-risk patients. Am J Psychiat 122:1265—1269, 1966.

Maxwell, R.D.H.: Electrical factors in electroconvulsive therapy. Acta psychiat scandinav 44:436, 1968.

McKenna, G., & others: Cardiac arrhythmias during electroshock therapy: Significance, prevention and treatment. Am J Psychiat 127:530—533, 1970.

Moore, M.T.: Electrocerebral shock therapy: A reconsideration of former contraindications. Arch Neurol Psychiat 57:693—711, 1947.

Zamora, E.N., & R. Kaelbling: Memory and electroconvulsive therapy. Am J Psychiat 122:546—554, 1965.

Zubin, J.: Memory functioning in patients treated with electric shock therapy. J Personality 17:33—44, 1948.

26...
Brief Psychotherapy

*The principles of brief psychotherapy are the same as for
any psychotherapy except that there is a preagreed limit on the
number of sessions. Goals are restricted, character problems are
avoided, and attention is confined largely to the here and now.*

Brief psychotherapy has evolved as a distinct psychiatric treatment
form as a result of the observation that many patients achieve marked relief
of symptoms and moderate character changes in a few interviews, whereas
continued therapy may produce little further progress. If the patient comes
to treatment in a crisis situation, his established defenses and behavior patterns are broken down, and this may prove to be an ideal time to develop
healthier defenses and better solutions to conflicts. Immediate therapy in a
crisis situation will prevent anxiety, depression, and other symptoms from
producing greater disorganization and psychopathology. An acutely suffering
patient is better motivated for change than one to whom chronic suffering
has become a way of life. The limited time available for clinic treatment, the
scarcity of psychiatrists, and financial pressure in private practice have
tended to encourage the development of brief psychotherapy, but the chief
reason for its emerging importance is that it is more effective than long-term
therapy for the management of acute psychiatric problems.

Brief psychotherapy is defined as a mutual undertaking by the patient
and therapist to change the patient's perception, thinking, feeling, and behavior within an agreed number (usually 10–15) of 50-minute interviews,
usually weekly. (Agreement on the number of interviews at the outset minimizes the problem of overdependence and motivates the patient to work
diligently to resolve his difficulties.) It differs from long-term therapy not
only in the number of interviews but also in its emphasis on the current
situation. Character problems are taken up only if very pertinent. If possible,
the patient's feelings for the therapist are kept positive and are not taken up
as an issue in treatment, and the therapist is more active in focusing the
discussion. Dependence and regression are discouraged.

SELECTION OF PATIENTS FOR BRIEF PSYCHOTHERAPY

Brief psychotherapy may be tried for any psychiatric condition, but
good results cannot usually be achieved in chronic psychotic illnesses, chron-

ic obsessive compulsive neuroses (and most are chronic by the time they come for treatment), and severe characterologic problems such as sexual perversion, alcoholism, inadequate personality, and passive-dependent personality. An acute episode of anxiety or depression occurring in a patient with one of the above-mentioned conditions may be treated provided the precise goals of treatment are stated so that the patient is not led to be overoptimistic. The patient with an acute symptom occurring in response to a maturational crisis (changing schools, graduation, marriage, increased job responsibility, etc) who has a previously sound character is best suited for brief psychotherapy. Others are patients with unexplained emotional or somatic symptoms or neurotic symptoms superimposed upon organic illness.

Patients must be motivated for treatment, and features that lead to a good prognosis are (1) a good reality situation, (2) stable relationships with people, (3) an ability to look at themselves realistically (ie, the ability to introspect), (4) no language barrier, (5) at least average intelligence, (6) willingness to accept personal responsibility for their difficulties; (7) the ability to tolerate anxiety, anger, and frustration without discharge through "acting out"; and (8) no significant "secondary gains" from their symptoms.

The psychotherapy discussed in this chapter is derived from psychodynamics of the psychoanalytic school. Behavior therapy by reciprocal inhibition as expounded by Wolpe is discussed in Chapter 28. Logotherapy (Frankel), hypnosis, and behavior therapy use a different technic stemming from a different theoretical basis, and there is no indication to combine them with brief psychotherapy as here described. They may be useful in certain cases such as isolated phobias.

If there is a marital problem, marriage counseling may be combined with brief psychotherapy. This is particularly indicated when the patient blames his or her difficulties on the spouse. Interviewing them jointly may help to clarify the rationalizations, distortions, and projections more rapidly; but it must be made clear that the fact that one partner is in therapy does not mean that there is a "healthy one–sick one" relationship in the marriage nor that all differences of opinion will be resolved in favor of the partner not in therapy.

When seeing a patient and spouse, the goals are (1) verbalization, to improve communication between partners and resolve ambiguities; (2) confrontation of the partners, by the therapist and by each other, with their maladaptive patterns of behavior; (3) clarification of the reactions, frequently tracing the behavior back to the family of origin; and (4) "working through" in the treatment situation difficulties that could not be dealt with otherwise, in the expectation that the partners will be able to make use of the technics learned.

In seeing couples, the therapist must be impartial. If he gives an opinion, he must give the reasons for it. Spouses who are not patients are much less likely to accept a psychiatrist's statements on faith than patients are.

It is time-saving in brief psychotherapy to see the spouse, since it makes the real situation much more clear and makes it possible to detect the patient's blind spots.

THERAPEUTIC FACTORS IN BRIEF PSYCHOTHERAPY

The therapeutic factors in brief psychotherapy may be summarized briefly as follows:

(1) **Suggestion** is an important therapeutic factor since the very fact that he is in treatment leads the patient to hope for improvement. Thus he is receptive to ideas deliberately or otherwise implanted by the therapist. Direct advice and guidance may be given, but the results are better if the patient's own ideas, solutions, and insights can be reinforced and authenticated.

(2) **Verbalization** consists of putting thoughts, wishes, fantasies, and feelings into words so that they can be examined. The act of putting things into words often makes it possible for the patient to deal with previously unrecognized matters in a therapeutically beneficial way.

(3) **The support** the patient receives from the therapist permits him to feel that something is being done for him and gives hope that in the future he will find another person to whom he can relate honestly and from whom he can expect an honest appraisal. Although the therapist accepts the patient's problems as real, he should also point out the patient's successes in life and not concur uncritically with those of the patient's self-criticisms that he feels are not justified. In successful therapy, the therapist will frequently serve as a model with whom the patient identifies.

(4) **Abreaction** is the recollection by the patient, with emotional discharge, of previously unconscious experiences and ideas, with the result that the patient gains awareness of the relationship between the undischarged emotion and his symptoms.

(5) **The "corrective emotional experience"** in the patient-therapist relationship makes it possible for the patient both to understand and to feel that the people in his present life are not identical with the pathogenic figures in his past life. In some cases the therapist may deliberately assume a role he feels to be opposite to the one the patient has been expecting of him, eg, be very strict in contrast to the patient's weak, yielding father.

(6) **Clarification** is the restatement by the therapist of previously unconnected facts which were unconscious or preconscious, with the goal of correcting misunderstandings.

(7) **Interpretation** is the explanation to the patient of his productions, resistances, and character defenses. This is best done by demonstrating patterns of responses using examples from the treatment or current reality situation.

(8) **Insight,** the intellectual understanding and emotional acceptance of the origin and development of symptoms, will help to protect patients from the repetition of previous conflicts. Patients should be helped to attain it only when they are able to tolerate it. The emotional response that comes with insight is one of the chief aims of interview therapy.

(9) **In "working through,"** the patient puts to use in real life situations what he has learned about himself in therapy. The satisfaction in mastery of once difficult situations serves as a stimulus to further progress.

STRATEGY OF TREATMENT

The natural sequence of events in brief psychotherapy is as follows: (1) The patient talks of ideas and feelings which then serve as the working materials of therapy. (2) The therapist attempts to understand what has been happening to the patient. (3) He communicates this understanding to the patient. (4) The patient uses this understanding to reorient and readjust his life. The foundation of treatment is the *therapeutic alliance,* in which the mature part of the patient works with the therapist to understand the immature part that is causing problems. This will be influenced by transference, which is a reaction to the therapist as though he were a previously important figure in the patient's life. If the transference is positive, it need not be touched (unless it becomes too intense or erotized); however, negative feelings must be worked out. Brief psychotherapy differs from long-term psychotherapy and psychoanalysis in that the transference is rarely investigated.

The therapist's feelings about the patient must also be considered, and the therapist should attempt to discover how the patient stimulates negative feelings and convey this understanding to the patient. If the therapist is unable to like and respect the patient, he should transfer him to another therapist.

PRECAUTIONS

The primary rule is to try to effect personality changes in the patient only when it is clearly for the best. The patient's equilibrium with society may change as a result of self-understanding, and some masochistic patients may seem to be made worse in the sense that they are no longer willing to tolerate the demands made on them. There are times when defenses—particularly denial, reaction formation, and intellectualization—are in the patient's best interests and should be supported rather than tampered with unless it is probable that a better solution can be found. Rash interpretation of matters in the unconscious must be avoided. If the defense is very obvious to the therapist and not to the patient, its purpose must be understood before any attempt is made to remove it. Overdependence may develop in any type of psychotherapy, but is minimized in brief psychotherapy because the patient understands from the beginning that the relationship is of a specified duration.

The therapist should (1) avoid making decisions that should be made by the patient; (2) frustrate the patient's unreasonable dependent demands; and (3) make use of the emotions generated by this frustration to clarify and interpret conflicts. However, he must realize that not all dependency is evil and must be able to tolerate the patient's dependency, particularly during crises, with the goal of working with it later at a more appropriate time.

When conflicts are uncovered, the patient may attempt to discharge uncomfortable feelings by actions. This "acting out" should be clarified and interpreted as soon as possible. If the acting out is dangerous to the patient, it should be discouraged with the statement that the objective of therapy is to solve problems by understanding rather than by unwise and premature action so that in the future, when the patient understands the reasons for his behavior, he will be free to make his own choices; but that until that time he should refrain from acting out. A specific form of acting out is regressive behavior with infantile actions (eg, sudden and continuous overeating or drinking), which may occur in therapy if a transference neurosis is allowed to flourish or if there is a serious reawakening of conflicts. Although some degree of regression may be useful in allowing patients to dissolve old defenses and substitute new and more useful ones, severe regression must be dealt with immediately and decisively. The therapist must simply condemn it and forbid it.

USE OF PSYCHOPHARMACOLOGIC AGENTS

Drugs may be useful, especially early in treatment, for the control of anxiety and depression or the relief of fatigue. The patient should understand that the purpose of the medication is to provide temporary relief of symptoms until understanding of the psychologic cause is achieved; that drugs are not "magic pills"; and that their use should be discontinued as soon as possible. Dependent patients easily become habituated to such drugs, with the rationalization that they were prescribed by a physician. They should be cautioned about the specific side-effects, particularly drowsiness, of most of the drugs. For neurotic anxiety, chlordiazepoxide (Librium), 10 mg 4 times daily, or diazepam (Valium), 5 mg 4 times daily, is useful. For psychotic anxiety, trifluoperazine (Stelazine), 2 mg 4 times daily, is more useful. The dosage of these drugs may be increased until the therapeutic effect is achieved or toxicity occurs. Trifluoperazine may cause motor restlessness, which is uncomfortable; if parkinsonism-like symptoms appear, benztropine (Cogentin), 1 mg twice daily, should be prescribed. Symptoms of depression may respond to amitriptyline (Elavil), 25 mg 3 times daily; imipramine (Tofranil), 25 mg 3 times daily; or desipramine (Pertofrane), 15 mg 3 times daily. Dextroamphetamine and similar drugs formerly used to combat fatigue or lack of energy are now forbidden in the USA for such symptoms. When difficulty in falling asleep is a complaint, a sedative such as chloral hydrate, 0.5–1 gm, is useful.

INTERVIEWING RELATIVES

Relatives and other significant persons in the patient's life may be interviewed if appropriate; however, the therapist should determine in advance what the meaning of such an interview might be to the patient. Particularly if there are paranoid trends—and generally when the patient is an adolescent—it is wise to have the patient present. The interaction between the patient and his relatives gives useful information on how the patient conducts himself outside the therapeutic situation, and the material gathered may help the patient correct his distortions. If the relatives are interviewed in the patient's absence, the factual material given by the patient must be kept confidential but the insights into family dynamics may be made use of. The relatives should be told that their information will not be kept secret from the patient.

STAGES OF PSYCHOTHERAPY

Brief psychotherapy is divided into 3 stages: initial, middle, and final.

Initial Stage

The initial stage, which is usually just the first interview, is crucial because at this time the chief problem must be identified and the plan for its solution made. The interview room should be quiet, soundproof, comfortable, and well lighted. The therapist should not take phone calls except in emergencies.

The interview is best started by setting the patient at ease and expressing an interest in him, with an introductory question such as, "How can I help you?" or, "What brings you to see me?" The patient should be permitted to tell his story in his own words. A complete and detailed history must be obtained, particularly of the present illness and precipitating causes. When the patient stops speaking, he can be encouraged to continue with questions such as, "Can you tell me more?" ... "How did you feel about that?" ... "What happened next?" In general, the questions should be phrased so that they elicit feelings as well as facts and so that they cannot be answered yes or no. The therapist listens for the precipitating events and for feelings about people important in the patient's life. It is crucial to ascertain why the patient comes for help at this particular time. He often gives a vague history, and the therapist must be persistent to obtain a specific and detailed history of the current illness, answering the questions *Who, Where, When, and What?* As a result of this information, the answer to the question *Why?* may be apparent.

The past history of similar (or different) illnesses and the circumstances surrounding them should be elicited. The family history, including a brief description of parents and siblings, with the patient's feelings about them and the family history of emotional problems, should be obtained. Reactions to maturational crises such as changing schools, graduation, employment, marriage, childbirth, and deaths are important, and the patient's adjustment to military life is an especially valuable source of information. Traumatic events should be looked for. The therapist should remember that emotional problems are usually due to multiple causes.

The patient's physical health must be inquired about, since his reaction to previous medical care will give an indication of the therapeutic alliance to be anticipated. Use of alcohol and drugs should be investigated. A brief mental status examination, including specific inquiries about phobias, obsessions, compulsions, depressive symptoms (such as crying, insomnia, anorexia, and guilt), depersonalization, and derealization, is usually indicated. Hallucinations and delusions need not be inquired about unless there is reason to suspect their presence. Suicidal ideation, if suspected, should be asked about with questions such as, "Do you ever feel life isn't worth living?" . . . "Have you ever thought of making away with yourself?" . . . "Have you made plans for suicide?" . . . progressing to, "Have you ever attempted suicide?" The questions should be asked in a nonjudgmental, uncritical manner. Many patients have unrelated phobias or obsessional thoughts which need not be taken up in treatment. Occasional mild suicidal ideation need not alarm the therapist; if the patient has current plans for suicide or has recently made a suicidal attempt, consideration should be given to discussing the situation with the relatives, and he should perhaps be hospitalized until the cause is understood and controlled. During the interview the patient should be observed for signs of anxiety, depression, sadness, and other feelings, and the point in the interview at which he develops them should be noted. Inconsistency between his apparent feelings and the facts he is discussing, as well as inappropriateness in dress or behavior, should be investigated. When the patient uses words such as anxious, worried, depressed, etc, he should be asked to explain exactly what he means.

Prior to the termination of the first interview, the therapist should ask the patient if there is anything he has not been asked about that he would like to tell the therapist and whether he has any questions. He should then review the findings in his mind, and, if there are any omissions or inconsistencies in the history, he should clarify them. The therapist should now be able to (1) identify the precipitating crisis, (2) make a descriptive diagnosis, (3) understand the basic character structure, (4) tentatively formulate the dynamics, (5) estimate the patient's motivation for treatment, (6) predict the transference, and (7) make his plan for treatment. Admittedly, this will take experience on the therapist's part.

The therapist next summarizes to the patient what he sees the problem to be and makes a recommendation for treatment, warning that there are rarely immediate solutions. The goals of treatment should be made explicit so that the patient and therapist are in agreement. A brief explanation of the process of treatment may be made—eg, the patient's task is to talk as freely as possible about his thoughts and feelings and the therapist's task is to listen, understand, and then help the patient understand what his problems are and to find better solutions than those previously used. Drugs should be prescribed if necessary, with attention being paid to the patient's sleep pattern. The therapist should make a decision about the degree to which he wishes to suppress (or, much more rarely, stimulate) anxiety in the patient and prescribe and act accordingly. An agreement should be reached about fees, and the next appointment made.

The therapist must keep in mind that many patients will repress or suppress, in the first interview, material they feel guilty or embarrassed about, especially sexual and aggressive. If the patient is extremely anxious, depressed, or having difficulty controlling impulses, the therapist may indicate that he is available by phone.

Middle Stage

The middle stage of therapy is directed toward resolving the chief problem. The second interview may be opened with an inquiry about how the patient has been since the previous interview. He should be asked if there was anything of importance he forgot or was unable to mention in the first interview, and the mechanics of treatment should be explained. The patient should be encouraged to talk about his chief complaint, and the focus of the interview should be kept on the present problem, making use of the past only as necessary to help the patient understand the origin of his reactions. When the patient presents material containing both facts and feelings, it is wisest to work chiefly with the feelings and then relate them to the facts. It may be explained that, although his reactions were useful and appropriate to his situation earlier in life, as an adult he is reacting inappropriately on the basis of these past experiences. Some patients have difficulty in feeling anger toward important people in their lives, and they tend to find a scapegoat (a person on whom hostility can be vented without guilt). The patient should be allowed to discover his previously unacceptable feelings gradually. If it is accepted without condemnation by the therapist, a confession of repressed ideas, feelings, and actions about which the patient feels guilty will help relieve superego anxiety (conscience), particularly if these can be understood and explained. The patient will be resistant to self-discovery, and this must be dealt with.

Patients often complain about the treatment they receive from others. The therapeutic task in such cases is to confront them with how they provoke this treatment and to uncover the motivation for such behavior. The individual defense mechanisms should be identified as material to document them becomes apparent. (*Examples:* When a patient reports that he feels his boss is angry at him in a situation in which the patient could reasonably be expected to be angry at his boss and there is no evidence that the boss is actually angry, the patient should be helped to see that he is projecting his own feelings of anger onto the boss. When a patient is angry with his boss but goes home and criticizes his wife, the displacement of hostility from boss to wife should be taken up. When the patient is angry with his wife but behaves in an overly kind manner, reaction formation may reasonably be suspected.) It should be pointed out that the patient is not the helpless victim of fate, and he should be encouraged to have confidence and a feeling of mastery over his life.

During the course of treatment the patient will usually identify with the therapist and take a personal interest in him. Reasonable questions about the therapist's professional background and interests may be answered, but if the patient asks highly personal questions the therapist should ask why the patient wishes to know—without rejecting him for having asked. By identifying with his therapist, a patient who formerly reacted on the basis of his conflicts will learn to ask himself the same questions his therapist would ask him in a situation that presents a problem. This use of intellectualization as a defense should generally be encouraged.

When a symptom occurs between therapeutic appointments, the patient should attempt to determine its cause and find a resolution for it. However, attempting to determine causes in the absence of symptoms is usually not helpful and may lead to excessive preoccupation with oneself; therefore, it should be discouraged. Dreams, when reported by the patient, should be interpreted in the light of the current situation.

Negative feelings about the therapy must be taken up immediately and, if justified, the cause corrected. In most cases, there will be a distortion on the basis of transference, and the patient should be helped to gain insight. Positive feelings should be left untouched unless they interfere with therapy.

A picture of the therapist's wife and family on the desk may reduce the sexualization of the situation by susceptible women patients.

During the course of treatment, repetitious patterns of behavior will become apparent. The patient should be confronted with these and the cause established. He should be stimulated to make use of what he has learned about himself in therapy by applying it to his daily life. He should be given credit for his accomplishments both in life and in therapy. His self-esteem must be maintained and, if possible, increased. The therapist might even point out that, "You know, you and I spend 90% of our time discussing only 5% of your personality, sometimes forgetting that the other 95% is trouble-free." Successful mastery of problems will act as a reward and encourage progress; failures should be viewed as opportunities for further investigation. Emphasis is placed on the fact that progress is due to the patient's hard work and his willingness to suffer in the process of improvement, and does not come from the magical words of the therapist.

The therapist must help the patient focus the discussions, and should keep the goals of therapy in mind at all times. Character problems which are not the chief complaint usually will not respond in the time limit, and it is unwise to become involved with them. The emphasis in treatment must be on "the here and now."

At the conclusion of interviews in the middle phase of treatment, a summary of the issues discussed, the conclusions reached, and how all this can be made use of by the patient may be useful.

Final Stage

The final stage of treatment is the most important, since in it the gains made in therapy must be solidified and separation anxiety mastered. It is further complicated because in psychiatric training many treatments are terminated artificially when the residents leave the clinic. Termination is taken up as an issue when the patient announces that he has achieved the results he wished, or 2 interviews before the maximum number of allowed sessions. This gives time to investigate and work with the patient's feelings about separation. When the goals of treatment have been thoroughly discussed and agreed upon, termination is usually not difficult.

When the patient feels he has made satisfactory progress and wishes to stop treatment, the evidence for his regarding himself as improved should be examined, the reasons for the change elicited, and the improvement supported. All patients should leave treatment feeling that they understand (1) what caused their difficulties, (2) how they achieved a current solution, and (3) how to prevent repetition of their difficulties. Specifically, they should be sure of their major defenses, the general issues the defenses have been erected against, and the tools they can use to prevent recurrences of past problems or the emergence of new problems. Patients should be more aware of themselves and their feelings, and should feel that therapy has been a rewarding emotional experience which they would be willing to repeat if necessary.

In well selected series, most patients who receive brief psychotherapy will feel they have benefited in the time allotted but may not have achieved all their desired goals. Their termination will be complicated by disappointment, which must be dealt with. Their negative feelings should be acknowledged and explained so that they are not guilty about their hostility. The gains that have been made should be pointed out, and this may present an opportunity to demonstrate to patients their ambivalence. Direct advice about how to minimize limitations may be given at this point.

Many (perhaps most) patients, regardless of the success of their treatment, will react to the prospect of termination (1) by having a recurrence of the original symptoms, which can be worked with as a response to separation anxiety; (2) by becoming angry with the therapist for terminating, which offers an opportunity to show them how they handle the anger and possibly the guilt they feel over it; (3) by experiencing panic at the prospect of being alone, which can be taken up in terms of dependency needs; or (4) by interpreting the termination in terms of their own worthlessness, at which point the therapist can demonstrate their sensitivity and the manner in which they interpret things personally in the light of their own self-esteem.

In general, patients should be seen for one or 2 interviews after termination has been agreed upon to work through the meaning of separation and loss. After the feelings aroused by separation have been resolved, the therapist should summarize the symptoms that brought the patient to treatment, their cause, what has been done in treatment, and what tools the patient now has to prevent future difficulties. As in the previous phases of treatment, the emphasis is on current reality. The patient should be warned that he will have problems in the future, but this warning should be put in such a way that regression is discouraged. The expectation is that the patient has learned something about himself and will be better able to cope with his problems henceforth.

Patients may resolve their immediate problems in brief psychotherapy and show an interest in long-term therapy for other problems. In general, it is wisest to allow the patient to work through the separation from therapy before starting further treatment. Although the patient is not prohibited from returning to therapy, he should not be encouraged to return by being told the therapist is always available in the future. The patient should be told to make a serious effort to resolve his future difficulties himself before considering further therapy.

Failures will occur in brief psychotherapy, and a recommendation must be made at termination. Psychoanalysis, long-term psychotherapy, drug therapy, or somatic treatments may be considered. One should remember that some problems do not properly fall into the province of psychiatry. When a psychiatrist has no special help to offer, the patient should be so advised rather than encouraged to waste his time and money in further treatment which is most unlikely to be beneficial. Too often, sad people are mistaken for sick people.

REFERENCES

Books and Monographs

Bellak, L., & L. Small: *Emergency Psychotherapy and Brief Psychotherapy.* Grune & Stratton, 1965.

Tarachow, S.: *An Introduction to Psychotherapy.* Internat Univ Press, 1963.

Wolberg, L.R.: *The Technique of Psychotherapy.* Grune & Stratton, 1967.

Journal Articles

Hansell, N., Wodarczyk, M., & B. Handlon-Lathrop: Decision counseling method. Arch Gen Psychiat 22:462–467, 1970.

Kubie, L.S.: The destructive potential of humor in psychotherapy. Am J Psychiat 127:861–866, 1971.

Lesse, S., & W. Wolf: Psychotherapy in the 21st century: An exploration of the basic determinants and trends of psychotherapy in our future and society. Psychother Psychosom 16:47–54, 1968.

Ruesch, J.: Psychotherapy in the computer age. Psychother Psychosom 16:32–46, 1968.

Uhlenhuth, E.H., Lipman, R.S., & L. Covi: Combined pharmacotherapy and psychotherapy: Controlled studies. J Nerv Ment Dis 148:52–64, 1969.

Wolberg, L.: Brief psychotherapy: Methodology in short-term therapy. Am J Psychiat 122:135–151, 1965.

27 . . .
Group Therapy

Group therapy offers, for the therapist, wider service and greater financial return; for the patient, less expense and greater opportunity for resolution of interpersonal and social problems. Patients should be screened for imminent psychotic or suicidal breaks. Leaders should be screened for proper education and training.

Group therapy involves processes that occur in formally organized and protected groups and are calculated to cause rapid improvement in personality and behavior of individual members through controlled group interactions. Methods of group therapy generally have similar counterparts in methods of individual psychotherapy, such as analytical, nondirective, existential, or directive approaches. Hence, to a large degree, group therapy is based on the same theoretical principles as individual psychotherapy. However, it has new dimensions and, as will be seen, addresses itself to problems not always met by individual therapy.

Traditionally, group therapy has been conducted by psychiatrists, psychologists, and social workers. In response to the growing demand for it, many clergymen, nurses, educators, other professionals and semiprofessionals, and even laymen have become involved as leaders of group therapy sessions.

There are many forms of group therapy. Various methods will be mentioned and defined below in the sections on History and Approaches. They can be broadly classified as *evocative, directive,* or *didactic.* The emphasis of this chapter will be upon evocative approaches, which encourage spontaneity and genuine expression of feelings by all members.

The criteria for success in group therapy are essentially the same as for individual therapy, eg, relief from distress, enhanced personal dignity, insight, and improved behavior and social relations. Individual therapy is sometimes preferable in achieving insight, but group therapy is often more effective. "To see ourselves as others see us" is a form of insight that groups provide.

The success of group therapy depends to a large extent on the degree of involvement of the therapist and the proper selection of patients. The therapist who considers group therapy to be an inferior form of psychotherapy tends to prescribe it for the least promising patients; if the results are then poor, his prejudice is reinforced.

407

Economy in money and personnel is perhaps the most obvious advantage of group therapy over individual treatment. This is not the only advantage, however, and it may not be as important as others. Group therapy, for example, offers a correction against social isolation engendered by technologic improvements in modern life.

The obvious advantages of group therapy in terms of the therapist's time and the cost per patient lead some to regard it as "cheap" treatment or as "diluted individual therapy." The therapist and his patients should both consider how the group can "multiply" therapy by bringing many minds and viewpoints to bear upon each patient's individual problem.

Group therapy offers the further advantage of providing each member with a safe human relations laboratory. Under its protection, one has the opportunity to test various ways of relating to others and to discover how others respond.

The patient's dignity is enhanced when he is a giver as well as a receiver of help. Truly valuable insights and interpretations are often given by one patient to another. Altruism is often fostered, sometimes in people in whom this quality has seemed to be lacking. In the atmosphere of mutual help, the patient also becomes a therapist.

Finally, there are conditions for which group therapy can be especially helpful. These will be noted later in the section on Special Indications.

History of Group Therapy

A. In 1905 **Joseph H. Pratt**, a Boston internist, introduced group therapy for tuberculosis patients, using the classroom method to instruct them in hygiene and to bolster their morale. Later he extended his method to patients with other illnesses.

B. In 1912, **Jacob L. Moreno** created psychodrama. He brought it to the USA in 1925 when he came to this country from Vienna. In this form of group therapy, patients express their feelings by acting various roles along with other patient-actors on a stage. Patients who are not participating form the audience. After a scene has been presented, the audience is asked to make comments and offer interpretations about what they have observed. Moreno's original method is quite elaborate and it has undergone many modifications by other therapists. For descriptions of roles taken and other details the reader should consult the literature on psychodrama. Moreno summarizes his approach in *The American Handbook of Psychiatry*, Vol II, Chapter 38.

Moreno coined the term *group psychotherapy* in 1931. He rebelled against orthodox psychoanalysis by treating a group instead of one individual and by making "therapy" rather than "analysis" the primary concern.

C. **Group psychoanalytic** methods were developed in the USA by Trigant Burrow in 1925; by Louis Wender, Paul Schilder, S.R. Slavson, and Alexander Wolf in the 1930s; and in England by S.H. Foulkes in the 1940s in order to apply the principles of individual psychoanalysis to the understanding and treatment of patients in groups.

D. **Alcoholics Anonymous** (AA) is a directive and inspirational form of group therapy for alcoholism. It was founded in 1935 in the USA by 2 physicians who were themselves alcoholics. Leadership is by the members. Many chapters of AA exist throughout the country. The movement has become strong in Canada, also, and chapters have been formed in Latin America, Europe, Africa, Asia, and Australia. Mutual help in time of stress or temptation is strongly emphasized, and the organization provides companionship for lonely members. A firm set of doctrines is set forth, including the belief that alcoholism is a specific disease; that an alcoholic will always be an alcoholic, even if he never drinks again; that sobriety can be maintained only by total abstinence; and that one must recognize and depend upon a "Higher Power." There are "twelve steps" for attaining management of one's life. Meetings consist mainly of talks by the members, who make a point of describing the extremity of their alcoholism and the desolation to which it led.

E. **Recovery, Inc.**, was founded by Abraham A. Low in 1937. It is for formerly hospitalized psychiatric patients, but the group also welcomes others with emotional problems. Like Alcoholics Anonymous, it has many chapters and is a directive and inspirational method of group therapy led by patient-members who use Low's book, *Mental Health Through Will-Training,* as a source of guidance.

F. **Group Dynamics Theory:** In the 1930s and 1940s Kurt Lewin introduced the scientific study of behavior in groups, which he termed "group dynamics." He was the originator of "field theory," by which he illustrated individual and group behavior with diagrams showing internal, social, and other forces acting as "vectors" of motivation. His ideas were used during World War II to improve group morale and effectiveness.

After World War II, Bach, Powdermaker, and Frank applied group dynamics to group psychotherapy. The emphasis is on promoting group cohesiveness, so that members sense enough basic mutual acceptance to allow honest expression of feelings about each other. The therapist focuses more on group interactions than on individual patients. The patient is helped to understand how his habitual ways of relating are perceived by others.

G. **The "Therapeutic Community" of Maxwell Jones:** In England in the 1940s Jones set out to make mental hospital care into a 24-hour-a-day treatment program. He opposed the notion that "therapy" can take place only during the short time that inpatients spend with a psychiatrist or other professionals. In his "therapeutic community" the hospital environment and policies, its nurses, attendants, and other staff members, and the other patients are all expected to be therapeutic agents. The movement spread to the USA and has fostered such trends as unlocked wards, frequent home visits, closer relations between the hospital and the patient's family and community, training of attendants to perform therapeutic rather than merely custodial functions, patient government and mutual responsibility, ward meetings of patients and staff, and greater democracy and freedom of expression between different staff echelons and between staff and patients.

As well as promoting "milieu therapy" within hospitals, the therapeutic community philosophy has been a stimulus to the more far-reaching movements of *social psychiatry*. (See Chapter 39.)

H. Existentialism in Group Therapy: Since World War II existentialist philosophy has extended into psychotherapeutic thinking. Its humanistic emphasis on patients as *lonely, feeling* people assigns to group therapy the task of relieving the patient's sense of alienation and of promoting a shared quest for *meaning* in life.

Like the practitioners of more traditional schools of psychotherapy, the existentialists encourage *spontaneity* in patients. They also encourage the therapist to express his feelings toward his patients spontaneously as long as he is sincere and admits his subjectivity. This is a departure from traditional teachings about the management of *countertransference,* which urge the therapist to guard against showing his personal feelings when treating patients.

I. Communications Theory and Family Therapy:

1. The "double bind"—In 1956 an interdisciplinary research team reported that the families of schizophrenics have a characteristic way of communicating which puts the "victim" in a "double bind," ie, unable to satisfy the "binder" (on whom he is dependent and whom he must please) because the latter habitually expresses 2 orders of message bearing conflicting demands. (*Examples:* "Assert yourself! I can't stand people who let others push them around!" [With the exception of *me,* of course. You jolly well better do what *I* say!] "Go ahead and do what you want. Don't worry about me." [Of course, I'll keel over and die if you don't let me run your life, and it will be all your fault.] "I'm going to let you run this thing. I'm giving you complete responsibility! Now the first thing you should do is . . ." [If you really think I'm going to let you follow your *own* way of doing it, you've got another think coming!])

2. *Family dynamics* and methods of *family therapy* have evolved from the work of the "double bind" team and have also been developed by Nathan Ackerman, Theodore Lidz, Carl Whitaker, Murray Bowen, and others. Family therapy continued to gain in popularity through the 1960s.

3. Eric Berne's "transactional analysis" focuses on the covert meanings in interpersonal communications and is oriented to group therapy. Berne found his approach especially useful for groups of married couples, in whom he pointed out "games" (repetitive, neurotic interactions with hidden meanings). His book, *Games People Play,* became a best-seller.

J. The T-Group (Training Group) Movement: T-Groups came into use as a method of training psychiatrists and other mental health professionals, especially those interested in becoming group therapists. Trainees participate as members of groups modeled after classical therapeutic groups. The method has been extended to business executives, clergymen, medical students, and others whose work demands special ability in dealing with people.

K. Encounter, Sensitivity, and Other Groups: Recently, some T-groups have developed a new function as a social movement for overcoming "alienation" or emotional distance between people in general. Membership in these groups is not limited to special professional and occupational groups nor to "patients" needing "therapy." Such T-groups, "sensitivity groups," or "encounter groups" sometimes take the form of "marathon sessions" lasting a weekend. At Bethel, Maine, in summer, T-groups are held intensively over 2-week periods, and the participants often report that they have been deeply moved and enlightened by the experience. Similar groups are held in several places in California and elsewhere in the USA.

In a few places, extremists have instituted *nude therapy,* in an avowed all-out attempt to help patients get rid of repressions.

APPROACHES

Evocative Group Psychotherapy

Evocative methods of group therapy are those that encourage spontaneous expression of feelings by patients in an atmosphere of acceptance and of effort toward understanding those feelings. In group therapy the evocative leader promotes mutual interaction among patients in preference to patient-to-therapist (and therapist-to-patient) exchanges. The leader avoids authoritarianism. He does not demand that patients express the *right attitude*; he wants them to feel free to express their **real** attitudes. Generally, in evocative groups, members and leader should be seated comfortably in a circle; the therapist is not placed in any special position that would make him the focal point of the group's attention. In some groups, members are encouraged to express their rage by beating the furniture or walls and vocalizing loudly. A few go so far as to permit amatory activity up to and including sexual intercourse; even rape has been countenanced.

Activity therapy as an evocative, analytically oriented group method for treating latency-age boys (about age 7–11) with disturbed peer relationships has been developed by S.R. Slavson. The group is carefully composed so as to achieve a balance of traits among the members (eg, aggressive, shy, compulsive). The setting provides for handicrafts, games, and noisy activity. The therapist is permissive–almost **laissez-faire.**

Group psychoanalysis for adolescents and adults carries the principles of individual psychoanalysis into the group setting. As when working with individual patients, the analyst remains quite passive. **Transference** and **resistance** take on new forms and complexity in groups. The patient develops transference feelings not only toward the therapist but toward other group members as well. The group may be perceived unconsciously as a reenactment of early family life, with the therapist as parent and the other members as siblings. At appropriate times the group analyst clarifies or interprets the transferences and resistances.

Other evocative approaches. Analytic, "nondirective," group dynamic, existential, "transactional," and other concepts are frequently combined in evocative group therapy. Psychodrama may be used.

Directive Groups

Directive methods are those in which the leader asserts his authority, especially as an expert on proper attitudes and conduct. Advice and commands may be given. In directive groups the leader stands or sits in a special position, such that he is the focal point of the group's attention (like a teacher before his class or a preacher before his congregation).

For ages **religious groups** have been used to inspire a shared sense of meaning and purpose in their members; to reinforce adherence to codes of belief and conduct; and to promote fellowship and solidarity.

Alcoholics Anonymous and **Recovery, Inc.**, are nonsectarian directive groups with a religious flavor, founded by physicians but run by the members (see p 408). **Synanon** is a similar group for narcotic addicts.

Didactic Groups

Didactic methods aim at educating patients, often with factual knowledge about their problems and what is known about their treatment. There may be an overlap between these methods and directive methods. When there is a distinction, the didactic approach seeks to **educate** whereas the directive approach seeks to **indoctrinate.**

Klapman and others have found that classes and seminars for institutionalized patients with psychoses, sex deviations, and other problems that respond poorly to less structured approaches can be of great value. Patients are taught about the nature, causes, and treatment of their condition. Their intelligence is thus acknowledged and enlisted. Through understanding, fear and hostility toward treatment are diminished and the patient is motivated to cooperate with other types of therapy.

Remotivation was designed by Dorothy Hoskins Smith, a mental hospital volunteer worker, for use by psychiatric attendants in the treatment of institutionalized chronic schizophrenics and other regressed groups. Group discussion of things in the world outside the institution is promoted by the leader. Introduced into Philadelphia State Hospital in 1956, the technic consists of a series of about 12 weekly or semiweekly meetings, each lasting 30 minutes to an hour, with 10–15 patients per group.

COMPOSITION OF GROUPS

Number of Patients

Evocative groups should be limited to 4–9 members (optimal, 6 or 7). Larger numbers of patients are feasible with directive and didactic groups. Allow for drop-outs and absentees by starting the group at about one-third more than the optimal number.

Types of Patients

The appropriate types of patients vary with the therapeutic approach (as described above). However, in all instances, and especially for evocative group methods, careful screening should be done to eliminate individuals so close to a psychotic or suicidal break that treatment of any kind is dangerous.

The most suitable patients for adult and adolescent evocative groups are those suffering from interpersonal maladjustments. Patients may have neuroses, psychophysiologic disturbances, or personality disorders (if they have sufficiently developed consciences). Overtly psychotic and sociopathic patients are generally not desirable for evocative groups.

Within the group, patients may vary with regard to sex, age, diagnosis, and other qualities provided that no individual is sharply set off from the others (eg, a solitary male among females; one 50-year-old among others in their twenties; one homosexual among heterosexuals).

Ideally, patients should have no previous acquaintance with one another. Exceptions occur with group therapy technics designed for families, married couples, and in certain training groups.

Special Indications

Many problems may be more amenable to group therapy than to individual therapy:

(1) For shy and lonely people (often diagnosed as schizoid or dependent personalities) the group process of "universalization" can be very helpful, ie, they discover they are "not so different from others after all." Such patients are typically reluctant to enter group therapy, protesting that groups are especially threatening to them. They can be told that this very fact makes group therapy promising.

(2) Patients who become too dependent upon an individual therapist may resist the idea of sharing the therapist's attention with others. Group therapy helps them to distribute their dependent transference around the group and mitigates their tendency to cling to the therapist.

(3) Group reinforcement gives added incentive to overcome phobias. In a group with more than one phobic, a healthy competition toward improvement may develop.

(4) Antagonism and fear toward parental and authority figures may cause the patient to withhold the expression of his feelings in individual therapy but he may overcome his reticence in a group, where hostility toward the therapist is more easily verbalized.

(5) Patients who have had unsatisfactory experiences with siblings, or no experience at all.

(6) Adolescent girls with confused sexual identification.

(7) Patients with difficulty in getting along with others—eg, patients spoiled as children, those who tend to demand much and give little, and those who have other unrecognized ways of alienating people—are likely to show their characteristic behavior in the group and to be made aware of it by the others.

(8) Patients with afflictions seen as shameful or unusual (eg, homosexuals, enuretics, alcoholics, narcotic addicts, obese persons) can be of great emotional support to one another.

(9) Group therapy with 3 or 4 married couples is a promising new approach. With 2 therapists (preferably a man and a woman), 5 couples may be feasible. It is sometimes difficult for a marriage counselor to maintain an unbiased role when working with one couple at a time. In couples' group therapy, the opportunity to "pass the buck" to others in the group makes it

easier to escape the judgmental role. Furthermore, in couples' groups, members discover that neither they nor their spouses are so peculiar after all. They find that disharmonies they had considered unique to their marriage are often present in other marriages also.

PROCEDURES

Recommending Group Therapy

Although the patient may have already acknowledged his need for some sort of psychiatric treatment, he may still be reluctant to accept a recommendation for group therapy. Typical objections are fear of ridicule, condemnation, or rejection by the others, as well as shyness, stage fright, and discomfort in groups and social situations. The therapist may tell the patient that group therapy is especially helpful for such problems. Other concerns may include fear of breach of confidentiality by other members and a desire for the therapist's individual attention. If the therapist is familiar with the indications and contraindications for this type of treatment and is personally convinced that group therapy will have specific advantages for the patient, he can usually persuade him to try it. After hearing the patient's objections, the therapist can explain the ground rules for group therapy and the specific benefits he feels it offers. A trial period of 6—8 sessions can be suggested, along with the reassurance that patients are not required to tell things they wish to keep secret. If the patient has very personal concerns which he wants to discuss only in private, the therapist may offer concurrent individual sessions. In them the therapist may consider that some of the material the patient brings up is appropriate for discussion in the group. If he does, he should encourage the patient to see what the group thinks about it.

Getting Started

A. Before the First Meeting: The therapist should see all members individually before starting them with the group. An explanation of how group therapy works, including the patient's and the therapist's roles, can be given at this time. Many group therapists provide their patients with printed "preparation sheets" before the first meeting.

B. First Meeting: Some therapists remain silent at the beginning of the first meeting, leaving it to the members to make introductions and to open the discussion. To help break the ice, the therapist may make an opening statement about why the group has met, possibly restating the procedural principles. He then may ask the patients to introduce themselves. As they do so they generally begin to tell something about themselves and their problems. If the group remains frozen, "going around" (see below) usually helps.

Problems and Resistances

A. Silence:

1. Of entire group—Silence of the entire group is less of a problem with voluntary outpatients than with institutionalized patients or those who have

been coerced into treatment. It is often an expression of group hostility toward the therapist, or a group reaction to a shocking revelation by a patient or to a remark just made by the therapist. The therapist can usually handle group silence by inquiring about the feelings behind it.

2. Of an individual member—If one member is habitually silent, other members will usually take the initiative and inquire about his silence, attempting to draw him out. If they fail to do so, the therapist may have to take action, eg, by "going around" or scheduling individual sessions with the patient.

B. Small Talk: At the beginning of group therapy, small talk may be part of the process of getting acquainted. If it persists, it is a formidable barrier to meaningful interaction. Examples include discussions of job and household details, books read, plays seen, psychiatric articles and theories, current events, and persistent joking and lighthearted chatter. Small talk in group therapy serves a function similar to resistive silence in individual therapy. In other words, whereas prolonged silence tends to be a common problem with individuals, prolonged small talk is a common problem with groups. Eric Berne refers to small talk as a "pastime." The therapist may need to point out how small talk is being used as a means of defending the members from the necessity to discuss personal feelings.

C. Monopolists: If a group is dominated by a monopolist, his removal from the group may be the only solution. A secondary monopolist may serve to challenge the monopolist's domination of the sessions. Supplementary individual sessions may offer some of the special attention the monopolist seeks while allowing the therapist to explore with him the needs behind his behavior in this particular group.

D. Attacks:

1. Against a member—Verbal attacks by one member upon another may be a displacement of hostile feelings toward the therapist. They may also be manifestations of other hostile feelings. The therapist needs to be alert to both possibilities.

2. Against the therapist—A group therapist must recognize that expressions of hostility toward himself are necessary to successful evocative therapy. Hence, he must be able to receive them without undue discomfort.

E. Interruption: If the group members fail to challenge a persistent interrupter, the therapist may intervene by saying he wants to hear the rest of what the interrupted member was saying, or he may wonder aloud about the meaning of the interruption or about how it makes the others feel.

F. Subgrouping:

1. In the meeting—Sometimes 2 or more separate conversations develop in a meeting, or a member will speak to another in a voice too low to be heard by all. The therapist should not allow such "subgrouping" to continue. He can interrupt to say that he can follow only one conversation at a time or that he cannot hear the (private) conversation and would they speak up.

2. Outside the meeting—Although many therapists approve of outside gatherings of the total membership of a group, social gatherings which exclude part of the membership are to be discouraged. Formation of a clique

which excludes any members damages the therapeutic effectiveness of the group. Members should be told that any contacts with one another on the outside are to be reported in the regular meeting.

G. Other Types of Resistance: These may include intellectualization, "quizzing the therapist" (demanding that he function as "expert" among "students"), playing "therapist's assistant," and many other defensive tactics.

Special Technics

A. Reflecting Questions and "Passing the Buck" to the Group: In new groups, members tend to set up the therapist as the "expert" from whom advice and answers to questions are sought. As in individual therapy, a question can be "reflected" back to the patient. It can also be handled by "passing the buck" to the group, ie, by asking for the opinions of other members. Thus, group interaction is promoted. It is occasionally useful for the therapist to give advice and "answers" based on knowledge that the patients do not have; in general, however, group interaction is discouraged if the therapist functions too often as a "higher authority" whose wisdom must be passively absorbed.

B. "Going Around": When a group seems to be bogged down in silence or small talk or to be dominated by a monopolist, or when other difficulties arise to prevent therapeutic interaction, "going around" can be an effective device for getting started again. Each member in turn, going around the room, is asked to express his feelings about something the therapist sees as relevant at the time. For example, the therapist might ask for each member's reaction to the person sitting at his right or left, to the group as a whole, or to the present predicament of the group. It often helps to ask everyone to state his basic purpose in life or what he hopes to gain from group therapy. Going around encourages chronically silent members to express themselves, and it often also encourages reticent members to voice opinions about the conduct of such members as monopolists.

C. Alternate Sessions: Opinions vary about whether alternate meetings of the group should be held without the therapist. Many therapists encourage such meetings if all members are included. Alternate sessions serve to speed up the process of getting acquainted and of developing group solidarity. Such sessions may immediately follow the regular session with the therapist, possibly over coffee. They may also take place in the home of a member or elsewhere. The group is asked to report on these proceedings at the next meeting with the therapist. In so doing, they may announce that they discussed deeper material than they ever did with the therapist present. If so, the therapist can explore the transference feelings involved.

D. Concurrent Individual Therapy: Individual therapy may proceed concurrently, either with the group therapist or with another therapist. Opinions vary about its desirability, but it is a common practice. Individual sessions allow the patient to discuss reactions and resistances to the group procedure, thus enabling the therapist to deal with them and to forestall potential dropping out. Monopolistic tendencies and problems too intimate for sharing may be dealt with individually. For discussion of the patient's feelings about the group and his conduct in it, the group therapist who sees the patient individually has an obvious advantage over another individual therapist. A patient who has been seen in individual therapy often finds it easier to express hostile feelings or negative transference toward the therapist in a group setting.

E. Detecting and Handling Transference: A myriad of transference manifestations develop in group therapy. Members develop transference feelings toward each other as well as toward the therapist. Such feelings tend to be expressed sooner and more easily in groups than in individual therapy, and this makes for very lively group sessions. The alert therapist can accomplish a great deal by recognizing and exploring them with the group. Sometimes the group may resemble the family—the therapist being cast in a parental role and other members as siblings. In group therapy with married couples, hostilities between husband and wife emerge rapidly and often are clearly related to experiences with their parents. Besides fostering insight, sound interpretations of the transference components of marital hostilities help prevent their reaching destructive levels.

Termination
A. By an Individual Member:
1. Drop-outs—If a member contemplates dropping out, he is urged first to discuss his wish to do so in a group meeting. The other members may dissuade him from quitting.

2. By agreement with the therapist—A patient may have improved enough to terminate, or the therapist may for other reasons feel that a patient will not profit from continuing in the group.

B. Termination of the Entire Group:
1. By prearrangement—A termination date may be agreed upon at the outset ("end-setting"). With a transient membership (such as students), or when the therapist anticipates his own departure, a prearranged termination date may be set. For practical reasons, training groups generally run for a predetermined period.

2. By attrition—If group membership dwindles to less than 4, addition of new members or termination of the group is in order.

3. By the therapist's departure—When the therapist finds that he must end his work with the group, he should give at least 3 weeks' notice. In the remaining meetings, feelings of abandonment are likely to be directly or indirectly expressed. Indirect expressions include discussions of loss, death, and previous abandonment, as well as expressions of rejection of and by the therapist and hostility toward him. If a new therapist is to take over the group, many members are likely to drop out during the transition period. The dependent transference toward the first therapist is usually such that the new therapist is seen as second-rate. The incoming therapist must expect this and encourage the group to ventilate its grief. The transition is eased if the new therapist participates in the final meetings with his predecessor.

SOCIAL MEANING AND IMPORTANCE
OF GROUP THERAPY

Alienation and the absence of close friendships are felt by many in this increasingly impersonal age. Group therapy may offer solutions for some. The T-group movement is gaining in popularity and is attracting people from many walks of life who want to get to know themselves and others. While traditional religious doctrine has become less convincing to many people, the need to get together, receive inspiration, and find meaning in life remains great.

Finally, developments in group psychotherapy appear to offer possibilities toward the resolution of conflicts—between individuals or between whole groups.

REFERENCES

Books and Monographs

Ackerman, N.W.: *The Psychodynamics of Family Life.* Basic Books, 1958.

Berne, E.: *Principles of Group Treatment.* Oxford Univ Press, 1966.

Edelson, M.: *Ego Psychology, Group Dynamics and the Therapeutic Community.* Grune & Stratton, 1964.

Foulkes, S.H.: *Introduction to Group Analytic Psychotherapy.* Heinemann, 1948.

Frank, J.D.: *Group Therapy in the Mental Hospital.* Monograph Series No. 1. American Psychiatric Association, 1955.

Hinckley, R.G., & L. Hermann: *Group Treatment in Psychotherapy.* Univ of Minnesota Press, 1951.

Howard, J.: *Please Touch.* Brunner/Mazel, 1970.

Kaplan, H.I., & B.J. Sadock (editors): *Comprehensive Group Psychotherapy.* Williams & Wilkins, 1971.

Moreno, J.L.: Fundamental rules and techniques of psychodrama. In: *Progress in Psychotherapy.* Masserman, J.H., & J.L. Moreno (editors). Grune & Stratton, 1958.

Pinney, E.L., Jr.: *A First Group Psychotherapy Book.* Thomas, 1970.

Powdermaker, F.B., & J.D. Frank: *Group Psychotherapy.* Commonwealth Fund, 1953.

Satir, V.: *Conjoint Family Therapy.* Science and Behavior Books, 1964.

Slavson, S.R.: *Analytic Group Psychotherapy with Children, Adolescents and Adults.* Columbia Univ Press, 1950.

Slavson, S.R.: *The Practice of Group Therapy.* Internat Univ Press, 1948.

Journal Articles

Bernstein, S., Wacks, J., & J. Christ: The effect of group psychotherapy on the psychotherapist. Am J Psychother 23:271–282, 1969.

Fleck, S., & others: Symposium on family research and family therapy. Psychother Psychosom 16:293–302, 1968.

Hampshire, A.: The use of groups in motivation for analytic group psychotherapy. Internat J Group Psychother 4:95–102, 1954.

Handlon, J.H., & M.B. Parloff: The treatment of patient and family as a group: Is it group psychotherapy? Internat J Group Psychother 12:132–141, 1962.

Hes, J.P., & S.L. Handler: Multidimensional group psychotherapy. Arch Gen Psychiat 5:70, 1961.

Igersheimer, W.W.: Analytically oriented group psychotherapy for patients with psychosomatic illnesses. Internat J Group Psychother 9:71, 1959.

Linden, M.E.: Group psychotherapy with institutionalized senile women: Study in gerontologic human relation. Internat J Group Psychother 3:150–170, 1953.

Linden, M.E.: Transference in gerontologic group psychotherapy: Studies in gerontologic human relation, IV. Internat J Group Psychother 5:61–79, 1955.

Lundell, F.W., & A.M. Mann: Conjoint psychotherapy of married couples. Canad MAJ 94:542–546, 1966.

Redlich, F.C., & B. Astrachan: Group dynamics training. Am J Psychiat 125:1501–1507, 1969.

Semrad, E.V., & J. Arsenian: The use of group processes in teaching group dynamics. Am J Psychiat 108:358–363, 1951.

Stoller, F.H.: Videotape feedback in the group setting. J Nerv Ment Dis 148:457, 1969.

Thompson, R.W., & E. Wiley: Reaching families of hospitalized mental patients: A group approach. Commun Ment Health J 6:22–30, Feb 1970.

28...
Behavior Therapy
& Hypnotherapy

Behavior therapy applies to human beings technics derived from experimental animal psychology (both operant and Pavlovian conditioning). In spite of enthusiastic and convincing reports in such inaccessable conditions as homosexuality, phobic and obsessive compulsive neuroses, alcoholism, drug addiction, and back ward schizophrenia, most psychiatrists remain unconvinced. Others concede that these procedures are in fact useful with certain patients suffering from these conditions.

The use of hypnotism in psychotherapy may cause more problems than it solves, but it may solve a few if properly and judiciously employed as an adjunct to other methods.

The behavior therapies have been gaining increasing acceptance as useful technics for the treatment of a variety of psychiatric conditions. The behavior therapies differ in several important respects from traditional psychotherapeutic procedures.

Perhaps the most important difference is that the behavior therapist views disturbed behavior as largely a psychologic rather than a medical problem. He thus addresses himself directly to the task of modifying maladaptive behavior—ie, the patient's symptoms—rather than attempting to identify the "underlying unconscious disease process" that most psychotherapists believe "cause" symptoms. For this reason the behavior therapist—most often a laboratory trained clinical psychologist or psychiatrist who thinks of himself primarily as a behavioral scientist—avoids psychodynamic formulations; does not deal with the unconscious, ego structures, or defense mechanisms; and does not employ insight as a prime treatment vehicle. He concerns himself only with maladaptive, inappropriate, or irrelevant kinds of *behavior* that can be measured and observed accurately and modified systematically. For the same reason, the behavior therapist selects his patients from among those who show a set of circumscribed behavioral difficulties rather than from those whose diverse symptomatology pervades their lives.

The 2 major types of behavior therapy differ in the kinds of behavior they endeavor to modify and in the procedures they use. The *classical conditioning therapies* employ unlearned, constitutional, physiologic reflex behavior to modify or eliminate unwanted, usually reflex (involuntary) behavior. The *operant conditioning therapies* employ operant (voluntary) environmental procedures to control the consequences of the patient's voluntary behavior; in so doing, they ultimately enable the patient to control the behavior itself.

Behavior therapists consider these technics to be effective in the treatment of all neurotic conditions, especially the anxiety and phobic reactions, and other functional psychiatric disorders, including the psychoses. They also assert that most behavior therapy is successful (ie, that all symptoms disappear) within 8–12 sessions and that subsequent "symptom substitution" occurs rarely.

CLASSICAL CONDITIONING THERAPIES

Counterconditioning

Counterconditioning, subvarieties of which are *reciprocal inhibition, desensitization,* and *aversive conditioning,* developed out of the fundamental behaviorist assumption that neuroses are simply persistent maladaptive learned habits associated with persistent anxiety. Carefully controlled experiments by Wolpe and others suggested to them that anxiety could be eliminated by inhibiting its expression with competing responses. Wolpe summarizes the concept as follows: "If a response inhibitory of anxiety can be made to occur in the presence of anxiety-evoking stimuli, it will weaken the bond between these stimuli and the anxiety."

The stimulus most commonly used to countercondition anxiety is the state of deep muscle relaxation. The therapist employing relaxation as a reciprocal inhibitor of anxiety usually spends 2–3 sessions training his patients in deep muscle relaxation. The patient then practices relaxation at home until he can consistently invoke the state on command. The most widely used technic for inducing relaxation is one derived from the Jacobson "progressive relaxation" procedures. The technic focuses successively on selected muscle groups, alternately requiring their contraction and relaxation. On relaxing previously contracted muscles, the patient is asked to "study the relaxation" in an effort to induce generalized relaxation of contiguous muscle groups. A session of relaxation training usually begins with relaxation of muscle groups in the arms and hands. Jacobson often commences such a session as follows:

> "Now I want you to get as comfortable as you can in your chair. If you feel more relaxed with your eyes closed, then close them. Now, try to concentrate your mind's eye on the most relaxing, pleasant thing you can think of. Perhaps it's sitting somewhere that's quiet, reading a book, occasionally looking out the window at some trees in the distance. Now, while you're relaxing, thinking of that pleasant, comfortable scene, I'd like you to tighten your left fist, just as tight as you can ... and hold the fist ... and now relax.... Let the relaxation spread from your fingers through your hand ... and up your arm ... and study the relaxation.... Now clench that left hand again and hold the fist ... tighter and tighter ... and now relax again and feel the release of tension spread through your arm.... Now I want you to do the same thing, only with your right fist. Clench your right fist as tight as you can and hold it.... Study the tension ... and relax.... Feel the tension dissolve and feel the relaxation spread through your fingers and your hand, your lower arm ..."

Relaxation training includes exercises designed to induce successive deep muscle relaxation in the arms, face, neck, upper and lower back, stomach and lower abdomen, buttocks, thighs, legs, and feet. It often takes 3 or 4 sessions before a patient can spontaneously induce relaxation through his body both in the therapist's office and at home.

Assertive training—in self-expression, self-control, and self-assertion in interpersonal situations—is given at the same time since successful assertive behavior, like relaxation, is thought to inhibit anxiety. Instruction in assertive training usually begins during an early session of behavior therapy. The patient is asked to emit an assertive response—usually a verbal statement of objection to or comment upon someone else's verbal behavior toward him which he would not otherwise make. The patient is reassured that an assertive response is not by definition a hostile one. It is, rather, a verbal expression of control and self-confidence, but one that he has not been willing to make of his own accord. The therapist asks the patient to make assertive responses only once or twice a day at first. Gradually, as therapy proceeds and the patient learns that a firm but not necessarily hostile statement of his own opinion about something of importance to him does not meet with counterhostility, he begins to make such responses more naturally. He also learns that assertive behavior and anxious behavior cannot coexist and that, if he can be self-confident enough to be assertive, he will have to spend less and less time being anxious.

While relaxation training is going forward, the patient and therapist together construct an anxiety hierarchy (or, if the patient is phobic, a fear hierarchy). These hierarchies list, in increasing order of capacity to elicit fear or anxiety, those situations that evoke anxious or fearful responses. Before such hierarchies are constructed, the patient is usually asked to complete several self-report forms, almost always including a Fear Survey Schedule (one of several checklists requiring the patient to grade the severity of his possible fear of a wide variety of environmental situations or objects, including various animals and inanimate objects, a variety of interpersonal situations, and other more abstract concepts such as death, sleep, and bodily restriction). The patient usually completes, in addition, the Life History Questionnaire (a self-report personal history procedure) and one or more short, objective personality measures (containing questions such as, "Do you cross the street to avoid meeting someone?") which are scored in terms of how often the patient shows such types of behavior. The forms enable the therapist to help the patient construct fear or anxiety hierarchies which include significant anxiety-evoking situations which the patient may not, for one reason or another, have reported to the therapist. The Life History Questionnaire also enables the therapist to trace the sequence of development of the patient's maladaptive behavior in case he wishes to employ other behavioral procedures such as aversive conditioning or positive reconditioning, which requires more extensive historical data preparatory to therapy.

The desensitization procedure itself is a relatively simple one. After the patient informs his therapist that he has been able to relax completely, the therapist asks him to imagine a neutral "control" or "reference" image to serve as a nonanxiety-producing image as counterconditioning proceeds. The therapist then describes that scene in the patient's hierarchy that causes least anxiety or fear. If the patient—now presumably completely relaxed—can experience this scene in his imagination without also experiencing anxiety (or fear), the therapist proceeds to succeeding scenes until the patient indicates that he does feel anxiety. The therapist then stops immediately and either backtracks to images in the hierarchy which the patient can successfully experience without anxiety or terminates the session.

Desensitization sessions continue until the patient can experience in his imagination the entire hierarchy without anxiety or fear. On completing the series, the patient usually finds that he can also experience the same situations in real life with little or no anxiety.

While counterconditioning is being carried out in the therapist's office, the patient is instructed to induce deep muscle relaxation when faced with potentially anxiety-provoking real life situations; he is also told to terminate these situations if he experiences anxiety.

According to Wolpe, desensitization of most anxiety- or fear-provoking stimuli can usually be accomplished in fewer than 15 sessions. Symptom substitution is said to be rare.

Reciprocal inhibition procedures have also been employed to eliminate other unwanted reflex behaviors. *Aversive conditioning* technics involve the repeated coupling of a negative stimulus (eg, an electric shock, an emesis-producing substance, a verbal admonition) and the behavioral sequence to be interrupted. They have been used extensively to treat drug and alcohol addiction and some types of sexual deviations. Whenever the patient behaves in an unwanted manner, he is punished immediately by an unpleasant stimulus until he cannot emit the maladaptive behavior without also experiencing the effects of the negative stimulus. The unwanted behavior eventually decreases and, as a rule, ultimately disappears.

Aversive conditioning has been used most often to treat male homosexuality. In one study, homosexual men who desired to extinguish their homosexual responses were shown a series of pictures of nude men. Whenever they experienced penile erection, they were given a painful electric shock so that, in time, whenever they saw the pictures, they experienced the painful memory of the shocks even though they were no longer being administered. These patients were instructed to initiate graded sexual contact with women. At the end of the study, a sizeable number of lifelong homosexuals had become practicing (if not completely enthusiastic) heterosexuals.

Alcohol addiction has also been treated by aversive procedures. Because these procedures have usually required permanent and total abstinence, a most difficult goal for any heavy drinker, they have not been very successful. A recent study, in which the treatment goal was "social drinking" rather than total abstinence, represents a more promising approach.* Patients were "reinforced" with additional drinks of beverage alcohol for requesting it whenever their blood alcohol levels were at or below 65 mg/100 ml and "punished" by painful electric shock and loss of subsequent drinks whenever

*See Lovibond & Caddy reference on p 431.

they requested alcohol with blood alcohols above this relatively moderate level. Patients gradually learned not to request beverage alcohol when they experienced the subjective sensations associated with higher blood alcohol levels. This sensitivity to internal bodily events gradually extended to real-life drinking situations, helping many of these patients become "social drinkers" rather than continuing to be "chronic alcoholics." In several cases, success continued a year after the original conditioning.

Positive Reconditioning

Positive reconditioning—the classical conditioning of new motor habits—has become less important as a treatment technic as more flexible operant technics for generating both voluntary and involuntary behaviors have evolved. Positive reconditioning is still used occasionally, however, to treat nocturnal enuresis. The technic employs an alarm set to awaken the sleeping patient, usually a child, as soon as he excretes the first drop of urine. Coupling the alarm with the first appearance of urine eventually decreases the child's tendency to urinate in response to bladder stimulation during sleep. Unfortunately, the technic has proved effective with only a small portion of the population of enuretics upon whom it has been tried.

Experimental Extinction

This type of classical conditioning therapy aims to weaken progressively an unwanted motor habit through repeated nonreinforcement (extinction) of the responses that manifest it. Tics and overeating have been most successfully treated in this way. In one classic application, Yates cured a patient with multiple tics both by systematically withdrawing attention from him for measured periods of time whenever he spontaneously produced a tic, and by requiring him to evoke deliberately a very large number of unreinforced tics whenever he did not produce them spontaneously. After repeated periods of experimental extinction, the patient's tic rate decreased significantly. Eventually, his tics disappeared completely.

Because this technic requires careful identification of the reinforcers that maintain the unwanted behavior, its utility is limited to fairly simple behavior problems with a limited and identifiable number of reinforcers. It should be used only with patients whose inappropriate motor habits are not maintained by nonspecific "internal" variables (like motivational states) that cannot be readily extinguished.

THE OPERANT CONDITIONING THERAPIES

Behavior Modification

The complex of therapeutic technics that go by the generic name behavior modification all aim to modify or eliminate inappropriate modes of operant (voluntary) behavior by systematically altering their consequences. All of them require as a first step an accurate frequency (baseline) count of the "target" behavior or set of behaviors to be modified, along with complete identification of all environmental variables that appear to "control" (reinforce) them. Although behavior modification technics are best known for the successes they have achieved in altering psychotic behavior patterns on mental hospital wards, they have also been used effectively to treat less formidable behavior and educational problems. Behavior modification technics are the treatment of choice for many ward management problems and a variety of other relatively circumscribed learned behavior problems.

One of the earliest reports on the use of behavior modification technics in an institutional setting involved the psychiatric nurse as a behavioral engineer, since behavior modification procedures in institutions require that behavior be under continuous observation and control and depend in large part on the cooperation of ward nursing personnel. The study, by Ayllon & Michael, presented behavior modification data on 19 patients—14 schizophrenics and 5 mentally retarded. A variety of procedures were employed to alter maladaptive behavior patterns in these patients. One patient, whose frequent visits to the nursing station usually succeeded in disrupting nursing activities, gradually decreased the frequency of these visits over a period of 8 weeks when attention was systematically withdrawn from her each time she appeared. Another patient who habitually produced only "psychotic talk" (largely delusional in character) was systematically punished by withdrawal of attention whenever she talked "crazy" and reinforced with praise and interest whenever she produced nonpsychotic talk. Over the course of 12 weeks, the frequency of psychotic talk decreased and that of nonpsychotic talk increased significantly. Other psychotic behaviors modified by operant technics in this group included psychotic posturing and withdrawal, anorexia, and hoarding. A variety of procedures were used to effect the systematic withdrawal or modification of the consequences (reinforcers) that had served to maintain these unwanted behaviors.

The behavior of psychotic children has also been treated with operant technics. Wolf and his colleagues successfully treated an autistic child's severe temper tantrums, bedtime problems, unwillingness to wear glasses, mutism, and eating problems with a variety of operant technics. The usual procedure was first to extinguish inappropriate behavior, eg, by placing the child in a room by himself whenever he began a tantrum or threatened to take off his glasses. More appropriate behavior was then established by "shaping" procedures, eg, socially appropriate verbal behavior was instilled at first by rewarding with food when the child repeated appropriate words, and later when he used the words without prompting.

"Normal" educational problems have also been dealt with successfully by operant conditioning procedures. Efficient study habits were instilled in college students by operant shaping technics. Of 5 students chosen for inclusion in the study, 2 were above and 3 below the college achievement average. All were required to prepare a careful analysis of their daily study schedules. Inappropriate and maladaptive study habits such as daydreaming, difficulties in concentration, partial learning, and inefficient use of study time were altered by operant shaping procedures designed at first to force the student to concentrate intensively for limited periods on circumscribed units of school work. Only when he could do so was he then scheduled to spend longer and longer periods on a greater variety of material, as he grew able to make more and more efficient use of his time.

Four of 5 students responded positively to these control procedures by making higher grades the semester following institution of the technics.

Social Imitation

Bandura and his colleagues have performed a variety of studies in support of the hypothesis that social imitation can be used to control behavior. Children can be taught to evaluate their own performance of a particular set of tasks by reference to an adult model performing the same tasks. One group of nursery school children was exposed to aggressive adult models and a second group to models who displayed inhibited and nonaggressive behavior. A control group was exposed to neither. The aggressive model exhibited unusual forms of physical and verbal aggression toward a large inflated plastic doll, whereas the nonaggressive model sat quietly, totally ignoring the doll and the instruments of aggression that had been placed in the room. The children in the first group displayed a great number of precisely imitative aggressive responses. Such responses rarely occurred in either the nonaggressive model group or the control group.

While these procedures have not yet been widely used to alter maladaptive behavior or to reinstate appropriate behavior in individuals with behavior problems, recent studies suggest that procedures for "teaching" socially appropriate behavior to persons who lack it may well be the next major area of interest in the behavior therapies.

ADVANTAGES AND DISADVANTAGES
OF THE BEHAVIOR THERAPIES

If the extensive confirmatory literature of behavior therapy can be believed—and many therapists have come to believe it—then it is clear that the principal advantages of these technics is that they succeed where other therapies have failed. The behavior therapists claim consistent success with patients who have been burdened for years with phobias, severe and intractable anxiety, and obsessional thinking. They also report success in the treatment of sexual disorders of all kinds and, with less conviction, in the treatment of drug addiction and alcoholism.

Back ward psychotic patients who have been restricted to locked wards for years because they lack elementary social skills and competencies are often able to leave the ward following behavior modification procedures which teach them the rudiments of these skills. While they may not be able to leave the hospital, they are able to spend their days in much happier circumstances, perhaps sitting under a tree instead of on a ward bench.

Behavior modification procedures are easily taught to persons unsophisticated in psychologic theory and technic. Psychiatric aides, parents, and public school teachers have been taught the principles of behavior modification with such success that they are able to assume responsibility for treatment within a few hours of instruction. The procedures are clear-cut, unambiguous, and consistent—all qualities which make for ready transfer of skill from professional to nonprofessional therapist.

Another advantage of these procedures over conventional ones is the much shorter period of time they require for a positive outcome. Patients who would have spent years in psychoanalysis are said to be helped greatly by treatment lasting only a few weeks. At the same time, the behavior therapists claim success equal to or greater than that of older procedures, with only rare instances of symptom substitution or reappearance of old symptoms.

Finally, these procedures offer many more opportunities for objective, scientific inquiry into modes of action and degree of therapeutic success than older procedures, notably psychoanalysis, which are relatively inaccessible to such inquiry.

At this point, the major shortcoming of behavior therapy lies in the enthusiasm with which its adherents "sell" the technics as a "cure-all" for all the world's ills. In many ways, such dedication to a single therapeutic point of view, accompanied as it is by selective inattention to other methods and points of view, is strikingly reminiscent of the early days of the psychoanalytic movement.

The behavior therapies have not yet proved effective in the treatment of most psychotic disorders and most personality disorders. Although Wolpe, among others, does claim that they are applicable to almost all psychiatric disorders, objective evidence supporting this claim does not yet exist.

Behavior modified on a hospital ward or in a therapist's office often does not carry over completely into the patient's life because all of the relevant "controlling stimuli" may not be present. The procedures may lose effectiveness because the patient becomes "satiated" with the altered consequences of his new behavior; when this happens, periodic reconditioning may still be effective.

Finally, social (interpersonal) behavior, especially verbal behavior, is difficult to generate in seriously disturbed patients because potential reinforcers are often absent.

Most psychiatrists remain unconvinced by the data published thus far and feel that suggestion has been playing an important part in the results—although unrecognized by either the patient or the therapist.

HYPNOTHERAPY

Hypnosis is a mental state of heightened focal concentration and dissociated attention in a subject who, in effect, abandons self-control and submits nonrationally to the will of the hypnotist. It is now regarded as a legitimate form of psychotherapy when used by a properly trained physician on suitably selected patients.

The use of hypnosis in psychotherapy has had a checkered history. When Mesmer first used what he called "animal magnetism" in 1775, the spectacular reactions created widespread public attention. The "Svengali" and sensationalist aspects of hypnotism led to hostile skepticism and condemnation from the scientific community, but what came to be called "mesmerism" continued to intrigue such men as Liçebeault, Charcot, Janet, and Freud.

In modern times, hypnotism has become (1) a form of parlor or vaudeville entertainment, (2) a legitimate research method in psychologic experiments, (3) a method of producing "anesthesia," especially in dentistry, childbirth, and minor operations, and (4) an adjunct to some forms of psychotherapy. This section will be concerned largely with the last.

Advantages of Hypnotherapy

In hypnotherapy, the therapist utilizes the "trance state" to increase the speed and effectiveness of his particular form of psychotherapy or to further his special psychiatric interest. Psychoanalysts who employ hypnosis refer to their therapy as "hypnoanalysis" and emphasize the value of the technic in the recovery of deeply repressed memories. Hospital psychiatrists use the hypnotic state in cases of amnesia to bring to consciousness enough personal data to identify the patient and initiate therapy. Military psychiatrists sometimes use hypnotic technics as an alternative to narcosynthesis for the abreaction of the traumatic events that preceded an acute hysterical illness ("combat fatigue," "war neurosis"). Forensic psychiatrists may put a prisoner in a hypnotic trance to test the truth of his defensive story. Some psychotherapists, counselors, and guidance workers use hypnosis to increase their powers of suggestion and persuasion in the modification of symptoms or alteration of behavior. Hypnosis has been urged as a valuable adjunct to psychotherapy in the treatment of obesity, compulsive smoking, homosexuality, gambling, drug addiction, phobias, and obsessions.

The technics involved and their relationship to other aspects of psychotherapy vary widely. The hypnotic trance state is brought about through the use of one of many procedures for focusing the patient's attention, inducing him to disregard everything in his surroundings except the therapist and increasing his suggestibility by informing him of body feelings he is about to have. The patient is given emphatic posthypnotic directions about how his future feelings and behavior are to be modified.

Disadvantages and Dangers of Hypnotherapy

Enthusiastic reports in the literature of the "cures" that have been effected through hypnosis have been lacking in controls and have not carried conviction. Objective studies have been disappointing. Many patients cannot be hypnotized; symptom relief, when it occurs, is often transient; behavioral changes are fleeting; and untoward (at times disastrous) reactions occur.

Hypnotherapy treats symptoms and not people or their illnesses. A patient may be induced to give up one symptom only to develop another. Chain smoking may change to obesity, or obesity to alcoholism, or alcoholism to depression. Specific suggestions may cause unexpected side-effects. One man gave up his bruxism (grinding teeth at night), but promptly had a nightmare in which he nearly throttled his wife. During hypnosis, a 40-year-old woman had a heart attack when she was told she felt cold because she took "cold" to mean "dead."

Relief of symptoms by hypnosis at best is palliative, not curative, and hypnosis fosters undue dependency on the therapist. The patient is encouraged in his already too great inclination to let the therapist do all his work for him—to regress to childlike belief in magic and hocus-pocus instead of facing up to the realities of life. Furthermore, the vaunted recovery of forgotten material involves reaching *behind* the patient's resistances—outwitting them, so to speak. The resistances remain and may spread or grow stronger in compensation. "Improvement" thus tends to be short-lived and disappointment long-lasting.

Hypnosis may also involve actual danger to the subject, the therapist, or others. A psychosis may appear either during an explosive abreaction or because of inability to bring the subject out of the hypnotic trance. Latent paranoid and homosexual conflicts may be liberated. Highly predisposed individuals—perhaps near the breaking point—undergo hypnosis at their peril. Other conditions presumably precipitated by hypnotic experiences include anxiety states, body image distortions, and a variety of psychosomatic symptoms.

Several therapists have suffered psychotic breaks while giving hypnotic therapy—largely as a result of exacerbation of latent megalomanic feelings. Some therapists have been physically attacked by acutely disturbed patients; others have been sued for malpractice, for assault and battery, or for sexual attack. Many have been hurt (and have hurt their patients) more subtly and indirectly by emphasizing the use of hypnosis to the exclusion of other therapeutic technics.

The danger to the public is in being misled by fallacious claims. Hypnosis is still little understood scientifically. Most research has been conducted on reasonably healthy volunteers, and extrapolation of results to sick patients is unwarranted. The interaction of the psychodynamics of therapy with those of hypnosis and the complicating effects of drug therapy are largely unknown. The literature reports successes more freely than failures and untoward reactions. People disposed to wishful thinking turn quickly to anyone offering apparently simple and easy "cures" for difficult problems.

The American Medical Association has issued standards whereby physicians may, with specific patients and for very specific treatment goals, make use of hypnotic technics—but only for goals and with technics that would be within the areas of their professional competence if they were treating these same patients in other ways, and then only after making an adequate physical and mental examination of the patient. The American Psychiatric Association has gone further, stating that the physician "must have sufficient knowledge of psychiatry, and particularly of psychodynamics, to avoid its use in clinical situations where it is contraindicated or dangerous." The APA refers to its "inappropriate use" as "particularly hazardous," and adds: "For hypnosis to be used safely, even for the relief of pain or for sedation, more than a superficial knowledge of the dynamics of human motivation is therefore considered essential."

The Committee on the Medical Aspects of Sports and the Council of the AMA issued in 1960 a "Joint Statement on the Use of Hypnosis in Athletics," condemning it because of the possibility of "irrevocable injury" to subjects. The British Hypnotism Act of 1952 is similarly condemnatory because of "severe adverse reactions." The British Broadcasting Corporation no longer permits hypnotism to be shown on television because members of the viewing audience may develop potentially harmful trance states. In 1960, a Texas court imposed a criminal sentence on a lay hypnotist who alleged to "cure" symptoms for violation of the state's Medical Practice Act. In other states, Better Business Bureaus have brought action against lay hypnotists for quackery. The Federal Drug Administration has taken similar action. In 1956, Pope Pius XII issued an edict proscribing the use of hypnosis by ecclesiastics except with special permission and asserting that hypnotism was not to be considered a plaything by laymen.

REFERENCES

Books and Monographs

Ayllon, T., & N. Azrin: *The Token Economy.* Appleton-Century-Crofts, 1968.

Bandura, A.: Social learning through imitation. Pages 211–269 in: *Nebraska Symposium on Motivation.* Jones, M.R. (editor). Univ of Nebraska Press, 1962.

Bandura, A.: *Principles of Behavior Modification.* Holt, Rinehart & Winston, 1969.

Bandura, A., & R.H. Walters: Aggression. Pages 364–415 in: *Child Psychology: The 62nd Yearbook of the National Society for the Study of Education.* Part 1. National Society for the Study of Education, 1963.

Franks, C.M.: *Conditioning Techniques in Clinical Practice and Research.* Springer Verlag (New York), 1961.

Franks, C. (editor): *Behavior Therapy.* McGraw-Hill, 1969.

Freund, K.: Some problems in the treatment of homosexuality. In: *Behavior Therapy and the Neuroses.* Eysenck, H.J. (editor). Pergamon Press, 1960.

Kanfer, F.H., & J.S. Phillips: *Learning Foundations of Behavior Therapy.* Wiley, 1970.

Tinterow, M.M.: *Foundations of Hypnosis: From Mesmer to Freud.* Thomas, 1970.

Wolpe, J.: *Psychotherapy by Reciprocal Inhibition.* Stanford Univ Press, 1958.

Wolpe, J.: *The Practice of Behavior Therapy.* Pergamon Press, 1969.

Wolpe, J., & A.A. Lazarus: *Behavior Therapy Techniques.* Pergamon Press, 1966.

Wolpe, J., Salter, A., & L.J. Reyna: *Conditioning Therapies: The Challenge in Psychotherapy.* Holt, Rinehart & Winston, 1964.

Journal Articles

Ayllon, T., & J. Michael: The psychiatric nurse as a behavioral engineer. J Exper Anal Behav 2:323–334, 1959.

Azrin, N.H., & J. Powell: Behavioral engineering: The reduction of smoking behavior by a conditioning apparatus and procedure. J Appl Behav Anal 1:193–200, 1968.

Bandura, A., & F.J. McDonald: The influence of social reinforcement and the behavior of models in shaping children's moral judgments. J Abnorm Social Psychol 67:274–281, 1963.

Colman, A.D., & S.L. Baker, Jr.: Utilization of an operant conditioning model for the treatment of character and behavior disorders in a military setting. Am J Psychiat 125:1395–1403, 1969.

Eysenck, H.J.: Behavior therapy: Unlearning neuroses. Med Opin Rev 3:68–74, 1966.

Fox, L.: Effecting the use of efficient study habits. J Mathematics 1:75–86, 1962.

Kanfer, F.H., & J.S. Phillips: Behavior therapy. Arch Gen Psychiat 15:114–127, 1966.

Lovibond, S.H., & G. Caddy: Discriminated aversive control in the moderation of alcoholics' drinking behavior. Behav Ther 1:437–444, 1970.

Mayer, D.Y.: A psychotherapist's note on behaviour therapy. Brit J Psychiat 115:429–434, 1969.

Paul, G.L., & R.W. Trimble: Recorded vs. "live" relaxation training and hypnotic suggestion: Comparative effectiveness for reducing physiological arousal and inhibiting stress response. Behav Ther 1:285–302, 1970.

Tighe, T.J., & E. Rogers: A technique for controlling behavior in natural life settings. J Appl Behav Anal 1:263, 1968.

Walters, R.H., & L.E. Thomas: Enhancement of punitiveness by visual and audiovisual displays. Canad J Psychol 17:244–255, 1963.

Wolf, M.M., Risley, T., & H. Mees: Application of operant conditioning procedures to the behavior problems of an autistic child. Behav Res Ther 1:305–312, 1964.

Wolpe, J.: Reciprocal inhibition as the main basis of psychotherapeutic effects. Arch Neurol Psychiat 72:205–212, 1954.

Wolpe, J.: Basic principles and practices of behavior therapy of neuroses. Am J Psychiat 125:1242–1246, 1969.

Yates, A.J.: The application of learning theory to the treatment of tics. J Abnorm Social Psychol 56:175–179, 1958.

29...

Psychiatric Social Work

The psychiatric social worker represents extra arms and legs (and brains) for the clinical psychiatrist. He can extend the services of the psychiatrist materially in intake, reception, case work with the patient and his family, and follow-up care. He is an essential member of the treatment team.

Psychiatric social work bears the same service relationship to psychiatry that medical social work bears to the rest of medicine. Medical social work was formalized as a new discipline in the United States in 1905 at Massachusetts General Hospital, and the first school of social work was established in 1918 at Smith College. There are now about 50 schools of social work in the United States, graduating about 6400 students yearly, and current membership in the National Association of Social Workers is over 44,000. About 25% of graduating students enter psychiatric social work, and about 25% of the members of the National Association are now employed in psychiatric social work.

The needs for the services provided by these specialists are so great that a number of available positions must be filled by persons who have not yet obtained the graduate training and the master's degree required for membership in the national organization. Estimates place the need for fully qualified social workers, both medical and psychiatric, at more than triple the number now available in the United States.

FUNCTIONS OF THE PSYCHIATRIC SOCIAL WORKER

Forty years ago, the functions of the psychiatric social worker were limited to assisting the psychiatrist in a mental hospital by gathering background historical data from the patient and his relatives at the time of admission. Today, his functions are as varied as those of the psychiatrist and actually overlap the psychiatrist's functions.

In general, the psychiatric social worker deals with people in 3 different roles: (1) In an individual relationship with one patient or one relative for purposes of so-called *case work* or *individual psychotherapy*. (2) In a group relationship with small groups of people for purposes of providing *group psychotherapy*. (3) In a group relationship with large groups of people for purposes of *community organization*. He usually develops his greatest skills in the area of case work, but the field now includes men and women whose considerable abilities and experience have made them expert in all 3 areas.

The psychiatric social worker usually works under the direction of a psychiatrist, who is considered the leader of the treatment team. Other members of the team may be a psychologist, a psychiatric nurse, an occupational therapist, a psychiatric aide, and perhaps a psychiatric volunteer or student (medical, social work, or occupational therapist). The purpose of the team is to administer psychiatric treatment as efficiently as possible by coordinated effort.

The psychiatric social worker is often a highly experienced member of the treatment team and provides, under the direction of the psychiatrist, psychotherapy or case work on an individual or group basis for the patient's family or, occasionally, for the patient himself. The types of problems dealt with in this way are largely environmental, eg, unemployment, financial problems, failure at work, poor housing, the need for medical care or housekeeping services, and the need for help with disturbed relationships with other people.

When the social worker understands the tensions his "clients" live with and knows how they feel and how they deal with their feelings, he can assist them by modifying stresses in their environments or by engaging their participation in more effective methods of coping with them.

From this description it will be obvious that much of his work is no different from what the psychiatrist spends part of his time doing in psychotherapy.

Social workers have been concerned about preserving a separate identity and a separate name ("case work") for the work they do so that psychiatrists would have no occasion to fear or resent an invasion of their province. However, psychiatrists know that the medical profession can never, by itself, meet the enormous psychotherapeutic needs of the American community, and additional qualified purveyors of the art are welcomed rather than resented. Unfortunately, since psychotherapy is not considered a medical discipline in many parts of the United States, it can be practiced by almost anyone with the inclination to do so, even without formal training or supervision. Some psychiatric social workers have paced their field by undertaking the private practice of psychotherapy and are now providing this treatment on a fee-for-service basis in "competition" with psychiatrists. The next decade may bring about the creation of state licensing boards for nonmedical psychotherapists to ensure that high standards are maintained. Well trained psychiatric social workers will probably lead this effort, and in so doing will add one more deserved credit to the list of their professional accomplishments.

One distinction often made between the work of the psychiatrist and that of the psychiatric social worker is that the social worker does not work with a patient's psychopathology as deeply as the psychiatrist. In practice, this may not be true. With many patients the social worker works with the same material, in the same way, and for the same length of time as the psychiatrist.

A third recognized feature of psychiatric social work is its emphasis on practical reality, or "here and now" psychiatry, as opposed to the "there and then" psychiatry of the probing psychoanalyst. Many psychiatrists, however, routinely do supportive psychotherapy in appropriate cases, emphasizing the same "here and now" features with the same purpose and effectiveness.

SCOPE OF ACTIVITIES

The social worker customarily works in all phases of the problem his team is approaching.

(1) **Intake:** (The initial contact by a patient with a psychiatric treatment resource, eg, an outpatient clinic or a mental hospital.) At this point the social worker gathers a discriminating social history pertinent to the development of the patient's mental illness.

(2) **Reception:** (A second phase that includes indoctrinating the patient or his family in the workings of the treatment resources.) At this point a social worker may be used to allay the anxiety of the patient and family over a forthcoming hospitalization or outpatient treatment.

(3) **Continued case work with patient or family:** (A phase during which case work is done with the principals in a treatment situation.) Often, in addition to doing case work, the social worker will serve a liaison function between the patient and his family, his community, or his employer. Reports on the patient's progress, as well as predictions of his needs in the community after treatment, may also be managed by the social worker during this period.

(4) **Aftercare:** (A final phase of treatment during which the social worker may be the only member of the psychiatric team still involved with the patient's care.) During this phase, supportive psychotherapy, family counseling, and continued liaison between the patient and his community may be provided by the social worker either alone or in conjunction with other treatment personnel or resources.

TRAINING AND SKILLS

The psychiatric social worker must have training in the areas of normal human behavior, psychopathology, family life, and community life. He must particularly acquire skills in utilizing community resources in the service of his client. He must also understand how clients feel about accepting help and how to help them manage these feelings. Finally, he must understand enough of his own feelings to be sure he will not let them interfere with his work (eg, he must not make a client unnecessarily dependent on him in order to satisfy his own need to feel strong).

The psychiatric social worker in case work helps his client ventilate feelings, recognize conflicts that are interfering with constructive action or provoking destructive behavior, and clarify decisions. He helps significant people in the client's life in such a way that the client will benefit.

Through the use of the skills and knowledge outlined above, the psychiatric social worker is an essential person in most psychiatric resources. Whether the resource is a child guidance clinic, school counseling service, court clinic, psychiatric consultation service in a general hospital, state mental hospital, community mental health center, psychiatric home treatment service, family counseling center, outpatient clinic, psychiatric inpatient unit of a general hospital, or a youth, neighborhood, or community center, the psychiatric social worker can make important contributions by applying his special talents for working with people individually or in groups.

REFERENCES

Journal Articles

Black, B.J.: Comprehensive community mental health services: Setting social policy. Social Work 12:51–58, Jan 1967.

Brotman, R., & J.A. Livenstein: A role model for social workers in community mental health practice. Social Work 12:21-26, Jan 1967.

Cohen, M.: Some characteristics of social workers in private practice. Social Work 11:69–77, April 1966.

Golan, N., Carey, H., & E. Hyttinen: The emerging role of the social worker in a psychiatric emergency service. Community Ment Health J 5:55–61, Feb 1969.

Ivey, A.E., & J.E. Hinkle: A study in role theory: Liaison between social agencies. Commun Ment Health J 6:63–68, 1970.

Jones, M.: From hospital to community psychiatry. Commun Ment Health J 6:187–195, 1970.

Miller, D., & C. Blanc: Concepts of "moral treatment" for the mentally ill: Implications for social work with posthospital mental patients. Social Service Rev 41:66–74, March 1967.

Olsen, K.M., & M.E. Olsen: Role expectations and perceptions for social workers in medical settings. Social Work 12:70–78, July 1967.

Wertz, O.T.: Social workers and the therapeutic community. Social Work 11:43–49, Oct 1966.

30...

Psychiatric Nursing

*The psychiatric nurse is an essential member of the psychi-
atric therapeutic team. She has unique opportunities to help her
patients in the ward therapeutic milieu. She also contributes to
consultations on medical and surgical wards and assists in teaching and research.*

Psychiatric nursing is a specialized branch of nursing in which the nurse
utilizes her own personality, her knowledge of psychiatric theory, and the
available environment to effect therapeutic changes in her patients' thoughts,
feelings, and behavior. Her ability to effect these changes varies according to
her experience and education. Registered nurses have a short experience in
psychiatric nursing, and graduates of baccalaureate programs have a broad
background in the social sciences as well. The nurse is considered a specialist
in this field only when she has completed a master's program in psychiatric
nursing.

Psychiatric nursing provides opportunities for patients to change their
maladaptive behavior responses in safe and comfortable surroundings where
anxiety-provoking situations can be controlled. For example, a patient filled
with anger who was raised in a home where expression of feelings was not
allowed can be encouraged to verbalize his anger after the nurse points out
that he has violated a ward rule. As he discusses the issue with the nurse, he
discovers that it may be all right both to feel anger and to express it. Later,
he may be able to admit to himself that he is filled with anger and work with
his therapist about it. Knowing that the nurses are concerned about him and
accept him even though he has angry feelings that seem to be unacceptable
in other settings may give this patient a grip on his self-esteem that he never
had before.

The *goal* of psychiatric nursing care is to encourage the patient to face
reality and resume independent action as soon as possible. The nurse must
permit appropriate expression of both positive and negative feelings, and the
patient must feel free to develop and use his own initiative and creativity.
The patient must have the opportunity to act both in his role as an individual with legitimate needs and as a member of a community with social
demands as well as rewards. An angry patient must be helped to see that his
explosive behavior is frightening to other members of the community, in
which case the nurse must help him to examine the appropriateness of his
reaction and its possible consequences to both himself (eg, retaliation or

isolation by the group) and others. During this discussion it must be made clear that the nurse's most immediate concern is for the patient, though there is no need to conceal the obvious fact that he is not her only concern on the ward.

As a member of the *therapeutic team* of psychiatrist, psychologist, social worker, occupational therapist, nurse, and auxiliary workers, the nurse assists in formulating and implementing a broad plan of care for each patient to meet his total needs. This plan is developed after some contact with the patient so that all team members can share their observations and outline some of the patient's most obvious needs. A depressed patient may require immediate supervision to prevent self-injury. The nurse providing this supervision could use the opportunity to help the patient bear his sadness and learn how to reach out to other people for help and comfort. She must also be aware of his underlying anger and begin to encourage him to face it. She may do so by sharing with him her annoyance at some situation. Offering assistance with physical care (bath, shampoo, obtaining clean clothing) may be a means of enhancing the patient's self-esteem. This type of care may open the door to discussion of the patient's view of himself.

Encouraging the patients to socialize in groups and take part in occupational, recreational, and social activities is a first step toward establishing a *therapeutic milieu.* As new patients face the problems of orientation to the ward setting and living with others on the ward—or when they are ready to return to the community—they may benefit from participation in group meetings. As the leader at such meetings, the nurse utilizes a problem-solving approach to reality situations and issues presented by the patients. She encourages open expression of feelings and attempts to facilitate communication as well as group cohesiveness. Other groups led by nurses (or by a nurse and a psychiatrist) may be concerned with such matters as patient government or ward activities. The psychiatric nurse is aware of and able to utilize relationships and situations in the light of therapeutic goals for each patient. The patient who has difficulty saying "No" to requests may find himself doing other patients' work assignments. The nurse may utilize this very real experience to help him learn to set limits. She may do this on an individual basis or in a group setting.

NURSING TEAM MEMBERS

The *nursing supervisor* is an experienced psychiatric nurse who has accumulated a fund of knowledge about the channels of communication and administrative workings of the hospital. It is her function to plan and administer the nursing service according to the principles and philosophy of the professional staff. Her concern is to provide high quality care for every patient. She offers guidance to the nursing staff to help each member develop to her full professional potential, and she supervises relationships with individual patients and groups. She plans ongoing educational programs of various kinds to meet the needs of the different levels of nursing staff. She serves as liaison between nurses and staff physicians on the service and as a consultant to nursing areas in the rest of the hospital.

It is the responsibility of the *head nurse* to provide efficient and effective ward administration. She assigns nursing duties, coordinates nursing team activities, provides individual supervision for some staff nurses' relationships with patients, and oversees the work of auxiliary personnel. She maintains communication with the medical staff and the residents.

The *psychiatric staff nurse* may serve either as team leader or as a team member in the nursing care of individual patients or groups of patients. She establishes and maintains effective relationships with other team members for the therapeutic care of patients. She assumes responsibility for the physical care of patients. She may lead and keep records for one or more therapy groups, and may also serve as a member of the psychiatric consultation team serving the rest of the hospital.

Licensed practical nurses (LPNs) function similarly to staff nurses depending on their ability and psychiatric training. The LPN cares for the physical needs of patients under the supervision of a staff nurse or head nurse.

The *psychiatric aide (orderly)* generally comes to the psychiatric service with less formal knowledge and experience in caring for the mentally ill than other members of the nursing team. Hospitals with large psychiatric inpatient censuses, such as VA, state, and some private and general hospitals, may have well organized, formal educational programs for the aides. However, in many psychiatric facilities, the recruitment and education of the aide continues to be less formally organized. The educational process consists of a 2-week orientation period, participation in ongoing in-service programs, and individual supervision by a qualified staff nurse.

The aide may come to the unit with preconceived ideas and prejudices about mental illness. Some of the attitudes and feelings of the aide that must be recognized and eliminated are fear and dislike of psychiatric patients; prejudice against people of a different race or religion; an exaggerated need to be a friend to patients rather than a therapeutic team member; and fear and distrust of authority figures, so that free communication with staff members may be limited.

The aide must receive initial instruction in and orientation to the problems of psychiatric ward care, and must continue to be supervised in his work with patients. He must be taught therapeutically effective ways of dealing with psychotic behavior and the emotional problems of ward patients. He is usually started with step-by-step procedures, and his interactions with patients are closely observed. He should be encouraged to think of himself as a member of the nursing team, and to share with other members his experiences with patients and his feelings about them. He may, for example, be badly frightened by a patient who attempts to escape during an escorted visit to the dental service, in which case he may need help in dealing with his resulting anger toward the patient and his feelings of inadequacy about the episode.

The aide participates in the discussion at meetings and conferences. He is expected to observe, report, and record patients' behavior and feelings and in a realistic, nonjudgmental manner to assist patients in dealing with personal issues.

Some patients find it easier to communicate with the aide than with the nurse because of similarities in regional, ethnic, or educational background. This may mean that the aide will be the only person on the service who knows what the patient is thinking or how he feels. This information can often be used to the patient's benefit. The aide can sometimes explain certain obscure features of the patient's history to other members of the team.

Since the aide is often the only male on the nursing staff, patients and nurses alike are apt to be reassured by his presence on the ward. He can be a deterrent to disorderly behavior on the part of patients and thus a comfort to the nurses and other patients.

The aide assists the nurses and LPNs in caring for the physical needs of patients, checks vital signs, feeds patients, and escorts them to diagnostic and treatment areas in the hospital.

A *public health nurse* in the community may have known the patient and his family and may be able to offer pertinent observations on the patient's attitudes toward medication or hospitalization. Her assessment of the stability of the family and its tolerance for deviant behavior may also be of value. Psychiatric nurses should maintain contact with public health nurses in the community to facilitate communication when a patient is admitted or discharged. If a public health nurse is asked to follow a psychiatric patient after discharge, her nursing tasks must be clearly delineated.

The psychiatric ward nurse may be asked to make home visits, either alone or with a social worker or doctor. The purpose may be to assess the advisability of returning a patient to his former environment; to encourage the family to take a more active part in the care of the patient; or to provide supportive therapy for family members and the patient upon discharge.

ROLES OF THE PSYCHIATRIC NURSING STAFF IN THE TOTAL HOSPITAL COMMUNITY

Consultation

In a general hospital, the specialized knowledge and services of the psychiatric nurse may be offered to the nursing staff of the other units whenever a psychiatric consultation is requested. When the psychiatrist sees a patient elsewhere in the hospital, she can help the nurses caring for the patient by assisting them to understand his problems and to find appropriate ways of relating to him. A cantankerous old woman whom no one can please and who therefore is neglected or avoided may become less shrill and unpleasant if the nurses on the ward can be encouraged to find out the reasons for her willful attitude. Simple solutions may suggest themselves after a few brief conversations, eg, a visit might be arranged with a favorite niece; a small light might be left on in her room at night; or the door may be kept closed—or left open. The psychiatric nurse can often help the staff to work more successfully with the patient by providing emotional support as well as medical and physical care.

The psychiatric nurse should become a familiar and unthreatening person to the other hospital nurses, ie, a colleague and an equal. She should attend general nursing meetings and acquaint the other nurses with the purposes and kinds of treatment available on the psychiatric service. For the psychiatric patient who needs attention in other departments of the hospital, the psychiatric nurse arranges appropriate referrals. She facilitates understanding and communication by bringing the patient to the other departments, introducing him to the staff there, and allowing time for conferences.

Research

The psychiatric nurse should make her skills and specialized knowledge available to qualified people who wish to initiate research projects on her ward. She should be consulted about the clinical aspects of the research design. For example, she may be able to point out that the rating scale for patient behavior is so long and complex that the nursing staff will have to hurry through it without sufficient thought. Being included in the planning also stimulates support and interest in the collection of data.

Nurses with research knowledge or interests should be encouraged to develop projects of their own such as defining and validating what kind of nursing interaction is most helpful to the patients being studied.

The purpose and design of the study should be shared with other members of the staff and appropriate progress reports offered.

Teaching

The psychiatric nurse should offer learning experiences to others with whom she is professionally involved. To the patient she offers help in finding alternative ways of adjusting to reality situations. With co-workers, she interprets her role, describes her observations, and seeks and gives validation of her nursing interventions. With nurses in the hospital and the community, she shares her knowledge of psychiatric nursing and assists in caring for the difficult patient on a medical or surgical ward and in the home.

REFERENCES

Books and Monographs

Alexander, E., & others: *Nursing Service Administration.* Mosby, 1962.

Barton, W.E.: *Administration in Psychiatry.* Thomas, 1962.

Fagin, C.H.: *A Study of Desirable Functions and Qualifications for Psychiatric Nurses.* National League for Nursing Education, 1953.

Georgopoulos, B.S., & F.C. Mann: *The Community General Hospital.* Macmillan, 1962.

Hospital Nursing Service Manual. American Hospital Association and National League for Nursing Education, 1950.

Peplau, H.: *Interpersonal Relations in Nursing.* Putnam, 1952.

The Psychiatric Nurse in the Mental Hospital. GAP Report No. 22. Group for the Advancement of Psychiatry, 1952.

Robinson, A.M.: *The Psychiatric Aide,* 3rd ed. Lippincott, 1965.

Schwartz, M.S., & E.L. Shockley: *The Nurses and the Mental Patient.* Wiley, 1956.

Weiss, M.O.: *Attitudes in Psychiatric Nursing Care.* Putnam, 1954.

Journal Articles

Atkinson, C.A., & others: Community psychiatric nursing. Canadian Nurse 63:31–33, June 1967.

Baggott, E.: Role of the hospital nurse in the wider psychiatric service. Nursing Times 63:993–994, 1967.

Johnson, D.: A philosophy of nursing. Nursing Outlook, pp 198–200, April 1959.

Lehman, K.: Supervision: Variation on a theme. Am J Nursing 67:1204–1206, 1967.

McCain, F.: Nursing by assessment. Am J Nursing 65:82, 1965.

Visher, J.S., & M. O'Sullivan: Nurse and patient responses to a study of milieu therapy. Am J Psychiat 127:451–456, 1970.

PART IV.
SPECIAL PSYCHIATRIC FIELDS

31 . . .

Psychoanalysis

Psychoanalysis is a form of psychotherapy based on Freudian theory: mental illnesses, especially neurosis and character disorders, result from unconscious conflict largely centered around an unresolved Oedipus complex. Improvement requires making the unconscious conscious. This is done by a technic necessitating hundreds of hours of free association (usually on a couch), dream interpretation, and utilization of the patient's transference reactions to the therapist.

To become a recognized psychoanalyst, a psychiatrist must undergo several years of additional education and training as well as a personal psychoanalysis.

Psychoanalysis is a special form of psychotherapy based upon an extensive theory of personality structure and development (both normal and pathologic) which holds that the major psychodynamic forces stem largely from the unconscious part of the mind. It originated with Sigmund Freud, a physician who specialized in neurology and the treatment of nervous disorders. Freud studied for a year with the French psychiatrist Charcot, who utilized hypnotism in the treatment of hysteria, primarily by the use of suggestion. Later, Freud worked with the Viennese physician Joseph Breuer, who also used hypnosis. Instead of using suggestion alone, Breuer sought to cure symptoms by having the patients talk about them ("talking out," catharsis). When Freud began to feel that sexual conflicts were a primary cause of hysteria, the more conservative Breuer parted company with him.

Finding that hypnosis was a very limited method of treatment, Freud developed the use of *free association* (saying whatever comes to mind without censorship or reservations) and the *interpretation of dreams* as technical tools of treatment.

He developed a number of complex theories of personality structure and psychopathology which he continuously expanded and modified from the 1890s until his death in 1939. Several of his early students elaborated and modified his theories and developed psychoanalytic theories of their own. The more important of these were Carl Jung, Alfred Adler, and Otto Rank.

In recent years in the United States 2 important groups of analysts have emerged: (1) Those who remain primarily Freudian—"orthodox" or "classical"—in their approach tend to adhere to the original Freudian concepts but continue to seek elaborations, modifications, and improvements on Freud's theories. Most of this group become members of the American Psychoanalytic Association. (2) The so-called "neo-Freudians" adhere to many of Freud's basic psychodynamic concepts but with marked theoretical differences—in general, deemphasis on the importance of sexual conflicts, increased emphasis on cultural and social forces in the personality, variations in the quantity and quality of the activity of the analyst in the treatment process, and greater stress on research, scientific principles, and the proper role of psychoanalysis as a branch of psychiatry and medicine. Most members of this group become members of the American Academy of Psychoanalysis.

Approximately 10% of the psychiatrists in the United States (less in other countries) are qualified psychoanalysts. At least half of the remainder (including practically all newly trained psychiatrists) are "psychoanalytically oriented," ie, they are deeply concerned with psychodynamics, in which they include unconscious motivation and conflict.

TRAINING OF THE PSYCHOANALYST

The psychoanalyst-in-training must first undergo complete residency training in general psychiatry—usually a 3-year program. The candidate must then have an extensive personal analysis by an experienced analyst (training analyst) in order to (1) eliminate "blind spots" in his personality that may interfere with his recognizing problems similar to his own in his patients and to maintain clinical objectivity when such problems do appear in his patients; (2) prevent undue anxiety when patients bring up unconscious material that may coincide with the analyst's conflict areas or that is fraught with basic id and infantile material; and (3) facilitate the recognition and effective handling of countertransference. Occasionally, a candidate may begin his personal analysis while he is still in residency training. The training consists of seminars and supervised analyses. The formal academic curriculum consists of readings, lectures, and discussions of the vast amount of literature on psychoanalytic theory and technic. Clinical seminars are concerned with individual case presentations, discussions of special types of clinical problems, and long-term continuous case presentations (the same case followed in detail over a period of months).

Each candidate must personally conduct at least 3 analyses under the direct supervision of a training analyst. There is usually a different supervisor for each case. The candidate must present a detailed account of the analysis to his supervisor—usually reporting once a week or every other week. Thus he reports on every 5–10 sessions with his patient at each supervised hour.

Graduation from a psychoanalytic institute requires the satisfactory completion of all these phases of training. The length of training is usually 5–8 years. It is not uncommon for candidates who are regarded as not fully satisfactory to be asked to withdraw from the training program.

FUNDAMENTAL THEORIES OF PSYCHOANALYSIS

The basic assumptions of psychoanalysis are (1) *psychic determinism or causality* and (2) the *theory of the unconscious.* The concept of psychic determinism holds that each psychic event is determined by events that preceded it, just as all physical events have causal determinants. Unconscious mental processes play a vital role in human behavior and thought processes although it may appear that other "causes" are operating or that the phenomena are "meaningless." Freud likened the mind to an iceberg in which the smaller part showing above the surface of the water is analogous to the region of consciousness, whereas the much larger part submerged below the surface represents the region of the unconscious.

Structure of the Personality

Personality is made up of 3 major systems which at times interact so closely with one another that it is difficult to determine which is playing the dominant role in behavior.

(1) The id: The id is the original system of the personality. It consists of all the psychologic components present at birth, including the instincts. It is from the id that the other 2 systems of the personality (ego and superego) develop. The id is the reservoir of all psychic energy and provides the power for the operation of the other 2 systems. It derives its energies from bodily processes. It operates according to the *pleasure principle,* seeking immediate gratification of instinctual needs and reduction of psychic tension regardless of the reality situation. Its characteristic way of functioning is via *primary process thinking,* ie, it seeks the direct and immediate response to an instinctual stimulus without distinguishing between reality and fantasy. In so doing, if a reality response is not possible, it will when necessary resort to dreams in healthy individuals and to hallucinations in the mentally ill. Such thinking, part of which appears in daydreams and fantasy life, is nonverbal, is not bound by logic or objectivity, is not interrupted by contradictions existing side by side, and is not restricted by time considerations. It is assumed to be the thinking of the infant and it surely constitutes much of the mental activity of the mentally ill.

(2) The ego: The ego is the executive part of the personality. It includes the conscious or aware parts of the personality, although parts of the ego are unconscious. It is the mediator between the id and the outside world, but must deal also with the superego, with past memories, and with the physical needs of the body. It operates according to the *reality principle.* The aim of this principle is to assess and evaluate the reality situation (reality testing) and, if necessary, to postpone the gratification of a need (the reduction of tension) until a satisfactory object and method have been discovered. The ego utilizes *secondary process thinking.* It attempts to satisfy id (instinctual) drives, but will do so, if necessary, by indirect and often delayed means while at the same time taking the demands of the environment into account. This type of thinking is verbal and is characterized by logic and objectivity. It is the principal type of thinking of the mature individual.

(3) **The superego**: The superego is the internalized representative of what the individual regards to be basically right or wrong, ie, the moral part of the personality. It has 2 parts: conscience and ego-ideal. (1) The *conscience* is based on those things of which the individual's parents and others who helped raise the young child disapproved or for which they punished him. Behavior or thoughts running counter to these proscriptions result in *guilt feelings*. (2) The *ego-ideal* represents those things of which the individual felt his parents and others strongly approved or for which they rewarded him. To conform to or satisfy the ego-ideal results in deep inner feelings of well-being and pride. The superego is formed principally at the time of the resolution of oedipal conflict (see below), when the child incorporates into his own personality what he believes to be the basic moral principles and ideals of his parents. He makes these things part of himself. At this point, self-control becomes a substitute for parental control. The superego also includes many of the basic values or traditions of the culture in which the individual is raised as these have been interpreted to the child by his parents and other authority figures.

Topography of the Personality

The *topographic* division of the psyche is into the conscious, the preconscious, and the unconscious.

(1) The *conscious* includes those parts of mental life of which the individual is readily aware at any given moment. It includes most, but not all, of the ego.

(2) The *preconscious* includes those parts of mental life which can be brought into consciousness with concentration and effort. It lies principally in the ego.

(3) The *unconscious* is unknown to the individual (totally outside of awareness). Its contents may remain permanently unknown, or parts of it may at times pass into the preconscious and from there be called up into the conscious. According to psychoanalytic theory, the contents of the unconscious, primarily id and superego, are of great significance in determining behavior and thought. The part of the ego which produces the mental mechanism of defense and symptom formation is unconscious.

Dynamics of Personality

Psychic energy is the subjective experience of power and enthusiasm. It is universally recognized but largely untranslatable into physiologic terms as yet. In psychoanalytic theory it may also be present but unconscious. It is the hypothetical driving force responsible for all psychologic action (*psychodynamics*).

The bridge between the energy of the body and that of the personality is the id and its instincts.

A. Instincts: All stem from the id.

1. Sexual instinct (*libido*, life instinct)—This includes those instinctual energies that produce individual gratification and racial propagation. The principal part of this is connected with the sexual drive, which has its source in the erogenous zones of the body (genital, oral, and anal) whose stimula-

tion or manipulation can produce pleasurable feelings. Derivatives of this instinct include affection, love, the desire to reproduce, the need for other people, and creativity in work and art.

2. Aggressive instinct—At one time much of the aggressive instinct was referred to as the death instinct. It includes all of the destructive and hostile forces in the human psyche, and derivatives include the impulse to self-assertion, ambition, competition, the desire to win, and the drive to succeed. There are often fusions between sexual and aggressive drives—eg, competition for the object of one's love and active measures of self-protection such as fighting to protect one's home and loved ones. Overt sadistic and masochistic activities are pathologic fusions of the 2 sets of instincts, with the aggression directed toward others in sadism and toward oneself in masochism. There is release of sexual tension in both activities.

3. Energy concepts—Psychic energy is distributed among the 3 systems—id, ego, and superego—in different ways in different individuals. Originally, all of the energy belonged to the id. The other 2 systems are formed from the id and derive energy from it. *Cathexis* is the theoretical amount of psychic energy that is directed to or invested in an object (person or thing) or function (such as one's work) with the purpose of gratifying an instinct or its derivative. The ego needs psychic energy in order to deal with the id and superego and in maintaining its defense mechanisms. The more psychic energy that is tied up in this manner, the less energy the ego has available to deal with the problems of the outside world. (*Example:* A college student whose ego is involved with neurotic conflicts, eg, conflict over whether to engage in sexual activity, is expending psychic energy in the attempt to resolve conflicts between opposing forces in the id and superego by excessive use of defense mechanisms. He thus has reduced stores of psychic energy available for his studies and may get into serious academic difficulties.) One of the main goals of analysis is to enable the ego to resolve conflicts on a realistic or objective basis. This lessens the need for defense mechanisms so that less psychic energy will be used in maintaining these defenses. Psychic energy is thus made available to the ego for use in a more constructive and creative manner.

B. Anxiety: Under normal circumstances anxiety warns of impending danger. When anxiety is aroused, it motivates the person, usually, toward "fight or flight." There are 3 kinds of anxiety. *Realistic anxiety* is a fear of real dangers in the external world, ie, if one smells smoke, one may be afraid of fire. *Neurotic anxiety* is a fear that the instincts will get out of control and cause the person to do something for which he will then be punished. This is the type of anxiety experienced by an individual when he becomes annoyed with his boss and then unaccountably finds himself very anxious (because of an unconscious fear that his anger may get out of hand—that his aggressive instincts may overpower his judgment and result in violence). *Moralistic anxiety* is the fear of conscience. The individual who has a well developed superego feels guilty when he does something or even contemplates doing something that runs counter to the moral code which he has made part of himself.

Sometimes neurotic anxiety takes the form of *free-floating anxiety:* the anxious feelings which actually stem from a specific conflict become spread to many apparently neutral or irrelevant situations so that the individual is unaware of any causality between the anxious feelings and any specific situation. This functions to prevent the conscious part of the ego from recognizing the actual specific conflict situation, in a pathologic attempt to "protect" the ego from the conflict.

Anxiety that overwhelms the ego and cannot be dealt with by effective action is referred to as *traumatic anxiety.* It is a state of intolerable discomfort (fright, tension, somatic distress, helplessness) that must be relieved. When the ego cannot cope with anxiety by rational measures, it falls back upon other methods—the so-called defense mechanisms, normal or abnormal.

Signal anxiety is the term used for the early preconscious perception of anxiety by the ego which causes the ego to initiate protective measures to prevent development of a full-blown anxiety state.

DEVELOPMENT OF THE PERSONALITY

The terms character and personality both refer to the aggregate of the individual's basic and distinguishing behavioral characteristics, and they may usually be used interchangeably. The former is more often used to designate what an individual actually is, while the latter may imply what he seems to be to others.

The early years of infancy and childhood are decisive in forming the basic character structure of the person. The personality develops in response to 3 major sources of tension: (1) physiologic growth processes, (2) external frustration of drives, and (3) internal conflicts between dynamic forces. These result in threats to the ego, and the infant and child must develop ways to reduce these recurring tensions. This process constitutes personality development.

The age limits noted below are only approximate, and there is much overlap from one stage to the next.

Pre-Oedipal (Birth to About Age 4)

(1) **Oral (birth to age 1—2):** The infant's primary interest is centered on the mouth and what it can do. Sucking and taking in are of the greatest importance. Later, biting becomes important. There is a desire to put everything into the mouth. Mouth movements and sounds are gratifying—gurgling, spitting, etc. Objects (persons) are not recognized at first. The breast is the desired object (partial object), not the mother as a whole person. The infant is almost totally narcissistic. Pleasures are auto-erotic. The infant regards himself as the whole universe. It is only later that he gradually learns that he is not "everything"—that the breast is separate from him and can be removed despite his desires, and later that there are many parts of the world which he cannot control. From this experience the individual learns the limitations of his own body and the fact that it is a separate entity. This separate entity concept becomes the original ego—a "body-ego."

The oral stage contains the basic elements of many later partial drives: to eat, drink, or talk excessively; oral aggression ("biting" sarcasm, verbal nastiness); to be taken care of passively (fed like an infant); to incorporate or "swallow up" people. Opposites also occur: inability to eat, reluctance to speak, etc. These are due to conflicts over the original drive or attempts to overcompensate (*reaction formation*) for the original drives.

(2) **Anal (age 1–3):** In this stage the libidinal energies are centered on the retention and expulsion of feces. Much attention is directed toward the control of the anal sphincter (bowel training), and a great deal of pleasure and a feeling of accomplishment are involved in this. The ability to control one's own body and the parent—to please or displease the parent by controlling or not controlling the sphincter—are satisfying experiences. This is still a narcissistic, auto-erotic stage of development. The roots of obsessive compulsive behavior are present in the ability to control and regulate, to hold back, or to release at will. The roots of sadistic trends are here also—the ability to soil or defecate (to "shit on you") as an act of aggression, defiance, and even of pleasure. The important mechanism of projection starts at this stage—to propel the "bad stuff" out of one.

At this stage we also see the beginning of the phenomenon of *ambivalence*—the existence of strong opposing feelings side-by-side, ie, the strong desire to expel feces and the strong desire to retain them. Ambivalence later appears in other mixed feelings (positive and negative)—to love and hate the same person, to accept and reject, to deny and affirm.

(3) **Phallic (age 3–5):** During the phallic stage, the penis or clitoris becomes the focus of libidinal energies. Boys evince great interest in the size and consistency of the penis (erect or not); in the ability to direct the urinary stream; and in the pleasurable sensations derived from touching it; and there is a great concern with the fact that half the people in the world (females) do not have one. This is the beginning of concerns with power, strength, masculinity, and size; the desire to be stronger, bigger, and more powerful than others; and to possess objects that symbolize these things, eg, powerful automobiles. Drives toward making oneself outstanding or exceptional in the eyes of others begin during this time. *Sublimated drives* may lead to career, athletic, or creative accomplishments. Unsublimated drives may be expressed in more direct (id) ways, eg, excessive sexual drives or Don Juanism. The latter usually includes a reaction formation, an overcompensation for feeling sexually inadequate.

The phallic stage is initially auto-erotic, but sexual interest is gradually directed toward the parent of the opposite sex. This is the beginning of the oedipal period.

(4) **Urethral (age 3–5):** This stage coincides in time with the late anal and phallic stages. It is characterized by interest in and concern with bladder control. The pleasures and conflicts with regard to retention and release of urine are similar to those of the anal period. The anatomic relationship of the urethra to the penis (and clitoris) gives the act of urination a special sexual significance. The phenomenon of shame (over urinary "accidents") may play an important part in character development. Ambition (and even competitiveness) may stem from a strong desire to overcome shame—to over-

compensate. There is also a passive-submissive element—to relax and let flow. The ability to direct the urinary stream (a matter of pride for boys, envy for girls) may be important as a symbolic forerunner of control and power. Setting fires and putting them out (with a stream of urine) occurs in fantasy and sometimes in reality. Children are fascinated at this stage even more than usual by fire engines and fire fighters. Bedwetting in later life may be due to conflicts during this stage, and it may have aggressive (urinating on the parents) or masturbatory elements in it.

Oedipal (Age 3–4 to 6–7)

Freud felt that the oedipal stage was the most vital stage of development of the personality. The child is seen as developing a sexual interest in the parent of the opposite sex and consequently a strong feeling of rivalry toward the parent of the same sex. There is a desire to displace (get rid of) the latter.

The child then learns that his sexual desires are forbidden, and has both feelings of love and hate toward the parent of the same sex. This leads to feelings of anxiety and guilt, and fear of punishment for the "crime." In fantasy (often largely unconscious), this takes the form, in males, of a fear of castration (*castration anxiety*). The punishment symbolically takes place at the site of the offending member (*talion principle*). In females, there is a fear of further genital damage or mutilation since, theoretically, the female already has a sense of inferiority due to having a "very small" (clitoris) or absent penis. Theory provides that the female wishes to have a penis (something that protrudes, that you can see, that does things—becomes erect, directs the urinary stream). Later in life, *"penis envy"* is manifested as one element in the female envy of masculine prerogatives and privileges and may partly explain the tendency of some women to emulate men in dress and appearance and to compete with them in jobs.

The intensity of the fear of castration becomes so intolerable that the child is forced to yield to the powerful rival and give up his or her sexual wishes toward the parent of the opposite sex. The sexual feelings are thus repressed. While renouncing these feelings (sexual toward the parent of the opposite sex; aggressive toward the parent of the same sex), the ego compensates by taking over and "identifying with" parts of each parent, making part of each parent part of himself. The part that is taken over forms the child's superego. The superego consists of the child's view of what is most important in the moral and idealistic values of each parent. One section of the superego consists of conscience—the ultimate of what the individual will regard as basically (morally) right or wrong, good or bad. The second section consists of ego-ideal—the supreme characteristics or types of accomplishment that one must attain to be fully approved of and praised by the parents. The superego is largely an unconscious part of the psyche.

In the resolution of the oedipal conflict and the formation of the superego, it is as if the ego were saying (in the male), "I cannot literally have Mother for my own, but I can make part of her (conscience and ideals) become part of me. Then I will possess her in this safe way. Likewise, I cannot do away with Father, whom I both love and hate, but I can become like him (by taking over his conscience and ideals), and then he will like me and no longer see me as a rival and hence will not castrate me. Mother will even like me more since in this nonsexual manner I have become more like Father, who is her real lover."

Girls go through a similar process. The daughter's attraction to the parent of the opposite sex is also referred to as oedipal although it formerly was called the *Electra complex*. The resolution of the oedipal period is somewhat more complicated for the female than the male. The male, although he must give up his sexual attachment to the original mother, eventually, if mature, forms a sexual bond with a mother substitute, a female. The female, on the other hand, who as an infant was attached to her mother, becomes attracted to her father in the oedipal phase. With resolution she gives up the original father and with maturity ends up with a father substitute—a male. However, the healthy woman is not able, as the male is, to find a substitute for the original infantile attachment to the mother. The compensation for this is that she can become a mother herself and in this reverse manner regain the gratifications of the mother-child relationship.

If the oedipal period is not satisfactorily resolved, a variety of emotional disorders may occur. Overattachment to one parent or the other may interfere with the ability to transfer positive feelings to persons other than the parents. Overidentification with the parent of the opposite sex may be associated with the development of feminine characteristics and homosexual tendencies in the male or masculine characteristics and homosexual tendencies in the female. Undue fears of the parent of the opposite sex may impair the individual's ability to deal with persons of that sex later in life. A poorly resolved oedipal phase will also result in a poorly formed or deficient superego which may be a factor in various disorders such as sociopathic character disorders and neuroses. In general, psychoses seem to stem from earlier pre-oedipal problems, at least insofar as their psychologic aspects are concerned.

The reasons for a poorly resolved oedipal period may include the following: (1) Entering the oedipal phase with too many unresolved pre-oedipal conflicts (oral, anal, phallic), so that not enough psychic energy is available to deal effectively with this new phase; (2) absence of either parent (without a good substitute) during this phase due to death, divorce, or prolonged separation (military, chronic illness); or (3) severe psychopathology in either parent, such as parental problems which cause the parent to be overly seductive, rejecting, cruel and threatening, or too inconsistent in attitude, behavior, and warmth toward the child. Serious defects in the parent's superego or sexual identification (eg, very effeminate father) make it very difficult for the child to identify with that parent and to form a stable, reasonable, or consistent superego.

The oedipal period also marks the beginning of what is often called the *genital phase*. The primary interest during this time is in genital experience, with the trend being toward the union of the genitals with those of the opposite sex, ie, more directed toward another person and not primarily auto-erotic, as in the phallic phase. In this stage the individual is not so narcissistic, and his genital interests are not aimed toward self-aggrandizement, as in the phallic period, but toward a love object.

Latency Period (Age 7–12 to 14)

Following the resolution of the oedipal period, there is a period of relative sexual quiescence called the latency period. Most sexual fantasies and activities are repressed during this phase.

Puberty and the Beginning of Adolescence (Age 12–15)

The relatively sudden surge of physiologic and endocrinologic activity in the body results in a renewed heightening of libido. At this point the individual begins to go through the phases of sexual development a second time, though much more rapidly. There tends to be a resurgence of oral, anal, and phallic drives, and a renewed sexual interest in and conflict with the parents, as in the oedipal phase.

Later Adolescence and Young Adulthood (Age 16–18 and Over)

At this period and through the remainder of life, one can observe the fixation points, the unresolved phases which leave their marks on the grown individual. This can be seen in terms of his character structure, his sexual identification, his emotional maturity, tendencies to regress in the face of stress, ability to form sound, lasting relationships, the degree of maturity of his sexual drives, and, where healthy growth has been seriously interfered with, the appearance of neurotic symptoms.

A more complete discussion of the psychodynamics of adolescence may be found in Chapter 34.

Bisexuality

Evidences of bisexuality are present in normal human embryology, anatomy, endocrinology, and psychology. For example, the clitoris is the analogue of the penis. There are male and female hormones present in varying proportions in individuals of both sexes. Similarly, in human psychology, everyone entertains some desire to be like the opposite sex; no male is devoid of some feminine type wishes and vice versa. Some individuals are much better able to accept their desires to be like the opposite sex than others. For those who cannot accept these desires or urges within themselves, a conflict exists that must be dealt with by some form of repression or symptomatology in order to keep them out of consciousness. Examples of feminine type desires in males are to be passive, to be taken care of, to be maternal to others, to prepare food, and in some individuals more extreme desires such as to dress in feminine fashion, behave with feminine mannerisms, and attract other males sexually. There are counterparts of these wishes in females—desires to be aggressive, controlling, not to appear feminine in dress, behavior, or hairdo. The definition of what is feminine or what is masculine in dress and appearance varies from culture to culture and from generation to generation. Whatever it may be at any one time, the desires of the individual contain elements which are bisexual.

FIXATION AND REGRESSION

Fixation may occur at any phase of development where there has been a great deal of difficulty and conflict, with the result that an inordinate amount of psychic energy is utilized in attempting to solve the problems of that phase. The result is that less energy is available for dealing with the problems of subsequent phases of development. The difficulties that result in fixation are usually caused by (1) overfrustration at a particular phase, eg, too early weaning in the oral phase; (2) overgratification, eg, too much and too long use of bottles, pacifiers, thumb-sucking; or (3) gross inconsistencies on the part of the parents, eg, in the anal phase, alternating periods of cruel and excessive efforts at bowel training with periods of laxity and indifference to training.

Regression consists of retreating to the behavior of an earlier phase of development when faced with a stressful situation. A 5-year-old, previously well trained, involved with oedipal conflicts, responds to the birth of a sibling by soiling his pants, ie, by regression to the anal phase. Regression takes place only to a point of fixation. The child in the example must have had a partial fixation at the anal phase in order to regress to that point instead of to the oral phase.

In explaining regression, Freud used the analogy of an advancing army that has a certain number of troops at the beginning of the expedition. As the army advances and takes over each town in its path, it leaves a few troops at each point to maintain the captured position. The number of troops left depends on how much difficulty or opposition was encountered at that town—the greater the difficulty, the more troops that are left there (fixation). If the advancing army then meets a severe reversal in a forward area, it will retreat (regress) to the town where it had left the largest number of troops (fixation point).

This illustration can also be used to demonstrate the principle of psychic energy—the troops representing units of psychic energy.

DEFENSE MECHANISMS OF THE EGO

The ego must deal not only with the demands and pressures of the id and superego but with memories of the past and with the outside world as well. It functions best when it is aware of all the facts, pressures, and drives with which it must contend and when it can be totally objective, logical, and rational. However, in situations that provoke strong feelings of anxiety or guilt, the ego cannot operate in this manner; signal anxiety (see above) unconsciously activates a set of defense mechanisms to protect the ego against imminent psychic pain. These mechanisms operate with varying degrees of success and in some cases are constructive and moderately efficient. Some are better than others in that they do not waste too much psychic energy and do not interfere too greatly with the other functions of the ego; but all are less satisfactory than unfettered ego functioning in full awareness of objective reality, and all require some expenditure of psychic energy.

All emotional illnesses are characterized by the use of one or more of the defense mechanisms with the exception of sublimation. So-called normal individuals utilize the defense mechanisms to lesser degrees. The mechanisms that are commonest in psychotic individuals are projection, denial, distortions of reality, and regression.

The following defense mechanisms are listed in approximate order of their frequency and importance. It will be noted that there are many places where the mechanisms overlap.

Repression

Repression is the underlying basis of all of the defense mechanisms. Through repression the ego keeps threatening impulses, feelings, wishes, fantasies, and memories from becoming conscious. As the undesirable impulse presses toward consciousness, the ego expends energy (countercathexis) to prevent it from emerging. A simple example of repression is "not hearing" the alarm clock the morning after a late night. Another is "forgetting" a repugnant work assignment. The other defense mechanisms listed below are essentially various types of ego activity which assist in maintaining repression.

Rationalization

Rationalization is the substitution of "good" reasons—acceptable to the conscious ego—for the real reasons for a piece of behavior. (*Example:* "It was my duty" is a "good" reason for reporting a friend's infractions to his superior, where the desire to outdo the friend or to express hostile feelings toward him is the "real" reason.)

Sublimation

Sublimation is the most efficient and creative of the defense mechanisms. It redirects libidinal drives (sexual and aggressive) into socially acceptable channels. For example, the infantile anal drive to play with feces may be sublimated into sculpturing with clay (deodorized "feces"), blocks (also dehydrated), or money (condensed, "filthy lucre"); sex drive may be sublimated into athletic activity, work, poetry, music, etc (to a limited degree).

Projection

Projection is the mechanism by which the ego refuses to acknowledge an unacceptable id impulse by relocating it onto someone else. (*Example:* A wife with strong but repressed illicit sexual wishes claims that all husbands are unfaithful and not to be trusted.)

Displacement

Displacement is a process whereby a whole may be represented by a part, or vice versa. Also, one idea or image may be substituted for another which is emotionally associated with it—although not always logically. (*Example:* If a woman has had a very unpleasant experience with a man with red hair, she may react strongly against all men with red hair. The part has come to symbolize the whole.) This phenomenon is important in dream interpretation, where one thing or a part often represents something else. It is also important in *transference,* whereby feelings about some important person in the patient's past are displaced or transferred onto the psychoanalyst.

Identification

Identification is the process by which an unacceptable impulse may be rendered acceptable by denying the impulse itself but identifying with (feeling a part of) someone who personifies this impulse. Examples of this are persons who repress strong aggressive drives but identify with powerful, aggressive leaders such as Hitler ("identification with the aggressor"), or women who repress strong sexual drives but identify with movie actresses who lead lurid lives.

A strong wish to possess a person, have him all for oneself (ie, "I want my daddy all for my own") may be followed by a desire to be like him.

Incorporation and introjection are primitive forms of identification. *Incorporation* is a general primitive process of symbolically taking a desired object or person into oneself so that one can always have the object. An example would be cannibalism in a symbolic sense. If I eat you, you are inside of me, you are part of me, I always have you. This is thinking most common to the very young child. *Introjection* is usually regarded as the same as incorporation. It is a term used as the counterpart to projection.

Identification with the aggressor refers to the process whereby an individual who is being persecuted or mistreated by someone takes on the characteristics of the persecutor, as in the case of the Jew who may take on the characteristics of the storm trooper. In becoming like the oppressor, the ego feels allied with him and hence less threatened by him.

Regression

In regression the ego retreats from conflictual situations at advanced levels of personality development to an earlier level. (*Example:* Overwhelming genital sexual problems may cause a retreat to the oral stage by overeating. Regression always goes back to a stage of fixation.)

Turning Against the Self

If one cannot tolerate an aggressive impulse toward a respected person (eg, parent or teacher), he may hurt himself instead. Introjection (an early form of identification) is used here. The person against whom the anger is originally directed is first "taken in," and this other person can then be hurt by self-punishment. This is less dangerous than hurting the other person directly.

Isolation

Isolation is the process whereby the affect or feeling that should go along with a painful memory, thought, or experience is excluded from consciousness. The person can recall the painful event or thought but without the emotional affect that should accompany it. This is commonly seen in obsessive neuroses, where an objectionable thought is isolated; eg, "I might stab someone," breaks into consciousness but without the true aggressive feelings that should accompany such a thought. Another example of isolation is the German refugee who can describe in detail how he was persecuted, members of his family killed, his property confiscated, and yet express no rage or resentment at the Nazis. The appropriate affect has been isolated (removed) from the ideas expressed.

Reaction Formation

Reaction formation is the mechanism whereby an undesirable impulse is kept unconscious by a strong emphasis on its opposite. (*Examples:* A person with strong sadistic trends may become an ardent antivivisectionist. Preoccupation with dirt may result in a "crazy-clean" housewife.)

Counterphobic behavior is a related phenomenon. In order to avoid the conscious recognition of a deepseated fear, the person actively engages in the feared activity. (*Example:* A girl who has a great fear of being hurt by males may become involved in promiscuous sexual activity as a means of attempting to deny her fear.)

Substitution

This is a process by which one object that is highly valued emotionally but that cannot be possessed for psychologic reasons is unconsciously replaced by another object that is acceptable psychologically and that usually resembles the forbidden object in some manner. (*Example:* A young woman who is very much attached to her tall, blond, blue-eyed brother may become quickly and much involved with boyfriends who are tall, blond, and blue-eyed.) This is a form of the process of displacement.

Restitution

This is a special form of substitution in which a highly valued object that has been lost (through departure, rejection, or death) is replaced by another object. (*Example:* A devoted husband whose wife dies may remain chronically unhappy until he finds another woman who can fulfill his ungratified unconscious as well as conscious needs.)

Resistance

Resistance is a phenomenon that occurs periodically during psychoanalysis or psychotherapy. The resistant patient does not cooperate in the therapeutic process, although he consciously avows his intention to do so. Resistance is an unconscious process by which the ego avoids revealing more about itself because the material that has been coming into consciousness is too distressing or anxiety-producing. The forms which resistance may take are multiple—such as silence, failure to free associate, failure to remember dreams, forgetting external events, undue annoyance with trivial aspects of the treatment situation (room is too cold, chair not comfortable, etc). Resistance must be resolved each time it appears so that the treatment process may proceed.

Dreams

Dreaming is a process by which forbidden or conflicting wishes of waking life may be partially fulfilled in a disguised fashion while one sleeps. If the dream is successful it allows the individual to remain sleeping. If unsuccessful, the dream causes such anxiety that the individual wakes up. If the anxiety is great on awakening, it is called a nightmare. Dreams, like thoughts, may also have other functions (anticipation, rehearsal, attempts at mastery, etc).

Fantasy

Fantasy is a process by which an individual makes up a story in his mind (daydreams) that satisfies a need or wish that cannot be satisfied in reality. (*Example:* A husband who is attracted to the wife of his best friend may have a detailed and lurid sexual affair with her in fantasy but never engage in any untoward behavior with her in real life.)

Symbolization

This is a process by which an apparently neutral object with certain characteristics represents another object which has a forbidden aspect to it. The symbol object is often held in common by the unconscious part of the mind of many people—*universal symbol.* Familiar examples of this are the so-called phallic symbols whereby tall, elongated, or projecting objects (skyscrapers, snakes, fire hose nozzles) represent the penis in the unconscious mind. Symbols commonly appear in dreams. It may be less distressing to the sleeping ego if a young girl dreams about being chased by a snake than being sexually attacked. Symbols are present in waking life as well as dreams. They may appear in daydreams, jokes, art, and literature.

Other frequent symbols are those for the female genital (opening, hole, bush, purse), mother (nurse, teacher, ship, ocean, department store), father (boss, tyrant, king, God, lion), sexual intercourse (various forms of fighting, dancing, games, rhythmic activity), castration (mutilation, loss, wound, absence).

Symptom Formation

Symptom formation, also called compromise formation, is a pathologic defense mechanism whereby the ego attempts to satisfy (partially) both the forbidden impulse and the ego reaction against it. (*Example:* Pathologic vomiting of pregnancy, which may express a forbidden desire to get rid of the pregnancy but is also a "physical symptom" by which the destructive impulse is rendered unconscious.)

Repetition Compulsion

A common feature of emotional illnesses is the "repetition compulsion," a strong tendency to repeat the pathologic process—symptoms, behavior pattern, disturbed thinking, involvement in a "sick" or troubled situation or with the same type of neurotic relationship (eg, women attracted to alcoholic males)—again and again. Experience does not teach anything when the determinants are largely unconscious. As the same unconscious needs keep arising, the ego, as if it were a "creature of habit," makes the same unsuccessful attempts to deal with them over and over.

Conversion

This is a process by which a psychologic conflict is "converted" into a physical symptom. An example of this is the man who is concerned that his anger may get out of hand and cause him to punch the boss in the nose, and develops a paralysis of his right arm (punching arm). Another is a woman who desperately wants a child and develops a protruding abdomen and the conviction that she is pregnant (*pseudocyesis*).

Dissociation

Dissociation is a process by which a whole segment of behavior may be separated in consciousness from the normal or usual personality or behavior pattern of the individual. Striking examples of dissociation are the so-called multiple personalities exemplified in literature, eg, *Dr. Jekyll and Mr. Hyde, The Three Faces of Eve*. As a rule, one personality is very proper, conservative, and moralistic whereas the other is wild, impulsive, and pleasure-seeking.

Other examples of dissociative behavior are somnambulism, sleep talking, amnesic episodes, and fugue states.

Compensation

This is a process by which an individual makes up for a deficiency in his image of himself (personality, intelligence, or physique) by strongly emphasizing some other feature of himself that he regards as an asset. This may be seen in the "little man syndrome," in which men of small physical stature compensate by being very aggressive, forceful, and controlling in their business and social dealings ("Napoleon complex").

Denial

Denial of reality is a pathologic mechanism by which the ego flatly refuses to see something that is obviously true because to recognize the reality would cause the ego much pain. (*Example:* Insisting that mother is not dead, but just "out of town for a few days.") This mechanism may also involve *distortions* of reality (misinterpreting reality). It is often seen in psychotic states, and a brief form of it is sometimes seen in normal persons.

BRIEF PSYCHOANALYTIC FORMULATION OF THE PRINCIPAL PSYCHOPATHOLOGIC STATES

In this section our attention will be confined solely to psychodynamics in classical psychoanalytic terms.

Clinical psychopathology implies the appearance of symptoms which are beyond the range of normal for individuals living within a particular culture. The symptoms may be obvious to others or they may be purely subjective. Symptoms are usually considered serious enough to require medical attention when they cause sufficient distress to the individual or to those associated with him to be regarded as "intolerable." What is "intolerable" to one individual may be tolerable to another. Differences in tolerance to one of its member's symptoms varies from family to family and from community to community.

Symptoms may interfere in varying degrees with an individual's daily functions—work, creativity, family and social relationships. The subjective symptoms which are most prominent are those of anxiety (tension, restlessness, apprehension, "queasy" feelings, insomnia, loss of appetite, irritability, etc); depression (sadness, melancholy, feelings of worthlessness, futility, hopelessness, feelings of guilt without specific reason, etc); and various psychophysiologic symptoms, ie, those which are located in bodily organs but are precipitated by emotional stress: headache, backache, upper or lower gastrointestinal distress, various skin eruptions, and disorders of any of the body's organ systems. There must be careful medical evaluation of any supposed psychosomatic symptoms since the primary cause may be physical instead of emotional and since it is possible that long-standing psychophysiologic symptoms may result in physical damage to various organ systems. Combined medical and psychotherapeutic management is often indicated.

Emotional illness is the resultant of several factors. The ego at all times attempts to cope with 3 sources of stress that constantly place pressure on it. One is the id with its constant push for instinctual gratification, a second is the superego with its constant reminder of what is good and what is bad, and the third is the ever-present force of outside reality with its multiple demands, obstacles, standards, temptations, and unpredictability. The ego attempts to deal with the many problems that confront it from these sources by the best and most efficient methods at its command.

First, the ego tries to handle the problems with a fully conscious, logical, and rational approach based on all its learned knowledge and benefiting from previous experience.

Second, the ego utilizes the various defense mechanisms it has acquired in its development. These are brought into play by the unconscious part of the ego. They can be valuable and useful but they are not as efficient as the first approach. Some of them, such as sublimation and reaction formation, can be very helpful in allowing the individual to cope with his problems. However, others such as projection and denial are not so useful in a socially constructive sense and may lead to problems of their own. The more primitive or inefficient the mechanisms called forth and the more exclusively these are used in contrast to the higher level defenses and conscious logical approach, the closer the individual approaches emotional illness.

Third, the ego utilizes symptom formation—anxiety, depression, phobias, obsessions, conversions, etc. This is a pathologic attempt of the ego to deal with problems after other methods have failed.

Thus, when psychopathology appears, we know that persistent or recurrent serious conflicts, problems, or stresses are facing the ego. The term conflict is used to emphasize that the problem usually involves 2 or more opposing forces (between id and superego, between id and reality, or among all three). An example of a conflict between the id on the one hand and the superego and reality on the other would be a highly respected, religious, conscientious married man who develops strong and persistent sexual urges towards the wife of an associate. The ego at first attempts to cope with serious conflict with more efficient methods; when this fails, it regressively resorts to more primitive methods and finally develops symptom formation.

The manner in which the ego attempts to cope with problems and the degree of success or failure depends first on the individual's early psychologic history (the difficulties or ease with which he passed through the various stages of development). This in turn depends on the presence or absence of and the types of personalities of the parents and siblings and the interaction between these and the individual—the psychologic milieu in which the young individual was raised. Certain ill-defined constitutional factors (hereditary or not) also make for differences in ego structures. Some people's egos seem predisposed to emotional illness—if faced with sufficient persistent stress—whereas others raised in similar psychologic environments seem able to cope reasonably well with the same degree of stress.

Psychoanalytic theory deals primarily with the factors involved in the development of the individual ego in its particular psychologic milieu rather than with constitutional factors.

From our knowledge of fixation points in the early developmental history of the individual (see analogy of the advancing army in the previous section), we know that regression in the face of stress to certain early stages of development results in typical clinical entities. In other words, a massive regression to a particular stage results in a type of thinking and a type of symptomatology which is characteristic for that stage. The following are characteristic syndromes (mental illnesses) that are observed when there is a large-scale regression to a particular stage of development. There is always some overlap of one stage and the next.

(1) **Schizophrenia.** There is a regression to the early oral (sucking) stage. Typically there is a great deal of narcissism, total involvement with the self, primitive grandiose fantasies, open demands for complete dependency, absence of logical thinking, great need to be loved and nurtured like an infant without giving anything in return, and presence of infantile thinking and behavior.

(2) **Manic-depressive psychosis.** This involves regression to the late oral (biting) stage. In addition to many of the features that may be seen in the early oral stage, in this stage there are more demanding and aggressive elements. The same degree of narcissism is present but there is a more direct demand on the environment to satisfy the needs. An aggressive type of elation is present or the aggressive element may be turned inward in the manifestation of depression.

(3) **Paranoia.** This involves regression to an early anal-expulsive stage. There is much concern with projection—getting rid of the "bad stuff" (feces). There is a great deal of aggression present—"defecating" on the adversaries. There is also great preoccupation with being controlled by perse-

cution (like the parents who control and regulate bowel movements) or with controlling others, if the patient is a grandiose type of paranoid. Psychoanalytically, the latter involves controlling the parents through the child's control of his anal sphincter.

(4) **Obsessive-compulsive neurosis.** There is regression to the late anal-retentive stage. In this stage, there is preoccupation with controlling, regulating, scheduling—as with bowel control. There is involvement with neatness and cleanliness, being proper or perfect, with saving and thrift (retaining feces). All of these are involved with various aspects of bowel training. The aggressive punishing element is always present also. Intellectual control is prominent at this stage.

(5) **Hysterical neurosis.** This involves regression to the phallic stage. The important element here is the great development of the mechanism of repression. The individual here learns to deal with problems—like the oedipal situation—by pushing them out of consciousness. The offending aspects of a situation are rendered innocuous by not being aware of them. A gross example of this is the amnesic episode for a very traumatic situation: A young girl is raped and is unable to recall anything of the entire day on which the episode occured.

The following are brief theoretical formulations of psychopathologic reactions (as opposed to illnesses):

Depression

Depression is aggression turned inward. Guilt and self-punishment are its most prominent features. The following steps take place: (1) Loss of a highly regarded object or ideal. (2) Ambivalence toward the object (both loved and hated). (3) Incorporation (taking in) of the lost object and then venting aggression against it and hence against the self.

Paranoia

In paranoid reactions, strong but highly undesirable drives (usually homosexual, but not overt) plague the ego. The projection mechanism is a prominent feature. The ego cannot accept the idea that, "I [a man] love him [another man]," but the reverse emotion, "I don't love him, I hate him" is acceptable. On an unconscious level, this is then projected, before entering consciousness, into its converse, "He hates me." Later this becomes, "He persecutes me." A whole system of persecutory delusion then develops. Following this, another trend may begin with the thought that one must be very important to have all of this attention (even though persecutory) directed toward him—the beginning of *grandiose delusions.*

Conversions

The emotional conflict, instead of being consciously experienced, is expressed through the voluntary musculature or the special sense organs, eg, hysterical paralysis or anesthesia. The symptom usually expresses both sides of a conflict—partially gratification and partially punishment. Paralysis of the hand used in masturbation, for example, draws special attention to and interest in the hand and at the same time renders the hand unable to perform the forbidden act. As in all emotional illnesses, there may be *secondary gains*, eg, the patient with the paralyzed hand is unable to work and hence can stay at home and be cared for by others. The *primary gain* is the ego's relief from the basic anxiety-producing conflict (masturbation).

In the case of a hysterical anesthesia or paralysis, the area affected does not conform to actual anatomical nerve distribution. The area affected is outlined by the individual's "idea" of his hand or foot. This results in a so-called "glove" or "stocking" anesthesia in which the area involved terminates in a pattern that is a straight line circumference around the wrist or ankle rather than the irregular outline of an actual nerve distribution. Such a hysterical anesthesia or paralysis is accompanied by *la belle indifférence,* a remarkable degree of indifference or unconcern about the rather startling and gross symptom. This is due to the ego's real concern with relieving the psychologic conflict that is repressed with the aid of the symptom. The ego is unconcerned by the apparent defect in the physical structure, a defect which it knows (unconsciously) does not exist.

Phobias

The underlying mechanism in the phobias is displacement of anxiety from its original internal source (eg, fear of a threatening father) to a specific external object (eg, horses). The anxiety can then be evaded by staying away from horses, which is easier than trying to deal with the internal fear. The external object selected has a special relationship in unconscious association to the original object. It *symbolizes* or represents unconsciously the source of the fear. For the patient in the example, the horse, by its gross size, size of phallus, gleaming teeth, snorting, etc, represents the father. There are no standard symbolic meanings. As in dreams, symbols may mean different things to different people. However, some symbols do occur in common for many people (see p 459). The best way to determine the meaning of a particular symbol for a particular person is by having him give his associations to it.

Obsessions and Compulsions

In this group of disorders, anxiety is manifested by unwanted but insistent and repetitive thoughts (obsessions) or urges to perform acts (compulsions). In spite of all efforts to control them, obsessions keep breaking through into consciousness. Compulsions are defensive substitutes for forbidden and repugnant acts, usually of a sexual or aggressive nature. Fixation in the anal stage is common in this group of individuals. Problems about bowel training and the relationship with the mother during the bowel training age are prominent. There is much concern with control, being controlled, soiling and cleanliness, and "magical thinking." For the young child, to want mother to go away and leave him alone is connected with the fear that his wish might be too powerful and she might actually disappear altogether.

Three mechanisms are operative in the obsessive-compulsive neuroses:

(1) **Ambivalence:** Strong contradictory feelings about the same person.

(2) **Isolation:** Separation of the true emotional tone from an idea or act (see p 457).

(3) **Undoing:** This is a prominent part of compulsive rituals. It is an act done symbolically to remove or expiate the destructive aspect of the compulsion. Doing and undoing are often combined: The individual first turns on the gas jet of the stove (doing) and then turns it off (undoing) to demonstrate that he really wants to make sure it is off so that his "loved" ones will not die.

PRINCIPLES OF TREATMENT
BY PSYCHOANALYSIS

Therapeutic Goals

The therapeutic goals of psychoanalysis are the reconstruction or major modification of the basic personality patterns and defenses of the patient as well as the relief of symptoms.

To attain these goals, earlier analysts strove primarily to reach so-called *id material*—early life experience with basic drives (sex and aggression), repressed memories ("infantile amnesia"), eg, *primal scene* memories (witnessing sexual relations of parents), etc. Modern psychoanalysis is much more involved with *ego psychology*—understanding the basic character structure of the individual and the defense mechanisms most frequently employed by him in handling anxieties. In either form of psychoanalysis there must be considerable interest in the events of the past, primarily because of their influence on the current emotional life of the patient.

Insight

Insight is the recognition of relationships between 2 or more sets of experiences, memories, behavior patterns, emotional responses, or trains of thought which had not previously been regarded consciously as related. True insight must not only be acknowledged on an intellectual or logical level but also accepted on an emotional or feeling level. It is only then that insight can be regarded as meaningful and useful in understanding emotional problems and in altering attitudes or resolving conflicts.

An example of intellectual insight which was not true insight is the following brief case history: A young man sustained a nerve injury in the war which resulted in partial paralysis of his right arm. Despite extensive physiotherapy and retraining, the arm was virtually useless to him. Shortly after entering analysis, he announced that he knew why he could not use his arm. It was like being castrated and he was castrated because he was afraid of his deceased father, of being more successful than his father. This "insight," although containing several elements of truth, resulted in no improvement in the function of his arm. Only many months later, after going into his relationship with his domineering mother, his fear of her, his attachment to her, his desire to remain a child in order to be dependent on her, to be disabled so she would have to care for him, did he begin to have true insight into the reason for his disabled arm. This culminated in a dream in which he clearly saw his disabled arm as a defective penis. He then recognized it with feeling as being a real symbol of castration—not just on an intellectual level. Following this, his arm recovered.

Corrective Emotional Experiences

"Reliving" during the analytic sessions of the feelings of previous traumatic or difficult emotional situations is part of emotional catharsis. Since the reliving takes place in the therapeutic situation, it can now be seen in a more accurate, objective manner in terms of the present as well as the past. Thus, with the aid of the analyst, there is a "corrective" element—not just a pure repetition—in the reliving. The traumatic event is seen in its true perspective, and this has therapeutic value in enabling the patient to re-orient his feelings about it.

"Working Through"

This is the process by which changes in emotional viewpoint about a particular person, set of experiences, or conflict situation take place gradually over a long period of time by frequent repetition of the same material. Different aspects of the same situation or the same situation recurring at different times in the patient's life are gone over repeatedly before being fully accepted emotionally and made part of a new outlook. The mere fact that a new discovery or insight about oneself seems to make sense does not mean acceptance of it. It must be thoroughly examined, studied, and digested a number of times before it is actually made part of oneself, ie, incorporated into the ego.

Analysis of Transference and the Transference Neurosis

Transference is the unconscious process whereby certain characteristics of significant persons out of the patient's past—usually parents—are transferred (displaced, projected) onto the analyst, whereupon the patient reacts to the analyst as if he actually were that person. For example, if the patient had a harsh, aggressive father (or saw his father in that way when he was a child), when he develops a father transference toward the analyst he will see him as a harsh, aggressive person and react to him accordingly. This is why it is crucial for the analyst to maintain a relatively anonymous, neutral role, so that it will be clear, when the time comes for interpretation, that the analyst is not actually a harsh, aggressive person but that the patient has transferred these characteristics onto him from out of the past. The analysis of the transference consists of convincing the patient that he must be doing the same thing in varying degrees in his relationships with other persons in his life, eg, his boss, his father-in-law.

Transference neurosis is a further development of the transference. After the development of the transference, the patient reacts to the analyst as he did to his parent. Gradually he develops a set of conflicts and defenses in his relationship to the analyst which is a repetition of his childhood (infantile) neurotic relationship with the significant parent. The original memories reappear in a new setting—in the analytic situation. This is the transference neurosis. All this must be gradually and with appropriate timing interpreted (pointed out) to the patient. The patient can then resolve the original neurosis by resolving its present version in the analytic situation. This is called analyzing the transference neurosis.

Countertransference
Countertransference consists of the feelings that the analyst may develop toward the patient because the patient represents a significant figure from his own remote past. Like transference, it is an unconscious process. The analyst must be alert, with the aid of his own personal analysis, to the development of this phenomenon so that he can prevent it from interfering with his clinical objectivity and his own reactions to the patient.

Both transference and countertransference should be distinguished from "reaction" and "counterreaction." The former 2 are unconscious, the latter 2 conscious. It is not transference if a patient reacts to a realistically oversevere analyst, nor is it countertransference if an analyst reacts to a seductive, attractive patient. In the latter instance, to be successful, he must inhibit, suppress, conceal, and control his reactions appropriately.

Attainment of Emotional Maturity
The analyst must allow the individual to continue his natural growth toward emotional maturity by removing obstacles and disentangling fixations which have interfered with this natural process. Unfortunately, in some individuals this natural drive toward maturity is not strong.

TECHNICS OF PSYCHOANALYSIS

Frequency and Duration
Psychoanalysis usually requires 3–5 visits per week lasting 45–50 minutes each over a period of 2–5 years. The length is due to several factors. The main goal is to modify the basic personality structure, not merely to eliminate symptoms. This means that efforts are directed toward altering the ego's characteristic use of defense mechanisms. This can only be done through exploring the various phases of development and points of fixation in the patient. The ego is resistant to changing its characteristic defenses since they have become habitual to the ego regardless of how undesirable or inefficient they may be. Treatment is constantly beset with resistance on the part of the ego. There is a running conflict between the ego's conscious desire to gain emotional maturity and free itself from the shackles of neurotic traits on the one hand and the unconscious resistance of the ego to any change in its characteristic defenses on the other. The repetition compulsion and the necessity of "working through" also add to the length of analysis.

The technic has evolved pragmatically. There was a great deal of art as well as science in the early days. It is in recent years that increased study is taking place to validate the methods and to explore the possibilities of briefer procedures, short-term psychodynamic therapy, analytic group psychotherapy, and combined analytic and drug therapy.

It is a costly, time-consuming procedure. There are some low-fee clinics, and some low-fee analyses are available. It has been noted that a seriously intentioned patient with a strong desire to be analyzed often manages to obtain an analysis even on a fairly modest income. Of course, a degree of sacrifice is involved. Economic sacrifice, if not extreme, is regarded by many to be a motivating factor to encourage the patient to work hard at his analysis in order to hasten it.

Use of Couch

Most analyses are conducted with the patient (analysand) lying supine on a couch and the analyst sitting so that he is not within view of the patient. This is because lying down and not seeing the analyst tend to facilitate projecting feelings onto the analyst (development of transference) and to encourage the free expression of fantasies and associative material, and because varied thoughts and feelings are more apt to enter into consciousness with the patient in a relaxed position. Not being able to see the analyst minimizes the inhibiting effect of objective cues such as the expression on the analyst's face. The couch encourages the patient to fantasize and day-dream (as one might do while lying in bed before falling asleep) and not to be shackled by reality factors.

The couch should not be used with patients who are borderline psychotics, whose grasp on reality is already tenuous. The passivity and symbolic vulnerability (to sexual or aggressive assault) implicit in the supine position may be a serious problem with some patients and must be dealt with to some extent in all patients.

The Basic Rule

The fundamental rule of psychoanalysis is that the patient must say whatever comes to mind, without any censoring, regardless of its nature or content—good or bad, flattering or otherwise—and no matter whom it is about, including the analyst, or whether he regards it as significant or trivial. The reason for the rule is to promote free association. Since all associations are actually predetermined, "free" association means that removal of conscious censorship allows the associations to be determined by the unconscious. This is an important way in which we can learn about the individual's unconscious and how it controls his thoughts, feelings, and behavior.

Resistance to the Basic Rule

Even though he knows what the basic rule is and agrees that it is valid, there are times when the individual has emotional blocks that prevent him from saying whatever comes to mind. This is called *resistance.* The reasons for its occurring at that particular time must be determined and interpreted (analyzed). The patient can then proceed, following the basic rule, until the next resistance occurs. This must then be analyzed, etc. Resistance is analyzed before content.

Activity vs Passivity of the Analyst

The analyst should avoid giving direct support and suggestions about how to handle reality situations. The patient must learn to deal with these on his own. Part of the purpose of analysis is to understand one's motivation and behavior, not to receive advice and guidance. However, the patient should avoid making major life decisions (marriage, career, etc) until the emotional factors involved are thoroughly understood, and he must be cautioned not to act impulsively.

The analyst therefore plays primarily a passive role, while the patient does most of the talking. This encourages the patient to project his feelings onto a neutral figure and to develop a transference relationship, and it fosters self-discovery. The analyst should be human and understanding—not a cold, unfeeling robot—but he acts principally as a catalytic agent in the patient's process of self-discovery; as a screen for the transference; and as an interpreter to assist the patient in gaining insight and overcoming resistance to self-understanding.

In order for a patient to accept an interpretation or to gain insight, he must feel within himself that it is correct, that it fits. It is similar to the sudden flash of recognition shown in cartoons by a light bulb glowing in the balloon over the character's head—an "Aha!" experience. It is not sufficient for the analyst merely to state the fact or try to be insistent about or persuade the patient to accept a piece of insight. The patient must be helped to discover the insight for himself in order for him to incorporate it, make it a part of himself.

Acting Out

"Acting out" is a form of resistance to analysis whereby the patient performs actions in his daily life—eg, quits his job, gets into fights, engages in risk-laden sexual activities—instead of talking about and analyzing the reasons for such impulses during therapeutic sessions. Because the content of the unconscious must be dealt with on a verbal and feeling level and not transformed into behavior before being understood, "acting out" is a type of resistance which must be discouraged.

Interpretation

From time to time during the course of analysis, the analyst drops his passive role and points out a relationship or connection between 2 or more sets of events or an aspect of a situation which the patient has not recognized. This is called interpretation. However, it is not sufficient merely that the interpretation be "correct." It must also be well timed, ie, it must be given at a time when the patient is capable of accepting it as meaningful. There are several ways to know if an interpretation that has been accepted is valid. The validity of an interpretation is confirmed (1) if there is an immediate emotional response, eg, laughing, crying, exclaiming, expression of surprise; (2) if the patient brings up other material that confirms the interpretation, eg, similar situations in his life in which he reacted in the same way as was pointed out in the interpretation; or (3) if the patient subsequently reports dreams that verify the interpretation.

The timing and correctness of interpretation is one of the primary skills of the analyst. When the patient is ready to accept an interpretation, he will gain insight and then he will be able to proceed a step further in his self-understanding. Interpretations are more valuable when they are given succinctly and only when highly pertinent. When the analyst does not talk "too much," the patient listens more acutely and with more attention when he does speak.

Examples of interpretation: An obese young lady could not understand why it was so difficult for her to diet. One day, she told of having an argument with her mother. She felt that her mother did not like her and had never liked her. On leaving her mother's home, the patient went on a shopping spree. She said, "I didn't need all the things I bought but I just had to have something of my own—Mom wouldn't give me anything." The interpretation was then made that she perhaps overate in the same manner. As a child, when she felt that her mother didn't give her anything, she ate a great deal to get something for herself. The patient suddenly realized that this was so and was later able to go on her first sustained diet.

A young man who had been progressing fairly well in analysis had several successive sessions where he said very little. He knew of no reason for this. Resistance was obviously prominent. Then he began to talk about how angry his wife had been with him on the preceding night because he had come home late for dinner. He could not understand why she made such an issue over it. She wouldn't even talk to him when he left for work next morning. The interpretation was then made that a week before, the analyst had been late for the patient's appointment and, although the patient had said nothing about it at the time, he had been more or less silent since then. Then, as with the wife who had been angry over the patient's lateness and not spoken to him the next day, so the patient must have been angry because the analyst had been late and instead of expressing his anger had become silent in his sessions. The patient then admitted that he had indeed been angry at the analyst over the latter's lateness. The resistance subsided and the patient began to talk about his difficulties in expressing anger.

Dream Interpretation

Dreams are the analyst's most direct route to the unconscious. They occur when the mind is not on guard, as it is in the waking state, so that more unconscious material comes to the surface. The "manifest" dream is the actual reportable content. The "latent" dream material, which is of much greater significance, is that which is learned by having the patient "associate to" his own dream material, ie, what the parts of the dream remind the dreamer of in his past and recent life experiences.

Although there are some universal dream symbols, eg, insects representing siblings, house representing the body, coming out of water representing birth, a cave representing the womb (also see above, p 459), the important part of dream interpretation is the individual's own associations to it at the particular stage of analysis he is in. In simplified terms, a dream is a disguised wish fulfillment. Patients are encouraged in a general way to bring in dreams but not exhorted to do so. One can often judge the presence of resistance by the patient not bringing in dreams. Recent technical studies of dreaming (REM—rapid eye movements—take place while a person is dreaming) indicate that most people dream about 5 times a night for 10—15 minutes each time. Interpretation of daydreams (fantasies) and of parapraxes (slips of the tongue) are also of value in psychoanalysis. It is in the patient's associations to these that we learn most about their meaning.

Variations From Classical Technics

Some patients, particularly those with more serious illnesses or ego defects (eg, borderline psychotics), respond better to variations in technic, eg, analyst being more active, talking more, being more giving, letting the patient sit up.

An example of a variation in classical technic is the case of a patient who has formed very few if any trusting, friendly relationships in his life. To encourage trust, the analyst drops some of his more usual anonymity and reveals things about himself to the patient—size of his (analyst's) family, favorite hobby, place of his vacation, etc—with the idea of transmitting to the patient the human element in the analyst.

Another example of a variation in classical technic is the occasional use of drugs, principally tranquilizers or antidepressants. While anxious or depressed feelings of a certain degree can be motivating forces in a patient's desire to learn about himself, they also can be so strong as to impair his functioning both outside and inside the analytic situation. In these instances, the judicious use of drugs facilitates analysis and may even prevent hospitalization. When drugs are prescribed, it is often necessary later to analyze the meaning of being given medication by the analyst, ie, being fed or not fed (when medication is stopped), being given "bitter" medicine by the parents when the patient was a child, feelings toward the pediatrician, feelings that "magic" rather than self-understanding can resolve problems, etc.

INDICATIONS FOR PSYCHOANALYSIS

Disorders That Are Amenable to Psychoanalysis

Some psychiatric illnesses are not amenable to psychoanalysis. Those in which psychoanalysis is particularly contraindicated are active psychoses (schizophrenias and manic-depressive psychoses in active stages), sociopathic character disorders, and some psychosomatic disorders during active stages of the physical aspect of the illness, eg, exacerbation of chronic ulcerative colitis. During remissions, some of the psychoses and psychosomatic illnesses may be analyzed but this must be done carefully to avoid exacerbations of the illness. Psychoanalysis is contraindicated in individuals whose grasp on reality is already tenuous, ie, psychotics. Analysis encourages fantasy life, daydreaming, bringing the unconscious to the foreground. In psychoses, the unconscious is already too much on the surface and needs to be regulated better by the ego, not less regulated as in analysis.

A. Neuroses: Of all psychopathologic entities, neuroses usually respond best to analysis. Those which are apt to respond best are the hysterias and anxiety reactions. Phobic reactions and the obsessive compulsive reactions tend to be more difficult. The depressive reactions tend to be difficult also, except for the immediate episode, which may subside fairly rapidly. The easier it is for the patient to form a transference relationship to the analyst, the more one can expect a favorable result. The more advanced (in the development scale) are the patient's points of fixation and characteristic defenses, the better the prognosis, ie, a patient whose problems center around the phallic level has a better prognosis than one whose fixation is primarily at the anal or oral level.

B. Personality Disorders: The results of psychoanalysis may be good in well motivated patients. However, there are many persons in the dyssocial categories (sociopathic personalities) who refuse to enter into such an extensive treatment program. This is also a problem in alcoholism and drug addiction. "Acting out" is a major problem in this category and a great obstacle to successful analysis.

C. Sexual Aberrations: Homosexuality and other sexual problems may respond to analysis providing there is a high degree of genuine motivation and a reasonable capacity for abstinence (not necessarily total). Court directives do not constitute sufficient motivation for successful analysis in these individuals.

D. Psychophysiologic Reactions: These may be susceptible to analysis if there is sufficient conscious recognition of emotional problems to motivate the patient. In many of these patients, the anxiety is so bound up with the physical aspects of the illness that the patient is almost totally unaware that he has emotional conflicts (except, in some sophisticated individuals, on an intellectual basis). The awareness must extend beyond pure intellectualism to be useful in motivating the patient in analysis. Trial may be made in doubtful cases.

E. Psychoses in Remission and Some Borderline Psychotic Patients: Some of these patients may be successfully analyzed. A great deal of skill and careful clinical judgment are required to avoid precipitating a psychotic episode. Variations from the classical technics are often introduced in these cases. They may vary from having the patient sit up to direct interactions with the patient, as in the so-called "direct analysis" method developed by John Rosen.

Patient Factors

A. Age: In general, aside from the special field of child analysis, young adults have been considered the ideal age group for analysis. In recent years more analytic work has been done with the late adolescence age group. Some analysts feel, however, that too many natural changes are taking place at this stage—that the ego is undergoing normal growth changes with which analysis may interfere, or that the ego cannot benefit from analysis at this stage. Middle age (35—50) is a fairly common time to be analyzed. The important factor here seems to be the degree of ego flexibility.

B. Flexibility of the Ego: Although this is a difficult personality variable to evaluate, it is more important than age in determining suitability for analysis. The rigid, restricted individual whose ego seems to maintain its integrity by being totally unchanging and unbending is not a good candidate for analysis.

C. **"Psychologic Mindedness"**: The capacity to think in psychologic terms, to see relationships between sets of ideas and feelings, and to form insights is more important than native intelligence as a determinant of the success of analysis. Some persons of very superior intelligence do not have this capacity and are poor candidates for analysis; on the other hand, there are individuals with modest IQs who do have this capacity and are therefore much more apt to benefit from analysis.

Psychologic testing, particularly projective tests such as the Rorschach and the thematic apperception test, may assist in evaluating a patient's personality assets and liabilities. However, at all times, clinical judgment based on experience and training take definite precedence over psychologic testing in evaluating and diagnosing patients. On some occasions, a trial of analysis itself may be the most accurate way of evaluating the patient.

D. **Capacity to Form Meaningful Relationships**: It is difficult for an individual to develop a satisfactory transference if he never in his life has shown the ability to form a reasonably meaningful relationship with another person. Without this capacity, analysis is not possible. However, some analysts would be willing to work with a patient on a trial basis if they thought there were some chance of his developing a transference, or, prior to that, the development of a *therapeutic alliance*—a genuine "working together" attitude (real feelings of working together with the analyst toward the goal of understanding the patient's psychic life), which is essential for successful analytic progress.

The *therapeutic contract* is the mutual commitment of the patient and the analyst which should be understood at the outset of analysis. The *contract* is made for the sole purpose of helping the patient to understand himself better in order to alleviate symptoms and to enable him to mature emotionally so that he will be able to free his ego's strength to be used in any constructive way that he desires. The contract for the patient is that he will present himself regularly, on time, and for whatever duration is necessary; that he will attempt to conform to the basic rule at all times; that he will attempt to cooperate actively in learning all that he can about his behavior and motivations. The analyst's part of the contract is that he will attempt to help the patient reach the goal of self-understanding by seeing the patient regularly for as long as necessary, to accept with clinical understanding the patient's anxieties, fears, and guilt, and actively to help— through searching interest—the patient to his goal by skillful interpretations, attempts to understand the patient, and assistance to the patient in understanding himself.

The *therapeutic alliance* is a feeling state which, hopefully, develops during the course of analysis. It is a conviction on the part of the patient that he is working together with the analyst on a mutual project of understanding himself. It is an alliance between the "observing part" of his ego and the analyst. The analyst is not regarded as one who is doing something therapeutic to the passive patient as in other forms of medicine, but rather they are actively working together on a joint project of discovery. A therapeutic alliance is essential for successful analytic or psychotherapeutic progress.

E. **Ability to Tolerate Anxiety**: The ego must have the capacity to tolerate a certain degree of anxiety in order to be successful at analysis. If the ego resorts to pathologic defenses at the first sign of anxiety, it will never have the opportunity to look at the feelings or thoughts which give rise to the anxiety.

F. **Motivation**: Although transient episodes of ambivalence are unavoidable, a fairly strong degree of conscious motivation is necessary to carry the patient through psychoanalysis. The patient's desire for analysis must be sufficient to carry him through the unpleasant, difficult, and at times slow-moving parts of his analysis, which is a long-term, time-consuming, and expensive process.

RESULTS OF PSYCHOANALYTIC TREATMENT

The results of psychoanalysis—as of any of the psychotherapies—are difficult to evaluate. The judgment of results depends on the subjective feelings of the patient and the objective views of those close to him. However, other elements are present also. One is the question of what one started with—what basic constitutional, physical, intellectual factors, what kinds of realistic traumas (early death of parents, etc). One cannot ignore the axiom of not being able to make a silk purse out of a sow's ear. Another very important issue is the test of time. Does the patient feel better not for a day or a week but in general over a period of several years and how does he function over a period of time? How does he handle stressful situations which previously upset him greatly and provoked symptoms? Life may also present new problems which were entirely unforeseen at the time of treatment. Analysis is not a vaccination against all of the ills which life may deal. Favorable results should mean that over an extended period of time the patient feels better about his life in general, is felt to be more mature by those close to him, is able to be more giving in close relationships (less narcissistic), is able to utilize more of his constructive abilities in his work and enjoy his leisure more, and is able to handle stressful situations more efficiently with less subjective distress. The point at which analysis should terminate should be when it appears that the patient has approached as near to these goals as he is likely to do—with any further increments seeming to be unduly time-consuming—and has shown evidence of being able to maintain these improvements. One must differentiate the condition known as a "flight into health," when there is a sudden great improvement in the patient's condition—temporary in duration—without any known cause. This latter is a type of resistance which the ego resorts to rather than risk further discussion of material which it feels is too uncomfortable.

Occasionally, life presents problems which distress a patient who has "finished" analysis so that he finds it worthwhile to resume analysis. Also, sometimes patients are able to deal with problems in a second analysis (with the same or a different analyst) which they could not deal with the first time. Unfortunately, a statistical survey of the results of psychoanalysis is not available. However, psychoanalysis is believed by many to be the best known way of achieving reconstructive personality changes. It makes possible the most far-reaching improvements of any known type of psychotherapy. With well selected patients, one-third of patients will probably be much improved, one-third will show moderate improvement, and one-third little or no improvement.

Results involve modification of personality structure as well as alleviation of symptoms. The patient who has undergone analysis is able to handle future stresses more efficiently and with less distress. Improvements are usually more lasting than with other types of psychotherapy.

OTHER USES OF PSYCHOANALYSIS

There are other uses of psychoanalysis besides that of being a therapeutic instrument. The principal use is that the psychoanalyst can often make unique contributions by relating psychoanalytic theory to particular projects. Psychoanalysts play a major role in teaching theory to psychiatric residents, clinical psychologists, psychiatric social workers, medical students, and persons in counseling fields. They can help these professionals in the understanding of personality and motivation and in learning psychoanalytic psychotherapy. Psychoanalytic theory has been helpful in certain aspects of community mental health projects and in school counseling programs. There is also an active program of multidisciplinary studies in medicine (eg, correlation of studies of asthmatic patients from the physical and psychoanalytic viewpoints; correlation between menstrual irregularities, endocrine disturbances, and psychoanalytic findings in the same patients) and in sociology. There are some pure psychoanalytic research programs (eg, correlation between observed early infant and childhood development and later childhood personality development). There have also been a number of attempts to evaluate and interpret historical figures and classics of literature from a psychoanalytic viewpoint.

PSYCHOANALYTIC PSYCHOTHERAPY

Psychoanalytic psychotherapy differs from psychoanalysis in that it is less intensive, less concerned with unconscious material, and has more modest goals. It is now widely used for the following reasons: (1) Less time and money are involved per patient treated than in psychoanalysis. (2) Less extensive training is necessary for the therapist, which means that many more therapists are available. (3) A greater variety of psychiatric disorders can be treated with this technic than are usually regarded as suitable for formal psychoanalysis—particularly the functional psychoses (schizophrenias, affective psychoses) and the borderline psychoses. (4) More flexibility is permitted in the use of adjunctive or combined treatment procedures, eg, use of drugs (tranquilizing or mood elevating), group therapy, counseling other members of the family ("family therapy"), environmental manipulation, and direct suggestion and support.

GOALS OF TREATMENT

The primary goal of psychoanalytic psychotherapy is the relief of symptoms. Undesirable personality traits and defense patterns can often be modified, but the aims are more modest than with psychoanalysis. The patient usually can be helped to handle mental conflicts and anxiety-producing situations in a more efficient manner and with less distressing side-effects.

TRAINING OF THE PSYCHOANALYTIC PSYCHOTHERAPIST

Complete psychoanalytic training, though desirable, is not necessary. Personal psychoanalysis or psychotherapy is desirable to lessen the effects of any personal problems the therapist may have that might impair his clinical objectivity and judgment. A therapist with unresolved or unrecognized emotional problems is apt to react with undue anxiety, bad judgment, or "blindness" to similar problems in his patients.

Formal training in psychoanalytic theory and therapy consists of lectures, readings, case presentations, and clinical demonstrations by experienced therapists and analysts. The extent and depth of the training here is usually not as great as in the full training of the analyst.

The psychiatric resident should conduct therapy with a number of patients over an extended period of time under the direct supervision of experienced psychotherapists or psychoanalysts.

TECHNIC OF PSYCHOANALYTIC PSYCHOTHERAPY

Psychoanalytic psychotherapy usually requires 1 or 2 visits a week lasting 45–50 minutes each over a period of 1–4 years. It is uncommon to use a couch. The patient usually faces the therapist directly, or chairs may be placed at angles so that the patient need not look directly at the therapist unless he wants to do so.

The length of treatment in psychoanalytic psychotherapy depends on many of the same factors that were discussed under length of treatment in psychoanalysis. The duration depends largely on the goals that the patient and the therapist set for themselves. Often these goals, particularly those of the patient, have to be modified to conform to reality. The patient's capacity to respond favorably to treatment is in part determined by innate constitutional factors but mainly by the type of early development which he has had—the points of fixation and the characteristic defenses which he has developed. The degree of flexibility of his ego may govern how far he can expect to go in therapy. His real-life situation must be considered also, eg, if he is likely to remain married to a very difficult spouse.

The important goal is the elimination or great reduction of symptoms. An attempt to modify the characteristic defense patterns is also made. It is hoped that the patient will be better able to tolerate previously symptom-producing stresses and to cope more efficiently with them.

Treatment should continue as long as the therapist and patient feel that some reasonable degree of progress toward the goals is taking place. When it appears that further effort, time, and money are not producing reasonable increments in progress, therapy may be interrupted. The door should always be left open; if the patient finds himself unduly distressed over a period of time, he should feel welcome to return. Therapy should not be construed as a protection against all of the obstacles and frustrations of life. However, one should be able to handle them better after therapy.

As in psychoanalysis, an important goal is to help the patient develop insight into his problems and motivations. Some corrective emotional experiences may also occur.

Transference develops in psychoanalytic psychotherapy almost as frequently as in psychoanalysis. It tends to be more difficult to resolve. The reasons for this are 2-fold: (1) Since the therapist is seen much more as an actual person than is the analyst, it becomes more difficult to convince the patient that his feelings about the therapist are transferred from past figures rather than being based on current reality. (2) Less unconscious material in terms of dreams and fantasies occur in therapy. It is this material that is often very useful in showing the patient his transference and hence in resolving it.

If some small degree of positive transference remains after psychotherapy (and it always does—in analysis to a lesser degree), this is not unfavorable. If it is excessive, it will not be beneficial since too much dependency on the therapist will exist which will make it difficult for the patient to function well without the therapist being available.

Free association is extensively used. The patient is encouraged to speak freely and openly about anything that comes to mind.

Dream interpretation is less extensively used than in psychoanalysis, but dream material may be used to a certain extent.

One of the main differences between psychoanalysis and psychoanalytic psychotherapy is that in the latter the therapist plays a more active role. Psychoanalysis is primarily a listening type of therapy—allowing the patient to "talk out" his problems with occasional interpretation, clarification, and elaboration. The psychoanalytic psychotherapist is usually more active than the psychoanalyst in directing the choice of subject matter and deciding how deeply or extensively a given subject should be pursued. The therapist uses more suggestion and more direct support than is usually considered desirable in psychoanalysis. The therapist lets his own personality and feelings be known to the patient both for purposes of suggestion and as an object of identification. Drugs are more frequently used to alleviate anxiety or depression. Although interpretations are based on the same theoretical considerations, there is a tendency to make them earlier and with less accumulated evidence than in psychoanalysis.

An important goal in psychoanalysis and psychoanalytic psychotherapy is "uncovering" (to allow the patient to look into his unconscious motivations). In psychoanalytic psychotherapy the therapist may also use reinforcing technics (covering up) to strengthen existing defenses in areas where it is felt that uncovering may create overwhelming anxiety (more than is desirable to facilitate the treatment).

Overall positive feelings of the patient toward the therapist are desirable and even necessary for best results.

INDICATIONS FOR PSYCHOANALYTIC PSYCHOTHERAPY

This type of therapy has the widest application of any of the psychotherapies. It is useful in nearly all psychiatric disorders that are generally considered to be amenable to verbal treatment: neuroses, functional psychoses, personality disorders, and psychophysiologic reactions. Variations of it may be used with almost any age group from childhood to old age. Because less time and money are involved, it is often a more "practical" approach than formal psychoanalysis. "Psychologic mindedness"—the ability to form insight—is, as with psychoanalysis, an important factor in the success of treatment.

RESULTS OF PSYCHOANALYTIC PSYCHOTHERAPY

With reasonable selection of patients, psychoanalytic psychotherapy produces essentially the same degree of "success," in terms of its somewhat more limited goals, as does psychoanalysis in its more far-reaching goals. This means, roughly, a marked improvement in about one-third of patients and a moderate improvement in another third, with less favorable results in the remainder.

Good results may be prevented by unalterable environmental stresses; basic—perhaps constitutional—defects in personality structure; inability to tolerate any degree of anxiety and consequent inability to look at oneself at all; or lack of capacity to utilize insight or to be genuinely cooperative. Symptom relief is the most common favorable result; modification and improvements in personality characteristics are the next most common; extensive personality modification and an enduring capacity to withstand serious future psychologic stresses are less common. The prognosis is most favorable in patients who showed evidence of good social and personal adjustments prior to the current emotional illness; in those whose illness was acute rather than insidious in onset; and where there was a definite external precipitating cause for the illness, eg, the death of a close family member. If the patient has been able to form a prolonged positive relationship with another individual, the likelihood of forming a therapeutically advantageous positive relationship with the therapist is greatly increased; hence, the prognosis is more favorable.

REFERENCES

Books and Monographs

Alexander, F., & others: *Psychoanalytic Therapy: Principles and Application.* Ronald Press, 1946.

Altman, L.L.: *The Dream in Psychoanalysis.* Internat Univ Press, 1969.

Brenner, C.B.: *An Elementary Textbook of Psychoanalysis.* Doubleday Anchor, 1957.

Colby, K.M.: *A Primer for Psychotherapists.* Ronald Press, 1951.

Deutsch, H.: *Psychoanalysis of the Neuroses.* Hogarth, 1951.

Eidelberg, L.: *Studies in Psychoanalysis.* Internat Univ Press, 1952.

Ekstein, R., & R.L. Motto: *From Learning for Love to Love of Learning: Essays on Psychoanalysis and Education.* Brunner/Mazel, 1969.

Fenichel, O.: *The Psychoanalytic Theory of the Neuroses.* Norton, 1946.

Ferenczi, S.: *Further Contributions to the Theory and Technique of Psychoanalysis.* Hogarth, 1950.

French, T.M.: *Psychoanalytic Interpretations.* Quadrangle Books, 1970.

Freud, S.: *Complete Psychological Works.* Standard edition, translated by James Strachey. 24 vols. Hogarth, 1953–1966.

Fromm, E.: *The Crisis of Psychoanalysis.* Holt, Rinehart & Winston, 1970.

Fromm-Reichmann, F.: *Principles of Intensive Psychotherapy.* Univ of Chicago Press, 1950.

Galdston, I. (editor): *Psychoanalysis in Present-Day Psychiatry.* Robert Brunner, 1969.

Glover, E.: *The Technique of Psychoanalysis.* Internat Univ Press, 1955.

Harper, R.A.: *Psychoanalysis and Psychotherapy.* Prentice-Hall, 1959.

Hollender, M.H.: *The Practice of Psychoanalytic Psychotherapy.* Grune & Stratton, 1965.

Kris, E.: *Psychoanalytic Explorations in Art.* Chap 14. Internat Univ Press, 1952.

Lennard, H.L., & A. Bernstein: *The Analysis of Psychotherapy.* Columbia Univ Press, 1960.

Lorand, S.: *Technique of Psychoanalytic Therapy.* Internat Univ Press, 1948.

Mendel, W.M., & G.A. Green: *The Therapeutic Management of Psychological Illness: The Theory and Practice of Supportive Care.* Basic Books, 1967.

Rank, O.: *The Trauma of Birth.* Robert Brunner, 1952.

Rapaport, D. (editor): *Organization and Pathology of Thought.* Columbia Univ Press, 1951.

Reich, W.: *Character Analysis,* 3rd ed. Parts 1 & 2. Orgone Institute Press, 1949.

Roheim, G.: *Psychoanalysis and Anthropology.* Internat Univ Press, 1950.

Thompson, C.: *Psychoanalysis: Evolution and Development.* Hermitage House, 1951.

Zetzel, E.: *The Capacity for Emotional Growth.* Internat Univ Press, 1970.

Journal Articles

Arlow, J.A.: Anal sensation and feelings of persecution. Psychoanal Quart 18:79–84, 1949.

Beres, D., & S.J. Obers: The effects of extreme deprivation in infancy on psychic structure in adolescence: A study in ego development. Psychoanal Stud Child 5:212–235, 1950.

Bibring, E.: The development and problems of the theory of the instincts. Internat J Psychoanal 22:102–131, 1941.

Blau, A.: In support of Freud's syndrome of anxiety (actual) neurosis. Internat J Psychoanal 33:363–372, 1952.

Dyrud, J.E., & C. Donnely: Executive functions of the ego. Arch Gen Psychiat 20:257–261, 1969.

Freud, A.: Problems of infantile neurosis. Psychoanal Stud Child 9:16–74, 1954.

Freud, A.: The widening scope of indications for psychoanalysis. J Am Psychoanal Ass 2:607–620, 1954.

Frosch, J.: Psychoanalytic considerations of the psychotic character. J Am Psychoanal Ass 18:24–50, 1970.

Greenson, R.R.: The exceptional position of the dream in psychoanalytic practice. Psychoanal Quart 39:519–549, 1970.

Hartmann, H.: Comments on the psychoanalytic theory of instinctual drives. Psychoanal Quart 17:368–388, 1948.

Hartmann, H.: The metapsychology of schizophrenia. Psychoanal Stud Child 8:177–198, 1953.

Hartmann, H., & E. Kris: The genetic approach in psychoanalysis. Psychoanal Stud Child 1:11–30, 1945.

Hartmann, H., Kris, E., & R.M. Loewenstein: Comments on the formation of psychic structure. Psychoanal Stud Child 2:11–38, 1946.

Hartmann, H., Kris, E., & R.M. Loewenstein: Notes on the theory of aggression. Psychoanal Stud Child 3-4:9–36, 1949.

Hoffer, W.: Development of the body ego. Psychoanal Stud Child 5:18–23, 1950.

Kaplan, A.H.: Joint parent-adolescent interviews as a parameter in the psychoanalysis of the younger adolescent. J Nerv Ment Dis 148:550–558, 1969.

Kernberg, O.F.: Factors in the psychoanalytic treatment of narcissistic personalities. J Am Psychoanal Ass 18:51–85, 1970.

Levitan, H.L.: The depersonalization process: The sense of reality and unreality. Psychoanal Quart 39:449–470, 1970.

Marmor, J.: Current status of psychoanalysis in American psychiatry. Am J Psychiat 125:679–680, 1968.

McGuire, M.T.: Repression, resistance and recall of the past: Some reconsiderations. Psychoanal Quart 39:427–448, 1970.

Schlesinger, H.T.: The place of forgetting in memory functioning. J Am Psychoanal Ass 18:358–371, 1970.

Taylor, F.K.: Prokaletic measures derived from psychoanalytic technique. Brit J Psychiat 115:407–420, 1969.

Van Ophuijsen, J.H.W.: On the origin of feelings of persecution. Internat J Psychoanal 1:235–239, 1920.

32...

Child Psychiatry

Children express their psychiatric problems in behavior. Parents must be involved in their treatment, as they already are in their cause.

Child psychiatry has evolved through many phases and has been enriched by the contributions of countless dedicated men and women. Today it is becoming ever more involved with the fields of pediatrics, neurology, child psychology, education, and the social services. Current foci of interest include the development of the child; the role of the family; work, play, and school ability; and the changing role of the maturing child in society.

CHILDHOOD DEVELOPMENT

The following is a brief description of the principal emotional, psychologic, and behavioral characteristics of the major stages of childhood development according to Sigmund Freud, Erik Erikson, and Jean Piaget.

Infancy (Birth to Age 1)

(1) **Freud (oral phase):** The mouth is the principal focus of pleasure, both in connection with feeding and with sucking per se. Two types of dependency are a prominent feature of this period: a parasitic, passive type in the first 6 months; and an aggressive, active type, based on increasing motor ability, eruption of teeth, and vocalization, in the second 6 months and the following year.

(2) **Erikson (stage of basic trust):** Satisfaction of the infant's needs for warmth, comfort, and food by the mother permits increasing tolerance of frustration. The signal achievement of this stage is the ability to accept the absence of the mother.

(3) **Piaget (sensory-motor period):** The child learns to retain images of objects not immediately in the sensory field and develops an elementary form of deductive logic in manipulating them.

Toddler Years (Ages 1–3)

(1) **Freud (anal phase):** The primary "erotic" zone is the anal area and, by extension, the urethra, bladder, rectum, and lower gastrointestinal tract.

Special pleasure is found in elimination and retention. Obstinacy, conflict with parental expectations and demands, messiness, selfishness, sadism, and ambivalence characterize the emotional aspects of this phase.

(2) **Erikson (stage of autonomy):** Increased mobility and control of body functions offer the child a new set of capabilities with which to interact with his environment. He can choose between 2 modes of social behavior—holding on and letting go—both of which are influenced by affective states. Active aggression, exploration, and manipulation of the environment, as well as experimentation with his new abilities, bring the child to a series of points of decision and choice in what had been a benign or at least neutral universe. Parental attitudes about such matters as obedience, schedules, and propriety come into conflict with the child's hunger for experience and power. Parents are faced with decisions about firmness or permissiveness and the need to let the child learn from experience. The emotion of shame is learned from parental prohibitions and incorporated into the child's ego. The child learns to modify his drive for independence in exchange for parental approval.

(3) **Piaget:** See next section.

The Pre-school Years (Ages 3–6)

(1) **Freud (phallic phase):** The primary site of erotic pleasure is now the genitalia. Handling the genitals is the main source of erotic stimulation, and there is intense curiosity about pregnancy and sexual intercourse. The *Oedipus complex* becomes established during this period, with possessive feelings towards the parent of the opposite sex and rivalry toward the parent of the same sex. The child wants all of the love, attention, and time of the desired parent and believes that he is sufficiently powerful to achieve this goal. Resolution of the complex differs for boys and girls because of anatomic differences as well as cultural traditions. In boys, resolution normally occurs when the child relinquishes his erotic attachment to the mother in the face of the threat of severe retaliation from the father (*castration anxiety*) and instead develops the ambition to grow up like the father and to marry someone like the mother. The girl usually relinquishes her sexual attachment to the father and her rivalry with the mother by accepting her lot. In both boys and girls, as the Oedipus problem is solved, a cohesive superego is established and the child is ready to enter the latency phase.

(2) **Erikson (stage of initiative):** Attack and conquest of persons, things, and skills are the keynotes of this stage, along with the incorporation of cultural values and restrictions. The sexes become differentiated in terms of basic modes of orientation, ie, intrusiveness and "maleness"; receptivity and "femaleness." The culmination of this period is "that specifically human crisis (the Oedipus conflict) during which the child must turn away from an exclusive, pregenital attachment to his parents to the slow process of becoming a parent, a carrier of tradition." The child now has a notion of past and future and of consequences.

(3) **Piaget (pre-operational period, 2–6 years):** The elaboration of the function of symbolization is marked in this period by the acquisition of language, the appearance of dreams and night terrors, and the beginning of

symbolic play and of drawing and other kinds of graphic representation. The child progresses from *animism* (in which inanimate objects can be invested with life) and *concretism* (in which adventitious properties such as names, temperature, etc are believed to be intrinsic to the object) to *abstract thinking,* in which names and words are seen as symbols detachable from the objects they denote and as objects to be manipulated mentally.

The Elementary School Years

(1) **Freud (latency phase):** With the resolution of the Oedipus complex, libidinal and aggressive drives diminish and mental energy becomes available for the task of learning. The superego is internalized, and the defense mechanisms become established. The child's interests turn largely to fields outside the family, ie, school, peers, and other persons. An important emotional activity is identification, basically with the parent of the same sex, with emphasis on social relations with members of the same sex. Partial or total identification with other individuals, male and female, occurs.

This phase can be divided into *early latency,* characterized by almost total absence of genital sexual concerns and extinction of masturbation; and *late latency* (prepuberty), in which the orientation becomes more heterosexual, and sexual interests and curiosity reassert themselves.

(2) **Erikson (stage of industry):** Accomplishment and the search for success mark this stage. A sense of inadequacy and inferiority may result from partial or complete failure or from inability to disengage from the family.

(3) **Piaget (period of abstract operations):** While the previous period was characterized by magical and concrete thinking, this period witnesses the development of thinking on the level of abstractions. The child can now perform mental operations "in his head" rather than with objects, eg, he can count mentally, as opposed to using his fingers or touching a number of objects. He can think about things, about classes of things, and about relationships between classes.

Adolescence (Ages 11–18)

Adolescence includes the period of puberty (11–14), which is marked by the appearance of secondary sexual characteristics and the onset of menses in girls and the production of semen in boys. It also includes the period beyond that—a long, often stormy process of psychologic and emotional maturation. While special attention is paid to adolescence in Chapter 34, the following characteristics of this period should be emphasized here: (1) *Vacillation,* often between widely divergent moods, points of view, and relationships, is frequent. (2) *Dependency* and a wish to return to (or not leave) childhood comes into conflict with wishes and abilities to be independent. (3) *Increased instinctual drives* must be dealt with in the face of internal and external prohibitions and modifiers. Erikson characterized adolescence as the *age of identity,* in which an alignment of the biologic and the psychologic identities must be made around vocational, familial, and social roles. Piaget calls adolescence *the stage of formal operations,* during which, along with biologic and emotional changes, there is an important change in style of thinking involving a higher degree of abstraction which permits thinking about thoughts, construction of ideals, and planning realistically about the future. Reasoning about propositions which are contrary to fact and the comprehension of metaphors are examples of formal operations. In general, the kind of thinking employed by adults characterizes the intellectualism of adolescence.

EVALUATION OF FACTORS AFFECTING PSYCHOLOGIC DEVELOPMENT

Each child is born with an intrinsic endowment of physical and psychologic abilities, limitations, and potentialities. This endowment is then modified by interaction with the environment, especially the parents.

Intrinsic factors are principally heredo-constitutional and are the matrix for the child's future development. Extrinsic factors are those that from birth onward impinge on the organism and affect its adjustment and development. The principal ones include maternal attitudes and attention, family climate, the father's role in the family, birth order and siblings, ethnic, racial, and religious background, socioeconomic level, and the myriad developments in the life of any person.

Symptoms may appear as a result of disordered internal development or disturbed interpersonal relationships and are manifested often by behavior that is upsetting to parents or others. The physician in his evaluation of the problem should proceed from several directions.

The Presenting Problem

Children and their problems are seen by general practitioners and pediatricians as well as psychiatrists. The investigation and management of most psychologic problems are within the scope of any physician who is willing to apply the time, patience, and wish to understand.

The physician should ask the parents to elaborate on their description of the presenting problem in respect to precipitating, exacerbating, and mitigating circumstances, duration of the problem, their reactions to the child's behavior, and their attempts to control or modify it. During this interview, other significant issues will be brought out about the child's development and current behavior, the parents' attitudes, and the parents' relationship to one another. It cannot be emphasized too strongly that the presenting problem, although stated in generalities, may be the event that has precipitated a specific family crisis at a particular time, but it often represents one aspect of a larger problem that is expressed also in a variety of other ways.

Developmental History

The child's development is reviewed systematically with the parents, beginning with the circumstances in which conception took place. (Was the child planned or desired at the time? What was the economic and emotional situation of the family?)

The pregnancy and delivery are investigated from the medical and emotional points of view. The various aspects of feeding in infancy are next explored (breast or bottle feeding, weaning, and special problems such as colic and food sensitivities or idiosyncrasies). The ages at which the major developmental "milestones" were reached and the child's facility with them are then considered (sitting up unaided, walking, first words, talking, etc). This is followed by a consideration of toilet training (age at which begun, measures used, child's reactions, behavioral characteristics during that period, ages and manner in which day and night bowel and bladder control were completed, and any persistent problems concerning elimination).

MEDICAL HISTORY AND EXAMINATION

The child's medical history should be reviewed to determine the care received and the nature of special problems. Hospitalizations, major or repeated injuries, and any history of seizures should be especially noted. The child's school history should be taken. When did he start? How did he react? How has his attendance been? What is his current grade placement, performance, and adjustment? What comments have teachers made? The child's sexual curiosity and behavior, as well as parental attitudes and policies toward them, should be explored.

Family History

Basic demographic information should be collected about the family and its members, as well as any other individuals living in the household: age, educational background, occupation, race, religious affiliations. The date and duration, circumstances, and problems of the present marriage, and whether there have been previous marriages and how they were terminated should be noted. Information should be gathered about the parents' upbringing, their present relationships with their parents and siblings, and their relationship with one another. An assessment should be made of the interrelationships between the patient and siblings. It is well to have a clear picture of the physical layout of the home and the sleeping arrangements and family routine, as well as some idea of the neighborhood and the family's social circle.

History From Other Sources

In most instances, information gathered from the child and his parents is sufficient for diagnosis. However, certain other sources of history (eg, records of diagnosis or treatment of the child at other psychiatric facilities, medical records) add the important perspective of professional impressions of the child and his situation at an earlier point in time, or over a long period. It may also be very illuminating to study pictures of the child in the family album.

In certain situations it is necessary to gather information (with parents' informed consent) outside the family, eg, if a symptom occurs almost exclusively in a certain setting such as at school. In such an instance, specific information should be elicited from the school social worker and the teacher; if necessary, the child should be observed in his classroom.

Examination of the Child

(1) **Pediatric examination:** A thorough pediatric examination should be performed by the child's physician or by a member of the clinic staff. (Some child psychiatrists with pediatric backgrounds prefer to combine the physical and psychiatric examinations.) A detailed assessment of the child's past and current medical status, growth, and development should be available. Special consideration should be given to evidence of brain damage, of the possible effects of physical abnormalities or illnesses on the maturational process, and of disorders of perception and motor coordination that may be affecting educational and social adaptation. The need for neurologic or other specialized examinations should be considered.

(2) **Psychologic examination:** In some clinics, psychologic testing is conducted routinely as a screening procedure. More often, psychologic examination is requested when certain differential diagnostic questions have been raised, specifically those concerning academic and learning disturbances, mental retardation, brain damage, and psychosis.

In general, psychologic testing supplies information about the child's assets and liabilities and provides a picture of the child's areas of difficulty and of his intrapsychic dynamics. The types of tests used are described in Chapter 7.

(3) **Psychiatric examination:** The purpose of the diagnostic interview with the child is basically the same as for adults, ie, direct observation of the patient's behavior, affect, ideas, and means of establishing relationships and coping with anxiety. Nevertheless, there are important and crucial differences which determine the amount and kind of diagnostic information that can be obtained as well as the success of any future therapeutic effort:

Because the child seldom explicitly requests or understands the necessity for psychiatric help, he needs and appreciates an honest, sympathetic preparation for his initial visit. The physician should prepare the parents by helping them to allay their own fears and to deal with possible misconceptions about the purposes and goals of his intervention. The child's most common fears center around notions that the psychiatrist will prescribe punishment for "bad" thoughts or behavior and around possibilities of physical pain or discomfort ("shots," etc).

Especially when the physician is a stranger to the child, he can win the child's respect and trust only if he earns them by a respectful, attentive, unhurried, and nonjudgmental hearing. It is often useful to conduct at least part of the first interview in the presence of the parents—not only to observe interactions but also to provide an opportunity for clarification of questions and to establish rapport. Condescension, "cuteness," and quizzing are poorly tolerated by children in a medical setting.

The younger the child, the less likely he will be to communicate information about his inner life by verbal means. Since play is the preferred means for the child to comprehend and master his experiences, both external and internal, simple toys, drawing materials, and games such as checkers or playing cards should be provided for playing out conflicts and feelings.

Close observation of the child's behavior and the interaction of the family members often brings to light attitudes and behaviors not reported or noted by the parents. Such items as the child's physical appearance, manner of speech and dress, and the characteristics of his adaptation to the clinical situation can provide important information about his difficulties and life style. For example, excessive neatness may suggest an obsessive compulsive "family culture," etc.

Diagnostic Formulation

The physician should attempt to formulate a diagnosis and a treatment plan based on the evaluation and synthesis of the information derived from the sources listed above, as follows:

(1) **Clinical-dynamic:** An assessment of the child's psychologic functions in the present. This is an elaboration of the presenting problem and related issues.

(2) **Developmental-genetic:** A longitudinal evaluation of the factors which prepared the ground for the child's present predicament.

SPECIAL PROBLEMS OF INFANCY AND THE PRESCHOOL YEARS

FEEDING DIFFICULTIES

Feeding problems are usually manifested by apparent lack of satisfaction with feedings, fretfulness, and signs of "colic." The most common feeding problems are due to the mother's insecurity about the adequacy or kind of feeding and to emotional turbulence that occurs when one or both parents lay extraordinary stress on the child's eating. Each change (weaning, beginning solid foods, etc) can become an area of conflict so that the infant and young child may use eating or not eating as a way of upsetting and opposing his parents. Feeding difficulties usually resolve themselves as parental concern about eating subsides.

Pica

This syndrome involves habitual ingestion of nonnutritive materials such as plaster, paint, dirt, etc. Although some children with pica may have nutritional deficiencies, many who are receiving a well balanced diet persist in the habit. Lead and other poisonings may result, but punishment does not eliminate the habit.

Pica often occurs in homes where the child is rejected and is given little affection. It seldom appears in the absence of other problems requiring psychiatric and medical treatment.

Thumbsucking

Finger sucking or thumbsucking may begin in the first year and continue with diminished frequency until the 5th or 6th year (seldom longer). Sucking usually occurs when the child is tired, upset, or insecure. When it manifests itself in exaggerated frequency, in a wide variety of circumstances, or into the school years, thumbsucking is considered pathologic and a sign of continuing oral dependent traits and insecurity. It usually will not cease without correction of the underlying causes.

SLEEPING DIFFICULTIES

As with eating, the development of normal waking and sleeping patterns depends on a stable emotional climate in the home as well as a sense of regularity in family habit patterns. However, at about age 2, children generally tend to resist going to sleep and awaken during the night. They thus avoid "missing out on things" and reassure themselves about continued contact with the parents. Refusal to give the assurance needed—or over-assurance in the form of taking the child into the parental bed—can carry the whole family into a vicious cycle of wakefulness and demands for reassurance.

Nightmares or fear of the dark in preschool children are not abnormal in themselves but may be associated with insecurity.

SPEECH PROBLEMS

Delayed Speech

Because speech is the most common method of interpersonal communication, anything producing a major disturbance of interpersonal relations will delay the acquisition of speech or its maturation. Most frequently, however, delayed speech is attributable to heredity, deafness (usually associated with middle ear and tonsil infections), or parental overprotection, ie, anticipation of the child's wishes in such a way as to obviate the need for speech. Early infantile autism, with its severely restricted capacity for relatedness, and mental retardation are other major causes of delayed speech. Maintenance of immature speech patterns such as lisping or "baby talk" often results from reinforcement by parents who refuse to allow the child to give up these "cute" ways of expressing himself.

"Sudden" loss of speech or arrest of speech development in young children strongly suggests psychosis, especially in the absence of deafness or of other organic conditions affecting cerebral function.

Stuttering

Transient periods of stuttering during ages 1–3 are common and are probably due to the fact that the child's vocal apparatus and vocabulary cannot keep pace with his thoughts when he is excited or under stress. Constant correction or supplying of words by the parents may tend to fixate the pattern and produce the type of stuttering which begins in the preschool years and is more constant, ie, is present even when the child is calm and increases in severity under stress.

Some believe that stuttering children have conflicts over passivity and aggressiveness. Speech is regarded as an aggressive function in which the child may attempt through hesitation to control both himself and his audience. The speech pattern eventually becomes habitual, ie, persists without constant emotional content, and the stutterer needs speech therapy and psychotherapy for help in resolving the emotional conflicts associated with the disorder. In some children the hereditary or constitutional factor may be so strong that all therapy remains ineffective.

ROCKING AND HEAD BANGING

These 2 forms of behavior usually occur together. Rocking begins in infancy and head banging at about age 1. The rocking may occur in any position and under any circumstance, but usually is first reported as occurring before sleep. Persistent rocking is found in children who are starved for affection and have little means of achieving pleasure aside from this kind of activity. Children confined to cribs or playpens for long periods may try to rock or bang their way out of their small prisons.

Head banging has a hostile and aggressive component, seeming to express the child's anger at his environment and fate.

Rocking and head banging persisting beyond infancy and early childhood are usually symptoms of severe psychopathology, probably of a psychotic disorder. However, they may occur occasionally in apparently normal children.

ABNORMAL MASTURBATION

Desultory masturbation without great frequency or interest is manifested by all children and generally is curbed in the toddler years as a "public" activity through parental disapproval. The child who masturbates frequently without regard for the presence of others—or even because others are present—usually has an environment with poor affective relationships. Criticism or punishment may increase the symptom in proportion to the child's underlying resentments.

PROBLEMS RELATED TO TOILET TRAINING

Fecal Smearing

Fecal play and smearing may be seen up to age 3 and is an expression of the interest younger children may exhibit in their excreta. Persistent smearing of feces on walls, cribs, etc is usually a form of revenge in a child who is rebelling against parents who are strict, rigid, and unloving in their attempts to train or in their general attitude toward him.

Encopresis
Under ordinary circumstances, "accidents" or fecal soiling occur during toilet training but rarely afterward. When a child persists in defecating frequently in his clothing even into the school years, he is said to have encopresis. This manifestation of a turbulent toilet training period is apt to be a more direct form of rebellion against the parents' attempts to train the child. When the symptom persists into the phallic phase and beyond, it may become the focus of fantasies about childbirth and related sexual matters.

Persistent encopresis is seldom due to organic gastrointestinal disease. Parental concern may lead to various anorectal examinations which only tend to increase everyone's focus on that portion of the child's body.

Enuresis
Enuresis (wetting) is one of the most common symptoms of emotional problems in childhood, but it occurs also in children with few or no emotional difficulties. Most enuretic children wet themselves in bed at night, during sleep; some are both diurnal and nocturnal enuretics, and others wet only during the daytime.

Attempts at treatment by conditioning, restriction of fluids, medication, etc have variable success, even under the best of conditions. The age at which treatment is started, the history of previous attempts, and the total affective atmosphere surrounding the child influence the outcome of treatment.

Proper treatment for enuresis, as for most behavior problems in children, involves consideration of the whole child. The primary goal is to strengthen the child's personality and his opinion of himself. To do this, unfavorable influences in his life, especially faulty parental attitudes, must be diminished and the force of the physician's personality used to build self-confidence in the child. Specific attention is given to the enuresis. Many physicians use a weekly chart and gold stars for dry beds in the case of younger children. Some use suggestion and persuasion for older children, sometimes by urging them to develop their "shut-off muscles" by starting and stopping the urinary stream several times during the day when they urinate.

Children should not be considered enuretic before age 4–5. Even though most children can achieve reasonable bladder control by the end of the third year, "accidents" do happen normally within the following year or so. Thorough medical examination is necessary to rule out the rare case of diabetes mellitus, diabetes insipidus, genitourinary tract infection, etc.

Several types of enuresis have been described. They may occur in "pure" or mixed forms.

(1) Revenge enuresis: This most common type of enuresis is similar to encopresis, certain feeding problems, and gross oppositional behavior in that it represents retaliation against excessive strictness in toilet training and other areas. There is usually a history of toilet training attempts before the child is physiologically mature and under stipulations with which he is unable to comply. The revenge motive is unconscious in the child but is well understood as such by the parents, especially the mother.

(2) **Regressive enuresis:** This type of enuresis may occur alone or in combination with other regressive symptoms after toilet training has been established. It occurs most often following the birth of a sibling. If the parents adopt a punitive or strict attitude toward the enuresis, further insecurity may ensue, with fixation and exacerbation of the symptoms.

(3) **Familial enuresis:** Some boys are enuretic because they have never been trained or because the family culture condones bedwetting as a family or, usually, "masculine" trait. They are unaware of any abnormality until they have to live away from home or are inducted into the armed services. A comparable condition is seen more rarely in girls.

The Struggle Over Control

Children may attempt to deal with excessive demands for conformity and insufficient love by developing symptoms related directly to the stage of development at which these struggles occur. Toilet training problems (see above) are the most common symptom. The child may also adopt total behavioral responses (characterologic maneuvers) that may persist as personality disorders. (See Chapter 17.)

(1) **Aggressive rebellion:** Some children enter into open, often destructive combat against anything or anyone who attempts to control or make demands on them. They respond poorly to punishment and become so self-centered as to be unconcerned about the rights or feelings of others.

(2) **Passive rebellion:** Passive resolution is characterized by procrastination and quiet obstructionism, with a superficial appearance of conformity and obedience. A child with this attitude is a source of exasperation to his parents because he is seldom reliable or true to his word although he is overtly agreeable and pleasant.

(3) **Pseudomaturity:** The child has given up the unequal struggle and has become inhibited, conforming, and "too good" but is emotionally brittle and easily upset.

Temper Tantrums

The temper tantrum is a violent, short-lived behavioral syndrome, usually caused by some seemingly minor frustration. Angry and worked up, the child loudly accuses the offending party of lack of love, of deprivation, or of unreasonable demands. He throws himself to the floor, bangs his head, holds his breath, etc, becoming oblivious to the world around him. Because he is temporarily out of touch with the environment, little can be done during the tantrum to control or calm him. Having exhausted himself after a few minutes, the child cries and may even apologize for his behavior.

Most preschool children have tantrums; they are considered pathologic only when frequent and severe. They are a means of releasing violent, pent-up feelings for most children, but they appear most often in 2 types of children. The *pseudomature child,* as noted above, has adopted a course of apparent conformity in the hope of achieving recognition or perhaps love from his parents. When something happens to upset the fine balance of forces inside him, all of his latent hostile and aggressive feelings explode violently in a tantrum. The *"spoiled"* child is one on whom few demands are made or who is overindulged. He retains a sense of infantile omnipotence and expects to be gratified constantly. When he is denied what he wants, he has a tantrum, and he may use tantrums or threats of them to blackmail his parents.

NEUROTIC DISORDERS

The disturbances of the preschool years are apt to be transient. Most of the syndromes or symptoms of those years are motivated by or are expressions of frustration. They may also be responses to excessive or ungratifying external demands. With the development of a conscience, the child's personality structure becomes more fixed and more like that of the adult. The psychiatric syndromes likewise become more structured and less apt to dissipate with time.

Neurosis-like disturbances do occur in the preschool years in the form of poorly differentiated phobic and anxiety reactions. In addition, "preneurotic tendencies" such as inhibition, fearfulness, and overconformity are manifested in that period. Children with neurotic disturbances lead marginal, distorted lives, and the energy required to maintain their defenses against unacceptable impulses and anxiety impairs their ability to grow and learn.

ANXIETY REACTION

Chronically anxious children are fidgety, hyperactive, and tense. They tend to move about rapidly, usually have short attention spans, and often present behavior problems in school. They adapt poorly to new situations and are generally fearful. Capacity to learn is impaired, and they relate poorly to other children. Sleep disturbances are common. These children frequently awaken at night or have nightmares, and may get up early looking for something to do. Unless the free-floating anxiety becomes either bound or relieved, the child may withdraw to avoid external stimulation.

PHOBIC REACTION

Transient phobias are common in young children and serve as attempts to project their unconscious concerns onto the world.

The phobic child is one in whom these fears persist and multiply so that he may be thrown into a state of panic when confronted with the feared object or situation. The content of the phobic child's fears may be little different from that of other children, eg, fears of the dark, animals, monsters, etc, but the affect is greatly exaggerated. The content of the phobias may be an important clue to the nature of the conflict the child faces. The classic example is Freud's Little Hans, whose fear of horses was related to fear of his father's retaliation for Hans's oedipal feelings toward his mother.

OBSESSIVE COMPULSIVE REACTION

Transient obsessions and compulsions are known to occur in otherwise healthy children, and are seldom incapacitating (eg, avoiding the cracks in the sidewalk, touching telephone poles). Obsessive compulsive neurotic children present certain typical characterologic and historical features. They are described as "good" or "little ladies and gentlemen" by parents and teachers because of their pseudomature attempts to please adults. They are polite, ingratiating, overly neat and clean, and, in fact, invest a great deal of energy in developing reaction formations (opposite reactions) to all the manifestations of their basic anality. Through the mechanism of isolation, they keep their feelings hidden from themselves and from others. Despite strong controls, however, the "model child" periodically blows up in a temper tantrum or occasional episodes of sadism directed toward a usually "loved" sibling or pet. These children have stern superegos, partly the result of the defense mechanism known as identification with the aggressor, ie, parents with rigid standards and excessive expectation of conformity. On the other hand, permissively raised children may be frightened by the absence of limits on their behavior and the potentiality for destructiveness this entails, and may therefore adopt stern obsessive compulsive countermeasures to protect themselves and others.

HYSTERICAL NEUROSIS

The personality characteristics of children who develop either conversion or dissociative reactions are roughly approximate to the hysterical personality, which does not appear in full bloom until adolescence. These children tend to be naive, immature, emotionally unstable, flighty, and suggestible. Although their psychosexual development may appear to be more advanced than that of other neurotic children, they seem more dependent and clinging, especially to the parent of the opposite sex. Such children seem to have become fixed, with the seductive help of one of the parents, in the midst of the Oedipus complex.

Clear-cut conversion reactions (eg, paralysis, blindness) are rare. Transient deafness or special concern over a long-healed surgical scar are examples of what may occur. More common examples are the pregenital conversion reactions such as stuttering and tics.

Of the dissociative reactions, somnambulism is the most frequent in children. Children who have been through an episode of somnambulism are seldom perturbed by it and are amnesic for the event. Although their eyes are open and they are capable of responding to stimuli, it is evident that they are neither awake nor alert. Injury during sleepwalking seldom occurs.

DEPRESSIVE REACTION

Opinion differs about whether true depression occurs in children, especially in the early years of childhood. René Spitz's classical studies of hospitalized infants attest to the development of apathy (often irreversible), retardation of growth and development, and "depression" following prolonged absence of mothering. This kind of reaction and depressive manifestations in the preschool and early school years have different intrapsychic dynamics from the transient episodes of sadness seen in older children or in the disturbances more closely akin to adult depressions.

There is no classical syndrome of depression in childhood similar to that in adults, although there are considerable similarities in dynamics. Children sometimes say they wish they were dead, but the statement does not have the same force or urgency as with the adult. Nevertheless, some children—usually psychotic—attempt suicide. The attempt represents hopelessness and despair in the face of insoluble conflicts.

Certain cases of obesity, hypochondriasis, accident proneness, and "running away" are manifestations of depression in childhood. To some extent, disorders such as ulcerative colitis and anorexia nervosa may be depressive equivalents. The intrapsychic conflicts in all of these entities are similar: an unconscious infantilism versus a strict, rigid, punitive conscience. The emotional hunger felt by such individuals is expressed in insatiable demands on the environment and in their self-imposed prohibition and hostile response to their repeated disappointments.

PERSONALITY DISORDERS*

Personality disorders are characterized by chronic or fixed maladaptive or pathologic patterns of behavior ingrained in the personality structure. Neurotic symptom formation seldom occurs, although the behavior patterns may be resolutions of earlier neurotic conflicts. The traits usually do not produce intrapsychic distress or anxiety. As structured entities, they do not usually make a clear appearance until late latency, although there are often

*The terminology in this section and the section on psychotic disorders is drawn from Report No. 62 of the Committee on Child Psychiatry of the Group for the Advancement of Psychiatry (GAP). DSM-II and other terms, when substantially different, are enclosed in parentheses.

earlier premonitory signs (see characterologic problems of the preschool years, above).

OBSESSIVE COMPULSIVE PERSONALITY

These children are tense, rigid, and chronically overconcerned with orderliness, cleanliness, and conformity. Their pseudomaturity and liveliness ingratiate them with adults. They often have some obsessions and compulsive rituals and feel tension and anxiety when their patterns are disrupted. However, they rarely decompensate into neurotic disorders, since they tend to see the environment as the cause of their occasional distress.

HYSTERICAL PERSONALITY

This disorder is seen principally in girls. They tend to be excitable, overemotional, dramatic, flamboyant, suggestible, and coy or seductive in behavior. In spite of their apparent social "poise" they are excessively dependent on their environments and, in spite of their overt sexual behavior, suffer unusual repression of sexual impulses and have difficulties in sexual identity and relationships. They may be masochistic and may tend to be manipulative or excessively demanding, but they rarely develop hysterical symptoms in situations of conflict.

ANXIOUS PERSONALITY

Although these children are chronically tense and anxious, especially in new situations, they seldom seem aware of their anxiety and, after an initial period of disturbance, tend to adjust well to new experiences. Because of their frequently overvivid fantasies, they perceive the environment as dangerous, but marked inhibitions or personality constriction do not occur.

OVERLY DEPENDENT PERSONALITY
(Passive-Aggressive Personality, Passive-Dependent Type; Immature Personality; Unstable Personality)

Grossly, these children are "babies" who are chronically helpless, clinging, and excessively dependent. Because of their difficulty in being autonomous or developing initiative, they tend to be controlling or demanding in an infantile way.

OVERLY INDEPENDENT PERSONALITY

These children seem bent on proving that they have no weakness, defect, or need. They are impatient to grow up and are overly responsible, active, ebullient, and pseudo-adult. They frequently are impatient with and have difficulty in accepting instruction and limit-setting by adults. When physically ill, they are unable to allow themselves to stay in bed or be taken care of, often rushing prematurely into full programs of activity. Some of these children have recovered from severe illnesses or handicaps, and this may play a causative role through unconscious denial of further trouble.

OVERLY INHIBITED PERSONALITY

These are the "pathologically shy" children who manifest passivity, inhibited initiative and motor action, and severe personality constriction, sometimes with diminished speech or elective mutism. Their "withdrawal" and inhibition usually are more marked in school or other extrafamilial settings. In contrast to isolated (schizoid) children, they seem to search for close relationships but are frozen with self-doubts related to fears of rejection or aggressive initiative. They frequently have problems in school around the assimilation and reproduction of knowledge.

ISOLATED PERSONALITY
(Schizoid Personality)

In contrast to the overly inhibited child, the isolated child tends not to seek affective relationships with other individuals and seems quite satisfied with his isolation and his preoccupation with his rich fantasy life, daydreams, and autistic reveries. This entity represents a life style rather than a preschizophrenic state, even though there may be sudden outbursts of bizarre aggressive, homicidal, or antisocial behavior that are seemingly unrelated to any reality situation. Such children may be shy, oversensitive, inhibited, and relatively unobtrusive in social settings. They are often able to achieve well in intellectual and other endeavors, although they may suffer from deviations in their thinking or concept formation.

MISTRUSTFUL PERSONALITY
(Paranoid Personality)

Suspiciousness and rigidity of thinking are characteristic of these children, who may also show some isolation. This pattern is primarily a phenomenon of later adolescence and is seldom seen before puberty.

OPPOSITIONAL PERSONALITY
(Passive-Aggressive Personality, Passive-Aggressive Type)

These children, although apparently conforming, continually provoke adults and other children by negativistic and stubborn behavior, dawdling, procrastination, inefficiency, etc. These patterns are most often passively expressed but may show actively aggressive elements. Some of these children develop learning disorders characterized by "blocking out," "not hearing," or passive resistance to authority.

TENSION-DISCHARGE DISORDERS
(Explosive Personality, Aggressive Personality, Antisocial Personality, Dyssocial Behavior, Unsocialized Aggressive Reaction of Childhood)

Children in this category habitually express their aggressive and sexual impulses without restraint. There are 2 types: impulse-ridden personality and neurotic personality disorder. Children in the *impulse-ridden* group act out their impulses or feelings toward individuals or aspects of society in destructive and antisocial ways such as stealing, physical attacks, truancy, and vandalism. They seldom are able to delay or inhibit gratification of wishes or expression of emotional states, and are unable to employ psychologic defenses or symptom formation. Relationships with other people tend to be shallow. Their conflicts are external, between society and their impulses, and they experience little or no anxiety or guilt. They do not seem to learn from experience, and have poor judgment and time sense, but there is no generalized disturbance of reality testing. Two basic defects in personality development interact in these children: a defect in impulse control, with poor capacity for storage of tension and delay of gratification; and a defect in superego formation, with the development of "lacunae," in which generally prohibited behaviors are approved of. These children frequently have a history of extreme emotional deprivation in infancy and early childhood, associated with frequent and prolonged separations from mothering individuals. The proportion of impulse-ridden children coming from lower socioeconomic levels is much higher than from other groups, but the disorder can appear in any level of society.

Children with *neurotic personality disorders* manifest the same behavior patterns as the impulse-ridden children except that their acting out is for the purpose of discharging tension resulting from repressed neurotic conflicts. They experience anxiety and guilt. Their antisocial behavior is repetitive, almost stylized, and symbolic, and their guilt seems to lead them to invite punishment or the establishment of limits. These children tend to have warmer—although ambivalent—interpersonal relationships, and have reasonably good impulse control during periods when conflict is reduced.

SOCIOSYNTONIC PERSONALITY DISORDER
(Dyssocial Reaction, Group Delinquent Reaction of Childhood)

This group includes children whose behavior patterns are consonant with the values and patterns of particular subgroups or subcultures within the larger social framework but are somehow different. One subcategory consists of children whose aggressive, destructive, or antisocial behavior is sanctioned by gang, neighborhood, or family ("hoods," "psychopaths"). The other subcategory includes certain patterns of personality derived from specific subcultures which hold beliefs or have experiences considered normal or desirable in the group but which are regarded as bizarre or peculiar by members of the majority culture (eg, "hippies").

SEXUAL DEVIATION

Few children can be included in this group, although disturbances of sexual identification such as effeminate traits in boys and transient sexual deviation such as exhibitionism or voyeurism are not uncommon.

JUVENILE DELINQUENCY*

Juvenile delinquency is essentially a legal term, not a psychiatric term. A juvenile delinquent is defined as a child who commits acts that would be considered crimes if committed by an adult. The upper age limit of childhood is usually taken to be 17 or 18, with a lower limit of 6 or 7. Children may also be adjudged delinquents for certain statutory offenses pertaining only to children, eg, truancy, running away, "waywardness," and, in some jurisdictions, disobedience toward parents or teachers. From a diagnostic standpoint, the majority of delinquent children fall within the group of tension-discharge disorders (see above). Since children with other disorders (mental retardation, brain damage, etc) may be involved in antisocial acts of various kinds, it is obvious that neither juvenile delinquents nor their offenses comprise homogeneous groups.

Outpatient psychiatric intervention is sometimes helpful, but many children with predelinquent tendencies or who are involved in delinquent or antisocial behavior are not referred to child psychiatric services until some crisis occurs which threatens to be resolved by school authorities, the police, or the courts. Because of the high incidence of juvenile delinquency under conditions of poverty, familial disorganization, and racial discrimination, questions of prevention and treatment often must be answered in social terms. If a child is brought to psychiatric attention before he becomes irrevocably involved with the authorities, placement in residential treatment centers or other group facilities may constitute the best treatment because it removes the child from a malignant environment and makes available reasonable controls and care.

PSYCHOPHYSIOLOGIC DISORDERS

The psychophysiologic disorders (see Chapter 18) are those conditions in which there are significant interactions between psychologic and somatic factors. They usually involve disturbances in organs or systems innervated by

*Not a GAP Committee on Child Psychiatry category.

the autonomic nervous system. The mechanisms are complex and poorly understood. Certain conflicts may predispose to certain types of illness, but attempts to distinguish type-specific profiles of personality, parent-child relationships, family patterns, social conditions, etc have been inconclusive. Often it is not clear whether the emotional disorder found in the child with a psychophysiologic disturbance is part of the illness, or its cause, or a reaction to it.

Some of the disorders considered by some authors to be due to psychophysiologic factors occur relatively frequently in childhood or early adolescence: certain types of obesity, "functional" constipation, eczema, bronchial asthma, anorexia nervosa, and ulcerative colitis. However, there is considerable evidence, for example, that obesity and anorexia nervosa may be "attitudinal" rather than "autonomic" disorders related to conflicts around eating.

The child psychiatrist is required to evaluate or treat a relatively unrepresentative sample of children with physical or psychophysiologic disorders. Some are referred because the attending physician believes the illness to be "psychological"; some because medical treatment has not succeeded in conditions considered severe or intractable; and others because they have obvious emotional or behavioral disturbances. All of these children should receive psychiatric evaluation and treatment appropriate to whatever emotional disorder is found, irrespective of the physical illness. A reasonable, realistic, and open relationship between the psychiatrist and the pediatrician or family physician can have only positive results for the patient.

PSYCHOTIC DISORDERS

The disorders included in this category are the so-called "functional" psychoses of childhood. The psychotic disorders of childhood cause severe, pervasive deviations from age-related behavioral expectations. The basic disorder appears to be extreme distortion of the process of personality development, with severe disturbances in functions related to thought, affect, perception, behavior, speech, and individuation and marked deficiencies in object relationships and reality testing. The specific manifestations of the psychotic disorders are determined very much by the age of the child. Clinically, such children exhibit most of the following symptoms or signs in varying degrees:

(1) Severe, continued impairment of emotional relationships with persons, together with aloofness and tendencies toward preoccupation with inanimate objects.

(2) Failure to develop speech or loss of speech development.

(3) Disturbances in sensory perception.

(4) Bizarre or stereotyped behavior or patterns of movement.

(5) Marked resistance to change in routine or environment.

(6) Outbursts of intense and often unpredictable panic.

(7) Lack of a sense of personal identity.

(8) Blunted, fragmented, or uneven intellectual development.

Differential Diagnosis of Childhood Psychotic Disorders

One of the most important and sometimes most difficult diagnostic decisions in child psychiatry is the differentiation of psychotic disorders from other disorders with some or many of the same clinical features. The practical issues of treatment, prognosis, and, particularly, institutionalization are crucial because the "strangeness" of such children sets them apart from other children and realistic plans must be made with their parents. When the diagnosis of a psychotic disorder is entertained, the following conditions should be considered.

(1) Deafness: Many deaf or partially deaf children tend to become autistic because of their isolation, and may be mute because of their inability to learn language. Psychotic children are usually inconsistent in their responses to audiometric examinations, being "deaf" at times and not at others. The reaction of truly deaf children to other persons is usually warm and responsive.

(2) Aphasia: When severe aphasia is compounded with early neglect or rejection, a child may become autistic, apathetic, unresponsive, and mute. Children with severe or intractable mutism often prove to be psychotic.

(3) Mental retardation: Psychotic children are sometimes diagnosed as mentally retarded because of their overall poor intellectual functioning. They may exhibit profound and unexpected inconsistencies in their responses to various tests, although most have severe difficulties in abstract reasoning. Retarded children, especially if they have been rejected and isolated from social contact, sometimes present full-blown pictures of autistic behavior that may resolve after a relationship is established with them.

(4) Brain damage: As is true of retarded and aphasic children also, brain damaged children with a history of early neglect, rejection, or isolation may simulate psychosis, with emotional lability, erratic responses, poor tolerance of environmental change, and autism. In general, however, these children tend to be overresponsive to external stimuli.

(5) Severe neurotic disorders: Psychosis should be strongly suspected in children with severe and multiple neurotic symptoms, especially if anxiety is not relieved by the symptoms and if reality testing is shown to be distorted. Withdrawal and mutism, the latter of which may be "elective," are not pathognomonic of psychosis in children and may occur in severe neuroses.

(6) Personality disorders with severe tension-discharge disturbances: Children with severe personality disorders frequently display bizarre, primitive behavior which is more apt to be due to failure of socialization than to psychotic thinking or relational incapacity. Such children are very disturbed and disturbing, but they have ego and superego defects rather than ego distortion or disintegration.

EARLY INFANTILE AUTISM

This disorder manifests itself as early as the first few months of life, most significantly through the infant's failure to develop any attachment to the mother, showing little or no apparent awareness of human contact. This entity, in which the autism is primary (as opposed to the secondary autism seen in brain damage and mental retardation), was first described by Leo Kanner in 1943. Associated symptoms include preoccupation with inanimate objects; absent or delayed speech, which, if it appears, may not be used for communication or used appropriately; resistance to change, to which the child responds with violent outbursts of temper or severe anxiety; severe problems with sleeping and feeding; and strange, stereotyped motor patterns.

INTERACTIONAL PSYCHOTIC DISORDERS

This term and the entity it describes are essentially equivalent to the symbiotic infantile psychosis first described by Margaret Mahler in 1952. These children usually develop adequately during the first and second years and subsequently manifest unusual dependence on the mother, with intensification and prolongation of the attachment. At some point between ages 2 and 4, the psychosis appears, precipitated by some real or imagined threat to the mother-child relationship. The child suddenly displays intense clinging and separation anxiety. Marked regressive symptoms then appear— particularly the relinquishing of communicative speech. Gradual withdrawal, aloofness, autistic behavior, and distortion of reality often lead to a picture little different from that of infantile autism. Beata Rank's preschool children with "atypical development" probably belong in this classification.

SCHIZOPHRENIA, CHILDHOOD TYPE

The onset of this disorder usually occurs between ages 6 and 11–12 and is often gradual, with neurotic symptoms appearing first. These are followed by severe and primitive denial and projection, looseness of associations, concrete thinking (literal interpretations and inability to form abstract concepts), low frustration tolerance, intense temper outbursts, and hypochondriacal concerns. The illness progresses to marked withdrawal, intense involvement in fantasy, autistic behavior, emotional aloofness, true thinking disorders, and defective reality testing. Other forms, in which the onset may be sudden and acute, involving crises with severe anxiety, uncontrollable phobias, and withdrawal, progress also to autistic behavior and loss of reality testing. Bizarre and stereotyped behavior (eg, whirling) and identification with inanimate objects are frequently present. Suicide threats and attempts or explosive outbursts of aggressive or self-mutilative behavior are also seen. Marked secondary mental retardation may occur, although this is not the rule.

Adult types of schizophrenia are seldom seen in children.

ORGANIC BRAIN SYNDROMES

Although young children seem to have great ability to compensate for the impairment of brain tissue, there may be profound effects on functions which develop at later stages, especially cognition and impulse control. The substance of the personality disturbances that occur in brain damaged children is related to the level of the child's development, predisposing personality patterns, current emotional conflicts and intrafamily relationships, and the nature of the organic disturbance and the attitudes of the child and family to it.

It too often happens that the diagnosis of "brain damage" (as well as of mental retardation) implies a kind of hopeless finality, so that a definitive diagnosis of these disorders should be made with considerable caution. (See also Chapter 15.)

Acute organic brain syndrome is manifested by delirium, which is usually reversible. Delirious children exhibit wildly agitated or confused behavior Subclinical forms may be seen also, with mild stuporous states, impairment of awareness, withdrawal, or irrational fears. In the absence of gross brain damage, children recovering from these disorders may have persistent perceptual and motor disturbances which affect learning ability in school.

Chronic disturbances of memory, judgment, comprehension, affect, learning ability, etc due to organic brain damage are persistent handicaps. Mental retardation may be present in some cases. There does not appear to be a "typical" personality disorder associated with these syndromes. Nevertheless, a *hyperkinetic syndrome* is seen frequently in preschool and younger school-age children, consisting of hyperactivity, distractibility, impulsiveness, and short attention span associated with diffuse EEG and EMG abnormalities. Such children also have difficulties in reading, writing, and abstract thinking (concreteness) as well as impairment of visual-motor coordination, spatial relations, etc. Because of the lack of specific neurologic defects and because young children with severe psychologic disturbances also exhibit similar manifestations, the differential diagnosis must be based on a documented history of early cerebral injury.

MISCELLANEOUS PSYCHIATRIC DISORDERS OF CHILDHOOD

SCHOOL REFUSAL
("School Phobia")

School refusal is a relatively common phenomenon manifested by anxiety, gastrointestinal symptoms (stomach ache, nausea, or vomiting), and expressions of dislike or fear of school or particular aspects of school. The symptoms usually take place in the morning before school, especially on Mondays or on the day of return from holidays.

Differentiation must be made between school refusal and truancy or malingering. School refusers usually look quite ill, so that their frequently overindulgent mothers send them right back to bed. Malingerers complain of being sick but rarely succeed in a perfect portrayal. Truants seldom insist on staying home, but rather pretend to go to school without ever getting there. School refusers generally are afraid to leave their homes, and especially their mothers.

Neurotic Type

This type of school refusal usually occurs in the early school years. It is associated with intense anxiety, usually over separation from the mother, and may be associated with other neurotic symptoms, especially phobias. The mother and her own conflicts may be a party to the problem.

Personality Disorder Type

This type usually is seen in the later elementary or junior high school years in children with persistent personality disturbances, and is associated with chronic argumentativeness, temper tantrums, and disobedience.

Psychotic Type

In school refusal with onset in adolescence, the existence of a psychotic disorder should be considered. In the psychotic type, there is severe, pervasive anxiety, often with paranoid trends involving suspicions and accusations against other students or school personnel. The syndrome is considered a manifestation of a need for close mothering and fearfulness of social contact and environmental change.

FIRE-SETTING

This symptomatic behavior, because of its potential for major damage and of its frequent association with psychotic and psychotic-like (borderline) disorders, is a significant cause of mandatory institutionalization of children. Boys, especially, normally play with matches and fires in the preschool and school years. Pathologic incendiarism is seen most frequently in the late latency or preadolescent periods, usually in association with aggressiveness and other types of antisocial behavior. Pathologic fire-setting is carried out in the context of fantasies of aggressive revenge against parents. Adolescent fire-setters often operate in pairs, plan their fires well, and arrange to view the conflagration while experiencing intense feelings of excitement, pleasure, and power, often with a strong erotic component.

READING DISABILITY
(Dyslexia, Etc)

Specific reading disability affects about 10% of all school children. It is seen in children of all levels of intelligence in whom reading ability is retarded in relation to intelligence. There is a tendency to familial occurrence. (Not included in this group are mentally retarded children or children with overall marginal academic performance resulting from personality disorders or social or familial disorganization and deprivation.) Boys are 4 times as frequently affected as girls. The correlation with tension-release, acting-out behavior disturbances (appearing first in the classroom and later elsewhere) is high, as is the correlation with neurotic disorders; these are associated with depression, low self-esteem, and a sense of futility and hopelessness. These children are soon classified by teachers as "slow learners" because they may have difficulties in writing and arithmetic as well as reading. It is likely that the other problems these children have are secondary to their sense of failure in reading.

Reading Disability Associated With Brain Damage

Reading potential may be impaired by brain damage with manifest neurologic deficits and with associated aphasias.

Primary Reading Disability

These children manifest defects in the ability to deal with letters and words as symbols, probably because of a basic disturbance in cerebral organization. There is usually no other evidence of gross neurologic disorder by history and examination.

Despite considerable speculation about the effects of methods of teaching reading and of emotional factors, genetic factors, etc, little is known about the causes of primary reading disability, despite its frequent association with left-handedness or crossed eye-hand dominance ("mixed brain dominance"). Remedial reading with special emphasis on phonics and training in spatial orientation, along with psychiatric treatment of associated personality disturbances, holds the greatest promise of help for children with the primary type of reading disability.

Secondary Reading Disability

A child may have a normal reading potential that is not being utilized because of neurotic, psychotic, or external social influences.

TREATMENT RESOURCES IN CHILD PSYCHIATRY

INDIVIDUAL OUTPATIENT TREATMENT

The type of therapy most often used in individual outpatient treatment of children consists of psychoanalytically oriented psychotherapy using play technics, in association with parallel psychiatric casework with the parents and environmental manipulation and modification. The major characteristics of psychotherapeutic work with children can be summarized briefly as follows:

(1) The therapist should attempt to develop a meaningful interpersonal relationship with the child and apply it to situations in the child's usual environment.

(2) He should control the child's behavior within the treatment context both by virtue of his position as an authority figure and his special relationship with the child.

(3) Therapy is a significant and unique occurrence in the child's life because of what happens within the process, the special circumstances under which it takes place, and the therapist's ability to make changes in the child's environment by influencing important adults.

(4) Child psychotherapy requires great expenditures of effort by the therapist, who must be an active, direct participant in the proceedings, always alert to the communications, affects, and behavior of the child.

(5) Child psychotherapy is almost exclusively oriented to the "here and now" and is located within an environmental context which contributes to and perpetuates the child's disorder and with which he must constantly cope.

OTHER OUTPATIENT THERAPEUTIC RESOURCES

Day School

Therapeutic day schools and day care centers have the advantage of permitting the patient to maintain continued contact with his family. They provide a specially oriented therapeutic milieu for children unable to cope with regular school programs. They are especially beneficial for younger children with behavior and learning disturbances.

Special Classes or Programs in Public School

Special classes are designed for emotionally disturbed youngsters who can remain at home and attend small classes at regular schools. The success of such programs depends on the maturity and background of the teacher, continuing psychotherapy, and a close working relationship between teacher and psychiatrist.

Group Psychotherapy

Two types of group therapy have been developed for children. *Activity group therapy* is a type of program in which children play and function together as a "club" or group, with the group leader, usually a psychiatrist, participating in the activities as coach or advisor while providing help in working through interpersonal and individual crises. *Analytic group therapy* may use any of the technics of activity therapy but involves also group interview technics similar to group therapy for adults, and is oriented toward older children and adolescents.

CHILD PSYCHOANALYSIS

Psychoanalysis is a costly and prolonged procedure that is seldom indicated as the treatment of choice in children. In general, the indications for psychoanalysis in the latency period apply also, with modifications, to other age groups:

(1) The classical neuroses (conversion hysteria, obsessive compulsive, and phobic reactions).

(2) Psychosexual regression, eg, regressive enuresis.

(3) Cases in which children consciously wish to be or behave as if they were of the opposite sex.

(4) Antisocial behavior associated with neurotic personality disorders.

(5) Pregenital conversion syndromes, eg, tics and stuttering.

(6) Sexual perversions.

RESIDENTIAL TREATMENT

Inpatient or residential treatment is indicated whenever it is necessary to remove the child from his usual environment because he cannot cope with it or because the environment is a major contributing factor to his illness, or whenever the child is in danger of seriously harming himself or others. There are situations also in which total milieu therapy (see below) is called for by the circumstances of the illness.

The distinction between the child psychiatric hospital or service as opposed to the residential treatment center should be clarified. Children's inpatient services have traditionally functioned similarly to mental hospitals for adults in that they have focused on the management of psychoses and severe behavioral disorders and have tended to be custodial rather than therapeutic institutions. Residential treatment centers have tended to be based on boarding school models with emphasis on education and group living but employing a variety of intensive psychiatric, vocational, and other therapeutic activities. In general, each residential treatment center establishes limited criteria for admission on the grounds of diagnosis, general behavior, and intelligence level, as well as on the types of treatment programs they provide. Both kinds of facilities are beginning to offer similar resources for disturbed children.

The practical therapeutic objective of *milieu therapy* is to provide an orderly environment in which corrective emotional and learning experiences can take place. It is an attempt at total reeducation of the child in new modes of behavior, feelings, and relationships which will persist after he leaves the center. Intensive psychotherapy is given by a psychiatrist, and other staff members provide emotional support and education with emphasis on the therapeutic work and insights.

PLACEMENT PROGRAMS

Foster and boarding homes, group homes, juvenile detention centers, boarding schools, and general and therapeutic summer camps fall into this category. These types of placement are similar to those provided by social agencies, sometimes for similar reasons, eg, family disorganization or pathology. Some children benefit immensely from being away from home in a reasonably favorable environment without formal psychotherapeutic treatment. This kind of treatment decision depends on a thorough study of the child, his family, and the placement facility. Juvenile detention centers are often more apt to be punitive institutions, although in some communities improvements in procedures, physical environment, and staffing (both professional and nonprofessional) have changed the old "reform schools" into useful therapeutic centers.

SOMATIC METHODS OF TREATMENT

Electroconvulsive Therapy

There is no longer any justification for the use of electroconvulsive treatment in children. Most of the earlier indications for it are now indications for pharmacologic treatment, especially with the phenothiazines and related compounds.

Psychopharmacologic Agents*

(1) Antipsychotic agents (phenothiazines): Chlorpromazine and related drugs have an important use in the modification of severely disturbed behavior, improving the ability of children to relate well to the therapist and to become involved in psychotherapy. They are used in outpatient and inpatient settings for the relief of anxiety, motor excitation, hyperactivity, aggressiveness, and impulsiveness.

(2) Antianxiety agents (also called minor tranquilizers): Benzodiazepines (eg, chlordiazepoxide, diazepam) and dicarbamates (eg, meprobamate) are frequently used by general practitioners and pediatricians in cases of mild anxiety states, night terrors, and similar disturbances. The use of these agents for the relief of mild anxiety states in children has had inconsistent results.

(3) Barbiturates: These drugs are used as mild sedatives and can be as effective as the antianxiety agents. The 2 groups have similar pharmacologic characteristics. Rarely, barbiturates may cause excitement in a child.

(4) Amphetamines: Dextroamphetamine and other amphetamines have a paradoxic "tranquilizing" effect when given to children with hyperkinetic syndromes involving hyperactivity, short attention span, impulsiveness, and emotional lability, and to children with hyperactivity due to brain damage. When effective, as it frequently is, amphetamine treatment of hyperkinetic children can continue for years without ill effect.

*All of these drugs are discussed fully in Chapter 24.

(5) Antidepressants: The antidepressants have been used primarily in severely disturbed hospitalized children and with variable effectiveness. Imipramine has been shown to be effective against nocturnal enuresis since one of the side-effects of the drug is urinary retention.

REFERENCES

Books and Monographs

Berlin, I.N.: *Bibliography of Child Psychiatry: With a Selected List of Films.* American Psychiatric Association, 1963.

Committee on Child Psychiatry: *The Diagnostic Process in Child Psychiatry.* GAP Report No. 38. Group for the Advancement of Psychiatry, 1957.

Committee on Child Psychiatry: *Psychopathological Disorders in Childhood: Theoretical Considerations and a Proposed Classification.* GAP Report No. 62. Group for the Advancement of Psychiatry, 1968.

Erikson, E.H.: *Childhood and Society.* Norton, 1950.

Finch, S.M.: *Fundamentals of Child Psychiatry.* Norton, 1960.

Ginott, H.G.: *Between Parent & Child.* Macmillan, 1965.

Kanner, L.: *Child Psychiatry.* Thomas, 1962.

Kliman, G.: *Psychological Emergencies of Childhood.* Grune & Stratton, 1968.

Pearson, G.H.J. (editor): *A Handbook of Child Psychoanalysis.* Basic Books, 1968.

Psychoanalytic Study of the Child. Internat Univ Press, 1945–present. [Annual. Various editors.]

Shaw, C.R.: *The Psychiatric Disorders of Childhood.* Appleton-Century-Crofts, 1966.

Wolff, P.H.: *The Developmental Psychologies of Jean Piaget and Psychoanalysis.* Psychological Issues, Monograph No. 5. Internat Univ Press, 1960.

Wolman, B.B.: *Children Without Childhood: A Study of Childhood Schizophrenia.* Grune & Stratton, 1971.

Journal Articles

Aird, R.B., & T. Yamamoto: Behavior disorders of childhood. Electroenceph Clin Neurophysiol 21:148–156, 1966.

Bender, L.: Childhood schizophrenia. Psychiat Quart 27:1-19, 1953.

Benedek, T.: The psychosomatic implications of the primary unit: Mother-child. Am J Orthopsychiat 19:642–654, 1949.

Blumenthal, M.D.: Experiences of parents of retardates and children with cystic fibrosis. Arch Gen Psychiat 21:160–171, 1969.

Bowlby, J.: The nature of the child's tie to his mother. Int J Psychoanal 39:350–373, 1958.

Buxbaum, E.: Technique of child therapy: A critical evaluation. Psychoanal Stud Child 9:297–333, 1954.

Conners, C.K., & others: Dextroamphetamine sulfate in children with learning disorders. Gen Psychiat 21:182–190, 1969.

Court, D., & M. Harris: Speech disorders in children. Brit MJ 2:345–347, 1965.

Eveloff, H.H.: Psychopharmacologic agents in child psychiatry. Arch Gen Psychiat 14:472–481, 1966.

Fish, B.: Drug use in psychiatric disorders of children. Am J Psychiat 124(Suppl):31–36, 1968.

Freud, A.: The concept of developmental lines. Psychoanal Stud Child 18:245–265, 1963.

Hingtgen, J.N., & D.W. Churchill: Identification of perceptual limitations in mute autistic children. Arch Gen Psychiat 21:68–71, 1969.

Kanner, L.: Problems of nosology and psychodynamics of early infantile autism. Am J Orthopsychiat 19:416–426, 1949.

Klein, M.: The psychoanalytic play technique. Am J Orthopsychiat 25:223–237, 1955.

Kramer, Y., & L.A. Rosenblum: Responses to "frustration" in one-year-old infants. Psychosom Med 32:243–256, 1970.

Lapouse, R.: Epidemiology of behavior disorders in children. Am J Dis Child 111:594–599, 1966.

Levy, S.: The hyperkinetic child: A forgotten entity—its diagnosis and treatment. Internat J Neuropsychiat 2:330–336, 1966.

Lurie, O.R.: The emotional health of children in the family setting. Commun Ment Health J 6:229–235, 1970.

Maurer, A.: What children fear. J Genet Psychol 106:265–278, 1965.

Menking, M., & others: Rumination: A near fatal psychiatric disease of infancy. New England J Med 280:802–804, 1969.

Munro, A.: Parent-child separation. Arch Gen Psychiat 20:598–604, 1969.

Pavenstedt, E.: A comparison of child-rearing environment of upper-lower and very low-lower class families. Am J Orthopsychiat 35:89–98, 1965.

Rexford, E.: A developmental concept of the problems of acting out. J Am Acad Child Psychiat 2:19–21, 1963.

Rexford, E.N.: Children, child psychiatry, and our brave new world. Arch Gen Psychiat 20:25–37, 1969.

Rochlin, G.: The dread of abandonment: A contribution to the etiology of the loss complex and depression. Psychoanal Stud Child 16:451–470, 1961.

Sperling, M.: School phobias. Psychoanal Stud Child 22:375–401, 1967.

Spitz, R.A.: The psychogenic diseases in infancy: An attempt at their etiologic classification. Psychoanal Stud Child 6:255–275, 1951.

33...
Mental Subnormality

Progress is being made in understanding and preventing this widespread affliction. Pediatricians and psychologists can help in diagnosis and therapeutic advice; management remains largely with parents and teachers. Parents need counseling at crises: first suspicion of diagnosis, time of diagnostic studies, school entrance, adjustment problems with siblings and peers, pubertal sex problems, job seeking, marriage, and institutional placement.

The American Association for Mental Deficiency defines mental deficiency as below average general intellectual functioning, originating in the developmental period, associated with impairment of adaptive behavior. According to the World Health Organization definition, mental subnormality consists of 2 categories: (1) that due to environmental causes with no CNS impairment (mental retardation), and (2) that due to CNS disorders (mental deficiency).

Intelligence is the ability to solve problems, adapt to new situations, form abstract concepts, and profit from experience. Apart from the regulation of internal homeostasis, the prime function of the CNS is adaptation of the organism to its environment. The adaptability of each species is determined in part by the form, structure, and function of its CNS. Man is born with the least differentiated and most adaptable CNS. Potentially normal humans trace their phylogenetic heritage from the level of reflex "intelligence" to levels of intellectual functioning characteristic of the species. The human potential for intelligence is inherited as a multifactorial genetic trait. Like similar traits, it follows an essentially "normal" frequency distribution curve, but the lower end of the curve is skewed by increased numbers of severely retarded individuals who may be regarded as "reproduction casualities." Statistically, 16% of individuals should have IQs below 85 and 2% below 70 (Fig 33—1).

FACTORS AFFECTING INTELLIGENCE

The undifferentiated state of the human infant's brain makes the infant dependent upon others for a long time. During this prolonged dependency, environmental factors play a crucial role in determining whether the individual develops his full intellectual potential. Intellectual potential is a reflection of biologic endowment; intellectual functioning is the summation of the interplay of endowment and environmental factors. An optimal environment may enhance intellectual functioning by 10-20 points as measured on IQ tests. An intellectually adverse environment may lead to profound or lesser degrees of mental subnormality. Early in development, intellectual subnormality due to adverse environmental influences may be corrected by providing an intellectually stimulating environment. As the child approaches maturity, his intellectual functioning becomes fixed. During early infancy and childhood, absent or deficient maternal care may be the major factor leading to varying degrees of mental subnormality. During later years, complex cultural and socioeconomic factors may result in a lower level of intellectual functioning. The biologic, sociocultural, and psychologic factors affecting intellectual functioning are illustrated in Fig 33–2.

CLASSIFICATION OF MENTAL RETARDATION

Mental retardation may be classified according to IQ, developmental characteristics, potential for education, or social and vocational adequacy. (See Tables 33–1 and 33–2.) There is no valid way of measuring social adaptability, but it is a far more reliable indication of the child's eventual outcome as an adult than his IQ. Many children with low IQs fit in well as adults because of their good social adjustment, whereas others with higher IQs end up in institutions because of their deviant behavior. Classifications have been based primarily on intelligence testing, but in assessing the potential for socially adequate adjustments in individual cases, the physician's observations and judgment are as important as objective ratings by IQ scores.

Previous concepts of mental deficiency in terms of diagnostic entities based upon clinical impressions and empiric observations have fortunately been discarded. The terms "moron," "imbecile," and "idiot" no longer serve a useful purpose and can actually be misleading. Mental subnormality is not classified according to cause (eg, hereditary, familial, or secondary to organic disease); and degrees of deficiency are expressed as "mild," "moderate," "severe," or "profound" according to the results of psychometric tests.

TABLE 33–1. Classification of mental retardation.

American Psychiatric Association		World Health Organization		American Association for Mental Deficiency	
IQ	Terminology	IQ	Terminology	IQ	Terminology
70–85	Mild mental deficiency	50–69	Mild subnormality	70–84	Borderline
50–70	Moderate	20–49	Moderate	55–69	Mild
0–50	Severe	0–19	Severe	40–54	Moderate

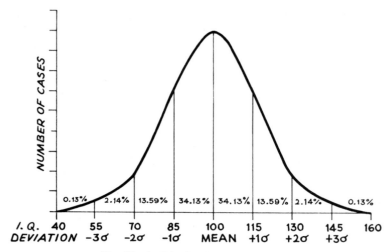

Fig 33—1. Distribution of intelligence.

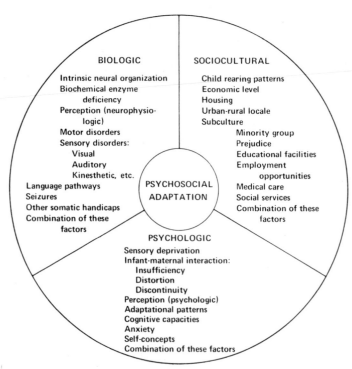

Fig 33—2. **Biologic, sociocultural, and psychologic factors influencing intellectual development.** (Redrawn and reproduced, with permission, from Richmond & Custman: J Med Educ 29:23, May 1954.)

TABLE 33–2. Developmental characteristics of the mentally retarded.* The table integrates chronologic age, degree of retardation, and level of intellectual, vocational, and social functioning.

Degree of Mental Retardation	Preschool Age 0–5 Maturation and Development	School Age 6–20 Training and Education	Adult 21 and Over Social and Vocational Adequacy
Mild	Can develop social and communication skills; minimal retardation in sensorimotor areas; often not distinguished from normal until later age.	Can learn academic skills up to approximately 6th grade level by late teens; can be guided toward social conformity.	Can usually achieve social and vocational skills adequate to minimum self-support but may need guidance and assistance when under unusual social or economic stress.
Moderate	Can talk or learn to communicate; poor social awareness; fair motor development; profits from training in self-help; can be managed with moderate supervision.	Can profit from training in social and occupational skills; unlikely to progress beyond 2nd grade level in academic subjects; may learn to travel alone in familiar places.	May achieve self-maintenance in unskilled or semiskilled work under sheltered conditions; needs supervision and guidance when under mild social or economic stress.
Severe	Poor motor development; speech minimal; generally unable to profit from training in self-help; little or no communication skills.	Can talk or learn to communicate; can be trained in elemental health habits; profits from systematic habit training.	May contribute partially to self-maintenance under complete supervision; can develop self-protection skills to a minimal useful level in controlled environment.
Profound	Gross retardation; minimal capacity for functioning in sensorimotor areas; needs nursing care.	Some motor development present; may respond to minimal or limited training in self-help.	Some motor and speech development; may achieve very limited self-care; needs nursing care.

*Adapted from Mental Retardation Activities of the U.S. Department of Health, Education, and Welfare, page 2. United States Government Printing Office, Washington, 1963.

TABLE 33–3. Incidence of mental retardation.

Age	Percentage of Retarded in Population	Comments
0–6	1%	Usually specific syndromes (eg, Down's syndrome) or major CNS insults.
6–16	3%	Peak at age 10–14 due to scholastic failures.
16 and over	1%	Functionally retarded as adults in society.

INCIDENCE OF MENTAL SUBNORMALITY

The incidence of diagnosed mental subnormality in preschool children is lower than in children of school age (Table 33–3). This is the result of several factors. CNS maturation continues from gestation until midadolescence. Many higher intellectual functions have not been differentiated in the preschool child. There is no way of predicting which children will subsequently develop higher intellectual functions and which will not. The peak incidence of mental subnormality during school years is a reflection of (1) the failure of some children to develop higher intellectual functions, (2) the educational system's emphasis on certain forms of abstract thought, and (3) the cumulative effect of environmental factors affecting intelligence.

The apparent decline in the incidence of mental retardation in the adult population can be attributed to the fact that many of the adaptational tasks of adulthood only require intelligence in keeping with a grade 5 education. Thus, the individual who was judged intellectually subnormal in a high school environment may be adaptationally adequate in his chosen occupation. Some mentally subnormal individuals continue to develop intellectually into adulthood.

Most mental retardation (87%) is mild, and these people usually remain in the community. The remaining 13% are moderately, severely, or profoundly retarded. Four percent of retarded people are in institutions, but this percentage is expected to decrease as alternative patterns of care in the community are developed.

ETIOLOGY OF MENTAL SUBNORMALITY

Many factors are to be found in the varied etiology of mental retardation. Certain maternal, obstetric, or fetal diseases or disorders as well as genetic factors play the most important part. A detailed list is given below.

High risk infants (those whose personal or family history has antecedent factors mentioned below) should be assessed at periodic intervals. Children showing developmental delays may merit more intensive investigation. About 3% of premature infants show later abnormalities of intellectual

Factors Associated in Some Degree With Mental Subnormality*

Family history

Presence of mutant genes
CNS disorders
Low socioeconomic group

Previous defective sibling
Parental consanguinity
Intrafamilial emotional disorder

Medical history of mother

Diabetes
Hypertension
Roentgen radiation

Cardiovascular or renal disease
Thyroid disease
Idiopathic thrombocytopenic purpuras

Obstetric history of mother

Toxemia
Miscarriage immediately preceding
  pregnancy

Unusual size of infants
High parity
Prolonged infertility

Present pregnancy

Absence of prenatal care
Maternal age ($<$ 18 or $>$ 38)
Multiple births
Polyhydramnios
Oligohydramnios
Out of wedlock pregnancy
Medications

Roentgen radiation
Anesthesia
Maternal rubella in first trimester
Diabetes
Toxemia
Fetal-maternal blood group
  incompatibility

Labor and delivery

Prematurity
Postmaturity-dysmaturity

Precipitate, prolonged, or complicated
  delivery
Low Apgar score 5 minutes after birth

Placenta

Massive infarction
Amnion nodosum

Placentitis

Neonatal

Single umbilical artery
Jaundice
Unusual head size
Infection
Hypoxia
Severe dehydration, hyperosmolarity,
  and hypernatremia
Convulsions

Failure to regain birth weight by
  10 days
Manifest congenital defects
Disproportion between weight or length
  and gestational age
Survival following meningitides, en-
  cephalopathies, and traumatic intracranial episodes

*Adapted from *Proceedings of the White House Conference on Mental Retardation.* Washington, DC, 1963.

functioning—either general mental subnormality or isolated intellectual deficits such as aphasia or dyslexia.

CLINICAL FINDINGS

The chief characteristics of mental retardation are delayed biologic development, immature social adaptation, and failure to develop the capacity for higher types of thought processes. Mild impairment of thought processes may be the only symptom of cultural or familial retardation. Numerous and complex disturbances of physical development and intellectual functioning result from specific genetic syndromes or brain injury.

Most cases of mild retardation represent a convergence of the factors listed in Fig 33–2. These children frequently come to the attention of psychiatrists because of learning or adjustment problems. The diagnosis and treatment of severe mental retardation is usually a pediatric rather than a psychiatric problem. Specific genetic syndromes are often responsible (see Chapter 8).

History

The pediatric medical and developmental history may reveal delayed motor, language, and social development. Mildly retarded children may develop normally before entering school. Anxious parents may present a falsely normal developmental history or may be unable to remember developmental milestones. Motor and language development parallel but are not synonymous with intellectual development, and this often leads to diagnostic errors.

Physical Examination

People with mild retardation are usually physically normal, but they may be dysplastic, ie, have unusual or coarse features, especially peculiar eyes, stubby fingers, and disproportionate body measurements.

Neurologic Examination

The pediatric neurologic examination is primarily an assessment of motor behavior. Much can be learned from comparison of fine and gross motor play patterns with normal children in settings such as kindergarten. In the more detailed neurologic examination, the retarded child often displays "soft" neurologic signs (strabismus, facial paralysis, unequal reflexes, altered muscle tone, clumsiness, poor coordination, and hyperactivity).

Speech, Language, and Hearing

Problems of differential diagnosis arise in these areas because both deafness and developmental aphasia may be confused with mental retardation and because many retarded children are partially deaf or have some type of language handicap, eg, peripheral speech impediments and central aphasic problems. Hearing and language tests are important in the evaluation of young children with delayed development. Delayed physical development may be the first cause of parental concern.

Testing young children is difficult. Serial assessments by psychologists accustomed to working with young children may be necessary.

Laboratory Studies

About 1% of severely retarded children have demonstrable inborn errors of metabolism. It has been estimated that possibly 10% of severely retarded children may have inborn errors of metabolism which cannot be proven as yet with contemporary laboratory technics. Apart from routine screening for phenylketonuria, other studies should be individually planned. Detailed metabolic investigations can be pursued in medical centers where equipment and personnel are available. EEGs may be of some assistance in cases of brain injury. Complex or hazardous procedures (eg, pneumo-encephalography) should be done only on specific indications.

In mild retardation, there are usually no abnormal laboratory findings.

Educational Assessment

Practice teaching sessions, wide range achievement tests, and diagnostic reading tests by specially trained teachers can be used to assess the educational level of retarded children of school age. Other tests (eg, Frostig and Kephart tests) are used to assess perceptual and motor skills which underlie educational tasks. From these, individual educational programs are developed based on the child's educational strengths and weaknesses.

Retarded children are divided broadly into trainable and educable, depending upon their ability to handle formal academic instruction.

Psychologic Assessment (Testing)

Mildly retarded children are often identified when poor academic performance leads to intelligence testing by a school psychologist. Diagnostic reliability depends in part upon the skill of the psychologist, and errors do occur. Even so, objective intelligence tests are more reliable than clinical impressions of intelligence. Where retardation is obvious, tests help to establish levels of functioning. The psychologist assesses the quality of thought processes, specific strengths and weaknesses, problem-solving approaches, and the presence of perceptual and motor deficits. Other tests measure specific abilities such as language development or motor skills. The type of test chosen will vary with the problem and the age of the child (see Table 33–4 and Chapter 7).

Psychiatric Interview

Factors related to intellectual and social development are emphasized in the comprehensive psychiatric interview (see Chapter 4). These include continuity and quality of maternal care during the early years, type of sensory, intellectual, and social stimulation offered the child, and socioeconomic and cultural patterns of the family and community. Emotional factors such as maternal depression, pathologic handling of aggression, fear of rivalry, and family secrets may result in neurotic inhibition of learning (pseudoretardation). Families relate to their children in ways that enhance (answering questions) or inhibit ("Don't touch!") intellectual curiosity. When a child is diagnosed as retarded, the parents may stop trying to educate him on the assumption that it is hopeless.

Because of varying reaction patterns, the parents and the child should be seen individually and together. Normal children can be separated from their parents for interview by age 4–5; the retarded somewhat later. The child's reactions to his parents, siblings, and other adults should be noted.

TABLE 33–4. Commonly used psychologic tests.

Test	Description	Comments
Catell Infant Intelligence Scale	Largely a test of neuromuscular development. Used up to 30 months of age.	Little predictive value for later intelligence. Good description of current functioning. Detects mental retardation and brain damage.
Gesell Developmental Schedule	Scale based on behavioral observations. Measures development from 4 weeks to 6 years.	Poor predictive value. Good measure of current functioning. Detects delayed development.
Vineland Social Maturity Scale	Individual interview schedule aimed at determining rate of development. Covers birth to maturity.	Easier to give and score than Gesell but based on mother's reports rather than examiner's observations. Gives a helpful picture of current social functioning.
Stanford-Binet Intelligence Scale	Used from age 2 up. Consists of variety of test items arranged as to difficulty. Individually given.	Reliable intelligence test. Heavy emphasis on verbal tests in older age groups. Correlates well with school performance. Because of language emphasis, affected by cultural factors and aphasia.
Wechsler Intelligence Scale for Children	Individual intelligence test for ages 5–16. Consists of 6 verbal and 6 nonverbal subtests. Gives a verbal and performance IQ.	Analysis of subtests allows determination of areas of intellectual strength and weakness. Performance tests less affected by cultural factors and do not rely as much on intact language skills as the Binet.
Bender Gestalt Test	Patient copies 8 geometric designs. Used from age 3 up.	Used in the differential diagnosis of brain damage. Used to assess perceptual motor development in children. Correlates highly with reading readiness.
Illinois Test of Psycholinguistic Ability	A test of expressive, receptive, and central language functions. Tests auditory, vocal, and motor responses alone and in combination.	Yields a profile of a child's language development. Helpful in cases of language immaturity. Many of the language skills measured are used in classrooms; results can be helpful regarding teaching approach.
Peabody Picture Vocabulary Tests	A series of pictures illustrating word meanings. Patient asked to point to picture showing meaning of word given orally by examiner.	Helpful in determining central language functions and intelligence in individuals with expressive language disturbances.

Other observations include the presence of sensory and motor defects, how the child compensates for handicaps, general level of social maturity, self-care skills (eg, buttons, shoelaces), language skills, degree of interpersonal warmth, certainty about the environment, level of anxiety, defense mechanisms used, level of self-esteem, establishment of sexual identity, aggressiveness, and manner of expression. Observations should also be made regarding attention span, freedom from distractibility and perseveration, environmental curiosity, drive to mastery, and frustration tolerance. Thought processes should be evaluated for cohesiveness, concreteness, and contamination by drives and irrelevant thoughts as well as for fund of knowledge, memory, ability to generalize, and level of intellectual functioning. Assessment of strengths is as important as identification of weaknesses since they represent assets in vocational or educational competition.

Mental Retardation and Allied Conditions at Various Ages
A. Infancy:
1. Major sensory deficits (eg, blindness).
2. Causes of delayed motor development (eg, amyotonia congenita).
3. Gross environmental deprivation (no stimulation).
4. Infantile depressions due to insufficiency, disruption, or distortion of mother-child relationship.

B. Early Childhood:
1. Partial sensory deficits (eg, myopia, high-frequency hearing loss).
2. Poor motor development (eg, maturational lag, minimal brain injury).
3. Developmental language problems (eg, aphasia, dysarthria).
4. Familial and cultural deprivation.
5. Childhood depression secondary to depression in the mother.
6. Maternal deprivation syndromes due to insufficiency, disruption, and distortion of the mother-child relationship.
7. Infantile autism (childhood schizophrenia).
8. Gross overindulgence and infantilization.

C. School Age:
1. Partial sensory deficits.
2. Maturational lags.
3. Minimal brain injury.
4. Perceptualmotor defects.
5. Developmental language problems.
6. Familial and cultural deprivation.
8. Childhood schizophrenia.
9. Neurotic underachievement.

D. Adolescence:
1. Partial sensory deficits.
2. Minimal brain injury
3. Perceptualmotor defects (diminishing).
4. Developmental language problems (diminishing).

TABLE 33–5. Approximate risk of mental defect in each child.*

	History in Relatives of Parents	Recessive (Usually Metabolic Defect With Normal Parents)	Dominant Disease (Often in Parent and Child)	Sex-Linked Recessive (Only in Males Related Through Females)	Unknown Cause†
No affected children	Negative	Parents related: under 3%.	Disease in parent's parent or in parent's sib and other relative: up to 25%. Parent partly affected: up to 50%.	Disease on father's side: no risk. Disease on mother's side: 50% for males (50% of females will be carriers).	Parents healthy: under 5%. One parent partly affected: up to 50%.
	Positive	Parents related or both have affected relative: up to 10%.‡			
One affected child	Negative	25%	Under 10% (see text)	50% for males, etc	Under 5%
	Positive	25%	50%	50% for males, etc	Up to 50%

*Reproduced, with permission, from Mental Retardation: A Handbook for the Primary Physician. American Medical Association, 1965.
†Mental retardation with somatic changes, and unknown cause.
‡No risk if biochemical tests show either parent not to be a genetic carrier.

5. Specific learning disabilities.
6. Familial and cultural deprivation.
7. Adolescent schizophrenia (increasing).
8. Neurotic underachievement (increasing).

PREVENTION

Preventive services give equal importance to the socioeconomic as well as biologic causes of mental retardation. Genetic counseling is becoming increasingly complex, but the family physician should know the genetic facts (Table 33–5) since parents often ask about the influence of heredity.

Since prevention is by far the most important aspect of management of mental retardation, all physicians should be familiar with the following facts about mental retardation and methods of prevention:

A. **Primary Prevention (With Parents):**

1. Public education—Causes and treatment of mental retardation.

2. Socioeconomic programs—Antipoverty campaigns, public housing, job training, educational services, day care.

3. Medical measures—Optimal obstetric and pediatric care.

4. Genetic counseling—Sex-linked or autosomal, dominant or recessive, with medical consultation as required.

B. **Secondary Prevention (With Children):**

1. Identification and treatment of phenylketonuria, galactosemia, hypothyroidism, and aminoacidurias.

2. Prompt treatment of bacterial meningitis, lead poisoning, subdural hematoma, hydrocephaly, craniosynostosis, and epilepsy.

3. Recognition of isolated handicaps (5% of school population), sensory and motor deficiencies, dyslexia, dyscalculia, dysgraphia, disturbances of attention span, aphasias.

4. Identification of culturally deprived children and treatment by means of Head Start programs.

C. **Tertiary Prevention (With Children):**

1. Treatment of behavioral and personality problems with individual and group psychotherapy, milieu therapy, and medication.

2. Parental counseling, including support, guidance, advice, homemaker service, holiday relief, group therapy.

3. Temporary institutionalization aimed at training, educating, and treating children whose needs cannot be met at home.

4. Vocational rehabilitation, stressing realistic vocational training suited to the individual, with placement and supportive services during the initial work experience.

5. Physical rehabilitation to overcome the physical handicaps associated with mental retardation.

6. Special education with preschool programs, individualized curriculum, remedial teaching methods, task analysis, operant conditioning technics, and psychiatric consultation.

MANAGEMENT

As is the case with normal children, the upbringing of the retarded child is primarily the task of parents and the schools. Specialists can only assist the child, his parents, and his teachers to solve problems they have not been able to manage. Periods of crises when families may need additional help include the first suspicion of the diagnosis, the period during which diagnostic studies are being made, school entrance, adjustment problems with peers and siblings, family crises, pubertal sexual problems, job finding, marriage, institutional placement, and guilt feelings following placement.

Management of Parental Reaction

Treatment begins when the diagnosis of mental retardation must be conveyed to the parents. This is a period of maximum stress. More must be done than report the facts; the parents must be given help with their feelings. The anxiety caused by a diagnosis of mental retardation results in a period of emotional disintegration. Later they learn to accept the diagnosis and resolve to help the child (period of reintegration). Residual feelings may hamper their efforts to rear the child in the most appropriate way. Most parents ultimately accept and love the retarded child and deal with him constructively without significant emotional stress (period of mature adaptation).

Except in readily recognizable conditions such as Down's syndrome, it is wise not to make lifelong predictions. The physician should convey only what he is certain of, ie, that the child's development is slower than normal. The parents will want to know why, and possible causes should be discussed. The investigation should be thorough enough to satisfy the parents that everything possible has been done to arrive at an accurate assessment of their child's true potential. Negative results of tests for specific organic syndromes increase the likelihood of simple idiopathic mental retardation. Rather than using the term "mental retardation," the doctor may at first prefer to indicate that the child is so many months or years behind other children of his age. Parents can often accept "slow development," whereas they may be unable to face the term "mental retardation" if their image of a retarded child is too terrifying. If they then ask whether their child is retarded, the physician should find out what they mean by the term. Their impression may be realistic and they may be ready to discuss the diagnosis. If their image is of a totally disabled child, they may not be able to accept the diagnosis in view of the child's known capabilities. If the parents refuse to acknowledge the child's delay in development, argument is pointless because they are not emotionally ready to accept the facts. The doctor should sustain the relationship by agreeing that there may be room for doubt. Time will help clarify matters. He should arrange to see the child periodically for reexamination and use these periods to discuss the child's continuing development with the parents. Ultimately, most parents come to accept the diagnosis of mental retardation.

The parents of a retarded child who are able to accept the diagnosis emotionally may react with a period of *depression* (mourning for what might have been) or a mild degree of *guilt* which is ultimately resolved. Pathologic reactions are frequently seen. Parents sometimes refuse to accept the diagnosis in the face of irrefutable evidence (*denial*). This allows them to continue a "normal" relationship with their child but may expose the child to inordinate expectations and interfere with the parents' ability to deal effectively with their child's problem and may lead to *overprotection*. They may transfer their own guilt feelings to other individuals such as the obstetrician by the process of *projection*. Parents may displace their emotional needs onto the community, becoming active in movements to promote understanding of the retarded. Baffled by a deviant child, parents cannot call upon their own childhood experiences in deciding how to handle him, and this *uncertainty* may be reflected in overprotection or in unrealistic demands for better performance. Each new developmental stage leads to exacerbation of parental anxiety that may require counseling and reassurance.

Reactions of the Siblings of a Retarded Child

Well integrated and functional families can almost always adapt to a retarded child, but this is easier for families in the lower socioeconomic levels of society than for middle class families with social or professional aspirations. In poorly integrated families, preexisting personal or marital problems may be aggravated by the presence of a retarded child. Other children in the family usually accept the retarded child to the degree that their parents do. Excessive sacrifices may cause resentment. If the mother transfers responsibility for the care and supervision of a retarded child to an older daughter, the daughter may react with both resentment and guilt.

Some retarded children impose intolerable burdens of care sufficient to disrupt the healthiest of families.

Role of the Physician

Through his training and his ability to offer continuity of care throughout the child's development, the physician is uniquely equipped to obtain and coordinate the services required in the management of retarded children. The physician must be familiar with the applicable professional and community services available to him. Unfortunately, probably no community at present offers the complete spectrum of desirable services summarized in the next section.

Array of Direct Services for the Retarded*
A. Infant:

Specialized medical follow-up	Sensory stimulation
Special diets, medication,	Child welfare services
or surgery	Home training
Home nursing	Environmental enrichments
Residential nursery	

---

*Adapted from *Proposed Program for National Action to Combat Mental Retardation.* The President's Panel on Mental Retardation, Washington, DC, 1952, p 76.

B. Toddler:

Correction of physical defects
Physical therapy
Foster care
Trained baby-sitters

Nursery school
Classes for slow learners
Playground programs

C. Child:

Psychiatric care
Dental care
Homemaker service
Day care
Short stay home
Boarding school
Special classes—educable
Special classes—trainable

Religious education
Work school programs
Speech training
Day camps
Residential camps
Scouting
Swimming
"Disabled child" benefits

D. Youth:

Psychotherapy
Halfway house
Occupational training
Vocational counseling

Personal adjustment training
Youth groups
Social clubs
Health insurance

E. Young Adult:

Facilities for retarded in conflict
Guardianship of person
Long-term residential care
Marriage counseling
Selective job placement
Sheltered employment

Total disability assistance
Bowling
Sheltered workshops
Guardianship of property
Life annuity or trust

F. Adult:

Group homes
Boarding homes
Evening school

Social supervision
Evening recreation

G. Older Adult:

Medical attention to chronic conditions
Old Age Assistance
Old Age Security Insurance benefits

MANAGEMENT DURING VARIOUS DEVELOPMENTAL STAGES

Infancy and Early Childhood

The developmental tasks during this stage are development of awareness and control of the body, the establishment of interpersonal relationships, and the acquisition of basic social skills (feeding, toilet training, self-care, and recognition of hazards). Retarded infants need a period of prolonged dependency which can be provided only by the mother or a mother substitute. If home care is not possible, foster care is preferable to institutionalization. Severely retarded children may ultimately require institutionalization because of associated problems (eg, blindness, deafness, or failure to develop mobility). Most children benefit from home care. Day nursery care helps to develop necessary social skills and relieves the mother of the burden of care for part of the day. Training by an emotionally neutral person may be more successful than training attempts by a mother with a negative emotional response to the situation.

For example, such a mother may not be able to cope with a child's incontinence, whereas a nursery teacher may succeed. Parents' groups, volunteer associations, public health nurses, and social workers are able to provide concrete and specific advice about developmental problems. Motor and language training may enhance school readiness. Many children have medical problems that need periodic assessment and treatment. Intellectual assessment may help to determine educational readiness.

Children of School Age

The development tasks in this age group include the ability to be separated from home and to form relationships with adults and children outside the family, the acquisition of social and academic skills, the development of a sense of mastery, and heightened self-esteem. Retarded children do not achieve the normal degree of social and academic success, and special classes will help them learn at their own rate, with the support of and in competition with children of similar ability. Retarded children who have not had the advantages of neighborhood and community experiences can be helped by special programs that provide companions for group, social, and play activities. Much emotional disturbance stems from adverse community experiences, leading to anger or withdrawal, and attitudes toward the self that are developed in this period continue into later years. During the school years, careful examination is required in order to identify developmental handicaps (specific learning disabilities, language or motor problems) that may respond to remedial technics.

Adolescence

The developmental tasks of adolescence include establishment of personal and vocational identity, separation from the parents, and the beginning of heterosexual relationships. The retarded adolescent may achieve only a few of these developmental objectives. Failure to achieve social acceptance and purposeful employment creates a peak of emotional disturbance. Increased social rejection may turn the adolescent back to his family and increase his dependency. More characteristically, the retarded adolescent vents his anger on the family and community.

Vocational success is essential for self-esteem. School occupational programs may not provide realistic vocational training. Most do not provide work experience, vocational placement, or follow-up services. Many adolescents prove to be capable workers when they receive this training and support. Moderately retarded adolescents may need residential placement for training before moving into a sheltered workshop program and supervised group living homes.

Developmental problems, physical disabilities, and academic problems may have lessened, but the adolescent may be in greater need of psychiatric consultation and social services. If group social experiences are not satisfactory, adolescents may drift into association with delinquent companions who may exploit their willingness to please. Adolescent sexual interests should be supervised and channeled, not suppressed. Most mentally retarded people ultimately marry.

Adulthood

The developmental tasks of adulthood include work, marriage, child-bearing, and the search for personal happiness. Mildly retarded adults can achieve these objectives. Successful child rearing does not require superior intelligence. Retarded parents may produce children with greater intellectual potential than themselves.

Mildly retarded adults may be more vulnerable to social stress and should have access to counseling services as emotional, social, and vocational problems arise. The moderately retarded may require a sheltered workshop setting, income supplementation, and social supervision. Group living homes increasingly will take the place of institutions, providing social supervision and a suitable recreational program.

SPECIAL EDUCATION

As with the normal child, the influence of schooling is second only to that of family experiences in the maximal development of the retarded child. Trainable retarded children (IQ 30–50) cannot achieve literacy but can be helped with oral language, self-help skills, and socialization. The educable retarded (IQ 50–75) can achieve a degree of literacy that is helpful vocationally. Educational programs may include a simplified slow-paced curriculum, assistance from resource teachers, and highly complex individual programs for the brain-damaged. The latter may require understanding on the part of the teacher of perceptual and neurologic development, behavioral and emotional approaches, and special remedial educational technics (eg, concrete materials for arithmetic, tracing the shapes of letters for letter recognition). Above all, special education classes prevent retarded children from being crushed by the educational system and developing an enduring sense of personal inadequacy.

SPECIAL PROBLEMS

Physical Problems

Many physical defects are associated with mental deficiency. In the past, cosmetic surgery, orthopedic repair and bracing, and medical procedures were largely neglected. It is now recognized that all measures that enhance personal or social adjustment are worthwhile. Children with multiple handicaps are best cared for at comprehensive care centers for the mentally retarded. Improvement of motor, sensory, and language functions are particularly important.

Emotional Problems

Almost any type of psychiatric disorder may be present in the mentally retarded. The extent of emotional disturbance often determines the success of ultimate adjustment. Emotional disorders may add to family burdens and preclude attendance at school. Psychiatric facilities may refuse these cases for treatment, although the results of treatment are just as good as when retardation is not present. Emotional conflicts may be dynamically simple and are often environmentally determined. This, plus a limited ability to verbalize, leads to the choice of active therapy rather than the passive listening that characterizes some types of psychotherapy. Positive relationships, friendly acceptance, and assistance with environmental problems are effective. Denial and overprotection may prevent families from seeking help until the situation is critical, eg, until the mother can no longer cope with the problem and the child is suspended from school.

Puberty presents special problems which parents may introduce by means of a trivial presenting complaint. Infantile manifestations of sexuality (eg, peeping) may be reactivated, and this can be handled by further social training and supervision. Parents of mildly retarded children may forget that masturbation is normal for adolescents. They may not realize that many mentally retarded people eventually have reasonably successful marriages.

Dating should be supervised. If simple guidance and reassurance fail, unconscious parental problems may exist that require psychotherapy.

The parents are usually relieved to hear that severely retarded children do not have abnormally intense sexual drives.

Social Problems

Social inexperience may prove to be a handicap to the overprotected retarded child or adolescent. Successful social experiences are best provided through special education programs and through social activity groups sponsored by local associations for the retarded.

MEDICATION

Some retarded children—especially those suffering from brain damage— are hyperactive and irritable, with short attention spans and temper outbursts. These symptoms may respond to dextroamphetamine, 5–20 mg orally in a single daily dose at breakfast.

HOME CARE VERSUS INSTITUTIONALIZATION

The decision about whether to treat the retarded child at home or in an institution requires careful assessment of the needs of the child and the ability of his family, the community, and community agencies to meet those needs. In most cases, home care is far superior to institutional care.

Institutions can provide specialized services but have great difficulty in providing an approximation to the normal family environment necessary for personality growth. When the child's family is unsuitable, foster care may be substituted instead of institutionalization. If a child is to be maintained in his own home, a variety of services may be necessary (see above).

Many communities have not yet developed a sufficiently wide spectrum of services for the mentally retarded. Institutionalization may be necessary if the needs of the child cannot be met in the community. Awareness of the detrimental effects of institutional living has led institutions for the mentally retarded to attempt to develop more homelike atmospheres.

Indications for Institutionalization

Some retarded children cannot be managed at home. These include the following: (1) Children with multiple handicaps who require special medical treatment. (2) Chronically bedridden and incontinent patients requiring continuous nursing care. (3) Profoundly retarded children as they become older. (4) Mentally retarded children with severe emotional disturbances. (5) Children with special educational, vocational, and occupational needs.

Severely emotionally disturbed children who cannot be educated in special classes in the school system constitute an increasing number of admissions. Their stay—and the stay of children with special training needs—should be as short as possible. In future, the majority of retarded individuals are likely to be cared for in their local communities.

REFERENCES

Books and Monographs

AMA Conference on Mental Retardation: *Mental Retardation: A Handbook for the Primary Physician.* American Medical Association, 1965.

Baumeister, A.A. (editor): *Mental Retardation.* Aldine, 1967.

Bernstein, N.R. (editor): *Diminished People: Problems and Care of the Mentally Retarded.* Little, Brown, 1971.

Church, J.: *Language and the Discovery of Reality.* Random House, 1961.

Deutsch, M. (editor): *The Disadvantaged Child.* Basic Books, 1967.

Flavell, J.H.: *The Developmental Psychology of Jean Piaget.* Van Nostrand, 1963.

Frieson, E.C., & W.B. Barbe (editors): *Educating Children With Learning Disabilities: Selected Readings.* Appleton-Century-Crofts, 1967.

Goodman, J.D., & J.A. Sours: *The Child Mental Status Examination.* Basic Books, 1967.

Hoffman, L.W., & M.L. Hoffman (editors): Mental retardation: Current issues and approaches. Pages 107–168 in: *Review of Child Development Research.* Vol 2. Russell Sage Foundation, 1964.

Johnson, D.J., & H.R. Myklebust: *Learning Disabilities: Educational Principles and Practices.* Grune & Stratton, 1967.

Kessler, J.W.: Mental subnormality. Pages 166–168 in: *Psychopathology of Childhood.* Prentice-Hall, 1966.

Masland, R.L., Saranson, S.B., & T. Gladwin: *Mental Subnormality.* Basic Books, 1958.

Myklebust, H.R.: *Auditory Disorders in Childhood.* Grune & Stratton, 1954. [See Table 23, pp 352–353.]

Noland, R.L.: *Counseling Parents of the Mentally Retarded: A Sourcebook.* Thomas, 1970.

Paine, R.S., & T.E. Oppe: *Neurological Examination of Children.* Heinemann, 1966.

Peter, L.J.: *Prescriptive Teaching.* McGraw-Hill, 1965.

Phillips, I. (editor): *Prevention and Treatment of Mental Retardation.* Basic Books, 1966.

Vuckovich, D.M.: Pediatric neurology and learning disabilities. Chap 2, pp 16–38, in: *Progress in Learning Disabilities.* Vol 1. H.R. Myklebust (editor). Grune & Stratton, 1968.

Yarrow, L.S.: Interviewing children. Chap 14, pp 561–602, in: *Handbook of Research Methods in Child Development.* P.H. Mussen (editor). Wiley, 1960.

Journal Articles

Grossman, H.J. (editor): Mental retardation. P Clin North America 15:819–1046, 1968.

Lott, G.M.: Psychotherapy of the mentally retarded. JAMA 196:229–232, 1966.

Matheny, A.P., & J. Vernick: Parents of the mentally retarded child: Emotionally overwhelmed or informationally deprived? J Pediat 74:953–959, 1969.

Menolascino, F.J.: Emotional disturbances in mentally retarded children. Am J Psychiat 126:168–176, 1969.

Menolascino, F.J., & R.G. Osborne: Television consultation for the mentally retarded. Am J Psychiat 127:515–520, 1970.

Meyer, R.J., Stafford, R.L., & M.D. Jacobsen: Patterns of family follow-up: A study of children with mental retardation and associated developmental disorders. Commun Ment Health J 6:393–400, 1970.

34...

Adolescent Psychiatry

Normal adolescence involves emotional turmoil often only one degree removed from psychiatric illness. Young counselors, not identified with the Establishment, do well with adolescents but should be supervised. They must help the adolescent establish personal and vocational identity, separation from the parents, and the beginnings of healthy sexual relationships.

Adolescence—the period between puberty and young adulthood (approximately 12–20)—is marked by a great surge of physical development and major social and psychologic adjustments. It begins a year or so earlier in females than in males, and may end earlier in females since they mature sooner than males both physiologically and emotionally. There are marked endocrinologic changes during this phase of life. Hormonal variations may well contribute to the intensity and quality of feelings that the adolescent experiences. Hence, these hormonal changes may play a definite role in creating the disturbed inner climate that the adolescent must face.

Normal adolescence is characterized by a multitude of personality changes. These may prove to be quite distressing to parents, teachers, and other adults. Just as the young child's first attempts at walking may produce a number of awkward movements, false starts, and falls before a confident gait is established, the adolescent's strivings toward maturity may be characterized by awkward, often disconcerting physical and emotional blunderings before a stable adult personality is achieved. Much of this turmoil involves the adolescent's attempts to establish himself as an independent individual. His efforts are often of a rebellious and radical nature—similar, in fact, to those of many newly established nations. The previously quiet, well behaved, obedient youngster (age 8–12) may become rebellious, defiant, and aggressive; the previously conscientious student may neglect his studies and skip classes; the polite, courteous youngster may become rude and sarcastic; and the honest child who confided in his parents may become a fabricator of fictions and a mystery man about his activities.

The bizarre, frequently irritating behavior and performance of the adolescent stem from the individual's untutored and inexperienced attempts to assert independence without becoming completely independent. The young person usually lacks the skill and experience to be himself aware of the strangeness of his performance. Knowing this should assist the parents in making this period bearable.

The "normal" adolescent almost always shows evidence of emotional turmoil and personality change. The adolescent who shows no emotional upheaval is apt to be repressed and is actually failing to deal with the problems of this phase of life. The result may be the appearance of unresolved personality disturbances in adult life.

The question of whether one should seek professional assistance for a troublesome adolescent or wait to see if he will "outgrow" his disturbing behavior is difficult to answer in general terms. As in all emotional illnesses, a social factor is involved—namely, How tolerant will a particular family, school, or community be of an individual's unusual behavior? One set of parents may be willing to tolerate behavior that others would find beyond endurance. The latter may seek out professional assistance much sooner than the former.

Adolescent Problems Requiring Therapy

In most instances, disturbing behavior in the adolescent is apt to modify and improve (in terms of adult approval) with time. However, this is not a sufficient solution in some cases. When the behavior of the adolescent tends to be destructive to himself or others, to be repeated several times, or to be chronic in duration (lasting several days or weeks instead of a few hours or days), the question of whether to seek professional help must be seriously considered. Transient or infrequent behavior disturbances that do not adversely affect the individual's life or harm others may not require professional help but only understanding and tolerance on the part of the parents.

The following are examples of behavior that may require professional help:

(1) Repeated incidents of so-called delinquent behavior (activities that are apt to lead to repeated difficulties with law enforcement agencies), ie, stealing, vandalism, personal assaults, frequent and excessive use of alcohol or drugs.

(2) Repeated overt sexual behavior that is likely to lead to social or legal problems, ie, promiscuity, pregnancy, perversion, homosexuality.

(3) Persistent inadequate school achievement in an individual capable of doing well.

(4) Prolonged or repeated mood disturbances such as depressions—sadness, crying, insomnia, loss of appetite, loss of ability to perform daily routines, a feeling of "hopelessness," preoccupation with suicide.

(5) Prolonged or frequent episodes of previously uncharacteristic withdrawal and isolation from family and friends, with decreased productivity, ie, decreased interest in social activities, increased amount of time spent alone or in apparent preoccupation or daydreaming.

(6) Evidence of mental symptoms such as hallucinations, delusions of persecution, ideas of reference (people talking about him in, usually, uncomplimentary ways), or other bizarre ideas.

If these symptoms are present or if the adolescent himself wishes assistance, consultation with the family physician or school psychologist is a useful first step. If these professionals feel that the individual's behavior is outside the normal range, they may either attempt treatment themselves or recommend referral to a psychiatrist. The ability of the family physician, psychologist, or social worker to deal effectively with adolescents depends on several factors: the seriousness of the problem; the professional worker's experience in dealing with adolescents; and his ability to be patient and understanding and to form reasonably comfortable and close relationships with adolescents. If he finds this too difficult or if, after 3–6 visits, he fails to see any progress or the beginning of a close relationship with the adolescent, referral to a psychiatrist who specializes in this field is indicated.

Common Factors Which Produce Problems in Adolescence

(1) **Giving up childhood:** (Dependency, protection, etc.) There are many gratifications in being given to and protected by older people, particularly when one has to do very little in return. Hence, there is a conflict between the desire to be a grown-up and to remain a child, receiving favors without effort.

(2) **Establishing independence:** (Rebellion against parents and other authority figures.) In order to prove to himself and to the world that he is really an autonomous individual, the adolescent often seeks to show his independence in an exaggerated, sometimes antisocial, even self-destructive or bizarre manner. Even those acts that get him into difficulties with his parents or with community authorities may be repeated over and over as the adolescent strives to assure himself that he is his "own boss." Examples of these acts are argumentativeness with parents, staying out late, truancy, drinking, smoking marihuana, and failing to do assigned school work. There may also be more serious, clearly pathologic behavior such as aggravated personal assaults.

(3) **Drives toward sex and aggression:** These emotional drives are reinforced by endocrinologic and physical development. The adolescent becomes capable of actually performing sexual acts and acts of aggression that may have serious consequences. He is eager to exercise some of his new powers but is wary of the possible consequences—eg, pregnancy, venereal disease, injury, or death. Sexual taboos are culturally determined; hence other cultures that have more liberal or more stringent prohibitions may have fewer, more, or different problems and the adolescent must attempt to adjust his drives to the mores of his culture.

(4) **Reluctance to trust and confide in adults:** Adults are looked up to as models with whom to identify, but they are also the authority figures ("the enemy") who seek to keep the adolescent subservient.

(5) **Pressures toward conformity and achievement:** The adolescent is caught between the pressures toward achievement—academic, social, and economic success—and his desire to rebel and not conform even though rebellion is against his "own good."

(6) **Pressures from peers:** (Gaining approval and acceptance.) The adolescent may engage in antisocial acts in order to gain gang approval; may participate in daring and dangerous acts to prove his manhood; and may try to gain approval by adopting certain group standards or symbols such as long

hair, certain types of clothing, "hippie" behavior, etc. Gangs tend to provide mutual support and "strength through numbers" for ideas and actions that the individual may be unable to sustain on his own. They provide a setting both for leaders and followers, and a symbol with which to identify.

(7) **"Identity crisis"**: (Role in life; life goals.) In late adolescence the individual becomes preoccupied with philosophic questions concerning his role in life and the meaning of life itself. He must decide whether to devote his life to gaining wealth and power or to the "better things"—altruistic aims, making a better world, scholarship, art, religion, etc. An attitude of cynicism, hopelessness, and futility often develops. ("What is the good of it all?") Preoccupation with death and its meanings may be a paramount concern. The individual's sexual role must be determined—active or passive, heterosexual or homosexual. In addition to all of these, girls have other problems. They must decide what the female role should be—wife, mother, career woman, or a combination of roles. Other matters of concern include competition with males, the need for achievement in academic or occupational pursuits, acceptance or rejection of a subservient role in relation to men, the question of the "female sexual role" (active or passive), and responsibility for the next generation—how and whether to rear children in "this world today."

(8) **Facing military draft**: (Possible death.) The draft may provide a devil-may-care attitude ("for tomorrow we die") or self-doubts about physical adequacy, stamina, and bravery. Military life pushes some young men into adulthood before they are able to accept it (via separation from home, keeping up with the "men" in sexual activities), and may heighten the conflict with authority figures by placing the young recruit in constant contact with superiors who expect him to obey orders without question. On the other hand, military life provides security through a new dependent atmosphere where everything is taken care of—food, shelter, clothing, etc. Barracks living may place great stress on young men who are already having conflicts with regard to homosexuality.

(9) **First exposures to sexual activity, alcohol, and drugs**: Although the adolescent may have attained physical maturity, his psychologic maturity lags behind. First exposures to overt sexual acts with women may thus be quite frightening and disturbing. He has strong sexual drives and a great deal of curiosity, but he is not yet ready to accept his feelings as an integral, normal part of himself and to adapt his sexual behavior to his sense of values, morals, and superego demands (conscience). First exposures to alcohol or drugs are equally distressing because of the conflict between desire and curiosity on the one hand and their highly forbidden nature on the other.

Involvement in so-called aberrant sexual behavior (homosexuality, voyeurism, exhibitionism, sadomasochism) is common in adolescence for several reasons: (1) A strong revival of sexual drives of all kinds. (Sexual drives originally appear in early childhood and are then repressed at about age 5—6.—Freud) (2) A body newly capable of adult sexual expression. (3) Intense curiosity. (4) A period of psychologic floundering in the attempt to determine what the sexual role will be: active or passive, heterosexual or homosexual. (5) Intense fears of the consequences—real, imagined, and exaggerated—of sexual activity (pregnancy, venereal disease, being "evil," doing "terribly forbidden acts"). These may lead to aberrant sexual activities to avoid what the adolescent may feel are the more forbidden normal heterosexual outlets. The adolescent's concept of what is forbidden stems from his interpretation of parental prohibitions, which may never have specifically touched on subjects of aberrant sexual behavior.

In any event, whether sexual activity is carried out or not—and regardless of its nature—the adolescent tends to be much concerned and often quite distressed over his sexual desires, feelings, thoughts, and acts (including masturbation).

(10) Masturbation guilt: Masturbation is almost universal in both males and females. Concern about the imagined physical or mental damage resulting from masturbation contributes to feelings of self-consciousness, inadequacy, "badness," shyness, or withdrawal.

(11) Reaction to menstruation: The menarche brings a sudden confrontation with "womanhood." There are mixed feelings toward becoming a "real woman" capable of reproduction and the inconvenience, discomfort, and embarrassment that often occur. Menstruation emphasizes the girl's difference from boys. The extent of the reaction to menstruation often depends on the amount of knowledge imparted before menarche; on the girl's attitude to the female role; and on the mother's attitude—eg, Does the mother regard it as a "curse"? Does the mother have somatic complaints during her periods? What is the girl's reaction to delayed onset, irregular periods, heavy or prolonged menstrual flow, and missed periods?

(12) Overreaction to major or minor differences: Adolescence is an age of great sensitivity and self-consciousness about real or imagined differences from others in the peer group or immediate environment. Feelings are very easily hurt with regard to any physical, racial, or socioeconomic differences. The following are of particular concern: (1) Physical impediments, eg, severe acne, overweight, tall or short stature, delayed physical maturation. (2) Minority roles (color, religion, racial origin). (3) Extremes of economic status (poverty or wealth).

(13) Seeking outlets for vigorous emotional expression: The adolescent seeks outlets for his strong drives toward sex and aggression. He finds the status quo, the conformist, the conservative, the old-fashioned ways stultifying and boring, and may seek to express his drives through identifying strongly with (or vigorously opposing) progressive causes (civil rights, peace marches, demonstrations), or by behaving in an uninhibited, socially disapproved manner such as irresponsible sexual activity, conflict with civil or military authorities, or through the use of drugs or alcohol.

(14) Male and female attributes: Males are greatly concerned with being "sufficiently masculine" (strong, brave, virile, athletic, masterful, vs weak, cowardly, "feminine," ineffectual). Females are concerned with being "sufficiently feminine" (attractive, tender, maternal, sexually responsive, etc).

Diagnostic Categories and Symptom Complexes

(1) **Adjustment reaction of adolescence:** This includes transient reactions which are expressions of emancipatory strivings and fluctuating impulses and emotions. They may include a variety of symptoms, such as "acting out" behavior (antisocial, delinquent, passive-resistant), anxiety feelings, school problems—academic or disciplinary, hypochondriacal complaints, depression, turmoil states (agitated and confused), and suicidal gestures. The prominent feature of this condition is its transient nature— usually hours or a few days. It requires careful evaluation in order to distinguish it from more profound or serious (long-term) disorders, ie, psychoneuroses or psychoses. The actual symptom may be quite violent or intense but transient. There is often a distressing external event which precipitates the symptoms, eg, argument with a parent, loss of a girl-friend, ostracism by the gang, disciplinary action by the school, "loss of face" before peers. Such symptoms may respond to counseling by an understanding physician or professional worker (psychologist, social worker, guidance counselor) who concentrates on the precipitating event and lets the adolescent ventilate his feelings about it.

(2) **Common psychoneuroses:** (Anxiety reaction, conversion reaction, obsessive compulsive reaction, etc.) The symptoms are the same as those observed in adults with the same psychoneuroses. The symptoms form a pattern or complex which is more characteristic of a particular neurosis, although these may overlap with the symptoms of another neurosis. The symptom complex tends to be persistent in duration (months or years) in contrast to the transient symptoms of adjustment reaction of adolescence. There is often no discernible external precipitating event. However, the symptoms may become more intense after the adolescent has been faced with a traumatic situation. The onset of symptoms is often gradual but progressive; there may be fluctuations in severity, but the symptoms seldom subside completely for any period of time. Whereas some of the symptoms may be obvious to the family—eg, trembling with anxiety, crying, spells of depression—other symptoms (such as insomnia or phobias) may be elicited only by questioning the patient. Low-grade neuroses may not interfere with the adolescent's activities and may not require treatment, but moderate or severe psychoneurotic symptoms should be treated by a psychiatrist. Without treatment, these conditions are apt to interfere markedly with the normal social and scholastic development of the adolescent, lead to chronic depressed states, or develop into severe neurosis in young adulthood. Furthermore, individuals with moderate to severe psychoneuroses are more apt to make ill-considered major decisions in life, eg, early marriage with the wrong partner, leaving school, impulsive career choices.

(3) **Common functional psychoses:** (Schizophrenic reactions, manic-depressive reactions, etc.) The symptoms are the same as those observed in adults with the same disorders, eg, hallucinations, delusions, ideas of reference, thought disturbances, overactivity, push of speech. The main differential diagnosis is an adolescent turmoil state, which more properly belongs in the category "adjustment reaction of adolescence." The symptoms of an

acute turmoil state may be quite similar to those of acute schizophrenic psychosis. Hospitalization to control behavior may be necessary, but the turmoil state tends to subside quickly (1–2 days) with no psychotic residuals such as disturbances of speech, thinking, or affect. As with adults, the psychoses require treatment by a psychiatrist and perhaps hospitalization during the acute stages. When they subside, follow-up therapy by trained clinic personnel, which may include psychologists and social workers under the supervision of a psychiatrist, may be utilized. A prolonged course of psychotherapy by a psychiatrist after a psychotic episode may restore a more stable emotional pattern and reduce the chance of recurrence.

(4) Personality and character disorders: (Antisocial reactions, passive-aggressive personality, etc.) These diagnoses are established when the individual's behavior patterns show repeated evidence of the above—eg, antisocial acts, vandalism, delinquency, obstructionism. They do not seem to be isolated events but rather part of the individual's "characteristic" pattern of behaving. The individual seems to understand the differences between right and wrong, but this does not alter his behavior. He does not seem to feel distressed, anxious, or guilty about his antisocial behavior, and is not deterred by punishment. Such individuals usually come to the attention of persons in charge of school discipline, guidance counselors, and court workers (eg, probation officers). Evaluation by a psychiatrist and the use of psychologic testing are indicated to establish the diagnosis and to help differentiate it from the psychoses and psychoneuroses. Some of these individuals may respond to psychotherapy if there is a measurable degree of anxiety and some genuine self-motivation for help. However, most of them are poor candidates for psychotherapy and are best handled by court clinics, court officers, and social agencies where the staff has had experience in dealing with such cases. Their tendency to repeat offenses is high; if they can be kept out of serious difficulties with the law, this must be considered as success.

(5) Toxic and organic psychoses: Confusion, disorientation, slurred speech, memory impairment, delirium, etc are prominent symptoms of toxic or organic psychoses, but one must take care not to miss early or mild cases or confuse these with the functional conditions mentioned above (especially schizophrenia). Treatment is of course directed toward the removal of the noxious agent, if possible, and protection of the individual from harm when his mental capacities are seriously impaired.

(6) Drinking and drug abuse: In addition to alcohol, the drugs which are prominently used by adolescents are marihuana, LSD, the amphetamines, barbiturates, and narcotics. LSD may precipitate acute psychotic episodes of a schizophrenic nature; marihuana is not addicting in itself; use of LSD or narcotics can have serious effects, especially if used repeatedly. An individual who frequently seeks artificial sources of gratification or thrills ("kicks") has underlying emotional problems which require help. This applies to excessive drinking also. Treatment, both in terms of withdrawal as well as working out underlying emotional problems, is much more favorable if the individual has genuine motivation and genuine concern (anxiety, guilt) over his condition.

Contrariwise, the longer the duration of the drinking or drug abuse, the poorer the prognosis.

(7) **Psychophysiologic illnesses:** Adolescents are subject to any of the psychosomatic disorders: peptic ulcers, ulcerative colitis, asthma, migraine, etc. Combined medical and psychologic treatment is required for effective long-range results. Medical treatment alone may control the individual episode, but psychotherapy helps reduce recurrences.

(8) **Mental deficiency:** The diagnosis of mental deficiency should be established by psychologic testing as soon as possible so that counseling and training can be started. The mentally retarded adolescent should be directed into activities and schooling commensurate with his abilities. He should be protected from the frustration of tasks he cannot master and from the ridicule of others, and should be made to feel as self-sufficient and self-respecting as possible. This can often be accomplished through special schools and social agencies.

(9) **Suicide in adolescents:** Suicide is much more common in late adolescence (16–20) than earlier. Adolescents may also make suicidal gestures, attempts, or threats, or be preoccupied with thoughts of suicide. Suicidal preoccupation or attempts may be part of a neurotic or psychotic depression or of any psychosis or neurosis, or they may represent a hysterical (histrionic) or attention-getting mechanism. A suicidal threat or gesture is an attempt to communicate a message (the "cry for help"), and an attempt must be made to understand the message. Is this merely the cynical philosophic musing of an adolescent mind? An exaggerated response to some minor frustration or disappointment? An attempt to draw attention and perhaps get one's way? Or is it a more serious matter indicating severe depression or despondency?

The parents are often the first to become aware of a suicidal threat or gesture, and they must decide whether to seek professional advice. If overt signs of depression are present (sadness, crying, withdrawal, loss of interest in studies or work, self-deprecation, self-accusation, insomnia, loss of appetite), consultation with a professionally trained person is definitely advisable. Depression is of more concern in a youngster who has not previously shown frequent mood swings. Suicidal threats are also of greater concern in an adolescent who is not prone to histrionic behavior such as crying and temper tantrums.

The following evidences of suicidal intent are listed in increasing order of pathologic significance: (1) vague thoughts about suicide; (2) specific thoughts about just how to commit suicide; (3) obtaining the items with which to commit suicide (eg, sleeping pills); and (4) actual attempts.

Suicidal gestures are regarded as minor attempts, eg, scratching the wrists, ingesting a few aspirin tablets. Actual attempts at suicide are potentially serious acts which could be fatal, eg, use of firearms, cutting to depths of arteries or tendons; ingesting large overdoses of sleeping pills, poisons, or material generally considered to be lethal; jumping from dangerous heights, hanging, inhalation of illuminating gas. Carrying out such acts at a time and place where one is unlikely to be quickly discovered, or without warning someone in advance of one's intentions, increases the serious aspect of the attempt. Disfiguring or bizarre attempts (eg, enucleation of an eye, castration), if actually seriously attempted, usually indicate a psychotic process such as schizophrenic reaction or psychotic depressive reaction.

If there is a definite question of the possibility of suicide, evaluation by a psychiatrist is advisable. Parents often consult the family physician first. If he too thinks that suicide is a possibility, he should refer the patient to a psychiatrist unless he feels competent (by virtue of special training) to handle the situation himself.

MANAGEMENT OF EMOTIONAL PROBLEMS IN ADOLESCENCE

Referral Sources

Adolescents with emotional problems are usually identified first by parents or school authorities. Less often, they come to the attention of police and court officers, clergymen, youth leaders (coaches, settlement house workers, etc), or the family physician. These, then, are the individuals who are primarily responsible for referring the adolescent for psychiatric help. Persons outside the home who feel that action should be taken about a problem involving the behavior of an adolescent are apt to take the matter up with the parents. Parents tend to turn to (1) the family physician, (2) psychiatrists or psychologists whom they may know, (3) school psychologists or guidance counselors, and (4) the clergy. In many instances, parents are reluctant to take any action unless they are firmly convinced of a need for evaluation and treatment. If a troubled or troublesome adolescent is identified in a school situation, he is usually referred by the dean, teacher, or principal to the school guidance counselor, psychologist, or consulting psychiatrist. Where court officials are involved, the adolescent may be referred to a court clinic, court-appointed psychiatric consultant, private psychiatrist or psychiatric outpatient clinic, or, occasionally, to a social work agency (usually after psychiatric consultation).

Professional Persons Who Should Manage and Treat Adolescents

There are a number of categories of professionals who may work with adolescents. The adolescent is a difficult individual with whom to deal. Hence, the therapist should have specific training and experience working with this age group. He should be interested in their special problems, be patient and understanding of their viewpoint, firm enough not to be manipulated by them, and warm enough to be capable of forming a favorable working relationship with the adolescent. If the therapist has these qualifications, he can work with most adolescent problems regardless of his specific professional status. In general, however, problems which are of a recent or apparently transient nature, which have a known specific external precipitating cause (eg, recent divorce of parents), or which seem to require support or reassurance only during a period of crisis may be handled by the family physician (if he has the time and experience), school psychologist or guidance counselor, psychologically trained clergyman, or psychiatric social worker. Diagnostic evaluations, both for the purpose of establishing a diagnosis and determining the need for psychotherapy, are best done by a psychiatrist. Psychologic testing may be of value in this.

Where the emotional disorder of the adolescent is judged to be of long duration, moderate to severe in intensity, posing a reasonably serious threat to his future (psychotic, borderline psychotic, moderate to severe chronic psychoneurosis, psychosomatic illness, character disorders in well motivated individuals), therapy with a psychiatrist—preferably one specializing or at least interested in adolescents—is the treatment of choice. Occasionally, an individual therapist of exceptional talent who is not a psychiatrist (eg, a clinical psychologist or psychiatric social worker) may do well working with serious adolescent problems. In general, however, if intensive or prolonged therapy is indicated, a psychiatrist is the professional person of choice. Short-term (1–12 visits) and supportive type therapy in such cases may be done by nonpsychiatrists.

The Therapist in the Psychiatric Treatment of Adolescents

It must be borne in mind that the adolescent is no longer a child and not yet an adult; the physician must address himself to the emotional level of the particular patient. The patient is looking for a "good" parent figure— one who is understanding, consistent, moderately firm, not threatening or critical, and who respects the patient as an individual. The patient will repeatedly test the therapist. (Can the therapist be trusted? How much will the therapist put up with?) The therapist must therefore win the patient over, prove his interest in the patient, and be more active in discussions than may be necessary or desirable with adults.

The patient will look to the therapist with whom he develops a positive relationship as a model with whom to identify with regard to such traits as honesty, attitudes toward sex and self-assertion, general goals in life, and the importance of success. With younger adolescents, a therapist of the same sex as the patient may be desirable since the patient will often use this person as a model for what a male or female "should be like." In older adolescents, the sex of the therapist is not so important, since most of the basic sex identification has already taken place; furthermore, the sexual role can be more easily defined and accepted at a verbal level without needing an actual person of the same sex with whom to identify.

In referring the adolescent for treatment, care must be taken to make the referral as acceptable as possible and so minimize resistance. The patient must be convinced that the physician knows he is troubled and is really interested in helping him, not in censoring or disciplining him.

Types of Therapy Used in the Treatment of Adolescents
A. Individual Psychotherapy:
1. Supportive psychotherapy—This type of therapy is indicated for adjustment reactions of adolescence, mild psychoneurotic disorders, mild depressions, postpsychotic readjustment reactions, and conditions where it is

felt that external precipitating causes played a major role. It may also be useful in even more severe disorders if intensive psychotherapy is not feasible for practical reasons or if the patient is poorly motivated or unable to comprehend or psychologically accept insight therapy. Some individuals with borderline psychotic conditions may be further disturbed by intensive therapy. There are also patients whose mental defenses, while of a neurotic quality, served them reasonably well until a traumatic event occurred. Such patients may do better with supportive therapy, which can shore up their existing defenses, than with prolonged and perhaps unsettling attempts at insight therapy. Supportive therapy should be undertaken by trained persons only—psychiatrists or psychologists, and psychiatric social workers who have been carefully trained and supervised.

The function of supportive psychotherapy is to provide the patient with an understanding and sympathetic (but strong) figure who will listen, encourage, clarify, answer questions, and make suggestions during a stressful period until the patient can deal with external and internal problems without help. Therapeutic sessions may vary in frequency from once a week to once a month, and eventually can be scheduled on an "as needed" basis. The duration may be several weeks or months.

2. Intensive, depth, or insight psychotherapy—This type of therapy is indicated for moderate to severe psychoneuroses; functional psychoses (both during and after acute stages); personality and character disorders where there is sufficient anxiety or guilt to provide motivation for treatment on the part of the patient; and psychosomatic disorders where the patient is adequately motivated to improve and the patient's physical condition is not critical. This type of therapy should be done by psychiatrists who have been trained in dynamic psychotherapeutic technics or psychoanalysis.

The objective of intensive psychotherapy is to help the patient gain insight or understanding into why he reacts as he does to internal or external stresses and to utilize this insight in appropriate situations in daily living. This is usually done by attempting to understand, in terms of the patient's past experiences and emotional associations, the underlying meaning of a particular stress and of a specific reaction to it. The therapist may (and usually does) play a supportive role at the same time. The frequency of these sessions may vary from once to several times per week, and treatment may have to be continued for up to 2–3 years.

B. Group Therapy: (See also Chapter 27.) Group therapy may be used in most of the disorders of adolescence—psychoses, psychoneuroses, addictions, and personality and character disorders. The group may consist of similar types of patients (other adolescents, male and female) or the family unit (parents and siblings). Group therapy enables the patient to see that others have similar problems, to know what their feelings and thoughts are about these problems, and to participate actively in the dynamic interchange between members of the group, thus gaining insight into his own reactions to others. This type of therapy may be done by individuals trained in this technic—psychiatrists, psychologists, or psychiatric social workers. Group therapy may be used alone or in combination with individual therapy. The frequency of group sessions may be once or twice a week or every other week; the duration of treatment varies from a few months to a year or more.

C. Counseling: This type of management is indicated in the milder or more transient disorders of adolescence, such as some adjustment reactions of adolescence; some of the character and personality disorders; situations which seem to be precipitated by known external events; and mild to moderate academic and disciplinary problems. It consists of supportive and advice-giving measures as well as opportunities for the adolescent to ventilate his feelings to an understanding and respected adult. It offers identification with a "good adult." The counselor requires special training and interest in adolescents. However, his training need not be so extensive as is required for intensive psychotherapy. Counseling may be done by a trained person such as a physician, psychiatric social worker, psychologist, guidance counselor, clergyman, or others with special talents and training in working with this age group, eg, teachers, recreational leaders, and athletics coaches.

Counseling of the parents by a psychiatrist or by other trained professional personnel may be required in addition to any of the treatment programs outlined in this section.

D. Environmental Manipulation: This is indicated where environment seems to be a major contributing factor to the problem, eg, actively disturbed parents (overtly psychotic, repeatedly abusive in a physical or sexual manner), frequent association with delinquent companions, poverty, severe overcrowding in the home. Examples of environmental manipulation are special schools, "junior republics," foster homes, and organized constructive activities (athletic teams, workshops).

E. Drugs: (See Chapter 24.) Tranquilizing and mood-elevating drugs may be given in the same dosage as for adults if the body size is adult. Drugs may be used in adolescents for hyperactivity, marked anxiety, undue tension, depression, and in psychoses. They may be used in conjunction with psychotherapy. They may also be helpful during withdrawal from addicting drugs and alcohol.

F. Therapy for Psychoses: Treatment of psychoses, as in adults, may include hospitalization, psychotherapy, drugs, and somatic therapies. ECT may be used in any severe depression that fails to respond to psychotherapy and mood-elevating drugs, especially if there is concern about suicide.

ESTIMATING PROGNOSIS OF EMOTIONAL DISORDERS OF ADOLESCENCE

Most adolescents outgrow this very difficult phase of development without professional help; after a sometimes stormy course which may be distressing to older persons near them, they become reasonably stable young adults who can master and control their basic drives. They attain maturity, gain success of varying degrees in terms of career, family, and community— and then have the privilege of becoming parents and dealing with their own adolescent children.

However, the adolescent who develops any of the pathologic conditions described above does require professional help in trying to negotiate this difficult period. These conditions may well persist into adulthood if untreated, and when this happens the result is an adult with a serious emotional disorder or with marked emotional immaturity. With treatment, the outlook for the disturbed adolescent is better than for the adult with a similar illness since the younger person's personality structure is more flexible and still growing toward maturity.

The following factors are useful in estimating the prognosis in many of the disorders of adolescence.

More Favorable Factors

Symptoms which are acute in onset—even if severe in intensity—and those that are precipitated by an identifiable external stress imply a favorable prognosis.

The prognosis improves with the feasibility of modifying the environment (persons close to patient, living conditions, undesirable associates, and stresses).

The prognosis is better if the patient has formed a close, positive relationship of moderate duration with another person (parent, other relative, other adult, or a friend of his own age)—in other words, the prognosis is more favorable if the adolescent has felt loved by someone whom he regarded as important at some time in his life, and has been able to love in return.

Less Favorable Factors

Unfavorable prognostic factors are a history of gradual onset of symptoms; longer duration of symptoms; history of numerous or severe emotional symptoms in childhood (eg, extended bedwetting, temper tantrums, nightmares, bowel training problems); disturbed family history (eg, mental or emotional disorders in parents or siblings, broken homes, loss of a parent); absence of an identifiable external precipitating cause for the onset of the symptoms; impracticality of modifying the environment if the latter is regarded as particularly noxious; and lack of a history of a close, lasting relationship between the adolescent and another person.

REFERENCES

Books and Monographs

Aichorn, A.: *Wayward Youth.* Viking, 1948.

Blaine, G.B.: *Youth and the Hazards of Affluence.* Harper, 1966.

Blos, P.: *On Adolescence: A Psychoanalytic Interpretation.* Free Press of Glencoe, 1962.

Blos, P.: *The Young Adolescent: Clinical Studies.* Brunner/Mazel, 1970.

Caplan, G., & S. Lebovici: *Adolescence: Psychosocial Perspective.* Basic Books, 1969.

Considerations on Personality Development in College Students. GAP Report No. 32, Vol 2. Group for the Advancement of Psychiatry, 1955.

Deutsch, H.: *Selected Problems of Adolescence with Special Emphasis on Group Formation.* Monograph No. 3. Internat Univ Press, 1967.

Easson, W.M.: *The Severely Disturbed Adolescent.* Internat Univ Press, 1969.

Eissler, R.S., & others (editors): *The Psychoaalytic Study of the Child.* Vol 25. Internat Univ Press, 1970.

Erikson, E.H.: *Childhood and Society.* Norton, 1950.

Farnsworth, D.: *Mental Health In College and University.* Harvard Univ Press, 1957.

Ginott, H.G.: *Between Parent and Teenager.* Macmillan, 1969.

Hirsch, E.A.: *The Troubled Adolescent.* Internat Univ Press, 1970.

Holmes, D.: *The Adolescent in Psychotherapy.* Little, Brown, 1964.

Keniston, K.: *The Uncommitted: Alienated Youth in American Society.* Harcourt Bruce, 1965.

Lorand, S., & H.I. Schneer (editors): *Adolescents.* Hoeber, 1965.

Miller, M.V., & S. Gilmore (editors): *Revolution in Berkeley: The Crisis in American Education.* Dell, 1965.

Normal Adolescence: Its Dynamics and Impact. GAP Report No. 68, Vol 6. Group for the Advancement of Psychiatry, 1967.

Sex and the College Student. GAP Report No. 60, Vol 6. Group for the Advancement of Psychiatry, 1965.

Slansky, M.A., & others: *The High School Adolescent: Understanding and Treating His Emotional Problems.* Association Press, 1969.

Vedder, C.B., & D.B. Somerville (editors): *The Delinquent Girl.* Thomas, 1970.

Weiner, I.B.: *Psychological Disturbance in Adolescence.* Wiley, 1970.

Weiner, N.: *Ex-Prodigy: My Childhood and Youth.* Simon & Schuster, 1953.

Whittington, H.: *Psychiatry on the College Campus.* Internat Univ Press, 1963.

Zubin, J., & A.M. Freedman (editors): *The Psychopathology of Adolescence.* Grune & Stratton, 1970.

Journal Articles

Blaine, G.B., Jr.: Some emotional problems of adolescents. M Clin North America 49:387–404, 1965.

Blos, P.: Prolonged adolescence: The formulation of a syndrome and its therapeutic implications. Am J Orthopsychiat 24:733–742, 1954.

Blos, P.: Preadolescent drive organization. J Am Psychoanal Ass 6:47–56, 1958.

Cohen, I., & others: Study of early differentiation between schizophrenia and psychotic manifestations in adolescence. Israel Ann Psychiat 8:163–172, 1970.

Eggertsen, P.F.: Caprice: The "cool" rebellion. Canad Psychiat Ass J 10:165–169, 1965.

Eissler, K.R.: Notes on problems of technique in the psychoanalytic treatment of adolescents: With some remarks on perversions. Psychoanal Stud Child 13:223–254, 1958.

Erikson, E.H.: Reflections on the dissent of contemporary youth. Internat J Psychoanal 51:11–22, 1970.

Fraiberg, S.: Some considerations in the introduction to therapy in puberty. Psychoanal Stud Child 10:264–286, 1955.

Freud, A.: Adolescence. Psychoanal Stud Child 13:255–278, 1958.

Garber, B., & R. Polsky: Follow-up study of hospitalized adolescents. Arch Gen Psychiat 22:179–187, 1970.

Geleerd, E.: Some aspects of ego vicissitudes in adolescence. J Am Psychoanal Ass 9:394–405, 1961.

Hartmann, D.: A study of drug-taking adolescents. Psychoanal Stud Child 24:384–398, 1969.

Hilgard, J.R., & U.S. Moore: Affiliative therapy with young adolescents. J Am Acad Child Psychiat 8:577–605, 1969.

Isay, R.A.: The draft-age adolescent in treatment. Psychiat Quart 43:203–210, 1969.

Jacobson, E.: Adolescent moods and the remodeling of psychic structure in adolescence. Psychoanal Stud Child 16:164–183, 1961.

King, L.J., & G.D. Pittman: A 6-year follow-up study of 65 adolescent patients: Predictive value of presenting clinical picture. Brit J Psychiat 115:1437–1441, 1969.

Lampl-deGroot, J.: On adolescence. Psychoanal Stud Child 15:95–103, 1960.

Laufer, M.: Ego ideal and pseudo ego ideal in adolescence. Psychoanal Stud Child 19:196–221, 1964.

Loomis, L.S., Rosen, V.H., & M.H. Stein: Ernst Kris and the gifted adolescent project. Psychoanal Stud Child 13:44–63, 1958.

Masterson, J.F., & A. Washburne: The symptomatic adolescent: Psychiatric illness or adolescent turmoil? Am J Psychiat 122:1240–1248, 1966.

Miller, D.: Adolescents and the high school system. Commun Ment Health J 6:483–491, 1970.

Rogers, R.: The "unmotivated" adolescent patient who wants psychotherapy. Am J Psychother 24:411–418, 1970.

Schiff, L.: The obedient rebels: A study of college conversions to conservatism. J Social Issues 20:74–95, 1964.

Shamsie, S.J.: Youth in conflict: Explanation based on developmental approach. Laval Med 41:544–547, 1970.

Spiegel, L.A.: A review of contributions to a psychoanalytic theory of adolescence. Psychoanal Stud Child 6:375–393, 1951.

Spiegel, L.A.: Comments on the psychoanalytic psychology of adolescence. Psychoanal Stud Child 13:296–308, 1958.

Weider, H., & E. Kaplan: Drug use in adolescents: Psychodynamic meaning and pharmacogenic effect. Psychoanal Stud Child 24:399–431, 1969.

35...

College Psychiatry

Increasing numbers of college students seek professional help for mental and emotional problems, usually involving crisis situations. A few counseling visits often produce gratifying results.

About 7 million young men and women are now in college in the USA. In colleges that provide mental health services, about 10% of students seek and get psychiatric help each year, either voluntarily or by referral.

The available statistics show that 44% have neurotic disorders, 31% character disorders, 17% situational problems, and 8% psychoses. Depression is present in 30–40% of patients. Suicide—the third ranking cause of death in the 15–19 year age group, is threatened by 90,000 students every year, attempted by 20,000, and successful in 1000. Only 2% of students who seek psychiatric help while attending college are hospitalized. Of the 40% of students who leave college before graduation, it is estimated that half do so for psychiatric reasons.

Of the 2252 college campuses in North America, only 76 have student mental health clinics. Fifteen colleges employ full-time psychiatrists, and only 100 others have arrangements with a psychiatrist on a part-time basis. In Boston, 24 colleges have formed a centralized college mental health center. Elsewhere, many students seek help in private offices, community clinics, and hospitals outside the college.

Considering that emotional problems in this age group usually respond readily to therapy, provisions for mental health care by a college could reduce disruptions in academic careers, raise the level of intellectual and emotional maturity, and help prevent the later development of mental illness.

THE MAJOR UNDERLYING CONFLICTS

College spans late adolescence and young adulthood, and the presenting complaint of the student patient may not represent a crystallized disorder which is identifiable in the usual psychiatric terms. As an individual moves toward adult life, vague and fleeting symptoms of emotional turmoil are common. Mood swings are frequent and wide, and anxiety attacks, depressive states, and near-psychotic phenomena such as lapses in judgment or slippage into primitive wishful or magical thinking occur without necessarily indicating a pernicious process. Since college life tolerates eccentric behavior which elsewhere would bring the individual into conflict with the norms of his environment, psychic conflict can be readily acted out with a relative absence of emotional distress.

When the clinician encounters the troubled student, he must judge whether the problem is a relatively normal manifestation of the stress of development or the early sign of a neurotic or psychotic process. Theorists such as Erik Erikson have suggested several developmental tasks pertinent to this age group that can aid in understanding otherwise puzzling clinical material.

Identity Formation vs Identity Diffusion

According to Erikson, a sense of identity is a result of the person's ability to integrate his early partial and varied identifications, eg, his identification with each of his parents, with newly manifest sexual drives, intellectual and emotional endowment, and social roles. The consequence of this integrative process is a sense of rightness about what he is doing and a feeling of comfort about who he is. Barring extreme changes, he continues to feel a "sameness" within himself. The process of crystallization of the sense of identity, which began in puberty, accelerates during the college years.

"Identity diffusion" (poor self-integration) occurs when the individual cannot integrate varied identifications to the necessary extent, eg, when he is unable to make a definite choice of career, role, values, or sexual object. It is accompanied by anxiety, depression, confusion, a sense of alienation or loneliness, or even frank psychosis.

During the college years, various identities and activities are tried on for size, eg, love affairs or fighting for a cause (often one that is inimical to the parents' values). If the ego lacks integrative ability, if childhood identifications are highly ambivalent, or if the pressures from impulses or the environment are too severe, diffusion occurs.

Independence vs Dependence

Separation from the family—both physical separation and removal from one value system to another—demands of the student either the strengthening of an established system of thought and behavior or acceptance of an identification with a new system. The student must learn to trust and respect both the person he is and the person with new knowledge and greater skills that he will become. Established dependency roles must be redirected toward new authorities.

If the need to be dependent is too great or if accepting new values or developing a new identity seems to imply the rejection of greatly needed parents, separation anxiety or depression may be the result. Sexual acting out, suicidal gestures, overeating, use of drugs and alcohol, obsessive compulsive activity, failure to achieve, or running away can be regressive manifestations of intense conflict over dependency issues. If the student's ego is functioning pathologically as an extension of the ego of one parent, or if the bond with the parent has been excessive, college life can precipitate a psychotic reaction.

Intimacy vs Isolation

During these years, the student learns to replace long-established closeness within the family with new relationships that require an intimacy probably not experienced before. Such intimacy involves equality, acceptance of needs, and genital sexuality. A prerequisite is a strong sense of ego identity which allows the individual to be close to another person or to embrace an idea or acknowledge an impulse from within without fear of losing himself or having a sense of being overwhelmed.

The approach to closeness with other people may stimulate neurotic difficulties, eg, regression to pregenital sexual practices or schizoid withdrawal into defensive isolation. Aside from producing social despair and barrenness, fear of blurring one's ego boundaries produces intense anxiety and may interfere with accepting assignments and instruction or obeying regulations.

Sexual Indulgence vs Continence

Many students come from families where "how far one can go" is sternly limited and where exploring beyond those limits implies trespassing on "dirty" or morally restricted ground. The student at college is not only free of parental restrictions and watchfulness but is immersed in discussions of all varieties of sex, with emphasis on liberalized attitudes and experimentation. This is true for both male and female students. Aside from elements of identity, dependency, and intimacy, sexual behavior can engender severe superego-ego conflicts and intense feelings of guilt or total rebellion with overthrow of moral standards. The student who cannot participate—for moral or other reasons—in either the discussions or the behavior may feel strange, lonely, or unaccepted.

It is interesting that, while attitudes toward sex in general evidently have become more liberal during the past 40 years, the incidence of sexual intercourse during college is said not to have increased very much.

PROBLEMS OF THE NEW STUDENT

The Incoming Freshman

The freshman student may encounter for the first time a wide variety of values, mores, and attitudes that conflict with those of his family. The conflict may be understood by him as one of individuality vs family loyalty; and the natural pursuit of individuality may provoke guilt feelings about rejecting and devaluing his own family.

The entrance of a son or daughter into college is often assumed by the family to mean acceptance of adult responsibilities, and not all young people are prepared or willing (not always consciously) to give up their comfortable dependent status. They may feel that the family has abandoned them. At the same time, the family may not be tolerant of the new values that the student brings home. The student may be in a particularly difficult position if he commutes to school and thus must function at both levels in 2 quite different environments.

The family serves as a reinforcement for self-discipline and impulse control. At college, sexual morality, commitment to work, and self-regulated living—rather than conformity to the guardian parent—become the task of the individual. Insecurity in these areas produces anxiety.

A prominent freshmen complaint is the depression brought on by his first failures to maintain accustomed levels of accomplishment. The student who was outstanding in his secondary school finds himself at the university in competition with many others of equal ability or aptitude. He then must rebuild the basis of his identity and self-esteem and tolerate strong competition in social and academic areas. Most freshmen have some concerns about being accepted and competing successfully at higher levels of accomplishment.

Away from home, the student with highly ambivalent feelings toward his parents may have to face heretofore suppressed negative feelings as they begin to enter consciousness. Guilt, anxiety, and self-deprecation may accompany these feelings.

The student who has been part of a neurotic family relationship may not be able to tolerate the college situation. If he has served as an ego extension of one parent, his sense of accomplishment may be replaced by feelings of resentment or low self-esteem. If he believes that the separation is harmful either to himself or to his parents, he will not be able to tolerate independence but will return home frequently to reassure himself that nothing has happened. His parents may be equally concerned with the student's safety.

If the partners to a bad marriage have been waiting until the student entered college to separate or get a divorce, the student may feel his family is deteriorating because of his absence. On the other hand, his parents may get along better when he is out of the household, and the student may then feel puzzled about the apparent ease with which his absence is tolerated.

If symbiotic bonds have existed between the student and one of his parents, separation may symbolize destroying this parent—an extreme threat that may precipitate a psychotic reaction.

Transfer Students

Students who transfer in from other institutions may have based their transfer decision on reality issues such as change of career choice, a mismatching of character and college, or changes in life situation such as financial problems or marriage. On the other hand, many students with social or academic difficulties seek to resolve their problems by making meaningless transfers from one college to another. When the student finds that he has not left his inner problems at his other college, he may be in a better position to recognize that he has personal difficulties and seek treatment for them.

There is evidence that schizophrenic students transfer more often than nonschizophrenic students.

PROBLEMS DURING COLLEGE

Problems of Academic Performance

Difficulty with studying and underachievement are the most common chief complaints of student patients. Students who cannot break away from their books are also seen, but rarely.

(1) **Intellectual deficiencies**: Reading problems, organic deficits, and intellectual deficits are sometimes uncovered in college, although this usually happens earlier. It is important that these students receive specialized help for their disability. The psychiatrist may be needed to help the student deal with attendant depression or feelings of inadequacy.

(2) **Difficulties in concentration**: Some students sit at their desks for hours and yet cannot organize or direct their thinking to the task before them. Such students are probably displacing family or social concerns onto their studies or are prevented from studying by obsessive ruminations, sexual preoccupations, or guilt feelings. Clarifying the source of the distractions and dealing with the underlying problems are necessary to break the study block.

(3) **Inability to work**: Students sometimes do well in the extracurricular aspects of college life but not in their academic work. In one student the reason may simply be that adjusting to the new social environment is of more concern to him than his academic tasks. In another, previous failure to be autonomous and self-reliant may have left him overly dependent, and he may be hoping through failure to attract a new authority who will replace the parents and tell him what to do. Lack of concern and interest or outright failure in studies can serve as an effective way of spiting or rebelling against parents who have been too intrusive, domineering, or involved in the student's academic success. Finally, deep unconscious conflicts of an oedipal nature may have endowed working and learning with fears of retaliation by an enraged competitive father.

In cases where unconscious forces are affecting study habits or academic accomplishment, insight-oriented therapy is most valuable but usually not sufficiently available. Dynamically oriented therapy and limited-goal insight therapy alleviate the immediate problem for many patients in this group.

(4) **Test anxiety**: Anxiety about exams may signify that more is at stake than completing a course successfully. Parental love or rejection may ride on a grade. On the other hand, the student may unconsciously wish to fail in order to test or hurt his parents, and the conscious expression of this would be fear of failing. Also, doing well on an exam may arouse unconscious fears of besting the father and perhaps suffering retaliation.

(5) **Thought disorders**: As part of their generally poor adjustability, borderline schizophrenic or frankly schizophrenic students have a great deal of difficulty doing college work. The stress of being in college shifts the ego toward decompensation. The abstraction and organization needed for some studies may be replaced with concretized thinking and confusion. The subject material then becomes too symbolically personal to be acceptable to the student. For severely shaky egos, even reading what another person has written can precipitate a sense of identity loss and arouse anxiety.

Sexual Concerns

(1) **Virginity**: Concerns about virginity are a frequent source of conflict among both male and female college students. There often is a wide gap between the liberal attitudes toward sex that find verbal expression on campus and the student's own stricter moral standards. He then wonders if he is "normal" or "acceptable" and feels under pressure to behave as he imagines others expect him to.

The conflict over virginity may conceal a deep pathologic fear of sexuality, fear of closeness to others, or an unresolved sexual identity conflict. The issue of social acceptance can be expressed as despair over inability to participate in sexual activities which others seem to enjoy.

(2) **"Petting," "making out," and rules**: Concerns about love making either express a value conflict or are indicative of deeper concerns. Problems of sexual identity, pre-oedipal and oedipal conflicts, or intimacy and activity-passivity difficulties arise. New forms of sexual behavior are of concern because they weaken shaky impulse controls which until then had been supported by the home environment.

Displacement of the stern superego onto the administration or the rules of the institution is a way of expressing rebellion and avoiding intrapsychic conflict.

(3) **Promiscuity**: Intercourse with a number of partners in a series of affairs—often single encounters—is promiscuity, a term usually applied to female sexual behavior. The woman usually does not experience orgasm.

There is a positive correlation between promiscuity and mental disturbances in college women, since this behavior is often an expression of intense conflict over dependency and the need for nurturing and love. The student is unable to gain love through true intimacy in a mature relationship and seeks momentary emotional gratification in frequent brief sexual contacts. The resulting guilt and sense of isolation from society increase her loneliness and lower her self-esteem. Promiscuous sexual behavior may also be the borderline psychotic woman's means of warding off decompensation into psychosis.

While it is depression that usually brings the promiscuous college woman into treatment, pregnancy and venereal disease may do so, and the student health physician should be alert to the emotional factors in his patient's sexual behavior.

The promiscuous man may be running away from a commitment to a closer, more mature, and lasting relationship, unconsciously defending himself against homosexual feelings, or acting out a Don Juan series of "triumphs."

(4) **Pregnancy and contraception**: The sexual freedom of the unmarried college woman may cause her no difficulty until she gets pregnant, at which time she usually experiences shock, intense anxiety, guilt, and shame. Pregnancy almost invariably interrupts her schooling and involves her family. The psychiatrist may be able to help her in dealing with her parents and in deciding her course of action by helping her to consider alternatives and explore her motivations.

The recently relaxed sanctions against abortion, as expressed in position statements by the American Medical Association, American Psychiatric Association, and many other authoritative groups and by drastically revised legislation in many states, have resulted in much greater latitude and freedom of action in cases of unmarried pregnant women. It is no longer necessary for a psychiatrist (usually 2 psychiatrists) to examine the woman and report that the continuation of the pregnancy would constitute a serious threat to her mental health or her life. Therapeutic abortion is now widely considered a matter of concern only to the woman and her physician. Moreover, careful studies are demonstrating that abortions may be expected to be tolerated as well psychologically as they are physically.

The problem of prescribing contraceptive methods for unmarried young women is still complicated by both moral and legal considerations, although here also relaxed regulations are becoming the rule. Some college administrations continue to have strict established policies on giving out such information. However, the health of the patient should remain the primary concern. Until a promiscuous girl in treatment is able to stop her pathologic sexual behavior, every effort should be made to help her avoid pregnancy.

On the other hand, a prescription for "the pill" is sometimes understood by the student as a license to indulge in wider sexual activity and thus causes anxiety by seeming to resolve a value conflict which the student needs to resolve herself.

The possibility of pregnancy and the responsibility involved in facing either abortion or bringing another human being into the world should be stressed as reasonable deterrents to meaningless sexual behavior.

(5) Masturbatory concerns: Guilt over masturbation often is based on religious proscription or arises from the fantasies associated with the masturbation. Concerns about the supposed physical or mental harm caused by masturbation are still prevalent but give way readily to education by the psychiatrist. By and large, masturbation is accepted by most male college students as a reasonable substitute for unavailable sexual intercourse, but it is still not easily talked about.

Excessive masturbation (several times a day in a compulsive fashion, without much pleasure) is a means of dealing with anxieties and pressures of other aspects of life or of dealing with interfering sexual preoccupations. It is usually neurotic in origin, and it may signal an impending decompensation toward psychosis.

(6) Homosexual panic: Some panic attacks stem from an upsurge of unconscious homosexual feelings. These attacks are brought on by the close living situation in dormitories, unconscious attraction to a person of the same sex in the locker room, the formation of a close friendship, or an attempted seduction by a homosexual. Although less common, homosexual panic occurs in female as well as male students.

Some degree of conscious recognition of homosexual feelings may be present, in which case reassurance is generally helpful. Otherwise, interpretation is to be avoided without preparatory therapy.

The sexual content in these attacks as well as in conscious homosexual feelings can be a superficial sexualized expression of deeper conflicts over dependency or passivity. In such instances, to label and consequently treat the individual as having a "homosexual problem" would not be treating the real problem at all. It is also well to remember that homosexual panic sometimes represents an early manifestation of a paranoid or other neurotic or psychotic process.

(7) **Homosexuality**: The overtly homosexual male student who has firmly established this sexual orientation may require advice and support in controlling his sexual behavior so as to avoid friction with the administration and the local law authorities. He may already have been referred by them. An exploration of the realistic aspects of such behavior is helpful, and admonitions not to attempt to seduce nonhomosexual men are often necessary.

The student who is in conflict over homosexual impulses, fantasies, or behavior should receive exploratory therapy to attempt to overcome the block in development of his heterosexual identity.

A heterosexual adjustment may still be possible at this age both for male and female patients, particularly if a bisexual interest exists. Dependency or passivity longings in relation to members of the same sex may be the basic problem. However, if the therapist feels that the homosexual orientation cannot be changed, understanding, acceptance, and support are helpful in balancing the patient's feelings of being an outcast and in raising his self-esteem.

Difficulties in Interpersonal Relationships

A complaint of difficulty in interpersonal relationships may signify a wide variety of conditions. The student may seek help voluntarily—eg, because he has no friends—or he may come to the psychiatrist's attention at the suggestion of or on referral from deans, friends, college physicians, or others.

(1) **The alienated student ("alienation syndrome")**: Many students respond to the stimulus of college with an attitude characterized by apathy, boredom, lack of involvement and commitment, and unhappiness. In recent years, use of illicit drugs and meaningless sexual behavior have become common accompaniments. Many such students appear schizoid and depressed, but other diagnostic categories are represented also. As a rule, these students have little interest in psychotherapy or anything else and they can present quite a challenge to the psychiatrist since their poor academic and social performances cause great concern to their colleges. Such students sometimes become severely depressed and may attempt suicide for nihilistic philosophic reasons.

This syndrome often appears to be causally related to the absence or denial of an internalized value system, with elements of repressed rage and guilt concerning parental figures.

(2) **Hysterical rejected student**: Some students react melodramatically to situations involving rejection. A broken friendship, a bad grade, or a

critical remark by a teacher can produce panic, weeping, impulsive behavior, and even suicidal gestures. Fugues, dissociative states, and seizures may occur. The dramatic quality of these events invariably involves friends and college officials and occasionally the police. What the student wants, although he may realize it only dimly, is immediate rescue from what he conceives to be a hopeless situation.

Dramatic recovery can occur without treatment, or a single one-hour interview may be all that is required. In some cases a prescription for tranquilizers or a night in the infirmary is necessary. Follow-up interviews are of value in determining whether a more serious pathologic process exists. These students are not aware of the rage involved in their symptomatology; their premorbid personality should be assessed and further treatment considered.

(3) The depressed student: In most cases the depressed student is easily identified. The usual symptoms of depression—anorexia, sleep disturbances, feelings of worthlessness, listlessness, and general unhappiness—bring him to the office. Many, however, are identified by college officials. Somatic concerns may alert the school physician to a masked depression. Isolation, withdrawal, or a depressed appearance may attract the attention of a teacher or dormitory proctor.

The depression may be either reactive (to an external situation) or endogenous. The recent death of a parent is a particularly difficult emotional problem for the college student. Broken romances, disappointing grades, or family problems can also produce depressive reactions.

Endogenous depressions—those with no discernible outside causes—are particularly dangerous and require careful handling by all concerned. Suicide may already have been considered as a feasible solution to unhappiness and despair. The suicide rate in college is higher than that of the age group as a whole, and in many cases the student gives little or no warning. There is no significant correlation between suicide and cultural background or academic standing.

The management of depression in college students is the same as in the general population. Immediate help and support are often quickly effective in averting a severe depressive reaction in this age group. Antidepressant medication is usually indicated in endogenous depressions. Hospitalization and electroshock treatment may have to be resorted to in severe or suicidal cases.

(4) Borderline psychotic or frankly psychotic students: These students can be divided into those with chronic symptoms of psychosis and those manifesting acute psychotic reactions.

The chronically borderline or mildly schizophrenic student may manifest the same problems as any other student. However, his difficulty in concentration may stem from the intrusion of bizarre thoughts. He may complain of bewilderment or horrible nightmares. He may not be able to realize how odd or peculiar his behavior is. He may call attention to himself with inappropriate remarks in class or in examinations and other written material. Any situational pressure may stimulate paranoia, mania, or other frankly psychotic reactions.

These students need firm, supportive, and prolonged contact with the health service. Tranquilizers, especially phenothiazines, may be very useful. Relief from pressure by dropping a difficult course (or dropping out of school for a while) may be necessary.

An acute psychotic reaction is a psychiatric emergency. Early careful handling may have long-range beneficial effects. Most psychotic students are not difficult to work with, but occasionally paranoid episodes may have murderous content, and the patient may have to be restrained by the authorities. The parents or guardians must be informed. Their cooperation in hospitalization or leaving school is necessary.

(5) **Misuse of drugs and alcohol:** (See also Chapter 21.) Alcoholism per se is rare among college students. Occasional brief periods of alcoholism as a reaction to neurotic problems may occur and lead to destructive behavior. If school regulations are violated, drinking problems are usually handled by college officials.

The widespread use of hallucinogenic and other illicit drugs is at present a problem of greater seriousness. Current studies show that in many colleges the large majority of students have tried illicit drugs at least once. Most have done so experimentally or out of curiosity and have limited their use to one or two times. A large minority, however, smoke marihuana regularly or resort frequently to barbiturates or amphetamines. The drugs used most frequently are marihuana, dextroamphetamine, methamphetamine ("speed"), barbiturates, LSD, and mixtures and analogues of these drugs. Heroin and other narcotics are rarely used, but there is reason to think their use is increasing.

It is helpful to consider misuse of drugs as social, neurotic, or psychotic in origin. The social reasons for drug abuse have already been mentioned, ie, experimentation, curiosity, or to keep up with the peer group. Few students consider either the legal risks or the not inconsiderable medical risks (eg, accidents occur in the acute intoxicated state, psychosis may be precipitated in susceptible or borderline individuals, and contaminated needles may transmit hepatitis).

The neurotic drug user risks dependency or addiction since he is attempting to obtain relief from constant psychic discomfort. However, continued methamphetamine abuse may produce a toxic psychosis within 7–10 days. Persistent excessive use of marihuana over a period of months may create emotional dependency as well as a diminution in reality perception, so that these students ("potheads") subject themselves to a loss of involvement with the world around them. Cognitive and creative abilities decrease, affect is impoverished, and personality deteriorates.

In psychodynamic terms, the use of these drugs is often an effort to deal with depression, insecurity, identity problems, or compulsive ruminations. Unfortunately, their use eventually increases the difficulties they are being called on to relieve. The drug user does find some security in belonging to a group of similar individuals, but in this he forms an identification with an essentially unhealthy segment of society and his fundamental insecurity remains unresolved. His dependence on this group increases his difficulty in leaving drugs alone and favors escalation to stronger drugs.

The psychotic drug user may augment his withdrawal from reality by the use of a drug, or his continued use of it can stand as a suicidal equivalent. Seemingly minor psychedelic compounds such as marihuana or hashish can produce a decompensation to acute psychosis in such a person.

True addiction to narcotics, tranquilizers, and the barbiturate-amphetamine cycle occurs rarely in college. These students require hospitalization for withdrawal and treatment.

Aside from diagnosing and treating underlying disorders in the student drug users, psychiatrists can perform an essential service as educators in this area. Acquainting students with the physical, emotional, and legal risks of drug abuse is one of the most effective means of control, since it allows the student to form his own opinions and make his own decisions, thus avoiding the rebellion that might result from coercive control measures. In addition, the college psychiatrist should be able to assure the student that he can seek help for his drug problems without the threat of arrest.

LSD and methamphetamine psychoses need the same treatment as other psychotic reactions. Chlorpromazine, 50–100 mg IM, can terminate a "bad trip" in LSD users.

Insight-oriented and supportive therapy can help drug users deal with their anxieties and depressions in more rational ways.

CONCERNS ABOUT GRADUATION

During their senior year, many students face final decisions concerning career, military service, postgraduate education, and marriage. If college has functioned as a prolongation of dependency, impending graduation along with the need for making important decisions, usually on the basis of insufficient data, can arouse intense conflicts. Any type of reaction, from simple examination anxiety to psychotic reactions, may occur as a result of this stress.

Exploration of the emotional functions college has served and discussion of rational attitudes toward the future should be the focus of therapy.

DROPOUTS

Psychiatric Dropouts

Students who develop depressive or psychotic reactions have to leave school if the disorder is severe enough to require relief from all stressful activity. Others with milder disturbances leave because assistance is not available to them at college. If the college is not flexible enough to allow a modification of routine, still other students may have to leave. For example, some students could remain in school if they were night patients at a nearby hospital and attended classes during the day, or if they could receive more supervision or lighten their academic responsibilities.

The anxious or agitated student can sometimes be helped to remain in school by therapy that explores the conflicts aroused by college. The student who unconsciously wishes to retaliate against his parents or to gain masochistic satisfaction may begin to fail or ignore his work, thereby engineering the termination of a college career that means nothing to him personally. This student's problem is less amenable to brief psychotherapy, particularly if it is indicative of an underlying character disorder.

Unfortunately, many students leave school impulsively or during a panic, thus making impossible any intervention by either the school or the psychiatrist.

Dropping Out as a Moratorium

Some students find themselves facing extremely severe identity crises. They complain of a growing doubt about what they want or who they are. Interest in the career choice wanes. Remaining at school seems a waste of time, effort, and money. They express the need to find themselves because they feel lost, aimless, and anonymous. They feel they are only going through the motions of living at someone else's request and someone else's expense.

For such a student, a leave of absence can serve as a period of moratorium during which the developmental process of identity formation is allowed to continue. He may work for a year, or enter the military services. (On the other hand, the draft often acts as a deterrent to dropping out for some young men who otherwise could make valuable use of a moratorium.) This moratorium should involve doing something for and by oneself, taking care of oneself, and proving one's independence. In many cases, school is resumed after a year or so with the feeling that further education is now what the student wants for himself and not just something to do for his parents.

PROBLEMS OF THE GRADUATE STUDENT

The graduate student may express his conflicts in a more symptomatic fashion by virtue of his older age and more advanced emotional development. He may seek help for marital problems. In these ways he more closely resembles the general adult psychiatric patient not in college.

Several difficulties are characteristic of the graduate student. He may be under great financial pressures, or he may be coping with suppressed rage and depression concerning his prolonged dependency on his parents, his school, or his wife, which he may view as a humiliation. He may have difficulty functioning well academically in the unstructured graduate school environment although he did well in the more directive situation in undergraduate studies. He may also unconsciously wish to prolong his dependency by failing or not completing his graduate studies, or by prolonging them interminably.

METHODS OF TREATMENT

COUNSELING AND ANCILLARY SERVICES

Most colleges have counseling services staffed by people at various levels of professional training. The skill and competence of these departments largely determine the types of problems they can handle. By and large, counseling services limit their activity to study and career problems and only secondarily provide a listening ear for the disturbed student. These services usually include psychologic testing and technics for referring problems the staff is not prepared to handle.

Others on the campus may also assist in filling the students' need for help with their emotional problems. The disturbed student may seek help and support from a member of the psychology department, the chaplain, a dean, a master, a tutor, or other faculty member. If a disturbed student has formed a close and supportive relationship with a nonmedical college official, the psychiatrist should usually function in an ancillary role to that relationship. He may hold consultative or supervisory sessions with the faculty member—always with the knowledge of the student—or he may prescribe medication for the student and allow the relationship with the other man or woman to remain the major source of help.

If a teacher feels that he can no longer deal with the student's difficulties, the student must be told. Referral to the psychiatrist then may be voluntary or may be made a condition for remaining in school. Tragedies sometimes occur because a faculty member loses sight of the realistic basis for a student's request for trust and confidentiality. For example, the student may threaten to do something desperate if anyone else is told about his difficulties. In such a case, where the alternative is possibly suicide, the teacher must first overcome the student's objection as a simple matter of common sense; the teacher must be able to accept his own limitations and take the realistic course of seeking aid for the student, perhaps by hospitalization under appropriate professional supervision.

ENVIRONMENTAL MANIPULATION

Environmental changes do not cure mental disorders, but relieving the pressure of the environment on an already stressed personality system is often an important adjunct to treatment.

On-Campus Changes

For the student with study problems, a lighter course load is better than failure. If he proceeds at a rate commensurate with his capacities, he has a better chance of completing his education even though it takes longer.

Rooming changes can temporarily rescue many students with interpersonal problems. Some students seem to be unable to tolerate roommates and dormitory living. Others need help in moving away from home if that is the major source of conflict.

The shy, withdrawn, or schizoid student may need direct help in joining social groups to combat loneliness and isolation.

If hospitalization becomes necessary, the advantages of having it on or near the campus are many. Whether hospitalization needs to be brief for a situational reaction or long-term for a psychotic reaction, maintaining the student's ties to the school can counteract regressive trends and perhaps help prevent symptoms from becoming chronic. The concept of hospitalization should be broadened to include only day and only night hospitalization programs, or only weekends or vacation periods, with arrangements for tutoring, group therapy, follow-up, and intermittent brief stays.

Off-Campus Changes

The recommendation to leave school has been discussed above as being helpful or necessary for some students. Feelings of guilt and failure in both the student and the administrator may need consideration. Hospitalization away from the school or near to the student's home is sometimes appropriate for therapeutic or financial reasons or may be simply unavoidable.

SHORT-TERM PSYCHOTHERAPY

For the purposes of this discussion, "short-term" designates an upper limit of perhaps 15 visits, or about one interview a week for a school term. Most students who make use of college mental health facilities find it necessary to attend only 2 or 3 times. Since this group includes all diagnostic categories, it is apparent that college mental health services deal with many situational problems and that this population is highly receptive to psychotherapeutic intervention. Research may show this to be true only for those students who ask for help and not true for those who are referred by others.

College students respond exceptionally well to therapists who combine a dynamic orientation with being also partially directive. Students need genuine interaction with their therapists to circumvent the generation gap and the anxieties regarding identity that might cause them to terminate treatment soon after it has begun. They come to the therapist to talk with him and not just to talk to him. Viewing the therapist as a "real person" in the beginning may provide ego support or even ego sharing against the forces that threaten to overwhelm or diffuse the ego.

At the same time, most students are introspective, sensitive, and curious. After rapport is established, exploration is usually intriguing and rewarding to them. Transferences develop easily, but in the time available a transference is rarely resolved. Instead, the so-called "transference cure" is sufficient. The average student has a multitude of interests and activities and does not want treatment prolonged beyond the relief of acute discomfort. The unveiling and clarification of a major conflict is often sufficient to clear the roadblock so that development can then proceed normally by itself without further psychiatric intervention.

GROUP THERAPY

Group therapy for the socially inept and withdrawn as well as for the socially abrasive student provides a situation wherein feedback and encouragement come from peers in a protective setting. It is also one answer to the scarcity of available professionals necessary for long-term individual therapy.

On the other hand, group therapy does not guarantee the anonymity of the individual, and if the group is composed of students from various colleges, different vacation and academic schedules may disrupt the continuity of the group experience.

PSYCHOACTIVE DRUGS
AND OTHER SOMATIC THERAPY

Drug therapy has limited use in college psychiatry. Phenothiazines are called for in psychotic reactions, and other sedatives, such as chlordiazepoxide (Librium) and meprobamate (Equanil, Miltown), may be useful on a short-term basis for panic and acute anxiety reactions. A brief course of antidepressants can help a depressed student mobilize his own energies to cope with his problems. Many students, however, come to a college physician or psychiatrist after trying to deal with their conflicts and feelings by the use of alcohol or psychoactive drugs. The physician's basic function is to help the student find more realistic methods of handling his problems. Some students view a prescription as a brush-off or another example of dishonesty in the "Establishment."

Other somatic therapies, mainly electroconvulsive treatment, have limited application and then only in a hospital setting. A student cannot function properly at school while receiving ECT.

INTENSIVE PSYCHOANALYTICALLY
ORIENTED THERAPY

Because of the expense and the time required, intensive psychotherapy and psychoanalysis are generally not available to college students. College students may also not be suitable candidates for intensive therapy because they usually do not have crystallized and established neuroses or character disorders. If they do have these, intensive dynamic therapy would be indicated if available.

LIAISON PSYCHIATRY

The role of the psychiatric consultant or psychiatric liaison physician to a college is still in an early stage of development. The liaison psychiatrist does not deal primarily with the treatment or disposition of students with mental disorders. He works with the social processes that tend to produce or stimulate conflicts, anxiety, or disorganization within an institution and thus aggravate intrapsychic disorders in the members of that institution. Thus he works with preventive measures, unfortunately often vaguely defined.

He may be asked to consult on an individual student, a group, or an administrative or disciplinary issue, but he is neither judge, administrator, nor disciplinarian. He may supervise or serve as a consultant to the counseling service, but he is not a counselor. He may be asked to help with intramural problems, ranging from long hair and bare feet to open revolution. He may meet with student groups or participate in education in a more formal sense as a lecturer. He must maintain his primary role as a consultant who deals with the clarification and alleviation of interfering emotional themes in the existent social processes, with the view to furthering the development of the many individuals involved. He is not a therapist in the individual sense, nor is he an advice-giver. He functions largely by helping his associates in the college work out their problems when they find themselves at an impasse.

REFERENCES*

Books and Monographs
Blaine, G.B., Jr., & others: *Emotional Problems of the Student.* Doubleday, 1966.
Caplan, G.: *Principles of Preventive Psychiatry.* Basic Books, 1964.
Chasell, J.O.: *Bennington Psychiatric Papers.* The Austen Riggs Center, 1967.
Douvan, E., & J. Adelson: *The Adolescent Experience.* Wiley, 1966.
Eddy, H.P. (editor): *Sex and the College Student.* Group for the Advancement of Psychiatry, 1966.
Erikson, E.H. (editor): *Youth: Change and Challenge.* Basic Books, 1963.
Farnsworth, D.L.: *Mental Health in College and University.* Harvard Univ Press, 1957.
Keniston, K.: *The Uncommitted.* Harcourt, 1960.
Pervin, L.A., Riek, L., & W. Dalrymple (editors): *The College Dropout and the Utilization of Talent.* Princeton Univ Press, 1966.
Wedge, B.M. (editor): *Psychosocial Problems of College Men.* Yale Univ Press, 1958.

Journal Articles
Allen, A.D., & J.F. Janowitz: A study of the outcome of psychotherapy in a university health service. J Am Coll Health Ass 13:361–378, 1965.
Baker, R.W.: Incidence of psychological disturbance in college students. J Am Coll Health Ass 13:532–540, 1964.
Council on Mental Health and Committee on Alcoholism and Drug Dependence: Dependence on Cannabis (marihuana). JAMA 201:368–371, 1967.

*See also references for Chapter 34.

Curran, W.J.: Policies and practices concerning confidentiality in college mental health services in the United States and Canada. Am J Psychiat 125:1520–1536, 1969.

Erikson, E.H.: Identity and the life cycle: Selected papers. Psych Issues 1:1–171, 1959.

Evans, J.L.: The college student in the psychiatric clinic: Syndrome and subcultural sanctions. J Am Psychiat 126:1736–1742, 1970.

Farnsworth, D.L.: Psychiatry and higher education: Practical applications of psychiatry in a college setting. Am J Psychiat 109:266–271, 1952.

Halleck, S.L.: Psychiatric treatment of the alienated college student. Am J Psychiat 125:642–650, 1967.

Halleck, S.L.: Sex and mental health on the campus. JAMA 200:684–690, 1967.

Halleck, S.L.: Sexual problems of college students. Med Aspects Human Sexuality 2:14–27, May 1968.

Hirsch, S.J., & K. Keniston: Psychological issues in talented college dropouts. Psychiatry 33:1–20, 1970.

Howe, L.P.: The application of community psychiatry to college settings. Internat Psychiat Clin 7:263–291, 1970.

Keeler, M.H.: Adverse reaction to marihuana. Am J Psychiat 124:674–677, 1967.

Krantz, J.C., Jr. (editor): Drug abuse: A symposium. CMD, 665–697, June 1968.

Kuehn, J.: Management of the college student with homicidal impulses: The "Whitman syndrome." Am J Psychiat 125:1594–1499, 1969.

Nicholi, A.M., Jr.: Campus disorders: A problem of adult leadership. Am J Psychiat 127:424–429, 1970.

Nicholi, A.M., Jr.: Harvard dropouts: Some psychiatric findings. Am J Psychiat 124:651–658, 1967.

Reifler, C.B., & others: College psychiatry as public health psychiatry. Am J Psychiat 124:662–671, 1967.

Smith, W.G., Hansell, N., & J.T. English: Psychiatric disorder in a college population. Arch Gen Psychiat 9:351–361, 1963.

Solomon, P.: Medical management of drug dependence. JAMA 206:1521–1526, 1968.

Sturgis, S.H., & others: Viewpoints on teenagers and the pill. Med Aspects Human Sexuality 2:6–14, Feb 1968.

Talbot, E., Miller, S.C., & R.B. White: Some antitherapeutic side effects of hospitalization and psychotherapy. Psychiatry 27:170–176, 1964.

36 . . .

Geriatric Psychiatry

Old people suffer the same problems that younger people do, plus aging. They respond to the same good care, especially if it is given with optimism and enthusiam and not with defeatism. The physician's task is to try to help them achieve a healthy perspective of their life as a whole and to accept advancing years with a healthy serenity.

Geriatric psychiatry is the study of mental disorders affecting older people. Perhaps unwisely, age 65 is traditionally accepted as the arbitrary dividing point between adult psychiatry and geriatric psychiatry. Some medical practitioners specialize largely in geriatric medicine, and some psychiatrists spend most of their time in geriatric psychiatry, often as consultants in homes for the elderly or to public agencies concerned with the welfare of old people.

Increasing attention is now being focused on this age group as greater numbers of people survive to old age. Functional and organic changes characteristic of old age may occur at any age but are most common after age 65. Chronologic age, however, does not necessarily coincide with biologic age; similarly, it may be difficult to differentiate the symptoms and signs of normal aging from those due to pathologic processes.

The increasing importance of this age group may be demonstrated by considering the following statistics.

In the USA in 1900, 3 million persons (4% of the population) were over age 65. In 1970, over 20 million persons (10% of the population) were over age 65, and further increases are anticipated.

Because of the higher death rate of men at this age, there are more elderly women than men in the USA. Half of elderly women are widows, whereas only 20% of elderly men are widowers. Of the families classified as poor, a third are headed by a person over 65 years of age.

Concurrent with the increases in this population, the medical and psychiatric needs of this group have also multiplied. The aged now form a significant number of first referrals to psychiatric hospitals (25%) and general hospitals, and they form a majority in nursing homes and rest homes. A large number of elderly persons also seek private medical and psychiatric care.

Most elderly psychiatric patients admitted to state hospitals have primarily organic disorders, whereas most of the elderly admissions to general and private hospitals—and those being seen by physicians and psychiatrists in the community—are suffering from functional disorders.

However, only about 4% of elderly people in the USA are in institutions at any given time. The remainder are in the community, usually living alone or with relatives. Of the patients in state hospitals, a significant proportion are elderly. In Massachusetts, over 40% of the state hospital population is over 65 years of age, and the percentage is increasing. Interestingly, as many as 20% of the elderly people in one community have been shown to be suffering from significant psychiatric illnesses.

Cultural Attitudes Toward Old Age

Social and ethical customs regarding the place of old people in society vary in different cultures and even in the same society vary in different eras. In some nomadic hunting tribes, where mobility is essential, the elderly who become a burden are often "left behind" to fend for themselves. By contrast, in some European and Asian cultures, the elderly have the respect of their children and are cared for by them without resentment.

With increasing industrialization and urbanization, the middle class family is more mobile, tends to live in apartments or small houses, and both husband and wife often work. The nuclear family thus becomes separated from the parental generation, with the result that caring for an elderly relative becomes realistically difficult even if the desire to do so is present. Old people who cannot afford private home care thus tend to seek or be directed toward public institutional care.

The increasing number of elderly people in the community has caused government to intercede with provisions for the care of the aged by means of social welfare programs, hospitalization and rehabilitation plans, insurance, nursing homes, and old age centers.

GENERAL FACTORS AFFECTING THE AGED

Old age does not imply pathologic decline in emotional balance or a trend away from mental health. The old person may continue to be energetic, alert, and confident to the moment of his death. However, many old people are less able than they once were to withstand the physical, psychosocial, and socioeconomic stresses operating in the environment. The cumulative effect of these stresses may interfere with function and lead to some of the common symptoms and signs of pathologic aging.

Physical Stresses

The following physical changes of old age may be considered normal: reduced vision, hearing, taste and odor perception; decrease in muscle mass and decline in motor strength; osteoarthritis; osteoporosis, with tendency toward hip fracture, and kyphosis; connective tissue changes and decreased elasticity of the skin; and general decline in function of the internal organs with an increased incidence of organic illness such as diabetes, heart disease, hypertension, and glaucoma. The elderly person may function adequately within these limitations until something happens that he cannot adapt to. Partial or advanced decompensation may then occur. The precipitating physical event may be an illness, operation, or accident.

Psychosocial Stresses

Certain psychologic changes occur with such frequency in the elderly that they may be considered a normal part of the aging process. A decline in intellect is common, although it appears that those with higher IQs and those who pursue creative and intellectual occupations into late life suffer the least decline. Impairment often appears first in novel situations or if abstract reasoning rather than experience is required for problem solving.

Another characteristic change is impairment of memory, more frequently for recent than remote events, and leading to other common behavioral manifestations. These include garrulousness, repetitiveness (forgetting what has already been said), dwelling on the past, losing things, etc. Often, however, the memory difficulty consists only of delay in recall. Names, words, and significant incidents may not come immediately to mind on demand as once they would, but they usually can be recalled a little later.

Other normal psychologic features in the elderly are narrowing of interests and inability to accept new ideas, suspiciousness, lack of enthusiasm, melancholy, pessimism, reluctance to acknowledge changes (improvement or decline) in physical health, possessiveness, selfishness, overcompensation due to awareness of diminished powers, and, not uncommonly, exaggeration of previous neurotic, hysterical, or hypochondriacal personality traits.

Previously well adjusted individuals may be able to compensate for their declining efficiency. Greater serenity, wisdom, judgment, and relief from the pressures of ambition are some of the more favorable attributes of aging.

The psychologic attributes of normal aging under stress merge imperceptibly into pathologic behavior and adjustment. Some threatening psychosocial situations that may lead to difficulties are a sudden forced change in environment, bereavement, diminution of social contacts (deaths of friends, retirement), concern over dwindling sexual potency (more pronounced in men than in women), difficulties in adapting to a changing cultural climate ("generation gap"), the fear of death; the feeling of loss of social status, prestige, and respect; and the frequent friction between the elderly and their children.

It has been said that, in a sense, mental health in old age begins in childhood. In general, the mature individual who retains a positive outlook on life adjusts better in senescence than the person who tends to be anxious and has a history of unsatisfactory interpersonal relationships or has tended not to be able to solve his problems. Lonely elderly people—the widowed, the divorced, the unmarried—also tend to have more difficulties in old age. Women usually adapt to old age more easily than men.

The effects of stressful events on the elderly may be minimal if coped with effectively. However, depression may develop and sometimes agitation, confusion, or even psychotic ideation. Feelings of helplessness and failure and decreased self-esteem and self-confidence may give rise to anger, which may turn inward, leading to depression, or outward, against the supposedly hostile environment. Transient gratification of angry impulses may result in guilt and realistic fears of retaliation, which only further diminishes the individual's sense of worth.

Depression is very common in old people and must always be taken seriously. Suicide threats should never be ignored. Statistically, the aged white male is most prone to be depressed or commit suicide.

Dependency is a common problem among old people suffering from feelings of low self-esteem and of physical weakness. The opposite of dependency—hyper-independence and cantankerousness—sometimes is observed.

Elderly people living with their relatives are often the cause of much discord. Resentment over the older person's demands may lead to premature institutionalization; conversely, guilt feelings may prevent the family from seeking hospitalization for a sick older member when all concerned would be benefited by such hospitalization.

Contrary to what is often thought, the older person is not always happy living with relatives. Elderly people with adequate incomes are often content to live alone, and are satisfied with few rather than many visits from relatives.

The attitude toward death presents a problem to all individuals. Feelings of fear and helplessness in the face of approaching death may be handled in many ways, depending on the strength and maturity of the personality. However, it appears that healthy elderly people use intellectualization as a major defense, whereas the ill tend to use denial. In general, people die as they have lived—fearfully or courageously, neurotically or realistically, cowardly or heroically. Dying is one's last job.

Economic Loss

In old age, financial security may be an even more important asset than good health. Realistic difficulties in obtaining and holding jobs and the fear of loss of employment are threatening to self-esteem.

Retirement calls for the ability to adapt to a new life style and to develop new outlooks and new interests. For men, it is analogous to the menopause in women, as a change of personal status is involved. The change commonly involves reversion to dependency, with reawakening of whatever dependency problems have gone unsolved or been repressed.

If the elderly are unprepared for it, retirement commonly becomes associated with feelings of uselessness, loss of interest, and loss of prestige. It may also result in depression, apathy, anxiety, or anger.

Reaction to retirement depends upon the degree of flexibility and ego strength of the individual and upon his previous economic status. The overly dependent person who holds a dull, routine job is likely to welcome retirement, whereas the man who is afraid of dependency with the resultant threat to his security does not. The authoritarian personality, feeling threatened by his subordinates, may also be loath to retire. Professional or executive individuals who have been immersed in their work may view retirement with reluctance. In many cases, rapid deterioration in physical and intellectual abilities with depression may occur unless the individual is helped to accept his new status with some grace.

MENTAL DISORDERS IN THE ELDERLY

Most of the psychiatric disorders occurring in the young adult may also occur in old age. A disorder may persist into old age, may recur in old age, or may manifest itself for the first time in old age. Chronic organic brain syndrome is a common finding only in elderly people.

The demarcation between normal and neurotic in old age is often as fuzzy as it is in young people. Simple *depression* is the most common psychiatric disorder in the elderly. The declining adaptability of the elderly and adverse psychosocial and socioeconomic factors contribute to depression. The patient may become quarrelsome, complaining, irritable, negativistic, agitated, apathetic, and verbally and physically threatening or assaultive, and he is a constant suicide risk. Hypochondriacal somatic complaints such as insomnia, anorexia, constipation, headache, fatigue, and general aches and pains are frequent.

The differential diagnosis between depression and early organic changes can be very difficult, as the early symptoms and signs may be similar. Unfortunately, there is a tendency to lump together as "senility" all emotional and behavioral difficulties in the elderly; however, since depression is usually reversible, the differentiation is important.

The psychoneuroses of old age, in declining order of frequency, are hysterical, anxiety, phobic, and obsessive compulsive (especially compulsive cleanliness).

Minor emotional disorders in the aged can often be viewed as goal-seeking attempts to manipulate an environment perceived as hostile. The dynamics of the clinging, demanding, and hostile behavior may become clear when viewed in the context of the individual's social and cultural framework.

Organic Brain Syndromes

Acute and chronic brain syndromes are discussed in Chapter 15. Two varieties of chronic brain syndrome—cerebral arteriosclerosis and senile deterioration—will be discussed briefly here.

Cerebral arteriosclerosis. Memory loss is an early sign but is often patchy (in contrast to senile dementias). Impaired ability to understand and concentrate and restlessness at night are common complaints. The patient's judgment and basic personality often appear well preserved. Deterioration is slower and more variable than in senile dementia. Episodes of severe depression often occur in the early stages as the patient perceives that he is "beginning to fail." Paranoid or manic traits are less often present. The diagnosis should be based on definite signs of cerebral arteriosclerosis, eg, strokes, vascular retinopathy, and focal neurologic signs; on the age at onset (commonly between 60 and 70 years); and on the intermittent course of the deterioration, with alternating periods of lucidity and confusion.

Senile deterioration (senile dementia) is characterized by parenchymatous atrophy of the brain. The cause is not known, but the syndrome is probably genetically determined. Symptoms and signs similar to those of cerebral arteriosclerosis may be present, but there are usually no focal neurologic signs nor evidence of strokes and cerebral arteriosclerosis. The intellectual deterioration usually starts later (after age 70) and is almost complete by age 80. The onset is insidious and the course steadily progressive, with the first symptom memory loss for recent events, followed by increasing inflexibility and loss of spontaneous mental activity. Early disinhibition with emotional outbursts occurs, with exaggeration of previous personality characteristics—eg, suspicious people become paranoid, often with sexual fantasies; and pessimistic people become depressed.

The patient may wander off, especially at night. Vocabulary diminishes, thought content becomes aimless and fragmented, and speech incoherent. Lack of concern for other people, deterioration in personal habits, incontinence, and antisocial behavior (eg, sexual misdemeanors) may occur, often to the acute embarrassment and consternation of the relatives.

In all types of organic brain disease, social preservation of the personality is maintained longer in better educated people who have held responsible, well compensated positions. Ultimately, however, most of these patients become totally unable to care for themselves, leading a vegetative existence and needing constant supervision.

Functional Disorders

Schizophrenic reaction, manic-depressive psychosis, and involutional depression also occur in the elderly. These have been dealt with in other parts of this book.

Miscellaneous

Drug dependence (notably alcoholism) is discussed elsewhere. Most patients who have had problems with alcohol are younger than the geriatric group, but some survive to old age and suffer from chronic brain syndrome.

Elderly people often become dependent upon sleeping pills and other favorite medicines.

Psychophysiologic disorders, eg, asthma or colitis, may be carried over into old age; and physical illness, eg, hypertension and diabetes, may be aggravated in the presence of neurotic disorders.

Mildly to moderately mentally retarded children and adults may survive to old age, but the severely retarded rarely do.

TREATMENT

The care and treatment of the elderly should not be viewed pessimistically. Even patients with irreversible organic brain disease can often be helped to make better adjustments to their environment, thus facilitating their management.

The ideal goals of treatment are to minimize the patient's suffering; to improve his behavior; to lessen interpersonal friction; to rehabilitate him for work or other vocational activity; and generally to make him more active and able to take pleasurable interest in his surroundings. To achieve these goals, attention must be paid to more than just the patient. His family, the community, social service agencies, and other special resources have to be considered. A combination of methods is used.

General Medical Care

Nowhere is the need for comprehensive medical care so urgent as in the treatment of the disabled elderly. They often suffer from general medical disorders, which may produce significant physical suffering and may contribute to psychiatric symptoms and signs.

A complete general medical examination with relevant laboratory investigations is essential. Correctable physical problems should be remedied, by means of aids and prostheses if necessary. The diet should be balanced and clearly adequate in vitamin content.

Personal hygiene should be attended to as indicated. Sympathetic, efficient nursing care is an asset, especially in the more severe organic disorders.

Recently, comprehensive multiphasic computer screening examinations for persons at risk (usually men over 45 years of age) have been introduced. Early detection and treatment of physical disorders result in diminished physical disability and hence improved mental health. Until recently, the screening examination has sought not only medical disease entities, but attention is now also being focused on emotional components as well. Those whose score deviates sufficiently from the norm are referred to an appropriate facility for further investigation.

Milieu Therapy

It is often difficult to decide how best to deal with an elderly patient in distress. Because of the stress associated with institutionalization and because a significant percentage of institutionalized old people never return to the community, hospitalization should be avoided if at all possible.

The patient may be seen as an outpatient and treated by a psychiatrist in his office or in the outpatient department of a general hospital, a community mental health center, or state hospital. Social workers and nurses should be used to evaluate the patient's home environment so that problems there can be dealt with as indicated. By all of these means, the patient can frequently be kept out of the hospital.

There are times, however, when it is not only therapeutically mandatory but less stressful, both to the patient and the family, for the patient to be hospitalized for medical and nursing care as well as for the supportive therapeutic relationships provided by the multidisciplinary staff. Treatment must be coordinated as a team effort by the physician, social worker, nurse, attendant, occupational therapist, rehabilitation counselor, and any others who may be required. The institutional environment should have pleasant decor and architecture and be designed for the comfort and safety of patients. It should serve as a setting in which congenial interpersonal relationships can flourish, and must have adequate facilities for physical exercise and for creative and stimulating vocational and recreational activities.

The relationships between the patient and the staff members is even more important to the patient than the medical and nursing care he receives. The attitude should be supportive, but the patient should not be "overprotected."

Elderly people frequently stay in the hospital longer than necessary. State hospitals have 2 main groups of patients over 65 years of age:

(1) One group has grown old in the hospital and consists mainly of "burned out" chronic schizophrenics who have become "institutionalized"– a term applied to patients who have spent many years in the barren state hospital atmosphere, with loss of outside contacts, loneliness, enforced idleness, and lack of responsibility. They become passive, apathetic, obedient, and lacking in initiative, and lose interest and individuality. Management of this group entails remotivation and resocialization and should be oriented toward breaking the ties with the hospital and working through the resulting separation anxiety before discharge to the community.

(2) The second group consists of recent admissions–patients who have decompensated in old age, usually for the first time in their lives. These patients almost invariably have active contacts with the community. They should be treated intensively by means of all available therapeutic technics, preferably in an acute admission ward. Improvement is usually rapid, and they often can be discharged back to the community within a few weeks.

For both groups it is important to maintain a link between the community placement and the hospital after discharge. This is usually done by providing a consultant to work between the hospital and the community. This supportive link also diminishes the likelihood of readmission to the hospital when and if the caretakers in the community have difficulty in dealing with the patient.

Community placements commonly available to elderly people are as follows:

(1) **Patient's own home:** The ideal disposition if the patient is able to care for himself or if others are available to assist him (family, friends, visiting nurses, etc).

(2) **Patient's relatives:** If available.

(3) **Nursing home:** Especially if physical disability is paramount.

(4) **Rest home:** When custodial care only is required.

(5) **Housing for elderly:** As above. The inhabitants may be reasonably well, mentally and physically.

(6) **Geriatric hospital:** Specialized hospital for the nonpsychotic elderly with primarily medical problems.

(7) **Family care home**: Private family providing a "live-in guest" arrangement for a fee.

(8) **Day hospital or day center**: Ideally, this should be located in the community, but it is often located on the grounds of a hospital. The patient spends the day, usually from 9:00–5:00, at the center for recreation or rehabilitation, and evenings at home or with relatives. This arrangement is suitable if the patient is unable to tolerate complete independence, and is usually a prelude to complete discharge.

(9) **Night hospital**: Similar arrangement as above, but the patient usually works or is otherwise active during the day and returns to the hospital at night. In such cases he needs the protective environment of a hospital ward before making a complete transition to the community.

Items (8) and (9) function as halfway houses for partial hospitalization and are staffed by professionals. This type of plan has been of considerable help in the resocialization and reorientation of the patient to the community. If the patient threatens to relapse, these facilities may also serve as resources for the prevention of complete hospitalization. Volunteer and visiting nurse associations are of great help in providing follow-up services.

Programs

The catchment area concept is now important in understanding community mental health and its relationship to the elderly. The catchment area is a geographically defined area with a target population which is served by a community mental health center or a unit of a state hospital. The center is responsible for the total mental health of all the citizens in its area, including the elderly. Thus it is no longer possible to have selective admissions (eg, below age 65) or other discriminatory criteria as a prerequisite for treatment by the center, and patients discharged from the center continue to be its responsibility. Thus, the elderly, who have long been neglected in terms of services rendered, are now coming more into their own.

Institutionalization is often not the answer to emotional disabilities. Increasingly, the full community health supportive network, including agencies such as home-health aides, homemakers, visiting nurse associations, etc, are being utilized to support patients in the community. On a planning level, collaboration is increasing between state and local as well as federal agencies to provide a coordinated group of services.

Programs to detect and treat emotional disorders early and thus prevent hospitalization are increasing in importance. Screening teams consisting of mental health workers frequently evaluate patients in their own homes, nursing homes, housing facilities for the elderly, etc rather than have the patient brought to the admitting room of a hospital. This type of consultation to care-givers increases the likelihood that the patient will remain in the community.

Psychotherapy

Psychotherapy is often of great benefit in the treatment of the elderly maladjusted and mentally ill—even those with organic brain syndrome.

One of the main obstacles in working with the elderly is the therapist's own dread of senility and death and his attitude to the failing, dependent parental figure. These may give rise either to undue pessimism or to unrealistic optimism regarding prognosis.

Fortunately, since there are not enough qualified psychiatrists to serve this expanding class of patients, it is not necessary for the elderly patient to undertake formal psychotherapy to obtain the help he needs; any person the patient sees in a parent surrogate and accepting role is potentially a therapist.

The goal of psychotherapy in this age group is not necessarily insight—although insight therapy may be possible if the patient is flexible, intelligent, and motivated. The principal goal of therapy is to provide emotional support by reducing anxiety and hostility and fostering a sense of security and self-esteem. Elderly patients—like younger ones—seek trusting relationships with parental figures; hence, they readily accept the role of the dependent (child) with the therapist if he is nonthreatening. Brief but frequent psychotherapeutic contacts with the elderly can produce remarkable results. Sometimes the patient is able to achieve a new and gratifying grasp of his whole life, its pluses and minuses, its successes and failures—perhaps a kind of "meaning" or integration or overall significance. This may lead to a sense of peace and serenity he has never experienced before.

Group psychotherapy can be of benefit as it encourages resocialization. It may be held as an open ward meeting, attended by all the patients and the ward personnel; or it may be conducted as a small closed homogeneous group for insight-oriented work.

Rehabilitation

Rehabilitation starts when the patient is first seen and continues throughout treatment and even after discharge. It may involve (as indicated) work by occupational therapists, recreational therapists, vocational counselors, music therapists, industrial workshop personnel, etc, as well as by the psychiatric team.

The patient undergoing rehabilitation therapy may be an inpatient or outpatient. Vocational or avocational work, especially if the patient gets paid, can considerably benefit self-esteem.

Apathy among elderly patients on the wards is common, and the above modalities are used to counteract it. It has been found that if beer or wine is served on the ward at a specific time and a ritual is permitted to develop in its distribution and consumption, the patients become more responsive, alert, socialize more, and grumble less. (Even incontinence diminishes.) If the wards are integrated for men and women, even greater improvements occur.

Work with the family or relevant caretaker is essential before a patient can be discharged from the hospital. After discharge, this link is maintained. Patients without family are the most difficult to move out of institutions. It is for this group that present community resources (some of which have been mentioned above) are often inadequate.

New programs are constantly being tried to make the life of the elderly more meaningful, eg, foster grandparent programs, in which the elderly volunteer their services to act as grandparents to young children or to children at orphanages.

Psychopharmacologic and Physical Therapies

The judicious use of drugs and electroconvulsive treatment (ECT) can be of benefit in the management of the elderly mentally ill. Although there is no primary treatment for chronic brain syndrome, the frequently coexisting secondary symptoms and signs (eg, depression or paranoia) are amenable to treatment.

ECT is definitely the treatment of choice in patients with severe depression, especially if suicidal. However, despite the muscle relaxants, the hazard of complications such as bone fractures, temporary increase in disorientation, and aggravation of physical disorders must be kept in mind.

The use of drugs in the elderly requires great caution as idiosyncratic side-effects and a tendency toward dependency are common. The patient may incorporate the side-effects of the medication into his symptom complex, thus complicating his emotional picture. The initial dosage should be small and gradually increased; rarely is it necessary to increase it to the full usual adult dosage.

For agitation and behavior disorders, moderate symptomatic improvement results with the use of the phenothiazine drugs such as chlorpromazine (Thorazine) and thioridazine (Mellaril). The initial dosage of either drug is 10 mg 3 times daily, and the dosage may be increased at intervals to about 50 mg 4 times daily. Postural hypotension is a not uncommon side-effect, especially at the higher doses.

The antianxiety drugs such as chlordiazepoxide (Librium) and diazepam (Valium), starting with 5 mg twice daily, are similarly helpful and cause few side-effects.

If depression or depressive-equivalent symptoms and signs are present, antidepressant drugs such as amitriptyline (Elavil) and imipramine (Tofranil) are of benefit, starting with 10 mg 3 times a day. Glaucoma and (in men) urinary retention are potential side-effects that have to be watched for.

Of the other drugs commonly used, hypnotics are the most frequent. Chloral hydrate (Noctec) and methyprylon (Noludar) are popular. The barbiturates should be avoided since they sometimes cause confusion or depression in elderly people.

INSURANCE AND BENEFITS AVAILABLE TO THE AGED

In the USA, funds are available to needy old people from several sources:

Social Security benefits are available to all citizens over age 65 who have completed a specified time in employment where Social Security deductions were made from the payroll. In 1969, the taxable base was increased to $7800, which makes possible maximum payments of $218 a month per person or $323 a month per couple when eligibility for maximum payments is reached. The individual rate also applies to the totally disabled person. If a person is not eligible for social security benefits, he will nevertheless receive $40 a month at age 72. Although for most elderly people this insurance program has been a great boon, inflation has diminished the value of the payments so that the amount available borders on the poverty mark.

Old Age Assistance (OAA) is a shared (half federal and half state and local) program, administered by the states along federal guidelines. The funds are available to all persons over age 65. The payments also include medical assistance. Assistance payments are sometimes used to supplement Social Security benefits for those recipients who receive only partial Social Security benefits. Massachusetts, a relatively liberal state, makes maximum payments of $169.70 a month per individual.

Medicare (Title XVIII of the Social Security Act) provides partial coverage for hospitalization for all citizens over age 65 and, upon a voluntary payment of a premium of $6 a month, extends the coverage to pay for some medical care. However, the psychiatric hospital coverage extends only to 190 hospital benefit days for a lifetime maximum. The plan was initiated to pay for hospital care primarily of acute illnesses. It also provides for some extended care benefits after discharge from hospital as well as some home health benefits.

Medicaid (Medical Assistance; Title XIX of the Social Security Act) introduced the concept of "medical indigence," where earnings are sufficient for everyday needs but not for the costs of serious illness. This is a federally sponsored and state administered program. The benefits are paid half by federal and half by state and local matching funds. Not all states have initiated this program. Medical Assistance may pay for all hospital and medical services without limit to eligible people under age 21 and over age 65, including long-term care in approved state hospitals for those over age 65.

In addition, a personal allowance of $40 a month is paid to all elderly recipients, to spend as they please. The hospital is required to conduct a quarterly Utilization Review Plan.

The financial criteria for eligibility vary from state to state. In Massachusetts, an income of $2160 annually or less (for an individual) provides the maximum benefits. The benefits then gradually decrease as the income increases.

This program is a boost to the care of the elderly in state hospitals. However, children have been the primary beneficiaries in the community.

Blue Cross—Blue Shield have recently introduced optional plans with their Master Medical Plan to provide, for the first time, psychiatric and psychologic coverage on an outpatient basis, either in a psychiatrist's office or in hospital and clinical outpatient departments. The limit, however, is $700 for both psychiatric care and psychologic services over a 24-month period.

All of the above programs are in process of constant change, for the most part in the direction of liberalization and increased availability, coverage, and protection. Application to care of psychiatric illnesses and disabilities continues to remain behind that of somatic conditions, but the difference is diminishing.

PREVENTION OF MENTAL DISORDERS IN THE AGED

The aim of all preventive programs ideally is **primary prevention**. This involves education, consultation, and counseling of community leaders such as legislators, social agency personnel, ministers of the church, and health professionals. The stresses and handicaps affecting the elderly are tackled, and a technic of crisis prevention and intervention is offered, eg, by counteracting loneliness through Golden Age Clubs and other group projects and diminishing the stress of forced retirement by pre-retirement counseling. The basic cause of aging is being studied by biochemical, neurologic, and genetic research, and this needs to be encouraged.

The work of McKay in the USA and Verźar in Switzerland postulates a molecular "cross-linkage" theory of senescence. This involves molecular changes in the cells of the body, notably collagen and perhaps DNA, in which, as the individual ages, molecules become linked and bound together, thus resulting in impairment of cell function. Certain intermediary products in the body, some chemicals, and ionizing radiations appear to accelerate the tendency. Some substances, especially enzymes, seem to retard the molecular cross-linking and hence resist the process of aging. A clinical example is the effect of estrogens on aging vaginal mucosa: the small, inelastic, and cracked vaginal wall can be returned to the youthful state with supple walls, lack of cracks, and normal size.

Further gerontologic research may produce approaches to the elusive "elixir of life," enabling us not only to prolong life but to increase the "youth period" percentage of the total life span.

Early recognition and prompt treatment of disorders is known as **secondary prevention**. This entails efficiently utilizing all of our present therapeutic resources and offering the best in treatment irrespective of age or socioeconomic standing of the sufferer. Feelings of usefulness and of self-esteem must be enhanced. Comprehensive computer screening for middle-aged people has recently been initiated and is being watched with interest.

Tertiary prevention is a community-wide effort aimed at reducing the rate of defective functioning caused by mental disorders. This requires that rehabilitation commence with the onset of illness and that continuity of patient care be available. The alienation of the mentally ill patient must be minimized by retention of community contacts and by short hospitalization, aided by halfway houses, clubs, etc.

In the future, it is hoped that research and study of the aging will be performed with an understanding of the problems facing the individual, with a concentration of effort, and with the full resources of the community.

REFERENCES

Books and Monographs

Agate, J.: *The Practice of Geriatrics.* Heineman, 1963.

Berezin, M.A., & S.H. Cath: *Geriatric Psychiatry: Grief, Loss and Emotional Disorders in the Aged.* Internat Univ Press, 1968.

Birren, J.E. (editor): *Handbook of Aging and the Individual.* Univ of Chicago Press, 1959.

Birren, J.E., & others (editors): *Human Aging: A Biological and Behavioral Study.* Publication No. 986. US Public Health Service, 1963.

Cumming, E., & W.E. Henry: *Growing Old.* Basic Books, 1961.

Death and Dying: Attitudes of Patient and Doctor. GAP Symposium No. 11. Group for the Advancement of Psychiatry, 1965.

Field, M. (editor): *Depth and Extent of the Geriatric Problem.* Thomas, 1970.

Hoch, P.H., & J. Zubin (editors): *Psychopathology of Aging.* Grune & Stratton, 1961.

Mental Health Problems of Aging and the Aged. Technical Report Series No. 171. World Health Organization, 1959.

National Clearing House for Mental Health Information: *A Comprehensive Review of Geriatric-Psychiatric Literature: The Post War Period.* Public Health Service Report No. 1811. US Printing Office, Washington, DC.

Psychiatry and the Aged: An Introductory Approach. GAP Symposium No. 59. Group for the Advancement of Psychiatry, 1965.

Stotsky, B.: *The Elderly Patient.* Grune & Stratton, 1968.

Tibbits, C.: *Handbook of Social Gerontology.* Univ of Chicago Press, 1960.

Toward a Public Policy on Mental Health Care of the Elderly. GAP Symposium No. 79. Group for the Advancement of Psychiatry, 1970.

Wolff, K.: *The Emotional Rehabilitation of the Geriatric Patient.* Thomas, 1970.

Journal Articles

Aldrich, C.K., & E. Mondkoff: Relocation of the aged and disabled: A mortality study. J Am Geriat Soc 11:185–194, 1963.

Barach, A.L.: The 65-plus distress syndrome. J Am Geriat Soc 12:262–265, 1964.

Berezin, M.A.: Sex and old age: A review of literature. J Geriat Psychiat 2:131–149, 1969.

Busse, E.W.: Geriatrics today: An overview. Am J Psychiat 123:1226–1233, 1967.

Busse, E.W.: Geriatrics: Some complex problems. Am J Psychiat 127:1078–1079, 1971.

Butler, R.N.: The responsibility of psychiatry to the elderly. Am J Psychiat 127:1080–1081, 1971.

Cohen, E.S.: Nursing homes, state hospitals and the aged mentally ill. Geriatrics 18:871–876, 1963.

Comfort, A.: Experimental gerontology and the control of aging. Geriatrics 25:176–184, 1970.

Daniels, R.: Psychiatric drug use and abuse in aged. Geriatrics 25:144–158, 1970.

Goldfarb, A.: Doctor-patient relationship in treatment of aged persons. Geriatrics 19:18–23, 1964.

Langley, A.E., & J.H. Simpson: Misplacement of the elderly in geriatric and psychiatric hospitals. Geront Clin 12:149–163, 1970.

Lipscomb, C.F.: The care of the psychiatrically disturbed elderly patient in the community. Am J Psychiat 127:1067–1070, 1971.

Lowenthal, M.F.: Social and related factors leading to psychiatric hospitalization of the aged. J Am Geriat Soc 13:110–112, 1965.

Markson, E., & others: Alternatives to hospitalization for the psychiatrically ill. Am J Psychiat 127:1055–1062, 1971.

Prehoda, R.W.: Retardation of aging. Med Opin Rev 64–72, 1970.

Rimoldi, H.J.A., & K.W. Vander Woude: Aging and problem solving. Arch Gen Psychiat 20:215–226, 1969.

Sloane, R.B., & F. Diana: The mentally affected old person. Geriatrics 25:125–132, 1970.

Volpe, A., & R. Kastenbaum: Beer and TLC. Am J Nursing 67:100–103, 1967.

Weisman, A., & T.P. Hackett: Predilection to death: Death and dying as a psychiatric problem. Psychosom Med 23:232–256, 1961.

Zimberg, S.: Outpatient geriatric psychiatry in an urban ghetto with nonprofessional workers. Am J Psychiat 125:1697–1701, 1969.

37...

Forensic Psychiatry

Many physicians and most psychiatrists appear in court at times as expert witnesses. They should know how to conduct themselves in court and should be familiar with such legal terms as competency, sanity, and various capacities (to testify, make a will or contract, live in the ordinary community). They should understand the safeguards and limits of privilege and confidentiality.

The problems of forensic psychiatry are "legal" problems as well as "medical" ones, and physicians, who are used to thinking in medical terms, may have difficulty thinking in legal terms. Specific knowledge of legal concepts and the legal framework and the uses to which those concepts are put is indispensable for a psychiatrist who wishes to function adequately in a forensic psychiatric situation.

An outline of the structure of the judicial system is beyond the scope of this handbook, although some of the more important specific principles are discussed below. The physician who is unfamiliar with the laws and procedures governing the relationships between him and the courts does well to discuss specific problems with his own attorney.

In general, the following discussion applies only to United States law.

PSYCHIATRIC TESTIMONY

Legal situations involving psychiatric testimony, whether they are civil or criminal, generally involve at least one of 2 major considerations regarding the individual whose psychiatric status is in question:

(1) Is (or was) he competent to perform certain actions? If not, he may be prevented from doing something he might want to do, or something he has done may be invalidated (testify in court, make a marriage contract or will, purchase property, etc).

(2) Is (or was) he responsible for the action which is at issue? If so, he may be forced to do something he does not want to do (pay money, go to jail, etc).

An incompetent person is not responsible for his actions in the area of his incompetence, and a person who is absolved from responsibility in some particular area is incompetent to act legally in that area.

The definitions and tests of competency and responsibility vary with specific legal issues. For example, responsibility for a crime is not the same as responsibility for a tort (civil wrong done to another). When an individual is wronged he may undertake his remedy in a civil proceeding. The tort-feasor—he who commits such a wrong—does not go to jail but usually pays monetary damages. Some torts are also crimes (serious offenses against society), and the individual may face both civil and criminal trials as a result of the same action.

PRACTICAL PRINCIPLES
FOR THE PSYCHIATRIST IN LEGAL WORK

Preexamination

Learn as much as you can about a case before you see the "patient" (defendant, accused, client, litigant, prisoner, etc). Talk with the lawyer and assemble any written material that is available (charges, police reports, copies of confessions, interrogations, professional opinions, medical examinations, laboratory data, etc). Be sure you understand exactly why you are being asked to examine the person, what kind of report you will be expected to write, and to what use it will be put. Inquire whether it is likely that you will also have to appear in court as an expert witness.

Examination (See Chapter 4.)

Be thorough and take complete notes. It is usually well to see the patient more than once. (Questions in cross-examination such as, "You saw him only once, doctor?" and, "How much time did you spend with him, doctor?" must be anticipated.)

If the question of mental retardation is likely to be raised, make a brief evaluation of the patient's intelligence (test simple reading, arithmetic, rote memory, current events, ordinary information, reasoning, judgment, and insight) and record verbatim as much of the patient's answers as you can.

In cases involving impulsiveness, loss of control, impaired consciousness, amnesia, fugue states, somnambulism, bizarre or dissociative episodes, or where there is a history of epilepsy, seizures or spells of any sort, severe migraine, or severe head injury or brain disease, inquire in considerable detail regarding indications of cerebral dysrhythmia and psychomotor epilepsy.

Postexamination

Arrange for special examinations if you think they would throw light on the patient's condition. The defense attorney, district attorney, and judge will almost certainly see that these are done if you offer reasonable arguments for them. Consider medical examination, neurologic consultation, x-rays of the skull, electroencephalography, psychologic and psychometric examination, social service investigation, and school report. You may wish to see the patient again in the light of reports of special examinations.

When your data are assembled, write a report that is as brief as you can make it and still include all relevant material. Give your opinion regarding the questions the authorities have raised and avoid anything further. (They usually are not concerned about matters of etiology, diagnosis, or prognosis, although such matters are often asked about during testimony at trial.) Give reasons for your opinion, and use as nontechnical language as you can.

Testimony in Court

Confer with the attorney in advance and be guided by his advice. Your attitude should be that of a calm, dispassionate professional who is confident of his competence in his field as it relates to the case at hand but does not claim to be infallible or omniscient. You are there to help the judge and jury administer justice, and you should make it clear that this is your intention. Feel free to admit that you are being paid for your professional services, but the source of your fee has nothing to do with the nature of your opinion, which is impartial and nonpartisan.

Speak clearly and use simple language. When you have to use a difficult word, spell it out for the benefit of the court stenographer.

Do not hesitate to say, "I don't know," and add, when appropriate, "and I don't think anyone else does either." If you are badgered in cross-examination, try to remain unperturbed. If you are pressed too far and the attorney on your side does not object in order to protect you, appeal to the judge and ask if you can try to explain your position in your own words. For example, if the cross-examiner insists that you answer a difficult question "yes or no," you may say, "Yes, but [turning to the judge] I should like to qualify my answer if your honor please." It is part of the judge's responsibility to help you help the court. He may well question you himself—and often does so more skillfully and sympathetically than the attorneys.

SPECIFIC LEGAL PROBLEMS INVOLVING PSYCHIATRIC TESTIMONY

Civil Proceedings Involving Competency

A. Contracts: A contract is an agreement (oral or written) between 2 or more parties (individuals, corporations, etc) to do or not to do some specific thing. A contract may not be valid if, at the time it was made, one of the contracting parties was incapable of understanding the nature of the transaction. If one party does not adhere to the contract, he may be sued by the other party to it.

The marriage contract implies the same requirements for understanding as in other types of contract. In this instance the party who was incapable of understanding the transaction usually is the plaintiff suing for an annulment. A person who is judged incompetent and who nevertheless gets married is usually considered to be married until the marriage is set aside. He must initiate procedures for an annulment.

B. Wills: A will is a written statement of a person's intentions regarding the disposition of his property after his death. The signature must ordinarily be witnessed by 2 or 3 persons. Generally the testator (person making the will) must know 3 things: that he is making a will, the nature and extent of his property, and the people who are his "natural" beneficiaries (spouse, children, etc).

The issue of competency to make a will ordinarily does not arise until after the death of the testator, when a dissatisfied relative sues to have the will set aside on the grounds that the testator was incompetent. The psychiatrist's testimony relates to that issue.

A person who is judged incompetent might nevertheless be able to execute a valid will if he has the requisite knowledge at the time of executing it. It is obviously wise in such situations to have a psychiatrist examine the individual to verify his competency for purposes of the will.

C. Capacity to Testify in Court: This is usually not in itself the subject of a court proceeding but arises in connection with other proceedings, both civil and criminal. In order to testify, a person must be able to (1) understand questions, (2) observe and recall situations, (3) distinguish between reality and fantasy, and (4) put his thoughts into words. Organic problems (eg, mental deficiency, senility) are likely to impair a person's ability to perform the first 2 functions or the last, whereas psychosis (eg, litigious paranoia) or severe neurosis (as in the case of a hysterical woman who makes the complaint of rape) is likely to affect the third function. This type of capacity is difficult to evaluate. It is presumptuous to challenge the competency of a witness who refuses to undergo a psychiatric examination; most are unwilling to do so when the occasion arises, and only rarely can an unwilling witness be ordered to submit to a psychiatric examination. Conclusions based on courtroom observations are notoriously unreliable. The issue of competency to stand trial arises most commonly in the case of defendants who plead not guilty by reason of insanity.

D. Capacity to Conduct One's Affairs (General Competency): It is difficult to specify the elements involved in ordinary conduct of affairs, and a judgment of incompetency is based on a total impression. A competency hearing is most often associated with psychiatric hospitalization, usually involving commitment, and the proceeding is usually initiated by a relative or friend or by the state. The determination of incompetency is made as a result of a hearing in court and is a legal decree. Psychiatrists do not judge incompetency; they only present evidence at a hearing. The patient may be represented at the hearing by an attorney and may try to rebut all evidence of his incompetency. Note that commitment and competency are separate issues and should not be confused.

When a person is judged incompetent, it usually entails at least the following: (1) Loss of voting rights. (2) Loss of right to contract (except for "necessities"). (3) Loss of right to practice a profession. (4) Suspension of driver's license. (5) Loss of right to adopt children or to prevent adoption of his own children. (6) Loss of right to convey (give or sell) property. (7) Difficulty in initiating a divorce, with associated difficulty in being sued for one.

Being judged incompetent is prima facie evidence of inability to execute a valid will, although the presumption may be rebutted by appropriate evidence.

A guardian (or "conservator") is appointed who controls the patient's property. Once a person has been judged incompetent, he remains so until a court certifies him to be competent; then he regains control over his affairs.

E. Psychiatric Disability: The person who alleges himself to be psychiatrically disabled, in a personal injury or workmen's compensation suit or in a suit against an insurance company, calls a psychiatrist as an expert witness to elucidate his disability or his "mental anguish." The other side may also call a psychiatric witness to counter the psychiatric testimony, and the court may order the plaintiff to be examined by a court-appointed psychiatrist.

Criminal Proceedings Involving Competency

A. Capacity to Be a Defendant in a Criminal Trial: An accused person must have the capacity to understand the nature of the proceedings against him and to cooperate intelligently in his own defense.

B. Capacity to Be Punished or Executed: A person may not legally be imprisoned or executed when he is grossly mentally ill. He is sent instead to a mental hospital or other treatment facility until he recovers, at which time the punishment is carried out.

C. Capacity to Act With Criminal Intent: The intent to commit the crime is an important element in the definition of most crimes. If at the time of an offense the accused was unable to form the requisite intent, he is not guilty. Thus, the allegation of inability to form intent is sometimes used as a defense in criminal trials, eg, to reduce a first degree murder charge (deliberate and premeditated) to a second degree charge (deliberate but not premeditated) or to a third degree charge (neither deliberate nor premeditated).

Criminal Proceedings Involving Responsibility

A. "Not Guilty by Reason of Insanity": Definitions of insanity vary among jurisdictions.

1. *M'Naghten Rule* (state and federal courts)—A person escapes responsibility for his action if at the time he labored under a defect of reason or mental disease such that he did not know the nature and quality of the act or did not know that it was wrong.

2. *U.S. Armed Services*—A person escapes responsibility for his action if at the time he had a mental disease, defect, or derangement rendering him unable to distinguish right from wrong or to adhere to the right.

3. *Durham Rule* (Washington, D.C.)—A person escapes responsibility if his criminal act was the product of his mental disease or mental defect.

4. *Model Penal Code* (suggested by American Law Institute)—A person should escape responsibility if, because of mental disease or defect at the time of committing the action, he lacked substantial capacity to appreciate the criminality of his conduct or to conform his conduct to the requirements of the law.

5. *Irresistible impulse* (much more variation among jurisdictions)—The definition of what constitutes an irresistible impulse varies, but the general notion is that the individual could not have resisted the impulse to commit the criminal action in spite of a high risk of detection or apprehension.

It is apparent that this defense is invoked only in cases of trials for major crimes. (Acquittal from a criminal charge by virtue of insanity may be less desirable for the defendant than an unqualified "guilty," for the person declared not guilty by reason of insanity is usually committed to a prison hospital for an indefinite period of time.)

B. In Mitigation After a Verdict of Guilty: Various extenuating factors, including mental illness and its consequences, may influence a judge to impose a lighter sentence on a convicted criminal. Psychiatrists may be called upon to present extenuating evidence at the time of sentencing.

The Pretrial Psychiatric Examination (See also Chapter 4.)

The following 9 examination points give some guides for approaching psychiatric legal questions.

(1) Was the examinee under the influence of intoxicants, and to what degree? Alcoholic intoxication, if severe enough, may render a person "unable to know what he is doing" or "unable to form a specific intent." An extreme degree of intoxication is generally considered to be necessary for these conclusions to be reached.

(2) Is the individual a mental defective, and how severe is the deficit?

(3) Is or was the individual suffering from delusions or hallucinations?

(4) Is or was the individual suffering from a mood disorder severe enough to compromise his ability to cope with reality?

(5) Is there a past history of epilepsy, hysterical fugues, or other amnesias? What are the EEG findings?

(6) Have there been head injuries or other organic brain disorders?

(7) If the examinee suffers from some specific mental illness, what treatment is recommended and what is the prognosis?

(8) Is the individual malingering?

(9) In a personal injury or disability case, what was the individual's pre-injury or maximum level of functioning?

Probably the 2 most serious sources of error in the area of forensic psychiatric evaluation are (1) attempting to evaluate an individual without knowing in advance the precise legal uses to which the examination results will be put and (2) forming premature opinions by the examining psychiatrist. A pretrial conference with the legal person calling for a psychiatric examination or opinion is desirable to ascertain the legal purposes attendant on it. Several interviews, psychologic tests, and even a period of observation in a hospital might at times be required in order to form a good opinion. On occasion, despite a thorough examination, there is still some uncertainty on the part of the examiner or disagreements among examiners.

THE PSYCHIATRIST'S CONCLUSIONS

From the foregoing it will be seen that critical legal issues involving psychiatrists are difficult to define and that the problems are difficult to evaluate in a reliable fashion, ie, so that evaluations by different competent individuals will lead to the same conclusion. Concepts of terms such as "knowledge," "understanding," "mental anguish," "ability," "disability," "intelligence," "impulse," etc cannot easily be circumscribed nor accurately delineated, nor can "right," "wrong," "nature and quality," etc. The problem is multiplied when those concepts must be related to an individual's "state of mind" at some time prior to the testimony and usually prior to an examination, if one can even be made. This is a difficulty inherent in psychologic processes and the legal system. Thus, to some extent, conclusions reached must be compromises and somewhat subjective.

There are no rigid procedural guidelines for these problems. The psychiatrist can only carefully approach the problem, consult medicolegal literature, and handle the situation in his own manner. Nevertheless, despite all the limitations of the legal framework and the intrinsic uncertainties of so many of the questions that must be considered, the testifying psychiatrist often is helpful to a jury in formulating its decisions. A diligent performance by the psychiatrist is satisfying both to himself and to those involved in the dispute.

For practical advice in examining psychiatric patients in medical-legal situations, see Chapter 4.

PSYCHIATRIC HOSPITALIZATION

Admission to a Psychiatric Hospital

Voluntary admission to a psychiatric hospital is similar in procedure and legal consequences to admission to any other hospital. Involuntary admission (commitment) is a serious infringement of the patient's liberties not to be undertaken lightly or without due consideration of alternative approaches. The conflict in involuntary mental hospitalization is between rival duties and rights: protection of the community from harm at the hands of a mentally sick person, protection of the sick individual from harm at his own hands, and the right of all individuals to conduct their own affairs without hindrance. The community has a right to protect itself and to protect the individual from his own sickness. Individuals who protest their own commitment usually feel that they are not sick and do not represent a threat to the community or to themselves. The evaluation of these issues constitutes the crux of a commitment decision. Since the stakes are high, it is important that the evaluation be made carefully.

Major defects in the laws and customs relating to commitment still exist in a few states of the USA. Voluntary admission is sometimes impossible by statute or is discouraged in fact, and a trial by jury is sometimes required (as opposed to being allowed if the patient wishes it). The mandatory appearance in court is unpleasant and often harmful to the patient, and criminal procedures are often used, making the patient appear (and feel like) a criminal. Most psychiatrists believe that the protection of rights afforded by a jury trial (with laymen deciding) can be obtained with a private hearing by a single judge or an appointed trained commission. Fortunately, admission on a voluntary basis, which is quite feasible in the great majority of cases, is rapidly gaining favor.

Psychiatric Hospitalization Provisions of Model Act (Suggested by American Law Institute)

   A. Voluntary Hospitalization:

   1. A mental hospital (of any type) should be able to accept patients who voluntarily apply for admission.

   2. A mental hospital should be able by itself to discharge a patient who voluntarily has sought admission (as opposed to needing a court order or some other agency's approval).

   3. If a voluntary patient requests release before he is medically regarded as ready, he may not be held more than 48 hours unless a request is filed in court for him to be held without his consent. This request must be acted upon within 5 days.

   4. A voluntary patient must be meaningfully informed of his right to request release (ie, not just in small print).

   B. Involuntary Hospitalization: (Four types.)

   1. Medical certificate (nonjudicial)—

   a. Application by relative, friend, police officer, etc.

   b. Certification by 2 licensed physicians, preferably psychiatrists, that the patient is mentally ill and likely to injure himself or others if allowed at liberty; or that he is in need of care and, because of his illness, lacks the capacity to make responsible decisions regarding hospitalization.

   c. Such a certificate authorizes a health or police officer to transfer the patient to a designated hospital (using a police car only in emergency) within 15 days.

   2. Medical certificate (emergency)—

   a. Application by any interested person.

   b. Certification by one physician that the patient is mentally ill and is therefore likely to injure himself or others if not immediately restrained.

   c. Police or health officer is authorized to transport patient to hospital within 3 days.

   3. No certificate (emergency)—Health or police officer (who believes commitment must be undertaken before an examining physician can arrive) may take the patient directly to the hospital.

   4. Court order (judicial procedure)—This would be the only way an individual involuntarily committed could be retained in hospital more than 5 days if he requests release.

   a. A responsible individual applies to court.

   b. Court gives notice to patient and his guardian, etc.

   c. Court appoints 2 examining physicians.

   d. A private hearing with opportunity for cross-examination of witnesses occurs after 5 days but before 15 days after the physicians' examination. (Patient need not be present but may be.)

   e. If court finds mental illness and need for hospitalization, it orders it for an indeterminate period, subject in 1 year to reapplication by the patient for another hearing (this provision is not in the Model Act but is desirable), or for an observational period not to exceed 6 months. If the court does not so find, the proceedings are terminated and the patient is released.

C. Status While in a Mental Hospital:

1. Commitment is different from an adjudication of incompetency. The 2 are sometimes confused. Even when committed to a mental hospital, a person ought to be able to exercise his civil rights, including those pertaining to disposing of property and voting, unless he has been properly adjudicated as incompetent.

2. Patients should receive humane treatment. Restraining apparatus must be kept under lock and key and used only with written authorization or in emergency. Treatment procedures must be kept separate from those required to maintain an orderly hospital atmosphere. (Electroshock, for example, must not be used as punishment.)

3. Unless expressly limited by a signed order, the patient must be allowed to communicate by sealed mail, to receive visitors at reasonable times, and to petition for a writ of habeas corpus.

4. Hospital records and other information about the patient must be kept confidential.

5. Patients should receive appropriate psychiatric treatment. (This provision is not in the Model Act, although it is obviously implicit in the situation of being hospitalized. Sufficient funds and facilities are of course required for implementation.)

D. Discharge From a Mental Hospital: The main points of the Model Act relating to discharge are these:

1. A hospital must be able to discharge a patient independently of a court order.

2. A patient has the right to petition the hospital for discharge, and he must be notified of that right. If he initiates such a petition, an examination and court order are required to keep the patient involuntarily for more than 5 days.

3. A patient committed by a court for observation should not be involuntarily held for a period longer than 6 months without reexamination and recertification.

4. A patient committed indefinitely by a court should be able to apply after 12 months for another commitment hearing.

5. Abuse of commitment procedures (eg, placing a patient involuntarily in a mental hospital to exploit or expropriate him) should be properly penalized.

PRIVILEGED COMMUNICATION OR CONFIDENTIALITY

It is considered fundamental to the nature of some relationships that one person be able in private to communicate freely with another without fear that the receiver of the communication will divulge the information to a third party or that other reprisal might occur. In such situations as the attorney-client relationship, the clergyman-penitent relationship, or (in some states) the doctor-patient relationship, the person who needs help must be able to speak freely about his problem, and the law recognizes his communications as having exceptional privileges. In some circumstances he may choose to waive it, though certain communication privileges may not be waived (eg, husband-wife conversations in divorce cases). **Privilege** is an option of the patient. He may relinquish it when he wishes, and he often does—when, for example, he wishes the psychiatrist to support his case against an insurance company for damages of a psychiatric nature. **Confidentiality** is an obligation on the psychiatrist, and in most cases he will breach it at his peril. In a court of law, however, he must yield it when the court insists (in most states) or cling to it at his peril.

Even if knowledge of such a communication might be relevant to settling a case at litigation, the court may not legally allow privileged information to be introduced in evidence.

A person who deliberately or unwittingly divulges confidential information without permission (notarized permission in writing is probably the safest form) is subject to a claim for damages or other penalties.

In order to qualify as privileged or confidential, a communication must be (1) not otherwise illegal and (2) communicated only to the recipient himself, functioning in his privileged role. A secretary or similar person functioning as the agent of the receiver or communicator constitutes an exception. If a third person is present who is not functioning as the agent of either (eg, a nurse incidentally present at an examination), the privilege is invalidated. An open door in the communication room may similarly invalidate the privilege.

The rules and restrictions on privileged communication refer only to testifying in court. A physician has no legal obligation to discuss a case with relatives of patients, the police, social or government agencies, the FBI, etc.

In some jurisdictions, certain acts of a patient constitute an automatic waiver of the privilege (eg, testifying about his disabilities in a personal injury suit). Psychiatrists are more apt to be involved in confidentiality situations where the psychiatric information is not the main thrust of the trial and the information might be detrimental to the patient. However, if the patient is suing for damages and alleges psychiatric injury, his entire relationship to his psychiatrist becomes nonprivileged.

Doctor-Patient Communications

In most states, communications between a patient and a doctor are not privileged. The doctor may legally be compelled to divulge them in open court or be subject to a contempt citation. This situation may occur in criminal trials where the patient is a defendant or in civil litigation where a person's statements may be important (eg, in a divorce case if he admitted adultery to his physician).

Even where the privilege exists, it does not extend to all situations in which the doctor sees the patient professionally. For example, if the doctor is appointed by a court to perform a diagnostic examination, the communications of the patient (if indeed the examinee must be called a "patient") are not privileged. Of course, the doctor should not try to make the examinee believe that what he says will be held in confidence or that the examination is for the patient's benefit.

Even in states with the privilege, if the patient has a disease or injury requiring the doctor to report it to authorities (gunshot wounds, etc), that is not privileged.

If the doctor does divulge facts without permission and the patient can show he was damaged by it, the doctor is subject to damage claims.

Psychiatrists' patients have no different communication privileges than other patients, though many authorities believe the psychotherapy situation is different from many medical situations and that there should be special rules to cover it. Actually, some states (eg, Massachusetts and Connecticut) now have laws permitting confidentiality privileges to psychiatrists.

Practical Considerations in Jurisdictions Without Doctor-Patient Privilege

The question arises whether a psychiatrist should tell a patient that he cannot legally keep the patient's communications confidential in a court-room. If he is a court-appointed psychiatrist examining a person accused of a crime, the examinee certainly should be told. In other situations that may reach a court, prudence suggests the psychiatrist warn the patient, even though medical effectiveness demands that confidence be preserved. Every psychiatrist must decide for himself how to resolve such dilemmas. Some psychiatrists have risked contempt penalties in order to preserve confidentiality, and others have divulged information damaging to their patients in courts, commissions of inquiry, etc. It is apparent that a psychiatrist in a courtroom dilemma of that sort ought to consult his own attorney. A satisfactory compromise can often be arranged by means of a frank discussion with the presiding judge.

Circumstances requiring that confidential information be divulged at times present a difficult and conflicting situation legally and morally. The basic considerations are similar to those involved in commitment proceedings. If the individual is a threat to himself or others or lacks the judgment to seek the help he needs, divulging the information may be in the patient's best interests. Balanced judgment is required to assess these situations. A responsible attending physician is reluctant to divulge information against the patient's wishes, but in some emergencies he must do so.

REFERENCES

Books and Monographs

Allen, R.C., & others (editors): *Readings in Law and Psychiatry.* Johns Hopkins Press, 1968.

Arens, R.: *Make Mad the Guilty: The Insanity Defense in the District of Columbia.* Thomas, 1969.

Curran, W.J.: *Law and Medicine.* Little, Brown, 1960.

Davidson, H.A.: *Forensic Psychiatry.* Ronald Press, 1952.

Disability and Social Security. [OASI-29f.] US Department of Health, Education, and Welfare, 1965.

A Draft Act Governing Hospitalization of the Mentally Ill. Publication No. 51. US Public Health Service, 1951.

Glueck, S.: *Law and Psychiatry: Cold War or Entente Cordiale?* John Hopkins Press, 1962.

Gutmacher, M.S., & H. Weihofein: *Psychiatry and the Law.* Norton, 1958.

Laws Governing Hospitalization of the Mentally Ill. GAP Report No. 61, Vol 6. Group for the Advancement of Psychiatry, (May) 1966.

Lindman, F.T., & D.M. McIntyre, Jr. (editors): *The Mentally Disabled and the Law: Report of the American Bar Foundation on the Rights of the Mentally Ill.* Univ of Chicago Press, 1961.

MacDonald, J.M.: *Psychiatry and the Criminal: A Guide to Psychiatric Examinations for the Criminal Courts.* Thomas, 1969.

Manning, G.P., Jr., Hollister, N.R., & F.M. Shultety: The components of post-traumatic disability. Chap 7 in: *Disability and the Law.* Manning, G.P., Jr. (editor). Williams & Wilkins, 1962.

Manual for Courts Martial, United States. Government Printing Office, 1951.

Psychiatry in Military Law. [Army TM 8-240; Air Force AFM 160-42.] Government Printing Office.

Robitscher, J.B.: *Pursuit of Agreement: Psychiatry and the Law.* Lippincott, 1966.

Simpson, K.: *Taylor's Principles and Practice of Medical Jurisprudence,* 12th ed. Churchill, 1965.

Journal Articles

Closson, W.G., Jr., Hall, R.A., & B.S. Mason: Confidentiality in psychiatry and psychotherapy. California Med 113:12–15, Oct 1970.

Goldstein, A.S.: Psychiatrists in court: Some perspectives on the insanity defense. Am J Psychiat 125:1348–1351, 1969.

Jablon, N.C., Sadoff, R.L., & M.S. Heller: A unique forensic diagnostic hospital. Am J Psychiat 126:1663–1667, 1970.

McGarry, A.L.: The fate of psychotic offenders returned for trial. Am J Psychiat 127:1181–1184, 1971.

Menninger, K.: The future of criminal law. Reflections 3:40–51, 1968.

Moore, R.A.: Legal responsibility and chronic alcoholism. Am J Psychiat 122:748–756, 1966.

Robey, A.: Criteria for competency to stand trial: A checklist for psychiatrists. Am J Psychiat 122:616–623, 1965.

Schroeder, D.C., Jr.: Malingering: Fact or fiction. Postgrad Med 40:A58, Oct 1966.

38 . . .

Psychiatric Consultation

Psychiatrists are increasingly asked to furnish opinions on the problems of individual patients, colleagues, and agencies. Successful performance at each of these levels involves special technics and precautions.

The demand for psychiatric services continues to increase out of all proportion to the supply. The public has learned that many forms of misery and unhappiness due to mental ill health can be relieved by treatment; physicians and workers in the service professions allied to medicine are recognizing their shortcomings in dealing with certain distressed patients and clients and are asking for psychiatric guidance; and the heads of many organizations, schools, industries, and institutions concerned about the well-being, morale, and efficiency of their personnel are requesting that a psychiatrist be added to the permanent administrative team. The new field of *consultation psychiatry*, which permits each psychiatrist to distribute his influence over a wider area, is the inevitable result of these developments.

Psychiatric consultation may be regarded as patient-centered, colleague-centered, or agency-centered, depending on who is intended to receive the major help. In *patient-centered* consultation, the patient, his family or physician, or perhaps some other interested party feels that help is needed. *Colleague-centered* consultation is often requested by social and welfare organizations, clergymen, schools and colleges, courts, penal institutions, and rehabilitation authorities. In *agency-centered* consultation, the physician is engaged to consult on problems of business, industry, and government. Certain considerations apply to all 3 types.

In his consultant capacity the psychiatrist represents not only himself but the entire field of psychiatry. He should emulate the ideal of the human, friendly professional person motivated to be helpful; should be confident of his skill and knowledge but aware of his limitations and of the importance of contributions from other fields; and should treat others with courtesy, respect, trust, and tact. He should not represent himself as infallible and omniscient nor as the self-appointed prophet of all things psychiatric. He should be neither overly critical nor unduly conciliatory.

The consultant should try as soon as possible to evaluate the problem and the difficulty the consultee is having with it. He should address himself—at least at first—to the problem he has been asked to solve, even though he may recognize other problems that might require psychiatric attention. He should try to identify with the values of the consultee or, in the case of an agency, with the basic purpose of its program. He should avoid jargon and unnecessary technical display, and adhere completely to confidentiality.

THE PATIENT-CENTERED CONSULTATION

This is the traditional consultation, usually implying that the patient's situation is serious.

The Request

In order to give the service that is needed, the consultant must receive an appropriate request and must know the reasons for the request, both alleged and actual. (For example, the desire of a referring physician to be rid of a troublesome patient may be the underlying motivation for a psychiatric referral.) Routine hospital requests are often inadequate, speaking only of "help in diagnosis and management." It is often wise to seek out the referring physician and discuss the case with him in advance, and to obtain pertinent information from ward personnel. In private practice, the first contact often consists of a phone call from the referring physician. An explicit understanding should be reached about whether the referring physician wishes the psychiatrist to take over the case for treatment if he thinks psychiatric treatment is indicated; there must be no competition for the patient and no feeling later that the patient was "stolen." The physician may merely be seeking reassurance or authoritative support for his own impressions; or he or the patient's family may be trying to shift a troublesome burden of management onto the consultant's shoulders.

The Examination

The nature and extent of the examination will depend on the realistic demands on the psychiatrist's time, his personal convictions in the field of psychiatry, and the circumstances of the individual case. Busy psychiatric residents with a daily handful of consultation requests must learn to work under the pressure of time. Many are able to conduct an interview in 20 or 30 minutes, keep it reasonably flexible as well as pertinent, allow for maximum affective expression, and yet cover a complete mental status examination that permits a definitive answer to the question underlying the consultation request. Fortunately, many of these hospital cases are not complicated.

In private practice the consultant may find that one session in the office is not enough to give him a full grasp of the case, and he may ask the patient to return again (or several times) before he feels ready for a discussion with the referring physician. He may feel he should explore the major forces (biologic, hereditary, social, etc) that play a role in the patient's problem. Some psychiatrists believe they should specialize their inquiries in the area of the unconscious, attempting to understand and interpret the patient's emotional conflicts in the context of his background, life experiences, significant relationships, and medical status. In this case, time spent discussing early memories, feelings toward key people, dreams, daydreams, and hopes and ambitions can be very helpful.

The diagnosis of psychosis as such is usually not difficult, but the question of commitability may be more complex and time-consuming. Much depends on the ability of the patient to cooperate in ambulatory treatment and on the willingness of the family to tolerate aberrant behavior. Neuroses, character disturbances, psychosomatic conditions, and behavior disorders are usually easy to identify, but prolonged study may be necessary before a recommendation regarding therapy can be given. Opinions regarding testamentary capacity, contractual capacity, mental ability to stand trial, and criminal responsibility may be easy to arrive at or very difficult indeed. As a rule, repeated examinations should be devoted to such cases in order to make sure of the findings and to enable the court to receive those findings with confidence. The psychiatrist must in all cases assure himself that the patient has had a physical examination and that the possibility of organic disease has not been neglected.

The Report

The report should be brief, clear, and helpful. All specific questions asked of the consultant should be answered succinctly or reasons given for not doing so. If the opinion is written in an open hospital record, intimate matters should be omitted. In urgent situations, a telephone call to the referring physician in advance of the written report is sure to be appreciated. Promptness is essential both in seeing the patient and in making the report.

THE COLLEAGUE-CENTERED CONSULTATION

The psychiatrist serving as consultant to other professionals must make it clear that he is working as one member of a team of colleagues. He has something special to offer but so do the others, and he respects their views. Just as the problems of war and peace are not solely the purview of military officers, the problems of mental health are not solely of concern to psychiatrists.

The psychiatrist must differentiate consultation from training, supervision, and psychotherapy and must not contaminate the former with any of the latter. Colleagues properly resent being underrated or patronized. The psychiatrist should not offer advice to a teacher on how to teach, involve a clergyman in religious disputes, or offer unsolicited criticisms of administrative procedures to an administrator.

The psychiatrist's approach should be helpful and not judgmental. He must remember that he is dealing with his colleague only as a professional person and not as a total human being. Nothing will destroy a psychiatrist's value as a consultant so effectively as a lapse into the therapist's role toward his colleague—even if, as sometimes happens, the colleague tacitly or openly seeks that relationship.

In continuing relationships, the consultant should wait patiently for the natural growth of his responsibilities in his role and for opportunities to make contributions. ("Fair and softly goes far.") Colleagues often test before they trust. In making suggestions, the psychiatrist should offer a choice if he can. People resent authoritarianism and should be permitted to retain as much independent action as possible.

Procedural Methods

While the psychiatric consultant will have to adapt his methods to the special requirements of each professional situation, certain general procedures are almost universally applicable. In preparation for working with the actual colleague consultee, it is well to start by enlisting the active support of the man at the top of the colleague's organization—president, chancellor, dean, director, manager, or superintendent. To this individual he should make it clear that he wishes to familiarize himself thoroughly with the organization. He should request sufficient time and opportunities for detailed observation and participation in field work, and ask for any reading matter that might be helpful to him.

He should then proceed down the hierarchy, meeting the important people at each level, discussing current problems, and being a good listener. Finally, when he gets down to the actual workers, he should make it clear that this is where he feels he belongs and has most to contribute. For example, after getting acquainted with and acquiring the backing of the principal of a school, the new school psychiatrist meets with various individual department heads, spends some time with each, and finally begins his real work with the teachers; these he gets to know personally as friends and colleagues until they trust him implicitly.

The psychiatrist usually can contribute most in group conferences. A case may be presented by one of the workers (eg, a teacher), but the patient himself (student) need not be seen. Others in the group are encouraged to comment, and the psychiatrist finally summarizes the discussion, offers his own opinion, and points out general principles that would apply to similar cases.

When a worker's personal problems are clearly interfering with his handling of a case, great tact must be exercised to avoid bruised feelings. For example, if a clergyman stresses the "evil" of alcohol or sex, the psychiatrist may mention the "nonjudgmental, scientific approach that all of us professionals in human behavior strive for" and counterstress such factors as organic illness, heredity, and environmental conditioning.

The psychiatrist should bear in mind that his goal is to improve the general mental health climate in the organization as well as to help individual colleagues. Crises should be looked at constructively as opportunities to promote individual growth and minimize regressive changes. Antisocial, maladapted, and deviant behavior should be regarded with tolerance and understanding while keeping in mind the importance of early casefinding and treatment in such cases as the neurotic, the prepsychotic, the psychosomatically ill, and antisocial character problems. The wide ranges of normal should also be recognized, particularly in adolescents and young adults, in whom adjustment problems tend to clear readily with simple, sensible changes in management. Certain high-risk individuals (the ungifted, the socially rejected, the physically handicapped) should receive special supportive attention because of their higher incidence of neurotic and psychosomatic symptom formation.

The psychiatrist should not take on private patients as an outgrowth of this type of consultation work, nor should he usually accept more than a part-time position and salary. He thus is better able to maintain an attitude of impartiality and unbiased integrity. Similarly, he must avoid participating in factional disputes (management vs employees, principal vs teachers, etc).

THE AGENCY-CENTERED CONSULTATION

Psychiatric consultation at the agency level is still new and relatively uncommon. In the previous section, the psychiatrist worked inside schools and other organizations as a consultant to his colleagues from other disciplines. In this section, the organization itself is considered the "patient" to be diagnosed and treated. The incentive may be underproduction or morale problems suspected of being on a faulty mental health basis (several large companies and corporations), or the desire to build sound mental health principles into an organization at its beginning (Peace Corps).

Most of the principles and procedures noted in the preceding sections apply equally well here. As the psychiatrist becomes known, respected, and trusted in an organization, he will be called upon more and more to participate in conferences concerning its well-being or future policies.

The history is taken by studying all available documents and by interviewing systematically down through the echelons of the organization. If there is a union, its consent must be obtained; it should be made clear that jobs are not in jeopardy and that no one will be interviewed who does not wish to be.

The examination should include investigations of morale, attitude surveys, statistics of illness, absenteeism, accidents, use of health insurance plans, worker turnover, and staff mobility. The purpose of the examination is to identify undue stress, unhealthy policies, faulty structure, widespread depressions, flagging morale, rebelliousness, and anything else that threatens the good of the organization. A kind of psychodynamic formulation can usually be arrived at for the "pathology" present in terms of clearly demarcated events in the development of the agency and in connection with the activities and attitudes of certain key individuals.

Reports and recommendations should be made to the top management and subsequently to all the workers in the agency.

REFERENCES

Books and Monographs

Caplan, G.: *Theory and Practice of Mental Health Consultation.* Basic Books, 1970.

Mendel, W.M., & P. Solomon: *The Psychiatric Consultation.* Grune & Stratton, 1968.

Journal Articles

Dumont, M.P.: Industrial psychiatry for the employer of last resort. Commun Ment Health J 6:411–417, 1970.

Hollender, M.H., & S.P. Hersh: Impossible consultation made possible. Arch Gen Psychiat 23:343–345, 1970.

Morrison, A.P.: Consultation and group process with indigenous neighborhood workers. Commun Ment Health J 6:3–12, 1970.

Rossi, A.M., Akins, K.B., & P. Solomon: Psychiatric consultation requests in a general hospital. Hosp Community Psychiat, pp 144–146, May 1966.

Schwab, J.J., & J. Brown: Uses and abuses of psychiatric consultation. JAMA 205:65–68, 1968.

Solomon, P.: The psychiatric consultation in private practice. Annals of the Medical Society of Washington, DC 37:322–324, 1968.

Tieman, G.R.: Toward collaborative mental health consultation. J Religion Health 9:371–376, 1970.

White, W., & others: Psychiatric referrals in a general hospital. Med J Australia 1:950–954, 1970.

39 . . .

Community Psychiatry

Many psychiatrists have left the ivory tower for the city streets, where they concern themselves with the mental health of all the people—blacks, browns, reds, yellows, and even the whites. Community mental health centers, store-fronts, and crisis clinics function around the clock with participation of neighborhood personnel in dealing with emergency situations such as attempted suicide, domestic violence, alcoholism, and drug addiction.

Community psychiatry is a new specialty—though a widely embracing one—within the field of psychiatry. It consists of the acceptance of responsibility by one or more psychiatrists and others working with them for the prevention, early detection, and short-term and long-term (including rehabilitative) treatment of mental disorders in a circumscribed population.

The community psychiatrist is professionally concerned with the psychologic well-being of this population as a whole. His aim is to enable its members to obtain the kinds of services they need in order to overcome mental illness and disability or to achieve positive mental health. The community psychiatrist and his colleagues provide or encourage others to provide these services in accordance with mandates received from the community's authorized spokesmen. Influencing the responsible leaders of the community in such a way as to elicit mandates that enable him to carry out his professional responsibilities effectively is one of the community psychiatrist's central and continuing concerns.

The term community can be defined either as a political (geographic) unit or as a functional unit. People qualify as members of a geographic or political unit by holding rights of citizenship within the boundaries of a specified territory or merely by living there. Functional communities consist of members of trade unions or professional associations; employees of a business, industry, or other organization; members of a military unit, students enrolled in a college, volunteers in the Peace Corps, etc. Except when individuals live apart from their families, the responsibility of community psychiatrists usually extends to family members as well as to persons directly involved in the functional community.

Whether as members of an organization or by virtue of territorial, political, religious, ethnic, or family ties, the individuals that make up a defined population constitute a community to the degree that they share a common heritage and destiny, a feeling of "being in the same boat," or an awareness of mutual identity. If these attributes are lacking, an aggregation of individuals constitutes simply a population and not a community. Communities affect the well-being of successive generations of individuals either indirectly, through the medium of families, or directly. The family is the principal "medium" by which the community's "message" is transmitted. While acknowledging the importance of biologic and other influences, the community psychiatrist places special emphasis on the fact that the emotional health of individuals and families depends on the healthy development and functioning of human communities.

Communities vary in *scope* and in *degree.* A nation is a community, and so is "the community of all mankind." A family is a small community, and each individual is a "community" of internalized relationships to his past, present, and future surroundings and associates. Whatever its scope, the community (nation, city, family, or individual) is valued for its own sake and as an end in itself.

In contrast to communities, *organizations* are formed for the sake of accomplishing definite objectives. Their structure entails a division of labor and a purposeful allocation of specific functional roles. To varying degrees, organizations may also have the attributes of communities, being then valued in their own right and not simply as means of achieving specified ends.

Medical responsibility is assumed by the community psychiatrist, whose therapeutic goal is to enable those for whom he is responsible to assume (or reassume) their own social and personal responsibilities. By assuming medical responsibility according to a *psychotherapeutic model* (not judgmental nor controlling but accepting, facilitative, reality oriented, and encouraging), the community psychiatrist and his co-workers also seek to strengthen the community's capacity to care responsibly for its citizens.

Catchment areas are bounded by lines drawn on a map. People living within such an area constitute the population for whose mental health a community psychiatrist and his colleagues accept responsibility. The boundaries of catchment areas may or may not coincide with those of communities, strictly defined. The term was at one time applied to the geographic area from which patients were committed to a given state mental hospital. Traditionally, the staffs of such hospitals had only minimal contact with nonhospitalized members of the population in their usually quite large catchment areas.

State mental hospitals, staffed with psychiatrists who were once called "alienists," served valuable functions when mental illness was widely feared and misunderstood. These hospitals have, however, contributed to the further alienation of patients from their communities. In their turn, communities have gladly surrendered responsibility (by commitment to mental hospitals) for members whose initial alienation may well have been due to pathogenic features of the communities themselves—eg, a high prevalence of poverty, unemployment, prejudice, crime, and inadequate housing, welfare, education, and recreation. The existence of large state institutions to which disturbed and disturbing people could be banished has enabled communities to remain unaware of the part they have played in creating—or failing to prevent—mental and emotional disturbances. Like some individuals, communities have thus been enabled to rely upon the defense mechanism of denial.

The *unit plan* is an application of community psychiatry to public mental hospitals. It furnishes a means of breaking down large, impersonal state hospitals or veterans' hospitals into relatively decentralized segments. In general, each segment nas its own catchment area, and a comprehensive range of services is offered to an area that is close by. Contacts between unit personnel and community agencies or practitioners located within each area are facilitated by the unit plan, as are visits by patients' families and helpful activities on the part of community volunteers. Patients who are rehospitalized return to familiar surroundings, so that the continuity of care is enhanced. Each unit contains a diversified group of patients whose therapeutic stimulus to each other is presumably greater than when patients are housed with others whose classifications (perhaps arbitarily defined) are the same.

Psychiatric services in general hospitals furnish another strategic application of community psychiatry. Here the hospital serves as the community. In this setting, psychiatric staff members can interact closely with their medical and paramedical colleagues. People turn more readily to nonpsychiatrist physicians for help with their psychologic difficulties than to anyone else. Furthermore, any illness is psychologically stressful both to the patient and to his family, and many physical illnesses are provoked at least in part by emotional tension. The psychiatrist in the general hospital can help his colleagues learn ways of responding psychotherapeutically to their patients.

For psychiatric patients who come to a general hospital instead of to a mental hospital, feelings of shame and stigma are minimized and the intensive care that can be given shortens the hospital stay. As in other psychiatric treatment settings, continuity of care can be maintained as people are transferred from outpatient to inpatient to partial hospitalization (night or day hospital) and then back to outpatient and perhaps halfway house or foster home status and discharge. Other hospital and clinic services (neurology, endocrinology, etc) are available to assist in diagnosis and treatment as indicated.

Community mental health centers are being established throughout the USA as a result of federal legislation enacted in response to President Kennedy's message to the Congress in February, 1963. The centers must include at least 5 elements: an emergency service; facilities for inpatient, outpatient, and partial hospitalization care so organized that patients eligible for treatment in one facility can also receive treatment in the others; and consultation and educational services to professional and other members of the community. The centers are designed to be comprehensive and multipurpose, providing service to all residents of the area regardless of ability to pay and giving assistance with a wide variety of problems related to mental health such as mental retardation, law enforcement, alcoholism and drug addiction, marital difficulties, child care, care for the aged, and rehabilitation of the handicapped.

This variety of responsibilities demands the services not only of psychiatrists but also psychologists, social workers, nurses, social scientists, and others. The part played by volunteers and other interested citizens and by subprofessional workers who can facilitate communication with certain groups within the population being served is increasingly being recognized. Ultimate medical responsibility remains, however, with the community psychiatrist, who must be intimately acquainted with the functions and capabilities of his co-workers, with other community resources, and with the ways in which major community decisions that affect the population's mental health are made.

Consultation and educational services provided by mental health specialists are designed to help other community agencies—churches, employers, schools, etc—to improve the mental health status of the people for whom they have assumed responsibility. Consultation with key people can often stimulate new approaches to problems that had previously seemed baffling and discouraging. In providing these services, the psychiatrist gives attention not only to influences directly affecting the psychologic well-being of individuals but also to those general problems of communication within groups and between groups that favor the emergence of emotional disorders. He is particularly concerned with ensuring good communication within his own organization and between it and other agencies, groups, and individuals in the community.

The fields of *child and family psychiatry* serve as models for much of what takes place in community psychiatry. The therapist treating an emotionally disturbed child recognizes that other members of the family play a part in his patient's disturbance. Parents may be urged to obtain individual therapy, or they may be regarded essentially as counsultees. The child's problems are then discussed with the parents in such a way as to ease the parents' tensions and enlist them as colleagues in treating the child. The psychiatrist may treat all members of the family together, with particular attention to the processes of communication; or he may elect to treat *only* the parents, anticipating that beneficial effects will be reflected onto the child.

In treating adults, it is not so obvious that immediate surroundings may play a significant part in causing or perpetuating emotional disturbances, or that treatment and preventive measures can be effective when the surroundings are dealt with rather than the patient himself. However, this point of view is becoming more widespread, and it clearly owes much to recent developments in child and family psychotherapy.

Treatment of the community or of society may be sought from a community psychiatrist. People often believe (and some psychiatrists agree) that his skill in treating patients enables him to solve the problems of war, draft protests, overpopulation, pollution, poverty, crime, sexual license, abortion, drug abuse, campus unrest, racism, rioting, and radicalism. The psychiatrist can respond helpfully to those who seek his advice in such matters, although he may not be able to solve these problems for them. The *first* step he can suggest is for people to clarify the issues involved, find out who is actively concerned, and see what resources are available. The *second* step is to consider fundamental values as they bear upon the issues: what people really want and care about most. *Third*, through reference to shared values, an agreement about goals of action can be reached; programs are then developed and associations are formed to carry them out. *Fourth*, necessary changes in laws or regulations are brought about through political or other means. *Fifth*, legal and other sanctions are used to overcome remaining opposition. *Finally*, community resources are reexamined and are now mobilized to achieve the goals on which agreement has been reached. As new issues emerge, the sequence can be gone through again.

This procedure differs from the usual method followed by social reformers or change agents, namely, first, plan a course of action; then collect facts to justify it; then either enlist support or overcome resistance from the community's power structure; and finally try to put the (now modified) plan into effect. By contrast, the sophisticated community psychiatrist relies on an approach that in many ways is comparable to his psychotherapy with patients.

RELATED CONCEPTS

The therapeutic and preventive point of view that sets community psychiatry apart as a developing specialty within the general field of psychiatry is also reflected in a variety of other psychiatric subspecialties and schools of thought. These are described briefly below and are dealt with more fully in other parts of this book.

Public health and epidemiology provide important models for community psychiatry. The public health physician accepts responsibility for safeguarding the health of a specified community through measures classified as primary, secondary, and tertiary prevention. The first has to do with reducing or eliminating health hazards so that illnesses and accidents can be prevented. The second refers to case-finding and early treatment. The third is concerned with rehabilitative measures to prevent long-term disabilities that may result from certain acute conditions.

Epidemiologic studies have to do with the rates and distributions of various types of disabilities that occur in a population. These studies show which age groups, occupational groups, etc are at greatest risk and in need of greatest protection or care. However, many epidemiologic studies of psychiatric conditions cover only patients receiving treatment; sometimes they deal only with those treated in hospitals. The few surveys of total communities that have been made show that untreated cases outnumber those that are treated and that many mental health care needs are not being met.

Systems analysis can be difficult to apply because systems exist at so many levels and because they can be abstracted in so many ways. The medical training of a psychiatrist ensures that he will be able to observe the physical organism as a system, noting its inputs and outputs. He can also see the human personality as a system, and sometimes he can extend his systems view to families and other kinds of groups. As he masters administrative skills, he further learns to see an organization as a functioning system. In addition to all of these, a firm grasp of the social sciences and of ecology (man's relation to his physical habitat) is essential for understanding the community in systems terms.

A systems approach is also essential for evaluative research. Procedures of cost-benefit or cost-effectiveness accounting and systems for planning and analyzing program budgets are increasingly being applied to obtain the data needed for evaluation, as well as for rational allocation of resources. A geographically or organizationally defined catchment area furnishes an appropriate unit for applying systems analysis to programs developed in the field of community psychiatry.

Community mental health is essentially a synonym for community psychiatry. The aim is to provide care for patients at centers located near their homes at a stage when their disorders have not yet become severe or chronic, so that disruption of their lives is minimized. In most cases these are patients whose prognosis is good. Both rehabilitative and primary preventive efforts are also emphasized, the latter through education and consultation. Nonpsychiatric members of the "mental health team" play a significant part in these efforts. Two potential dangers have been noted: (1) that centers may solidify into "little state hospitals"; and (2) that staff members may concentrate on those segments of the population they find most congenial, leaving the community's worst problems no better attended to than in the past.

Social psychiatry is regarded sometimes as identical with community psychiatry and sometimes as either broader or narrower in scope. In its narrow sense, the emphasis of social psychiatry is primarily on individual patients and the particular social networks in which they are involved rather than on the wider community. In the concrete process of treating patients, where the therapist often is in touch with others in the patient's surroundings as well as with the patient himself, the 2 approaches may coincide. Viewed more broadly, social psychiatry is concerned with the social sciences generally and with their contributions to the understanding of human psychology. From the latter standpoint, community psychiatry can be regarded as one segment of this much larger field.

Preventive psychiatry also may be regarded as synonymous with community psychiatry when the public health use of the term (primary, secondary, and tertiary prevention) is intended. As with community mental health, however, there is a danger that efforts to "prevent" mental disorder may result in the neglect of severe mental disorders or disabilities that already exist in the population or that may occur in spite of preventive programs. Preventive psychiatry also tends to focus on minimizing hazards to individuals, whereas community psychiatry includes efforts to improve the functioning of the total community.

Crisis intervention is strongly emphasized in community psychiatry. Emotional crises can occur in connection with major transitions such as leaving home, getting married, or starting a new job; or as a reaction to bereavement, physical injury, loss of a job, etc. During periods of crisis, individuals are regarded as being more receptive to help—or susceptible to harm—than at other times. Depending upon the response of those individuals who intervene, the crisis may be an occasion either for achieving greater maturity and an enhanced capacity to cope with trouble or for becoming psychologically more vulnerable than before. "Striking while the iron is hot" enables a little help to go a long way. Failure to act promptly in a constructive fashion may permit maladaptive (defensive) reactions to be established that will become harder to modify at a later time.

An understanding of how to intervene effectively can be passed on by mental health specialists to other community caregivers—clergymen, public health nurses, lawyers, and others to whom individuals turn for help. Crisis intervention can also be applied in working at the social system level. Organizational or community crises, like individual crises, pose both a threat and a challenge. Here, too, it is important for the specialist in community psychiatry to be in a position to intervene quickly, encouraging key people to confront the crisis as realistically and responsibly as possible.

Transactional psychiatry is concerned with sequences of response-arousing events that occur between a given person (patient) and his biologic, psychologic, social, and physical environment. These are examined in order to assess the impact of such events upon the processes of organization or disorganization taking place in the individual's personality. Primary emphasis is placed upon interpersonal transactions, and attention is given to the effects of the patient's actions upon the therapist (or upon other persons to whom the patient relates) as well as to the impact of the therapist's or other people's actions upon the patient. The formulations of transactional psychiatry appear to be quite compatible with those of social psychiatry, family psychiatry, and community psychiatry.

Existential psychiatry, in its emphasis upon the uniqueness of the individual's total being and his view of the world, would seem to represent the extreme opposite of community psychiatry. However, common ground can be found in the importance attached to social involvement, action, and responsibility. The existentialists hold that man's life can be humanized and rendered authentic or meaningful if the individual thoughtfully probes each conflict or crisis within himself, makes a choice about action, and then assumes responsibility for the consequences of his choice. The goals of the community psychiatrist are much the same in his "encounters" with individuals, groups, and community spokesmen.

The *therapeutic community* is an approach to treatment in a hospital or day hospital by which the active efforts of patients as well as those of all staff members are consciously mobilized to further the goals of treatment. Decisions regarding issues of daily living are reached democratically rather than by administrative fiat; communication is open and efficient; feedback and confrontation, with regard to staff as well as patients, is encouraged; and patients share in assuming responsibility for themselves, for others, and for the therapeutic community as such. To some degree, this approach can be extended out from the institution to the surrounding community; thereupon it becomes indistinguishable from the approach of community psychiatry.

Milieu therapy likewise attempts to mobilize institutional resources to further the goals of treatment in a hospital setting. Patients are not explicitly called upon to exert therapeutic influence upon each other, however, and decision making is less democratic than in the therapeutic community. Rather, through his understanding of psychodynamic processes, the psychiatrist prescribes the attitudes that ancillary staff members should take to the patients and the kinds of activities in which the patients should engage. The strategic contributions these staff members make to the patient's treatment is fully recognized, and the considerations behind the psychiatrist's recommendations are discussed with staff members as a basis for securing their full cooperation.

Community treatment generally refers to the placement of psychiatric patients in a foster home or halfway house within a receptive community environment. Resources for psychotherapy are available, as well as guidance for the persons in whose charge they are placed. This form of treatment has been most highly developed in the community of Gheel, in Belgium. The term has also been applied (with some negative overtones) to the routine outpatient treatment of persons who live at home with their families, even though the latter may be heavily burdened with the patient's care and frustrated in their attempts to secure adequate help with the problems he presents. An integrated and competent organization of various services in the community that can be mobilized for the patient's benefit represents community treatment in a more constructive form. This last is again indistinguishable from community psychiatry or community mental health.

Cross-cultural or comparative psychiatry is concerned with tracing the different rates and forms of mental disorders that occur in different social and cultural settings. Studies in this field explore the ways in which variations in the cultural patterning of sex roles, family structure, age distinctions, religious beliefs, modes of physical sustenance, etc may be reflected in varied patterns of psychiatric symptoms. What is constant is also revealed—the mental disorders or defects that evidently arise universally, regardless of cultural differences, from the nature of the human condition.

TRENDS—A BASIS FOR ASSESSMENT

A listing of recent trends in community psychiatric services provides a basis for judging the adequacy of such services—or at least their conformity to certain current views. These trends are toward the following goals:

(1) Treating many diagnostic categories of patients rather than just a few.

(2) Serving all age groups rather than principally children.

(3) Treating people of low socioeconomic status rather than predominantly the middle class.

(4) Working with families or others who are in close touch with patients rather than only with persons who have been defined as patients.

(5) Intervening promptly at the critical period when help is sought rather than imposing a waiting period.

(6) Beginning treatment at the initial contact rather than first requiring prolonged intake and diagnostic procedures.

(7) Providing brief therapy whenever possible rather than expecting long-term psychotherapy to be the technic of choice.

(8) Encouraging diversified and flexible approaches to patient care, including treatment in the patient's home, rather than holding strictly to any one model of treatment.

(9) Giving attention to primary prevention and to rehabilitative and aftercare services as well as to the actual treatment process.

(10) Ensuring maximum continuity of care rather than requiring transfers and referrals that sever therapeutically significant relationships.

(11) Broadening, rather than narrowing, the range of professional mental health skills.

(12) Cultivating close ties with resources that provide various medical and health care services rather than remaining aloof from other branches of medicine.

(13) Broadening the concept of the "psychiatric team" to include others besides the traditional psychiatrist, psychologist, and social worker.

(14) Accepting members of other professions as colleagues of the psychiatrist rather than as his subordinates; also, accepting nonprofessional and volunteer personnel as colleagues or potential colleagues.

(15) Working to enable both patients and others in the community to assume as much responsibility as possible rather than "taking over" in ways that deprive them of responsibility.

(16) Encouraging resourcefulness and effectiveness on the part of others through appropriate decentralization and through the fostering of democratic processes rather than seeking to maximize central authority and control.

(17) Developing contractual and other working relationships among public, private, and nonprofit resources in the community in order to enhance patients' freedom of choice rather than permitting a single bureaucratized "empire" to be formed.

(18) Accepting guidance from community representatives regarding policy decisions relating to mental health rather than serving merely as a source of such guidance.

(19) Relying on cost-benefit or cost-effectiveness accounting and systems analysis as a means of allocating resources and evaluating performance.

(20) Carrying out longitudinal and community-wide studies of mental disorders and disabilities rather than keeping track only of currently and locally treated cases.

(21) Consulting and collaborating with members and leaders of organized community groups from the standpoint of their interests and concerns rather than focusing simply on issues of patient care.

(22) Taking all possible steps to overcome the stigmatizing, degrading, or abusive handling of any groups or individuals within the community who are targets of hostile or punitive reactions rather than intervening only to secure greater respect and acceptance for psychiatric patients.

REFERENCES

Books and Monographs

Bellak, L., & H.H. Barten (editors): *Progress in Community Health*. Grune & Stratton, 1969.

Bergen, B.J., & C.S. Thomas (editors): *Issues and Problems in Social Psychiatry*. Thomas, 1966.

Bindman, A.J., & A.D. Spiegel (editors): *Perspectives in Community Mental Health*. Aldine, 1969.

Caplan, G.: *Principles of Preventive Psychiatry*. Basic Books, 1964.

Decentralization of Psychiatric Services and Continuity of Care. Milbank Memorial Fund, 1962.

Dimensions of Community Psychiatry. GAP Report No. 69 (vol 6). Group for the Advancement of Psychiatry, April 1968.

Duhl, L.J., & R.L. Leopold (editors): *Mental Health and Urban Social Policy: A Casebook of Community Action*. Jossey-Bass, 1968.

Dumont, M.: *The Absurd Healer: Perspectives of a Community Psychiatrist*. Science House, 1968.

Education for Community Psychiatry. GAP Report No. 64 (vol 6). Group for the Advancement of Psychiatry, March 1967.

Fairweather, G.W., & others: *Community Life for the Mentally Ill: An Alternative to Institutional Care*. Aldine, 1969.

Goldston, S.E. (editor): *Concepts of Community Psychiatry*. Publication No. 1319. US Public Health Service, 1965.

Greenblatt, M., & others: *From Custodial to Therapeutic Patient Care in Mental Hospitals*. Russell Sage Foundation, 1955.

Kaufman, M.R. (editor): *The Psychiatric Unit in a General Hospital*. Internat Univ Press, 1965.

Klein, D.C.: *Community Dynamics and Mental Health*. Wiley, 1968.

Lamb, H.R., Heath, D., & J.J. Downing (editors): *Handbook of Community Mental Health Practice: The San Mateo Experience*. Jossey-Bass, 1969.

Roberts, L.M., Halleck, S.L., & M.B. Loeb (editors): *Community Psychiatry*. Univ of Wisconsin Press, 1966.

Shore, M.F., & F.V. Mannino: *Mental Health and the Community: Problems, Programs, and Strategies*. Behavioral Publications, 1969.

Williams, R.H., & L.D. Ozarin (editors): *Community Mental Health: An International Perspective*. Jossey-Bass, 1967.

Journal Articles

Becker, A., Murphy, N.M., & M. Greenblatt: Recent advances in community psychiatry. New England J Med 272:621–625, 674–679, 1965.

Galdston, I.: Community psychiatry: Its social and historical derivations. J Canad Psychiat Ass 10:461–473, 1965.

Gottesfeld, H., Rhee, C., & G. Parker: A study of the role of paraprofessionals in community mental health. Commun Ment Health J 6:285–291, 1970.

Hutcheson, B.R., & E.A. Krause: Systems analysis and mental health services. Commun Ment Health J 5:29–45, 1969.

Jones, M.: Therapeutic community practice. Am J Psychiat 122:1275–1279, 1966.

Leeds, A.A., & others: Planning for mental health. Commun Ment Health J 5:206–214, 1969.

Leighton, A.H.: Poverty and social change. Sc American 212:21–27, May 1965.

Rogawski, A.S.: Community psychiatry and education of psychiatrists. Commun Ment Health J 5:129–139, 1969.

Rubin, B.: Community psychiatry. Arch Gen Psychiat 20:497–508, 1969.

Scherl, D.J., & J.T. English: Community mental health and comprehensive health service programs for the poor. Am J Psychiat 125:1666–1673, 1969.

Stubblebine, J.M., & B.J. Decker: Are urban mental health centers worth it? Am J Psychiat 127:908–912, 1971.

Zuithoff, D.: Community psychiatry and social action: A survey. Am J Psychiat 126:1621–1627, 1970.

Zusman, J.: Design of catchment areas for community mental health services. Arch Gen Psychiat 21:568–573, 1969.

Appendix

PSYCHIATRIC CLASSIFICATION

SUMMARY OF *DIAGNOSTIC AND STATISTICAL MANUAL OF MENTAL DISORDERS (DSM–II, 1968)**

I. Mental Retardation

310.	Borderline
311.	Mild
312.	Moderate
313.	Severe
314.	Profound
315.	Unspecified

With each: Following or associated with

.0	Infection or intoxication
.1	Trauma or physical agent
.2	Disorders of metabolism, growth, or nutrition
.3	Gross brain disease (postnatal)
.4	Unknown prenatal influence
.5	Chromosomal abnormality
.6	Prematurity
.7	Major psychiatric disorder
.8	Psychosocial (environmental) deprivation
.9	Other condition

II. Organic Brain Syndromes (OBS)
A. Psychoses
Senile and Presenile Dementia

290.0	Senile dementia
290.1	Presenile dementia

Alcoholic Psychosis

291.0	Delirium tremens
291.1	Korsakoff's psychosis
291.2	Other alcoholic hallucinosis
291.3	Alcohol paranoid state
291.4	Acute alcohol intoxication†
291.5	Alcoholic deterioration†
291.6	Pathologic intoxication†
291.9	Other alcoholic psychosis

Psychosis Associated With Intracranial Infection

292.0	General paralysis
292.1	Syphilis of central nervous system
292.2	Epidemic encephalitis
292.3	Other and unspecified encephalitis
292.9	Other intracranial infection

Psychosis Associated With Other Cerebral Condition

293.0	Cerebral arteriosclerosis
293.1	Other cerebrovascular disturbance
293.2	Epilepsy
293.3	Intracranial neoplasm
293.4	Degenerative disease of the CNS

*Prepared by the Committee on Nomenclature and Statistics of the American Psychiatric Association.

†These diagnoses are for use in the USA only and do not appear in ICD–8. (ICD–8 = International Classification of Diseases, adopted by the Nineteenth World Health Assembly in May 1966, to become effective in all member states in 1968.)

293.5 Brain trauma
293.9 Other cerebral condition
Psychosis Associated With Other Physical Condition
294.0 Endocrine disorder
294.1 Metabolic and nutritional disorder
294.2 Systemic infection
294.3 Drug or poison intoxication (other than alcohol)
294.4 Childbirth
294.8 Other and unspecified physical condition

B. Nonpsychotic OBS
309.0 Intracranial infection
309.13 Alcohol† (simple drunkenness)
309.14 Other drug, poison, or systemic intoxication†
309.2 Brain trauma
309.3 Circulatory disturbance
309.4 Epilepsy
309.5 Disturbance of metabolism, growth, or nutrition
309.6 Senile or presenile brain disease
309.7 Intracranial neoplasm
309.8 Degenerative disease of the CNS
309.9 Other physical condition

III. Psychoses Not Attributed to Physical Conditions Listed Previously
Schizophrenia
295.0 Simple
295.1 Hebephrenic
295.2 Catatonic
295.23 Catatonic type, excited†
295.24 Catatonic type, withdrawn†
295.3 Paranoid
295.4 Acute schizophrenic episode
295.5 Latent
295.6 Residual
295.7 Schizo-affective
295.73 Schizo-affective, excited†
295.74 Schizo-affective, depressed†
295.8 Childhood†
295.9 Chronic undifferentiated†
295.99 Other schizophrenia†
Major Affective Disorders
296.0 Involutional melancholia
296.1 Manic-depressive illness, manic

296.2 Manic-depressive illness, depressed
296.3 Manic-depressive illness, circular
296.33 Manic-depressive, circular, manic†
296.34 Manic-depressive, circular, depressed†
296.8 Other major affective disorder
Paranoid States
297.0 Paranoia
297.1 Involutional paranoid state
297.9 Other paranoid state
Other Psychoses
298.0 Psychotic depressive reaction

IV. Neuroses
300.0 Anxiety
300.1 Hysterical
300.13 Hysterical, conversion type†
300.14 Hysterical, dissociative type†
300.2 Phobic
300.3 Obsessive-compulsive
300.4 Depressive
300.5 Neurasthenic
300.6 Depersonalization
300.7 Hypochondriacal
300.8 Other neurosis

V. Personality Disorders and Certain Other Nonpsychotic Mental Disorders
Personality Disorders
301.0 Paranoid
301.1 Cyclothymic
301.2 Schizoid
301.3 Explosive
301.4 Obsessive-compulsive
301.5 Hysterical
301.6 Asthenic
301.7 Antisocial
301.81 Passive-aggressive†
301.82 Inadequate†
301.89 Other specified types†
Sexual Deviation
302.0 Homosexuality
302.1 Fetishism
302.2 Pedophilia
302.3 Transvestitism
302.4 Exhibitionism
302.5 Voyeurism†
302.6 Sadism†

302.7 Masochism†
302.8 Other sexual deviation
Alcoholism
303.0 Episodic excessive drinking
303.1 Habitual excessive drinking
303.2 Alcohol addiction
303.9 Other alcoholism
Drug Dependence
304.0 Opium, opium alkaloids and their derivatives
304.1 Synthetic analgesics with morphine-like effects
304.2 Barbiturates
304.3 Other hypnotics and sedatives or "tranquilizers"
304.4 Cocaine
304.5 *Cannabis sativa* (hashish, marihuana)
304.6 Other psycho-stimulants
304.7 Hallucinogens
304.8 Other drug dependence

VI. Psychophysiologic Disorders
305.0 Skin
305.1 Musculoskeletal
305.2 Respiratory
305.3 Cardiovascular
305.4 Hemic and lymphatic
305.5 Gastrointestinal
305.6 Genitourinary
305.7 Endocrine
305.8 Organ of special sense
305.9 Other type

VII. Special Symptoms
306.0 Speech disturbance
306.1 Specific learning disturbance
306.2 Tic
306.3 Other psychomotor disorder
306.4 Disorders of sleep
306.5 Feeding disturbance
306.6 Enuresis
306.7 Encopresis
306.8 Cephalalgia
306.9 Other special symptom

VIII. Transient Situational Disturbances
307.0 Adjustment reaction of infancy†
307.1 Adjustment reaction of childhood†
307.2 Adjustment reaction of adolescence†
307.3 Adjustment reaction of adult life†
307.4 Adjustment reaction of late life†

IX. Behavior Disorders of Childhood and Adolescence
308.0 Hyperkinetic reaction†
308.1 Withdrawing reaction†
308.2 Overanxious reaction†
308.3 Runaway reaction†
308.4 Unsocialized aggressive reaction†
308.5 Group delinquent reaction†
308.9 Other reaction†

X. Conditions Without Manifest Psychiatric Disorders and Nonspecific Conditions
Social Maladjustment Without Manifest Psychiatric Disorder
316.0 Marital maladjustment†
316.1 Social maladjustment†
316.2 Occupational maladjustment†
316.3 Dyssocial behavior†
316.9 Other social maladjustments†
Nonspecific Conditions
317 Nonspecific conditions†
No Mental Disorder
318 No mental disorder†

XI. Nondiagnostic Terms for Administrative Use
319.0 Diagnosis deferred†
319.1 Boarder†
319.2 Experiment only†
319.3 Other†

Fifth Digit Qualifying Phrases

Section II	**Section III**	**Sections IV through IX**	**All disorders**
.X1 Acute	.X6 Not psychotic now	.X6 mild	.X5 In remission
.X2 Chronic		.X7 Moderate	
		.X8 Severe	

SUMMARY OF TREATMENT
OF ACUTE POISONING

Those who call in on the telephone in cases of poisoning are usually panicky. Ask them to calm down and tell you exactly what happened as well as they can—including when, what material, how much, and in what way— and have them describe the patient's condition—behavior, consciousness, color, breathing, and perhaps temperature and pulse.

It may be possible to decide at once that there is no emergency and that the situation can either be ignored or that the patient can be seen later at some mutually convenient time and place. (*Example:* A woman calls late in the evening and says her 16-year-old daughter has told her that she just took 3 of her mother's sleeping pills [Seconal, 100 mg] and that she intends to have "a long sleep and maybe never wake up." The parents should be reassured, told to put the girl to bed and hide the rest of the pills, and bring her to the office the next day.)

The physician may recognize that the situation is potentially dangerous but not critical and elect to recommend immediate treatment measures at home to be followed by attendance at the hospital or office. (*Example:* A father calls to say that his son returned home from a party in a drunken state and just swallowed an unknown number of sleeping pills. He is staggering about and bemoaning his own fate and that of the world. The father is told to induce vomiting by the use of ipecac or other means and then bring the young man to the hospital emergency room.)

If the situation is more urgent or requires emergency measures that are not available or easily administered at home, the patient must be brought at once to the hospital. The physician should call the hospital himself and go there as soon as he can. (*Example:* A child has ingested a bottleful of Seconal tablets and is unconscious and cyanotic. He should be rushed to the hospital for immediate and vigorous treatment.)

If it appears that the patient may be at the point of death, call the fire department or police ambulance. (*Example:* A patient has imbibed unknown substances and is having repeated convulsions followed by periods of apnea and cyanosis. Call an emergency resuscitation squad immediately.)

When in Attendance

The following measures may be necessary. They are given in the order of relative urgency.

1. Maintain patent airway and support respiration and circulation.

2. Institute symptomatic treatment for shock, coma, convulsions, etc.

3. Take a brief history and perform necessary physical examination. Utilize the relatives or those who brought the patient to the hospital. If necessary, send the police out for a history of what happened.

4. Consider gastric lavage or induced emesis for orally ingested toxins unless the patient is comatose or convulsing. The value of lavage is not well established. Induced emesis is preferable. Give syrup of ipecac, 15–20 ml by mouth, followed by large quantities of fluid. Repeat once if emesis does not occur in 15–20 minutes.

Apomorphine acts more rapidly than ipecac. The dosage is 6 mg IM in adults and 0.05 mg/kg IM in children. The action of apomorphine can be terminated with levallorphan (Lorfan), 0.02 mg/kg IM.

5. Give specific therapy if available.

6. Increase the rate of excretion of poisons—eg, give fluids, osmotic diuretics.

7. Take a full definitive history and perform a complete physical examination. Identify the noxious agent if possible.

8. Collect laboratory samples for identification and determination of levels of poison, both for control of treatment and for medicolegal purposes.

GENERAL BIBLIOGRAPHY

See also lists of books, monographs, and journal articles accompanying the chapters. Many excellent works listed there are not repeated here.

Abraham, K.: *Selected Papers of Karl Abraham.* Basic Books, 1953.
Adler, A.: *The Practice and Theory of Individual Psychology.* Harcourt Brace, 1924.
Alcoholics Anonymous: The Story of How Many Thousands Have Recovered From Alcoholism. Cornwall, 1965.
Alexander, F., Eisenstein, S., M. Grotjahn: *Psychoanalytic Pioneers.* Basic Books, 1966.
Alexander, F., & Selesnick, S.T.: *The History of Psychiatry.* Harper, 1966.
American Psychiatric Association: *Impressions of European Psychiatry.* American Psychiatric Association, 1961.
American Psychiatric Association: *The Psychiatric Emergency.* Joint Information Service, Washington, DC, 1966.
Arieti, S. (editor): *American Handbook of Psychiatry.* 3 vols. Basic Books, 1966.
Balint, M., & E. Balint: *Psychotherapeutic Techniques in Medicine.* Lippincott, 1961.
Bandler, B.: *Psychiatry in the General Hospital.* Little, Brown, 1966.
Becker, E.: *The Revolution in Psychiatry.* Collier-Macmillan, 1964.
Bellak, L.: *Contemporary European Psychiatry.* Grove Press, 1961.
Bellak, L.: *Handbook of Community Psychiatry and Community Mental Health.* Grune & Stratton, 1964.
Bergen, B.J., & S.T. Claudewell (editors): *Issues and Problems in Social Psychiatry.* Thomas, 1966.
Blaine, G.B., Jr., & others: *Emotional Problems of the Student.* Doubleday, 1966.
Blum, R.H., & others: *Society and Drugs.* 2 vols. Jossey-Bass, 1969.
Breuer, J., & S. Freud: *Studies on Hysteria.* Basic Books, 1957.
Chasell, J.O.: *Bennington Psychiatric Papers.* The Austen Riggs Center, 1967.
Connery, R.H.: *The Politics of Mental Health.* Columbia Univ Press, 1968.
Cummings, J.N., & M. Kremer: *Biochemical Aspects of Neurological Disorders.* Davis, 1968.
De Reuck, A.V.S., & M. O'Connor: *Disorders of Language.* Little, Brown, 1964.
De Reuck, A.V.S., & R. Porter: *The Mentally Abnormal Offender.* Little, Brown, 1968.
Deutsch, H.: *Neuroses and Character Types.* Internat Univ Press, 1965.
Deutsch, H.: *Psychoanalysis of the Neuroses.* Hogarth, 1951.
Deutsch, M. (editor): *The Disadvantaged Child.* Basic Books, 1967.
Douvan, E., & J. Adelson: *The Adolescent Experience.* Wiley, 1966.
Dunham, H.W., & S.K. Weinberg: *The Culture of the State Mental Hospital.* Wayne State Univ Press, 1960.

Eddy, H.P. (editor): *Sex and the College Student.* Group for the Advancement of Psychiatry, 1966.

Elkins, H.K.: Psychiatry. Chap 21 in: *Current Medical References,* 6th ed. Chatton, M.J., & P.J. Sanazaro (editors). Lange, 1970.

Ellis, H.: *Studies in the Psychology of Sex.* 2 vols. Random House, 1942.

Engel, G.L.: *Psychological Development in Health and Disease.* Saunders, 1962.

Erikson, E.H.: *Identity, Youth and Crisis.* Norton, 1968.

Erikson, E.H.: *Insight and Responsibility.* Norton, 1964.

Erikson, E.H. (editor): *Youth: Change and Challenge.* Basic Books, 1963.

Ewalt, J.R., & D.L. Farnsworth: *Textbook of Psychiatry.* McGraw-Hill, 1963.

Eysenck, H.J.: *The Effects of Psychotherapy.* Internat Science Press, 1966.

Ferenczi, S.: *Further Contributions to the Theory and Technique of Psychoanalysis.* Hogarth, 1950.

Frank, J.D.: *Persuasion and Healing: A Comparative Study of Psychotherapy.* Johns Hopkins Press, 1961.

Freedman, A.M., & H.I. Kaplan (editors): *Comprehensive Textbook of Psychiatry.* Williams & Wilkins, 1967.

Freud, A.: *The Ego and the Mechanisms of Defense.* Internat Univ Press, 1946.

Freud, A.: *Introduction to the Technic of Child Analysis.* Allen & Unwin, 1931.

Freud, S.: *Beyond the Pleasure Principle.* Liveright, 1950.

Freud, S.: *Civilization and Its Discontents.* Cape & Smith, 1930.

Freud, S.: *The Ego and the Id.* Hogarth, 1927.

Freud, S.: *A General Introduction to Psychoanalysis.* Garden City, 1938.

Freud, S.: *Group Psychology and the Analysis of the Ego.* Hogarth, 1922.

Freud, S.: *New Introductory Lectures on Psychoanalysis.* Norton, 1933.

Freud, S.: *An Outline of Psychoanalysis.* Norton, 1950.

Freud, S.: *The Problem of Anxiety.* Norton, 1936.

Freud, S.: *Complete Psychological Works.* Standard edition, translated by James Strachey. 24 vols. Hogarth, 1953–1966.

Galdston, I.: *Historic Derivations of Modern Psychiatry.* McGraw-Hill, 1967.

Glasscote, R.M., & others: *The Treatment of Alcoholism.* Joint Information Service of the American Psychiatric Association and the National Association for Mental Health, 1967.

Glasscote, R.M., & others: *The Community Mental Health Center.* Joint Information Service of the American Psychiatric Association and the National Association for Mental Health, 1964.

Glover, E.: *The Technique of Psychoanalysis.* Internat Univ Press, 1955.

Goffman, E.: *Asylums.* Doubleday, 1961.

Gray, W. (editor): *General Systems Theory and Psychiatry.* Little, Brown, 1970.

Graylin, W.: *The Meaning of Despair.* Science House, 1968.

Greenacre, P.: *Affective Disorders: Psychoanalytic Contribution to Their Study.* Internat Univ Press, 1953.

Greenblatt, M., & others: *Mental Patients in Transition.* Thomas, 1961.

Griffith, C.R., & L.M. Libo: *Mental Health Consultants: Agents of Community Change.* Jossey-Bass, 1968.

Guilford, J.P.: *The Nature of Human Intelligence.* McGraw-Hill, 1969.

Haley, J., & L. Hoffman: *Techniques of Family Therapy.* Basic Books, 1967.

Harper, R.A.: *Psychoanalysis and Psychotherapy.* Prentice-Hall, 1959.

Hartman, H.: *Ego Psychology and the Problems of Adaptation.* Internat Univ Press, 1958.

Hartman, H.: *Essays on Ego Psychology.* Internat Univ Press, 1964.

Hartwich, A.: *Aberrations of Sexual Life.* Capricorn Books, 1962. [After Krafft-Ebing, R.: *Psychopathia Sexualis.* Albert Muller Verlag, 1937. First published in 1906.]

Hill, L.B.: *Psychotherapeutic Intervention in Schizophrenia.* Univ of Chicago Press, 1955.

Hinsie, L.E., & R.J. Campbell: *Psychiatric Dictionary.* Oxford Univ Press, 1960.

Hoffman, M.: *The Gay World.* Basic Books, 1968.

Hollender, M.H.: The need or wish to be held. Arch Gen Psychiat 22:445–453, 1970.

Hollingshead, A., & F.C. Redlich: *Social Class and Mental Illness: A Community Study.* Wiley, 1958.

Horney, K.: *The Neurotic Personality of Our Time.* Norton, 1937.

Isaacson, R.L.: *Basic Readings in Neuropsychology.* Harper, 1964.

James, A.E. (editor): *Parenthood: Its Psychology and Psychopathology.* Little, Brown, 1970.

John, E.R.: *Mechanisms of Memory.* Academic Press, 1967.

Joint Commission Report on Mental Illness and Health: *Action for Mental Health.* Basic Books, 1961.

Jones, E.: *The Life and Work of Sigmund Freud.* 3 vols. Basic Books, 1953.

Jones, M.: *Social Psychiatry in the Community, in Hospitals, and in Prisons.* Thomas, 1962.

Jones, M.: *Beyond the Therapeutic Community.* Yale Univ Press, 1968.

Jones, R.M.: *The New Psychology of Dreaming.* Grune & Stratton, 1970.

Jung, C.G.: *Contributions to Analytic Psychology.* Harcourt Brace, 1928.

Kahn, R.L., & others: *Organizational Stress: Studies in Role Conflict and Ambiguity.* Wiley, 1964.

Kanner, L.: *Child Psychiatry.* Thomas, 1957.

Kanno, C.K., & R.M. Glasscote: *Private Psychiatric Hospitals.* American Psychiatric Association, 1966.

Katz, B., & others: *The Psychology of Abnormal Behavior,* 2nd ed. Ronald Press, 1961.

Kaufman, M.R., & M. Heiman: *Evolution of Psychosomatic Concepts.* Internat Univ Press, 1964.

Keniston, K.: *The Uncommitted.* Harcourt Brace, 1960.

Kiloh, L.G., & J.W. Osse Hon: *Clinical Electroencephalography.* Butterworth, 1966.

Klein, D.C.: *Community Dynamics and Mental Health.* Wiley, 1968.

Knapp, P.H.: *Expression of the Emotions in Man.* Internat Univ Press, 1963.

Kolb, L.C., & others: *Schizophrenia.* Little, Brown, 1964.

Kolb, L.C.: *Modern Clinical Psychiatry.* Saunders, 1968.

Kotinsky, R., & H.L. Witmer (editors): *Community Programs for Mental Health.* Harvard Univ Press, 1955.

Krafft-Ebing, R.: See Hartwich, A.

Leighton, A.H., & others: *Psychiatric Disorder Among the Yoruba.* Cornell Univ Press, 1963.

Lennox, G.W., & M.A. Lennox: *Epilepsy and Related Disorders.* 2 vols. Little, Brown, 1960.

Lidz, T., Fleck, S., & A.R. Cornelison: *Schizophrenia and the Family.* Internat Univ Press, 1965.

Lidz, T.: *The Person: His Development Through the Life Cycle.* Basic Books, 1968.

Lindesmith, A.R.: *The Addict and the Law.* Indiana Univ Press, 1965.

Lisansky, E.T., & B.R. Shochet: Psychiatry in medical practice. Mod Treat 6:635–899, 1969.

Locke, S.: *Neurology.* Little, Brown, 1966.

Lorand, S.: *Technique of Psychoanalytic Therapy.* Internat Univ Press, 1948.

Marmor, J. (editor): *Sexual Inversion.* Basic Books, 1965.

May, R., & others (editors): *Existence: A New Dimension in Psychiatry and Psychology.* Basic Books, 1958.

Mayer-Gross, W., Slater, E., & M. Roth: *Clinical Psychiatry.* Cassell, 1954.

Menninger, K.: *The Vital Balance.* Viking, 1963.

Messer, A.A.: *The Individual in His Family.* Thomas, 1970.

Milbank Memorial Fund: *Decentralization of Psychiatric Services and Continuity of Care.* 1962.

Mullan, H., & I. Sanguilliano: *The Therapist's Contribution to the Treatment Process.* Thomas, 1964.

Murphy, J.M., & A.H. Leighton: *Approaches to Cross-Cultural Psychiatry.* Cornell Univ Press, 1965.

Mussen, P.H. (editor): *Handbook of Research Methods in Child Development.* Wiley, 1960.

Nemiah, J.C.: *Foundations of Psychopathology.* Oxford Univ Press, 1961.

Nunberg, H.: *Practice and Theory of Psychoanalysis.* 2 vols. Internat Univ Press, 1948.

Offer, D., & M. Sabshin: *Normality.* Basic Books, 1966.

Oversey, L.: *Homosexuality and Pseudohomosexuality.* Science House, 1969.

Padula, H.: *Approaches to the Care of the Long-Term Mental Patient.* Joint Information Service of the American Psychiatric Association and the National Association for Mental Health, 1968.

Pervin, L.A., Riek, L., & W. Dalrymple (editors): *The College Drop-out and the Utilization of Talent.* Princeton Univ Press, 1966.

Redlich, F.C., & D.X. Freedman: *The Theory and Practice of Psychiatry.* Basic Books, 1966.

Resnik, H.L.P.: *Suicidal Behaviors: Diagnosis and Management.* Little, Brown, 1968.

Riessman, F., Cohen, J., & A. Pearl: *Mental Health of the Poor.* Free Press, 1964.

Roberts, L.M., & others: *Community Psychiatry.* Univ of Wisconsin Press, 1966.

Rosen, G.: *Madness in Society.* Routledge & Kegan Paul, 1968.

Rubenstein, R., & H.D. Lasswell: *The Sharing of Power in a Psychiatric Hospital.* Yale Univ Press, 1966.

Ruesch, J.: *Therapeutic Communication.* Norton, 1961.

Rush, B.: *Medical Inquiries and Observations Upon the Diseases of the Mind.* Hafner, 1962.

Schwing, G.: *A Way to the Soul of the Mentally Ill.* Internat Univ Press, 1954.

Senn, M.J.E., & A.J. Solnit: *Problems in Child Behavior and Development.* Lea & Febiger, 1968.

Shapiro, D.: *Neurotic Styles.* Basic Books, 1965.

Shepherd, M., Lader, M., & R. Rodright: *Clinical Psychopharmacology.* English Univ Press, 1969.

Shore, M.F., & F.V. Mannino (editors): *Mental Health and the Community: Problems, Programs, Strategies.* Behavioral Publications, 1968.

Skinner, B.F.: *Science and Human Behavior.* Free Press, 1953.

Spence, K.W., & J.T. Spence: *The Psychology of Learning and Motivation.* Academic Press, 1967.

Spitzer, S.P., & N.K. Denzin: *The Mental Patient: Studies in the Sociology of Deviance.* McGraw-Hill, 1968.

Srole, L., & others: *Mental Health in the Metropolis: The Midtown Manhattan Study.* McGraw-Hill, 1962.

Steiger, W.A., & A.V. Hansen, Jr.: *Patients Who Trouble You.* Little, Brown, 1964.

Stone, A.A., & S.S. Stone: *The Abnormal Personality Through Literature.* Prentice-Hall, 1966.

Sullivan, H.S.: *The Interpersonal Theory of Psychiatry.* Norton, 1953.

Susser, M.W.: *Community Psychiatry: Epidemiologic and Social Themes.* Knopf, 1968.

Swanson, D.W., Bohnert, P.J., & J.A. Smith: *The Paranoid.* Little, Brown, 1970.

Szasz, T.S.: *Law, Liberty, and Psychiatry.* Macmillan, 1963.

Szasz, T.S.: *The Myth of Mental Illness.* Hoeber, 1961.

Thompson, J.S., & M.W. Thompson: *Genetics in Medicine.* Saunders, 1966.

Usdin, G.L.: *Psychoneurosis and Schizophrenia.* Lippincott, 1966.

Warner, L.: *Mirrors.* Knopf, 1969.

Wayne, G.J., & R.R. Koegler: *Emergency Psychiatry and Brief Psychotherapy.* Little, Brown, 1966.

Whittington, H.G.: *Psychiatry in the American Community.* Internat Univ.Press, 1966.

Williams, R.H., & L.D. Ozarin (editors): *Community Mental Health: An International Perspective.* Jossey-Bass, 1968.

Winters, E. (editor): *The Collected Papers of Adolf Meyer.* Vol 2. Johns Hopkins Press, 1951.

World Health Organization: *Mental Health Problems of Aging and the Aged.* Technical Report No. 171. World Health Organization, 1959.

Wyden, P., & B. Wyden: *Growing Up Straight.* Stein & Day, 1968.

Index

Psychiatric Emergency Routine

HISTORY

This may be vital. If the patient cannot supply it and there are no friends or relatives with him, query the ambulance driver or, if necessary, call the patient's home (or send the police) to get it. Be sure to ask about past mental illness and hospitalizations, recent accidents, injuries, serious illnesses, use of alcohol or drugs (dose, time, etc), and personal crises.

DIAGNOSIS AND IMMEDIATE TREATMENT

Patients presenting as psychiatric emergencies are usually *overactive, underactive,* or *suicidal.*

Overactive Patients

A. Violent: (Disturbed, unmanageable, psychotic.) Irrational, uncooperative, deluded, paranoid, assaultive, hallucinating patients are psychotic. Quiet them with a calm, firm, unhurried approach. Sedate with chlorpromazine, 100 mg IM. Admit to hospital and search for causes.

B. Anxious: (Agitated, panicky.) Patients who are rational and cooperative but restless, tremulous, profusely perspiring, and flushed, with rapid pulse and respiration, dilated pupils, and hyperactive reflexes may be psychotic, prepsychotic, or neurotic. Give reassurance first and search for causes later, both organic and psychologic. Sedate and arrange for psychotherapy.

C. Drunk: The drunken patient is usually flushed, reeks of liquor, and staggers. He may be belligerent, comatose, or lachrymose. Determine blood alcohol or alcohol content of expired air. Check for injuries and do a thorough physical examination, including neurologic status. Rule out head injuries, subdural hematoma, pneumonia, diabetes, acidosis, hypoglycemia, cardiac decompensation, Wernicke's syndrome, and peripheral neuritis. Treat by watchful waiting and symptomatic measures.

D. Drug Withdrawal:

1. Morphine type—The symptoms of drug withdrawal, in increasing order of seriousness, are: (1) Restlessness, anxiety, craving for the drug. (2) Yawning, lacrimation, sweating, rhinorrhea. (3) Gooseflesh, anorexia, muscle twitching, muscle and joint pains; dilated, sluggish pupils. (4) Fever, rapid pulse and respiration, increased blood pressure, nausea and vomiting, diarrhea, marked restlessness, insomnia, and psychotic behavior.

Estimate the type and degree of drug dependence by the history of drug abuse, duration, dose, frequency, and interval since the last dose. Watch out for the malingerer who wants only a "fix" (dose of his drug). At the first sign of pupillary dilatation and gooseflesh in morphine or heroin withdrawal, start substitution therapy with methadone, 5, 10, or 25 mg twice daily orally or, if necessary (patient vomiting), intramuscularly. If convulsions occur, watch airway and give diphenylhydantoin.

2. Barbiturate type—Barbiturate withdrawal is characterized by marked agitation, insomnia, and convulsions. Give 200 mg of pentobarbital orally and evaluate the sensorium in 1 hour. The nontolerant patient will be somnolent but arousable; one tolerant to 500—600 mg/day will have nystagmus, mild dysarthria, and ataxia; one tolerant to 700—800 mg/day will have some nystagmus; and one tolerant to 900 mg/day or more will show no signs of intoxication on a test dose of 200 mg.

After this evaluation, give the drug in a stabilizing dose and later withdraw it gradually.

3. Alcohol type—(Delirium tremens.) This is characterized by frenzied fear, tremors, hallucinations (usually visual), and sometimes by convulsions. Give sedation (phenothiazines, paraldehyde, chlordiazepoxide) and attend to fluid and electrolyte balance, vitamins, and nutrition. Arrange for constant special nursing.

Underactive Patients

A. Depression: Prominent symptoms are melancholy facies, manner, speech, tearfulness, self-accusation, and psychomotor retardation. Estimate seriousness by degree of impairment of ordinary activities (housework, job, school), by diminution of appetites (food, sex, sleep, activity), and by suicide threat. For the last: Has he *thought* about suicide? Has he thought about *how* he would do it? Has he taken any *steps in preparation*? Has he made or begun to make an *attempt*? The first 2 (thought) are usually not serious; the last 2 (action) are serious. Notify relatives or other responsible persons about seriously depressed patients. In most cases, they should be hospitalized. For the others, arrange outpatient care.

B. Catatonia: The patient is largely mute and motionless. He maintains postures he is put into. This is psychosis—he may be frozen with fear but is very alert and dangerous. Hospitalize at once and start phenothiazines.

Attempted Suicide

The history is crucial. Get details at once. Attend to airway, wounds, and surgical shock; then lavage and give antidotes.

Estimate the degree of suicide danger by the following, listed in descending order of seriousness:

1. Continued death threat	11. Alcoholism
2. Psychosis	12. Drug dependence
3. Marked depression	13. Hypochondriasis
4. Previous attempts	14. Male over 40
5. Previous psychosis	15. Homosexuality
6. Suicide note	16. Mild depression
7. Violent method	17. Social isolation
8. Chronic disease	18. Chronic maladjustment
9. Recent surgery or childbirth	19. Bankrupt resources
10. Recent serious loss	20. No apparent secondary gain

The presence of any of the more serious or 2 or 3 of the less serious items usually warrants hospitalization. Every patient should be followed on an inpatient or outpatient basis, and the responsibility should be shared with relatives, friends, or authorities.